Chemistry and Pharmacology of Anticancer Drugs

Chemistry and Pharmacology of Anticancer Drugs

Editor: Octavia Settle

AMERICAN
MEDICAL PUBLISHERS
www.americanmedicalpublishers.com

AMERICAN
MEDICAL PUBLISHERS
www.americanmedicalpublishers.com

Cataloging-in-Publication Data

Chemistry and pharmacology of anticancer drugs / edited by Octavia Settle.
p. cm.
Includes bibliographical references and index.
ISBN 978-1-63927-975-3
1. Antineoplastic agents. 2. Cancer--Chemotherapy. 3. Drugs. 4. Pharmaceutical chemistry.
5. Pharmacology. I. Settle, Octavia.
RS431.A64 C44 2023
615.798--dc23

American Medical Publishers,
41 Flatbush Avenue,
1st Floor, New York,
NY 11217, USA

ISBN 978-1-63927-975-3 (Hardback)

Contents

Preface

The purpose of the book is to provide a glimpse into the dynamics and to present opinions and studies of some of the scientists engaged in the development of new ideas in the field from very different standpoints. This book will prove useful to students and researchers owing to its high content quality.

An anticancer drug is a type of drug that is effective in the treatment of malignant or cancerous diseases. The four major groups of anticancer drugs are alkylating agents, antimetabolites, natural products and hormones. Chemotherapy is one of the major categories of medications that are used for the treatment and management of cancer. It involves the use of one or more anti-cancer drugs, as part of a standardized chemotherapy process. Alkylating antineoplastic agents are used to treat several types of cancer. They have the potential to alkylate many molecules, including proteins, RNA and DNA, which is the primary cause for their anti-cancer effect. This book is a compilation of chapters that discuss the most emerging trends in the field of anticancer drugs. It presents researches and studies performed by experts across the globe. This book is an invaluable resource for cancer researchers, medicinal chemists and other biomedical scientists involved in the development of new anticancer therapies.

At the end, I would like to appreciate all the efforts made by the authors in completing their chapters professionally. I express my deepest gratitude to all of them for contributing to this book by sharing their valuable works. A special thanks to my family and friends for their constant support in this journey.

Editor

1

Novel 11-Substituted Ellipticines as Potent Anticancer Agents with Divergent Activity against Cancer Cells

Charlotte M. Miller, Elaine C. O'Sullivan and Florence O. McCarthy *

School of Chemistry, Analytical and Biological Chemistry Research Facility, University College Cork, Western Road, T12 K8AF Cork, Ireland; charlotte.herstad@dynea.com (C.M.M.); elosullivan@hotmail.com (E.C.O.)

* Correspondence: f.mccarthy@ucc.ie;

Abstract: Ellipticines have well documented anticancer activity, in particular with substitution at the 1-, 2-, 6- and 9-positions. However, due to limitations in synthesis and coherent screening methodology the full SAR profile of this anticancer class has not yet been achieved. In order to address this shortfall, we have set out to explore the anticancer activity of this potent natural product by substitution. We currently describe the synthesis of novel 11-substituted ellipticines with two specific derivatives showing potency and diverging cellular growth effects.

Keywords: ellipticine; anticancer; heterocyclic chemistry; indole; NCI screen; topoisomerase II

---

1. Introduction

Cancer is a collection of diseases defined by the proliferation of cells in an unregulated and inappropriate manner leading to tumours and eventual mortality. Within this broad definition it is evident that the control of cell growth is a key mechanism as cell growth can be restricted, proliferation can be stopped and cells can be killed by multiple anticancer agents, one of which (ellipticine) is explored further here [1].

Ellipticine **1** (5,11-dimethyl-6*H*-pyrido [4,3-*b*]carbazole, Figure 1) is a natural product which was isolated in 1959 from a small tropical evergreen tree (*Ochrosia elliptica*) by Goodwin et al. [2]. The extract also contained a number of other alkaloids, including the related 9-methoxyellipticine **2**. Since its isolation, the planar tetracyclic structure of ellipticine has been the focus of extensive chemical and pharmacological research [3]. Over the last 60 years, ellipticine and its derivatives have been identified with potent anticancer activity and been subject to clinical trials. Celiptium (9-hydroxy-*N*-methylellipticinium acetate) **3** and 9-hydroxyellipticine **4** both progressed to phase II clinical trials though these were subsequently discontinued due to side effects and efficacy [4–7].

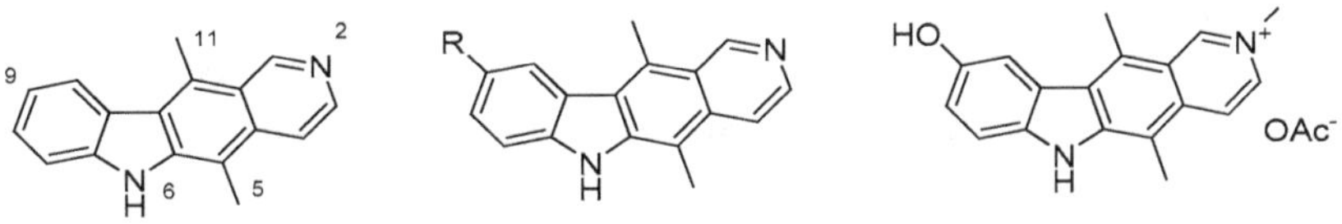

1

2 R = OCH_3
4 R = OH

3

Figure 1. Structures of Ellipticine **1** and related anticancer agents.

The mechanisms by which ellipticine exerts its anticancer activity are particularly diverse. These include topoisomerase II inhibition with associated DNA intercalation, well established in the literature and clinically relevant [8–10]. Cytotoxic ellipticine metabolites via biooxidation at a number of positions on the tetracycle and subsequent adduct formation have also been identified as responsible for some of the effects [11]. Recently, ellipticines have been described to interact with kinases such as c-Kit, AKT and CK2, and to influence the p53 tumour suppressor, all of which have key roles in cell growth and progression [12–14]. Ellipticines have also been discovered to disrupt RNA polymerase I transcription and stabilize pharmaceutically relevant G-quadruplexes and so there is significant and continued interest in the biological effects of this compound class [15,16].

It is therefore evident that ellipticine and its derivatives exhibit multimodal activity with simple substitutions on this template eliciting diverse effects. Despite their potency, there has been little exploration of the functional space in this natural product outside of the 1-, 2-, 6- and 9-positions in order to answer fundamental questions in pharmacology and effect on cells. A programme of research has been initiated in this group in order to evaluate the effect of novel substitution patterns on the ellipticine framework. This has led to the recent discoveries of substituted ellipticine and isoellipticines as new investigational probes with diverse pharmacology and exceptional in vivo activity (**5** and **6**, Figure 2) [17–20].

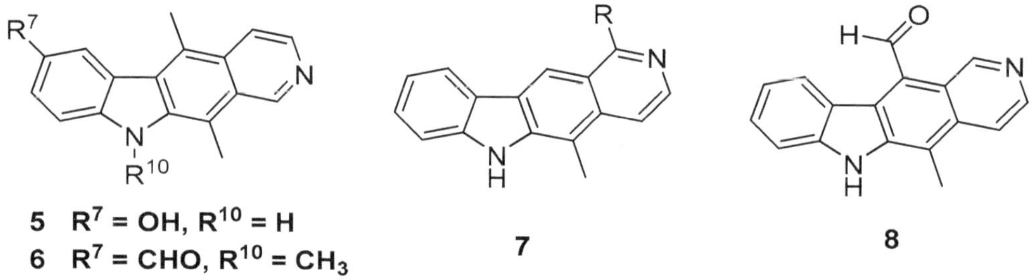

Figure 2. Substituted isoellipticines (**5** and **6**) with in vivo activity, Olivacine **7** and 11-formylellipticine **8**.

The 11-position of ellipticine has received little attention from medicinal chemists despite evidence that it may be a key position in order to affect the bioactivity and crucially selectivity of pharmacology [21]. The activity of the closely related olivicine series of compounds signifies that removal of the methyl group does little to affect the potency of the template especially in regard to topoisomerase activity and DNA intercalation (**7**, R = CH_3, Figure 2) [22,23]. An olivacine derivative, S16020 (**7**, R = carboxamide) has also progressed to phase I clinical trials before being discontinued [24]. Despite synthesis of 11-formyl ellipticine **8** (Figure 2) almost 30 years ago, no concerted effort to functionalise this position is recorded in literature other than a carboxamide and a methyl ketone (only four reported compounds in total with carbonyl at 11-position).

Molecular modelling of ellipticine in the active site of biological targets has postulated that 11-substitution with bulky or mobile functional groups would inhibit the intercalation process and may reduce a number of undesirable effects associated with treatment [25]. This position has also been implicated in the process of DNA adduct formation via oxidation [11].

To this end, we set out to functionalise the parent heterocycle and to exploit its known anticancer activity: it has obvious potency across numerous spheres of biology and affects cells from development to apoptosis [4]. Substitution of 11-position is an important step towards full SAR profiling of the cellular effects of ellipticine derivatives. We document here the initial scoping of this chemical space and probe of the anticancer activity through known ellipticine mechanisms.

2. Results and Discussion

2.1. *Synthesis of 11-Substituted Ellipticine Derivatives*

Since its isolation in 1959, the total synthesis of ellipticine has been accomplished many times and most recent work in the area has focused on preparation of analogues and derivatives of ellipticine [3]. At the outset of this work there existed relatively few examples of 11-substituted ellipticines. Gribble et al. had published a very versatile and efficient route in 1989, giving access to 5- and 11-substituted ellipticines [26–29]. This was further elaborated by Modi et al. to give 11-formylellipticine 8 and this compound was chosen as the starting point for the current synthetic work [30,31].

2.1.1. Modification of 11-formylellipticine

11-Formylellipticine 8 was synthesised as previously described and initially the focus was to provide a carboxylic acid handle for modification (Scheme 1) [30,31]. Hence, 8 was subjected to oxidation under a number of conditions with the most successful conversion to carboxylic acid 9 achieved using sodium chlorite and dimethylsulfoxide (73% yield). Subsequent conversion to acid chloride 10 allowed for introduction of amide functionality which was a key target in this series and the benzylamine derivative 11 was prepared in two steps in 30% yield. The methyl ester 12 was also prepared via similar methodology using carbonyldiimidazole.

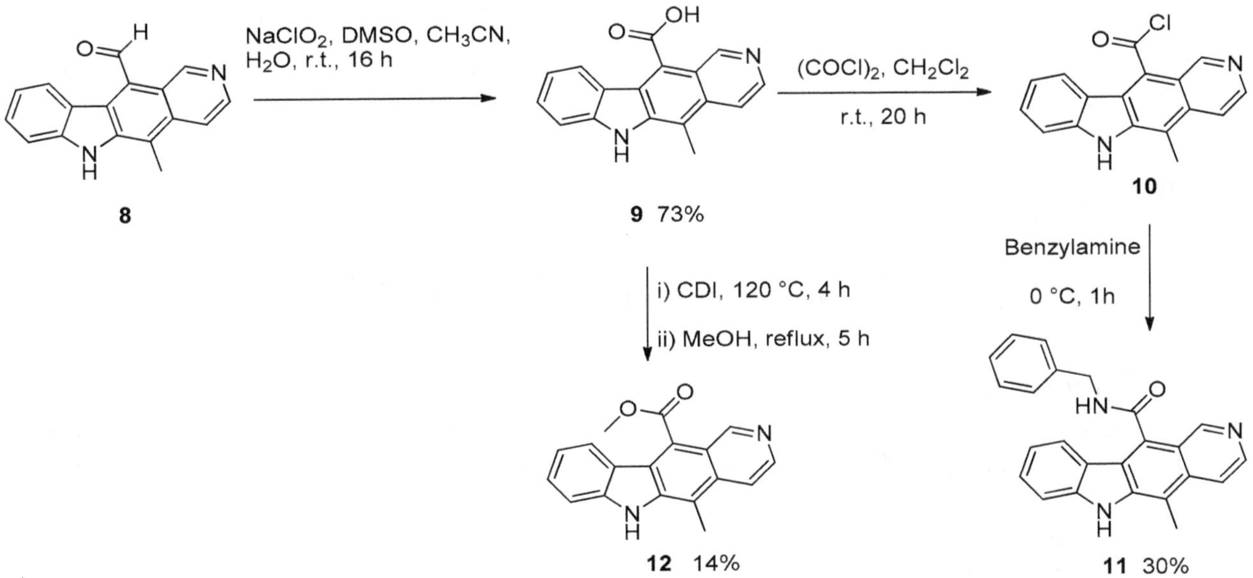

Scheme 1. Formation of 11-substituted ellipticine amide **11** and ester **12**.

Interestingly, while attempting to form the acid initially with other oxidants the expected product was not isolated. On treatment of 8 with potassium permanganate under standard conditions the reaction resulted in base condensation of acetone and isolation of the novel α,β-unsaturated ketone 13 in 87% yield (Scheme 2).

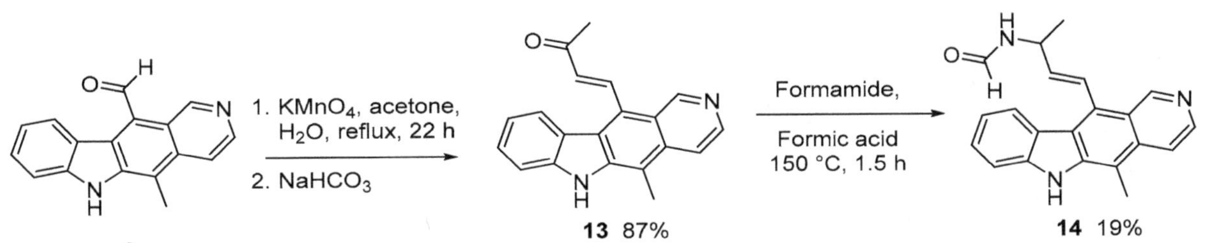

Scheme 2. α,β-Unsaturated ketone condensation product **13** from acetone solvent.

Attempts at cyclisation of compound 13 using aluminium chloride in dichloromethane or chloroform to form a new ring system were unsuccessful and unreacted starting material was recovered. However, a Leuckart reaction gave the formamide 14 in 19% yield, the low yield owing to difficulties in purification. However, the unsaturated ketone 13 provides an interesting template for potential covalent adduct formation and will be revisited in the future.

2.1.2. Modification of the 9-position of 11-substituted Ellipticines

Given the extensive literature background in 9-substituted ellipticines and the recent developments in this area we next turned our focus to functionalization of this position. Initially, carboxylic acid 9 was derivatised via a Duff reaction to give the aldehyde 15 in 82% yield (Scheme 3) [32].

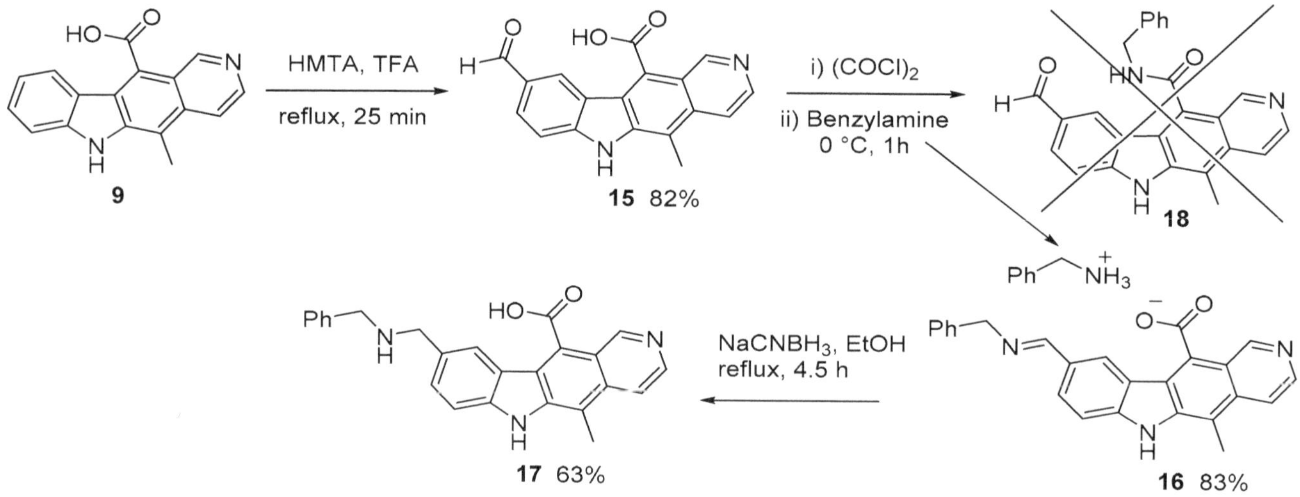

Scheme 3. Synthesis of 9- and 11-substituted ellipticines.

Subsequent reaction of 15 with nucleophiles opens up opportunities for potential synthesis at either the 9- or the 11-position (Scheme 3). To probe the 11-position further, acid chloride formation prior to the addition of benzylamine (as seen in Scheme 1) was undertaken with the aim of generating amide 18. In this reaction, the product isolated was the imine 16 (83% yield) which was identified after full characterization. Confirmation of structure was given by subsequent treatment with aqueous acid which hydrolysed the product to starting material 15.

Additional conformation of the imine 16 was provided by reduction of the imine with sodium cyanoborohydride in ethanol to give the novel amine 17.

2.1.3. 1H NMR Analysis of 11-Substituted Ellipticines

A summary of the ^{1}H NMR analysis is provided in Supplementary Materials (Figures S1–S3). Of note is the influence of conversion from aldehyde to carboxylic acid at the 11-position with corresponding upfield shift of C1 and C10 protons (reversed on formylation of the 9-position). The shift of the C10 proton is again evident on conversion of carboxylic acid to amide and ester.

2.2. Biological Evaluation of 11-Substituted Ellipticines

Given the interest in new ellipticines, several of the novel 9- and 11-substitued ellipticines were evaluated for their biological activity in cellular screens and by gel electrophoresis. In the first instance, inhibition of topoisomerase II (a well-known target of ellipticines) was assessed.

2.2.1. Inhibition of Topoisomerase II

Topoisomerase II inhibition is a clinically used cancer treatment and is considered to be a key mechanism of action for ellipticines [9]. Topoisomerase II has key functions in the change of topological structure of DNA and hence cell replication which can be evaluated using a decatenation assay. As expected, the planar ellipticine 1 and the simple 9-substituted ellipticines (2,4,19) all displayed excellent inhibition of topoisomerase II at 100 μM (Figure 3). On assessment of the 11-substituted ellipticines, the majority were inactive against topoisomerase II but compounds 13 and 16 showed the most promise. α,β-Unsaturated ketone 13 and 9-substituted imine 16 both represent new templates for discovery. Both compounds were evaluated in a subsequent three-fold dilution assay (at 100, 10 and 1μM) where it became apparent that activity reduced significantly below the initial test concentration.

Notwithstanding this, the emergence of two diverse templates for topoisomerase inhibition will be of keen interest to the field and future efforts will aim to increase the potency of this interaction.

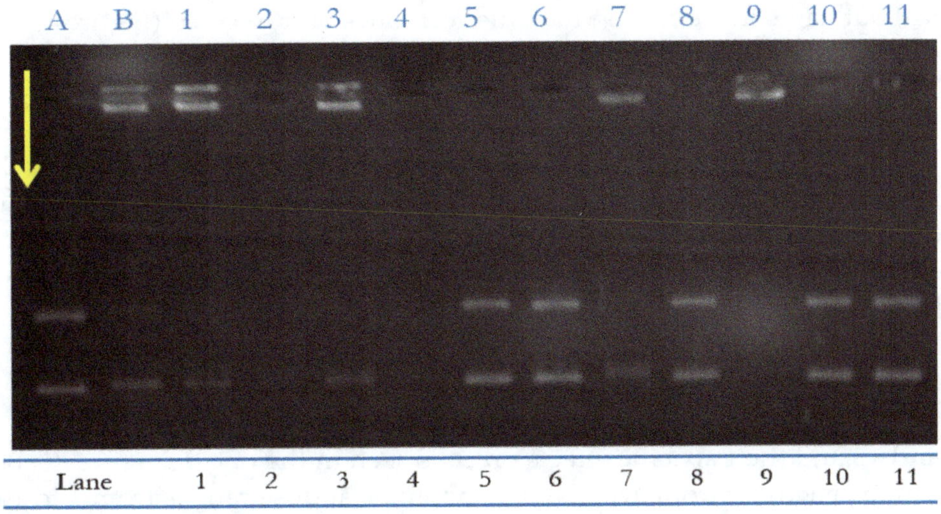

Figure 3. Screen of topoisomerase II inhibitory activity of the ellipticine derivatives at 100 μM. A = Positive Control (kDNA + ATP + Topo II); B = Negative Control (kDNA + ATP + Topo II + 100 μM Ellipticine); Consequent lanes all screened at 100 μM: 1 = Ellipticine 1; 2 = 9-Methoxyellipticine 2; 3 = 9-Formylellipticine 19; 4 = 9-Hydroxyellipticine 4; 5 = 8; 6 = 9; 7 = 13; 8 = 15; 9 = 16; 10 = 17; 11 = 11.

2.2.2. Inhibition of Cancer Cell Growth

Having identified some limited topoisomerase activity, screening of the 11-substituted ellipticine test set was next conducted by assessment of inhibition of cancer cell growth. Initial evaluation of anticancer activity at the National Cancer Institute focuses on the effect of each individual compound on the growth of up to 60 cancer cell lines at a specific concentration (10 μM). The results are summarised in Table 1 (see Supplementary Material for full data, Figures S5–S10).

Table 1. 11-Substituted ellipticine topoisomerase activity and National Cancer Institute (NCI) mean growth percent (single dose).

	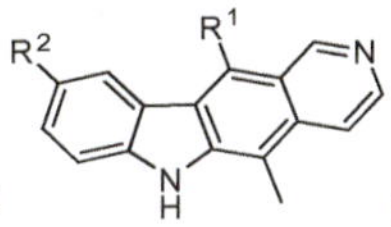 R^1	R^2	**Topo II Inhibition** [a]	**NSC No**	**NCI Mean Growth %**
8	CHO	H	–		Not tested
9	COOH	H	–	762124	99.92
11	$CONHCH_2Ph$	H	–	762144	21.22
13	CH=CH-C(O)Me	H	+	762123	17.83
15	COOH	CHO	–	762141	95.56
16	$COO^{-}\,{}^{+}NH_3CH_2Ph$	$CH{=}NCH_2Ph$	+	762142	106.19
17	COOH	CH_2NHCH_2Ph	–	762143	101.72

[a] R^1 = C-9 substituent; R^2 = C11 substituent (+) Inhibition observed at 100 μM; (–) no activity observed at 100 μM.

Inhibition of Cancer Cell Growth—One Dose Assay

National Cancer Institute (NCI) evaluation of 11-substituted ellipticines identifies significant effects on the growth of the 60-cell line panel with mean growth values ranging from 18% to 106%. The Mean Growth percent is a reference tool whereby screening at 10 μM concentration is used to filter active anticancer compounds. Of the six compounds tested, two (11-substituted amide 11 and conjugated ketone 13) achieved Mean Growth percentages of <25% and fulfilled the requirements for progression to the five dose assay (Table 1). Of the other four compounds growth percentages were between 96% and 106% and hence have no effect on the growth as an average across the 60 cell lines. Compounds 9, 15, 16 and 17 elicited very similar effects being most active against renal cancer cell line UO-31 (range 63%–76% growth) and breast cancer cell lines MCF7 and MDA-MB-231/ATCC (range 68%–87% growth) but have little effect on the other cell lines of the screen (Figures S5, S8–S10).

In contrast, benzylamide 11 and ketone 13 had significant anticancer effects with differing cellular profiles. Ketone 13 is associated with a non-specific pattern with the range of cell growths (lowest to highest) of 77% whereas benzylamide 11 has a range of 165% and there is an evident difference in cell line effects. At 10 μM, compound 11 is cytotoxic (negative growth percentage) to 15 of the 60 cell lines whereas compound 13 to only four cell lines. It is noticeable that a large number of cell lines are refractory to benzylamide 11 which suggests there may be a targeted effect. It is also obvious from this preliminary screen that there is chemical space at the 11-position of ellipticine to accommodate anticancer activity.

Inhibition of Cancer Cell Growth—Five Dose Assay

The progression to evaluation at five dose assay confirmed the potency of both 11-substituted ellipticines 11 and 13 and their specific effects on cells seen in the one dose screen. Benzylamide 11 exerts a broad range of activity from cytostatic to cytotoxic at dose ranges from 1 to 100 μM (Table 2; Figure S11). In specific, the activity of this compound against HOP62, SNB75, OVCAR-3, OVCAR-4 and 786-0 is exceptional with more than 50% cytotoxicity measured after 48 h incubation (at 10 μM). Growth is restricted across the other cell lines but there is clear selective cytotoxicity. In addition it can be seen (Figure S12) that a number of cell lines are refractory with no evident effect on cell growth of cancer subtypes, in particular melanoma: Leukaemia (HL-60), Lung (EKVX), CNS (SF-295, SNB-19), Melanoma (MALME-3M, M14, SK-MEL-2, SK MEL-28, UACC-257), Ovarian (OVCAR-5, NCI/ADR-RES) and Breast (T-47D).

Table 2. Selected GI50 and LC50 of the NCI 60 cell line panel for compounds **11** and **13** [1].

Cell Line	Cancer Subtype	11		13	
		GI50	LC50	GI50	LC50
HOP-62	Lung	2.15	>100	1.77	26.0
SW-620	Colon	2.86	>100	1.65	44.0
SNB-75	CNS	2.05	>100	2.65	34.8
OVCAR-3	Ovarian	2.33	<10	2.53	28.0
OVCAR-4	Ovarian	1.71	6.19	2.88	41.5
786-0	Renal	2.79	72.0	2.79	29.8
A498	Renal	50.5	>100	0.386	7.48
UO-31	Renal	2.73	>100	1.25	33.8
MCF7	Breast	2.71	>100	1.74	52.3
MDA-MB-231/ATCC	Breast	2.43	>100	1.74	41.3
HS578T	Breast	2.61	>100	1.96	48.4

[1] data reported in μM values from NCI 60 cell line five dose assay; GI50: Growth Inhibition 50%; LC50: Lethal concentration 50%.

Ketone 13 exerts a far more cytotoxic effect across all cell lines with consistent cell death evident at 10 μM as in the one dose screen (Table 2, LC50 column; Figures S13 and S14). Aside the exception of the leukaemia cell panel, all cells are killed by 100 μM of 13 which suggests a potent and common mechanism of action. The compound is exceptionally potent against the growth of A498 renal cancer cells with a GI50 of 386 nM and merits future investigation. In the design of compound 13, the Michael acceptor moiety is presumably involved in alkylation of the essential machinery of the cell and development of this is the subject of current work.

In comparing the global effect of both 11 and 13 (Figures S13 and S16) it is evident that they affect cell growth by different mechanisms as would be expected from their structures. In specific, compound

11 has the potential for use in ovarian cancers given its exceptional toxicity against the OVCAR-3 and OVCAR-4 phenotypes (LC50 6.2 and <10 μM respectively; OVCAR-4 value assigned due to inflection of graph). OVCAR-3 and OVCAR-4 are both mutant p53 status but have individual profiles with OVCAR-3 having known upregulation of BRCA2-interacting transcriptional repressor and cyclin E1. OVCAR-4 in turn has been identified as a good model cell line for High Grade Serious Ovarian Cancer (HGSOC) which make these findings significant from a clinical perspective [33].

2.3. *COMPARE Analysis of Compounds* ***11*** *and* ***13***

COMPARE analysis was performed on the NCI COMPARE algorithm in order to identify correlations with known anticancer agents within the NCI database. Both compound 11 and 13 were analysed and with a specific focus on two subsets of the database: synthetic compounds and mechanistic set. Compound 13 gave a number of correlations as high as 0.74 with the most relevant mechanistic hit being to Chrysanthemic acid (NSC 11779) but this must be seen in the overall non-specific profile of activity of 13 and its limited potency.

However, on analysis of 11 in the synthetic compounds set, the top ranked correlation (0.6) is to SCH1473759 (NSC 761691) which has recently been reported as a picomolar inhibitor of Aurora kinases [34]. Again, while an important finding and a good match of cellular activity profile, this result must be seen in the context of potency with SCH1473759 having >100 the potency of 11 in the NCI assay (Figure S17). Compound 11 also gave rise to a correlation of 0.58 to Aclarubicin (Aclacinomycin A, NSC 208734) being the top hit of the mechanistic compound set. Aclarubicin has known topoisomerase inhibitory and recently reported histone eviction from open chromatin activity so despite the lack of evident topoisomerase activity of 11, this result merits further evaluation in respect of its interaction with DNA and DNA interacting enzymes [35].

3. Materials and Methods

Solvents were distilled prior to use as follows: dichloromethane was distilled from phosphorous pentoxide; ethyl acetate was distilled from potassium carbonate; ethanol and methanol were distilled from magnesium in the presence of iodine; toluene was distilled from sodium and benzophenone; hexane was distilled prior to use; tetrahydrofuran was freshly distilled from sodium and benzophenone. Diethyl ether was obtained pure from Riedel-de Haën. Organic phases were dried using anhydrous magnesium sulphate. All commercial reagents were used without further purification unless otherwise stated. All samples were confirmed as >95% pure by use of high resolution LCMS analysis.

Infrared spectra were recorded as a thin film on sodium chloride plates for liquids or potassium bromide (KBr) disc for solids on a Perkin Elmer Spectrum 100 FT-IR spectrometer.

^{1}H (300 MHz) and ^{13}C (75 MHz) NMR spectra were recorded on a Bruker Avance 300 NMR spectrometer. ^{1}H (600 MHz) and ^{13}C (150.9 MHz) NMR spectra were recorded on a Bruker Avance III 600 MHz NMR spectrometer equipped with a dual CH cryoprobe. All spectra were recorded at room temperature (~20 °C) in deuterated dimethylsulfoxide (DMSO-d_6) were assigned using the DMSO-d_6 peak as the reference peak. Chemical shifts (δH and δC) are expressed in parts per million (ppm) relative to the reference peak. Coupling constants (J) are expressed in Hertz (Hz). Splitting patterns in ^{1}H NMR spectra are designated as s (singlet), br s (broad singlet), d (doublet), br d (broad doublet), t (triplet), q (quartet), dd (doublet of doublets), dt (doublet of triplets), ddd (doublet of doublet of doublets), ddt (doublet of doublet of triplets) and m (multiplet).

Low resolution mass spectra were recorded on a Waters Quattro Micro triple quadrupole spectrometer (QAA1202) in electrospray ionisation (ESI) mode using 50% acetonitrile:water containing 0.1% formic acid as eluent. High resolution mass spectra (HRMS) were recorded on a Waters LCT Premier Time of Flight spectrometer (KD-160) in electrospray ionisation (ESI) mode using 50% acetonitrile:ater containing 0.1% formic acid as eluent.

Melting points were measured in a uni-melt Thomas Hoover capillary melting point apparatus and are uncorrected. Thin layer chromatography (TLC) was carried out on precoated silica gel plates

(Merck 60 PF254) or aluminium oxide TLC paltes (Sigma). Visualisation was achieved by UV light detection (254 nm).

5-Methyl-6*H*-pyrido[4,3-*b*]carbazole-11-carboxylic acid 9. 5-Methyl-6*H*-pyrido[4,3-*b*]carbazole -11-carbaldehyde **8** (92 mg, 0.353 mmol) in acetonitrile (9 mL) was treated with dimethylsulfoxide (0.03 mL, 0.423 mmol) and conc. sulfuric acid (0.3 mL, 0.622 mmol). A solution of sodium chlorite (48 mg, 0.530 mmol) in water (3 mL) was added dropwise and the reaction mixture was stirred at room temperature overnight. The reaction was quenched with sodium sulfite (22 mg, 0.177 mmol) in water (1 mL). The acetonitrile was evaporated to leave an aqueous solution, which was carefully adjusted to pH 5 with saturated aqueous sodium bicarbonate to precipitate the product. The mixture was cooled to 0 °C, filtered and washed with water (3 mL), to give 5-methyl-6*H*-pyrido[4,3-*b*]carbazole-11-carboxylic acid **9**. The orange solid was dried at 0.02 mbar for 24 h (71 mg, 73.2%). m.p. >300 °C; vmax/cm^{-1} (KBr): 3161 (NH), 3010 (OH broad), 1689 (C=O), 1648 (C=C arom.), 1597 (C=C arom.), 1488, 1463, 1417, 1241 (C-O stretch), 1109; δH (300 MHz, DMSO-d_6): 2.88 [3H, s, C(5)CH_3], 7.26 [1H, t, J = 7.9, C(9)H], 7.55–7.62 [2H, m, C(7)H, C(8)H], 8.03 [1H, d, J = 5.9, C(3)H], 8.21 [1H, d, J = 7.8, C(10)H], 8.47 [1H, d, J = 5.9, C(4)H], 9.43 [1H, s, C(1)H], 11.64 [1H, s, N(6)H]; δC (75.5 MHz, DMSO-d_6): 12.3 [3H, s, C(5)CH_3], 111.5 [CH, C(7)H], 113.3 (C, aromatic C), 117.7 [CH, C(3)H], 118.5 (C, aromatic C), 120.0 [CH, C(9)H], 120.3 (C, aromatic C), 122.3 (C, aromatic C), 123.1 [CH, C(10)H], 124.9 (C, aromatic C), 129.1 [CH, C(8)H], 132.2 (C, aromatic C), 136.1 [CH, C(4)H], 141.9 (C, aromatic C), 143.1 (C, aromatic C), 147.9 [CH, C(1)H], 168.8 [C, C(11)COOH]; m/z (ESI+): 277 [$(M+H)^+$ 40%], 115 (100%); HRMS (ESI+): Exact mass calculated for $[C_{17}H_{13}N_2O_2]^+$ 277.0977. Found 277.0977.

5-Methyl-6*H*-pyrido[4,3-*b*]carbazole-11-carbonylchloride 10. 5-Methyl-6*H*-pyrido[4,3-*b*]carbazole -11-carboxylic acid **9** (99 mg, 0.358 mmol) in dichloromethane (50 mL), under N_2, was treated with oxalyl chloride (0.04 mL, 0.459 mmol). Slight fizzing was observed on addition and mixture was stirred at room temperature for 20 h. The bright orange suspension was evaporated under reduced pressure. IR analysis showed the carbonyl peak at 1785 cm^{-1} indicating acid chloride formation.

***N*-Benzyl-5-methyl-6*H*-pyrido[4,3-*b*]carbazole-11-carboxamide 11.** 5-Methyl-6*H*-pyrido[4,3-*b*] carbazole-11-carboxylic acid **9** (99 mg, 0.358 mmol) in dichloromethane (50 mL), under N_2, was treated with oxalyl chloride (0.04 mL, 0.459 mmol) and stirred at room temperature for 20 h. The mixture was evaporated under reduced pressure, cooled to 0 °C under N_2, and treated drop-wise with benzylamine (2 mL, 18.3 mmol). After stirring for 1 h, diethyl ether (40 mL) was added, the mixture was cooled and filtered to give a cream solid (220 mg) containing the desired product and residual benzylamine. This was stirred with diethyl ether and decanted (3 × 40 mL). Purification by column chromatography, eluting with dichloromethane:methanol (100:0–95:5), gave product **11** as a yellow solid (39 mg, 30%). m.p. 294–296 °C; vmax/cm^{-1} (KBr): 3159 (NH), 3051 (CH) 1731 (C=O), 1621 (C=C arom.), 1600 (C=C arom.), 1542, 1466, 1410, 1245; δH (600 MHz, DMSO-d_6): 2.79 [3H, s, C(5)CH_3], 4.65–4.70 [2H, m, CONHCH_2], 6.98 [1H, t, J = 7.4, C(9)H], 7.28 [1H, t, J = 7.2, N-benzyl-C(4)H], 7.36 [2H, t, J = 7.3, *N*-benzyl-C(2)H, C(6)H], 7.43–7.50 [4H, m, C(7)H, C(8)H, *N*-benzyl-C(3)H, C(5)H], 7.72 [1H, d, J = 7.8, C(10)H], 7.93 [1H, d, J = 5.9, C(3)H], 8.37 [1H, d, J = 5.1, C(4)H], 9.19 [1H, s, C(1)H], 9.41 [1H, t, J = 5.9, C(11)CONH], 11.46 [1H, s, N(6)H]; δC (150.9 MHz, DMSO-d_6): 12.2 [CH_3, C(5)CH_3], 43.1 [CH_2, C(11)CONHCH_2], 110.9 (CH, aromatic CH), 111.3 (C, aromatic C), 116.0 [CH, C(3)H], 119.1 [CH, C(9)H], 119.8 (C, aromatic C), 120.9 (C, aromatic C), 121.1 (C, aromatic C), 122.8 [CH, C(10)H], 127.1 [CH, N-benzyl-C(4)H], 127.2 (C, aromatic C), 127.9 (CH, aromatic CH), 128.0 (CH, aromatic CH), 128.2 (CH, aromatic CH), 128.4 (CH, aromatic CH), 128.5 (CH, aromatic CH), 131.7 (C, aromatic C), 138.9 (C, aromatic C), 140.4 (C, aromatic C), 140.7 [CH, C(4)H], 142.7 (C, aromatic C), 150.1 [CH, C(1)H], 167.1 [C, C(11)CONH]; m/z (ESI+): 366 [$(M+H^+)$, 100%]; HRMS (ESI+): Exact mass calculated for $[C_{24}H_{20}N_3O]^+$ 366.1606. Found 366.1615.

Methyl 5-methyl-6*H*-pyrido[4,3-*b*]carbazole-11-carboxylate 12. 5-Methyl-6*H*-pyrido[4,3-*b*]carbazole -11-carboxylic acid **9** (99 mg, 0.358 mmol) in dimethylformamide (8 mL) under N_2, was heated gently until the acid dissolved. Carbonyldiimidazole (70 mg, 0.430 mmol) was added and the solution was heated at 120 °C for 4 h. The mixture was cooled to 0 °C and diethyl ether (20 mL) was added. The resulting precipitate was filtered and washed (diethyl ether 10 mL). The solid was cooled to 0 °C and treated dropwise with methanol (10 mL). The mixture was stirred at r.t. for 1 h and heated to reflux for 5 h. On cooling, a precipitate formed which was filtered to give the methyl ester, methyl 5-methyl-6*H*-pyrido[4,3-*b*]carbazole-11-carboxylate **12** (14 mg, 14%). m.p. 247–250 °C; vmax/cm^{-1} (KBr): 3147 (NH), 3008 (CH), 1742 (C=O), 1634 (C=C arom.), 1589 (C=C arom.), 1457, 1422, 1246 (C-O stretch), 1095; δH (300 MHz, DMSO-d_6): 2.89 [3H, s, C(5)CH_3], 4.22 [3H, s, C(11)$COOCH_3$], 7.27 [1H, overlapping ddd, *J* = 8.0, 5.8, 2.3, C(9)H], 7.57–7.63 [2H, m, C(7)H, C(8)H], 7.99 [1H, d, *J* = 8.0, C(10)H], 8.04 [1H, d, *J* = 6.1, C(3)H], 8.50 [1H, br s, C(4)H], 9.38 [1H, br s, C(1)H], 11.73 [1H, s, N(6)H]; δC (150.9 MHz, DMSO-d_6): 12.4 [CH_3, C(5)CH_3], 53.1 [CH_3, C(11)$COOCH_3$], 111.3 [CH, C(7)H or C(8)H], 113.7 (C, aromatic C), 116.2 [CH, C(3)H], 119.6 [CH, C(9)H], 120.2 (C, aromatic C), 121.3 (C, aromatic C), 121.8 (C, aromatic C), 122.5 [CH, C(10)H], 128.7 [CH, C(7)H or C(8)H], 131.6 (C, aromatic C), 140.2 (C, aromatic C), 140.9 [CH, C(4)H], 143.1 (C, aromatic C), 149.8 [CH, C(1)H], 168.4 [C, C(11)C=O]; m/z (ESI+): 291 [$(M+H)^+$, 100%]. HRMS (ESI+): Exact mass calculated for $[C_{18}H_{15}N_2O_2]^+$ 291.1134. Found 291.1121.

(*E*)-4-(5-methyl-6*H*-pyrido[4,3-*b*]carbazol-11-yl)but-3-en-2-one 13. A stirred solution of 5-methyl -6*H*-pyrido[4,3-*b*]carbazole-11-carbaldehyde **8** (300 mg, 1.15 mmol) in acetone (70 mL) was treated drop-wise with potassium permanganate (364 mg, 2.30 mmol) in water (70 mL). The mixture was stirred at r.t. for 1 h and heated to reflux for 22 h. Sodium bicarbonate (244 mg, 2.30 mmol) was added and stirred for 20 min. The mixture was filtered through celite and washed with water (100 mL) and acetone (200 mL). The filtrate was concentrated under reduced pressure to remove the acetone and then acidified to pH 5 with 20% aqueous HCl. The aqueous layer was extracted with chloroform:methanol (90:10, 3 × 100 mL). Organic extracts were combined and washed with water (1 × 100 mL) and brine (1 × 100 mL), dried over magnesium sulphate and evaporated under reduced pressure to give an orange solid (300 mg). Analysis showed that the desired carboxylic acid **9** had not formed but instead the condensation product (*E*)-4-(5-methyl-6*H*-pyrido[4,3-*b*]carbazol-11-yl)but-3-en-2-one **13** (87.0%). m.p. 263–265 °C; vmax/cm^{-1} (KBr): 3149(NH), 3087 (CH), 2982 (asymm. CH_3 stretch), 2883 (symm. CH_3 stretch), 1664 (C=O), 1620 (C=C), 1592 (C=C arom.), 1464, 1404, 1383, 1243; δH (300 MHz, DMSO-d_6): 2.61 [3H, s, $COCH_3$], 2.84 [3H, s, C(5)CH_3], 6.75 [1H, d, *J* = 16.6, C(11)CH=CH], 7.25 [1H, overlapping ddd, *J* = 8.0, 6.6, 1.5, C(9)H], 7.53–7.61 [2H, m, C(7)H, C(8)H], 7.98 [1H, dd, *J* = 6.1, 0.7, C(3)H], 8.14 [1H, d, *J* = 8.0, C(10)H], 8.47 [1H, d, *J* = 6.1, C(4)H], 8.59 [1H, d, *J* = 16.6, C(11)CH=CH], 9.58 [1H, s, C(1)H], 11.57 [1H, s, N(6)H]; δC (75.5 MHz, DMSO-d_6): 12.2 [CH_3, C(5)CH_3], 27.8 (CH_3, $COCH_3$), 111.1 [CH, C(7)H], 111.7 (C, aromatic C), 115.9 [CH, C(3)H], 119.4 [CH, C(9)H], 120.5 (C, aromatic C), 121.9 (C, aromatic C), 122.4 (C, aromatic C), 123.6 [CH, C(10)H], 126.0 (C, aromatic C), 127.9 [CH, C(8)H], 132.3 (C, aromatic C), 135.9 [CH, C(11)CH=CH], 138.4 [CH, C(11)CH=CH], 140.2 (C, aromatic C), 140.9 [CH, C(4)H], 143.0 (C, aromatic C), 150.1 [CH, C(1)H], 197.8 (C, C=O); m/z (ESI+): 301[(M+H)+ 100%]; HRMS (ESI+): Exact mass calculated for $[C_{20}H_{17}N_2O]^+$ 301.1341. Found 301.1348.

(*E*)-*N*-(4-(5-methyl-6*H*-pyrido[4,3-*b*]carbazol-11-yl)but-3-en-2-yl)formamide 14. (*E*)-4-(5-Methyl -6*H*-pyrido[4,3-*b*]carbazol-11-yl)but-3-en-2-one **13** (91 mg, 0.303 mmol), formamide (0.2 mL, 5.03 mmol) and formic acid (0.1 mL, 2.65 mmol) were heated to 150 °C for 1.5 h, at which point TLC analysis indicated consumption of the starting material. On cooling, saturated aqueous sodium bicarbonate (8 mL) was added and extraction was attempted with dichloromethane:methanol (90:10), however the organic extracts contained no material. The aqueous layer was treated with 20% aqueous HCl to pH 1, stirred for 20 min and then adjusted to pH 10 with 20% aqueous NaOH. The aqueous layer was extracted with dichloromethane–methanol (90:10 3 × 30 mL and 80:20 4 × 30 mL), dried and evaporated under reduced pressure to give an orange solid (64 mg). Purification by column chromatography on alumina, eluting with dichloromethane:methanol (97:3–90:10) gave three fractions. The largest of these (34 mg) was repurified by chromatography on silica to give an orange solid (19 mg). This was found to be the formamide, (*E*)-*N*-(4-(5-methyl-6*H*-pyrido[4,3-*b*]carbazol-11-yl)but-3-en-2-yl)formamide **14**. δH (300 MHz, DMSO-d_6): 1.47 [3H, d, *J* = 6.9, C(11)CH=CH–CH(CH_3)], 2.83 [3H, s, C(5)CH_3], 4.88–4.95 [1H, m, C(11)CH=CH–CH(CH_3)], 6.14 [1H, dd, *J* = 16.2, 5.6, C(11)CH=CH], 7.21 [1H, overlapping ddd,

J = 8.0, 6.7, 1.4, C(9)H], 7.36 [1H, d, *J* = 16.5, C(11)CH=CH], 7.52 [1H, td, *J* = 7.4, 1.1, C(8)H], 7.56–7.59 [1H, m, C(7)H], 7.99 [1H, br s, NHCHO], 8.23 [1H, br s, C(3)H], 8.33 [1H, d, *J* = 7.7, C(10)H], 8.43 [1H, br s, NHCHO], 8.54 [1H, d, *J* = 7.5, C(4)H], 9.58 [1H, br s, C(1)H], 11.51 [1H, s, N(6)H]; m/z (ESI+): 330 [$(M+H)^+$ 60%], 169 (100%); HRMS (ESI): Exact mass calculated for $[C_{21}H_{20}N_3O]^+$ 330.1606. Found 330.1619.

9-Formyl-5-methyl-6*H*-pyrido[4,3-*b*]carbazole-11-carboxylic acid 15. 5-Methyl-6*H*-pyrido[4,3-*b*] carbazole-11-carboxylic acid **9** (497 mg, 1.80 mmol) in trifluoroacetic acid (60 mL), was treated with hexamethylenetetramine (2.522 g, 18.0 mmol) portionwise over 5 min and heated to reflux for 25 min. On cooling, the reaction mixture was concentrated to approx. one quarter volume, water (30 mL) was added and the solution was transferred to a large conical flask (500 mL). The solution was cooled to 0 °C and neutralized with solid sodium bicarbonate while stirring vigorously. The mixture was stirred at 0 °C for 1 h, readjusted to pH 7 and filtered to give a brown solid which was dried at 0.02 mbar for 2 days (449 mg, 81.9%). m.p. 315–317 °C; vmax/cm^{-1} (KBr): 3069 (OH broad), 1677 (C=O × 2, broad), 1583 (C=C arom.), 1472, 1404, 1349, 1242 (C-O stretch), 1128, 808; δH (600 MHz, DMSO-d_6): 2.88 [3H, s, $C(5)CH_3$], 7.72 [1H, d, *J* = 8.3, C(7)H], 8.04 [1H, d, *J* = 6.0, C(3)H], 8.10 [1H, d, *J* = 8.4, C(8)H], 8.50 [1H, d, *J* = 6.0, C(4)H], 8.80 [1H, s, C(10)H], 9.51 [1H, s, C(1)H], 10.04 [1H, s, C(9)CHO], 12.14 [1H, s, N(6)H]; δC (150.9 MHz, DMSO-d_6): 12.3 [3H, s, $C(5)CH_3$], 111.4 [CH, C(7)H], 113.0 (C, aromatic C), 116.2 [CH, C(3)H], 119.7 (C, aromatic C), 120.4 (C, aromatic C), 121.3 (C, aromatic C), 125.7 [CH, C(10)H], 128.5 (C, aromatic C), 129.8 [CH, C(8)H], 129.9 (C, aromatic C), 132.4 (C, aromatic C), 140.8 [CH, C(4)H], 141.1 (C, aromatic C), 146.9 (C, aromatic C), 150.7 [CH, C(1)H], 169.2 [C, C(11)COOH], 191.6 [CH, C(9)CHO]; m/z (ESI+): 305 [$(M+H)^+$ 70%], 155 (40%), 64 (100%); HRMS (ESI+): Exact mass calculated for $[C_{18}H_{13}N_2O_3]^+$ 305.0926. Found 305.0940.

Benzylammonium 9-((benzylimino)methyl)-5-methyl-6H-pyrido[4,3-b]carbazole-11-carboxylate 16. A suspension of 9-formyl-5-methyl-6*H*-pyrido[4,3-*b*]carbazole-11-carboxylic acid **15** (194 mg, 0.638 mmol) in dichloromethane (65 mL), under N_2, was treated with oxalyl chloride (0.08 mL, 0.917 mmol) and stirred at room temperature overnight. Additional oxalyl chloride (0.08 mL, 0.917 mmol), was added and the reaction was stirred for 4 h. The mixture was evaporated under reduced pressure, cooled to 0 °C under N_2, and treated drop-wise with benzylamine (2 mL, 18.3 mmol). After stirring for 1 h, diethyl ether (40 mL) was added, the mixture was cooled and filtered to give a yellow solid. Crude analysis showed this to contain residual benzylamine. Recrystallisation from dichloromethane followed by a second recrystallisation from methanol gave product still containing benzylamine in 1:1 ratio with product. To investigate whether an amide or imine had formed, the product (27 mg) was dissolved in dichloromethane:methanol (90:10, 10 mL) and washed with 1M HCl (10 mL). The organic layer was dried and evaporated under reduced pressure. NMR and MS analysis showed that the compound had hydrolysed to the starting material **15**, indicating imine rather than amide formation. Full analysis (along with subsequent reduction of the imine) confirmed the product as the imine salt, benzylammonium 9-((benzylimino)methyl)-5-methyl-6*H*-pyrido[4,3-*b*]carbazole-11-carboxylate **16** (208 mg, 82.9%). m.p. 241–243 °C; vmax/cm^{-1} (KBr): 3029 (NH), 2864 (OH, broad), 1598 (C=O), 1572 (C=C arom.), 1494, 1450, 1402, 1347, 1278, 1244 (C-O stretch); δH (300 MHz, DMSO-d_6): 2.81 [3H, s, $C(5)CH_3$], 4.06 [2H, s, benzylammmonium-CH_2], 4.74 [2H, s, $C(9)CH{=}NCH_2$], 7.23–7.29 [1H, m, iminobenzyl-C(4)H], 7.33–7.42 [7H, m, iminobenzyl-C(2)H, C(3)H, C(5)H, C(6)H, benzylammmonium-C(3)H, C(4)H, C(5)H], 7.48 [2H, dd, *J* = 7.7, 1.7, benzylammmonium-C(2)H, C(6)H], 7.56 [1H, d, *J* = 8.3, C(7)H], 7.91 [1H, dd, *J* = 6.1, 0.7, C(3)H], 7.97 [1H, dd, *J* = 8.4, 1.6, C(8)H], 8.38 [1H, d, *J* = 6.1, C(4)H], 8.52 [1H, s, C(9)CH=N], 8.73 [1H, d, *J* = 1.1, C(10)H], 9.50 [1H, s, C(1)H], 11.64 [1H, s, N(6)H]; δC (75.5 MHz, DMSO-d_6): 12.0 [CH_3, $C(5)CH_3$], 42.3 [CH_2, benzylammonium CH_2], 64.1 [CH_2, $C(9)CH{=}N{-}CH_2$], 110.6 (CH, aromatic CH), 115.7 (CH, aromatic CH), 119.2 (C, aromatic C), 119.4 (C, aromatic C), 122.2 (C, aromatic C), 124.3 (CH, aromatic CH), 125.1 (C, aromatic C), 126.7 (CH, aromatic CH), 127.3 (C, aromatic C), 127.9 (CH, 2 × aromatic CH), 128.2 (CH, aromatic CH), 128.3 (CH, 2 × aromatic CH), 128.5 (CH, 2 × aromatic CH), 128.6 (CH, aromatic CH), 128.7 (CH, 2 × aromatic CH), 131.3 (C, aromatic C), 132.1 (C, aromatic

C), 134.6 (C, aromatic C), 139.9 (CH, aromatic CH), 140.5 (CH, aromatic CH), 141.1 (C, aromatic C), 144.3 (C, aromatic C), 144.5 (C, aromatic C), 152.0 (CH, aromatic CH), 162.2 (C, C=O); m/z (ESI+): 394 [$(M+H)^+$ 20%], 305 (20%), 108 (100%); HRMS (ESI+): Exact mass calculated for $[C_{25}H_{20}N_3O_2]^+$ 394.1556. Found 394.1560.

9-((Benzylamino)methyl)-5-methyl-6*H*-pyrido[4,3-*b*]carbazole-11-carboxylic acid 17. A solution of benzylammonium 9-((benzylimino) methyl)-5-methyl-6*H*-pyrido[4,3-*b*]carbazole-11-carboxylate **16** (88 mg, 0.224 mmol) in absolute ethanol (12 mL) was treated with sodium cyanoborohydride (21 mg, 0.338 mmol) and heated to reflux for 4.5 h. The solution was evaporated under reduced pressure and water (10 mL) was added. The mixture was stirred for 15 min, cooled and filtered. The orange solid was washed with water (5 mL) and diethyl ether (10 mL) and dried at 0.1 mbar for 24 h (56 mg, 62.9%). m.p. >300 °C (without melting); vmax/cm^{-1} (KBr): 3370 (NH), 3188 (OH, broad), 3056 (CH), 1596 (C=O), 1565 (C=C arom.), 1482, 1403, 1348, 1247 (C-O stretch); δH (600 MHz, DMSO-d_6): 2.73 [3H, s, $C(5)CH_3$], 3.89 [2H, s, one of CH_2], 4.04 [2H, s, one of CH_2], 7.21–7.26 [3H, m, *N*-benzyl-C(3)H, C(4)H, C(5)H], 7.39–7.40 [2H, m, N-benzyl-C(2)H, C(6)H], 7.46 [1H, d, *J* = 7.3, C(7)H], 7.53 [1H, d, *J* = 7.5, C(8)H], 7.82 [1H, d, *J* = 5.6, C(3)H], 8.29 [1H, d, *J* = 5.6, C(4)H], 8.42 [1H, s, C(10)H], 9.44 [1H, s, C(1)H], 11.39 [1H, s, N(6)H]; δC (150.9 MHz, DMSO-d_6): 12.0 [CH_3, $C(5)CH_3$], 50.3 (CH_2), 51.4 (CH_2), 108.3 (C, aromatic C), 110.4 [CH, C(7)H], 115.6 [CH, C(3)H], 119.1 (C, aromatic C), 119.3 (C, aromatic C), 122.4 (C, aromatic C), 124.5 [CH, C(10)H], 127.7 [CH, *N*-benzyl-C(4)H], 128.1 (CH, C(8)H], 128.3 [CH, *N*-benzyl-C(3)H, *N*-benzyl-C(5)H], 129.0 [CH, *N*-benzyl-C(2)H, *N*-benzyl-C(6)H], 129.1 (C, aromatic C), 132.0 (C, aromatic C), 133.7 (C, aromatic C), 136.0 (C, aromatic C), 140.2 [CH, C(4)H], 141.3 (C, aromatic C), 142.2 (C, aromatic C), 152.2 [CH, C(1)H], 170.8 (C, C=O); m/z (ESI+): 396 [$(M+H)^+$ 80%], 306 (100%); HRMS (ESI+): Exact mass calculated for $[C_{25}H_{22}N_3O_2]^+$ 396.1712. Found 396.1729.

Topoisomerase II decatenation assay. The decatenation assay kit was obtained from Inspiralis, Norwich Bioincubator, Norwich Research Park, Colney, Norwich, UK. The kit comprised of the following: assay buffer (supplied as 10× stock) containing 50 mM Tris.HCl (pH 7.5), 125 mM NaCl, 10 mM MgCl2, 5 mM DTT and 100 μg/mL albumin; dilution buffer containing 50 mM Tris. HCl (pH 7.5), 100 mM NaCl, 1 mM DTT, 0.5 mM EDTA, 50% (v/v) glycerol, 50 μg/mL albumin; ATP 30 mM; kDNA (100 ng/μl); 10 U/μL human topoisomerase II in dilution buffer; 5× stop buffer containing 2.5% SDS, 15% Ficoll-400, 0.05% bromophenol blue, 0.05% xylene cyanol and 25 mM EDTA. Tris-acetate-EDTA buffer (supplied as 10X buffer) and agarose were obtained from Sigma Life Sciences (Dublin, Ireland) and Safe View Stain was supplied by NBS Biologicals, Cambridgeshire, England.

The topo II decatenation assay protocol involved initial incubation of each inhibitor candidate (100 μM) along with a stock solution containing water, ATP, assay buffer, kDNA obtained from the mitochondrial DNA of Crithidia fasciculate, and topo II, at 37 °C for 1 h. Following addition of stop buffer, agarose DNA gel electrophoresis was run at 50 V for 2 h using a Consort EV243 power pack, to determine the relative amounts of decatenated DNA bands obtained in each compound lane. Positive (water), as well as negative controls (ellipticine) were incorporated in order to validate the results of each run. The resulting gels were viewed under UV light using a DNR Bio-Imaging System and photographed using GelCapture software.

NCI-60 Anti-cancer screening. Tested compounds were initially solubilised in DMSO, diluted into RPMI 1640 and 5% fetal bovine serum/L-glutamine, and added to 96-well plates containing cell lines previously cultured for 24 h. After 48-h incubation, the media were removed, and the cells were fixed and stained with sulforhodamine B to determine overall percent growth/total protein content. Unbound dye was removed with five washes of 1% acetic acid, and the plates were allowed to air dry. The dye was then resolubilised in Tris buffer, and the colorimetric absorbance was measured (515 nm). Growth inhibition was measured relative to the response generated from proliferating cells cultured under identical conditions for 48 h. In the five dose study, serial 5 × 10-fold dilution from an initial DMSO stock solution was performed, prior to incubation at each individual concentration (10 nM, 100 nM, 1 μM, 10 μM and 100 μM).

Using seven absorbance measurements (time zero (Tz), control growth (C), and test growth in the presence of drug at the five concentration levels (Ti)), the percentage growth was calculated at each of the drug concentrations levels. Percentage growth inhibition was calculated as:

$[(Ti-Tz)/(C-Tz)] \times 100$ for concentrations for which $Ti \geq Tz$
$[(Ti-Tz)/Tz] \times 100$ for concentrations for which $Ti < Tz$.

Three dose response parameters were calculated for each experimental agent. Growth inhibition of 50% (GI50) was calculated from $[(Ti-Tz)/(C-Tz)] \times 100 = 50$, which is the drug concentration resulting in a 50% reduction in the net protein increase (as measured by Sulforhodamine B staining) in control cells during the drug incubation. The drug concentration resulting in total growth inhibition (TGI) was calculated from $Ti = Tz$. The LC50 (concentration of drug resulting in a 50% reduction in the measured protein at the end of the drug treatment as compared to that at the beginning) indicating a net loss of cells following treatment was calculated from $[(Ti-Tz)/Tz] \times 100 = -50$. Values were calculated for each of these three parameters if the level of activity was reached; however, if the effect was not reached or was exceeded, the value for that parameter was expressed as greater or less than the maximum or minimum concentration tested [36,37]. Data from one dose experiments pertains to the percentage growth at 10 μM.

COMPARE analysis. COMPARE analysis was conducted using the private access system provided by the National Cancer Institute (https://dtp.cancer.gov/databases_tools/compare.htm). Seed compounds were analysed using a number of target sets: synthetic compounds, mechanistic set, standard agents, marketed drugs and diversity set. While the minimum correlation was set to 0.4, correlations of less than 0.5 were discounted. All other criteria were unchanged. Experiments that were carried out at different concentrations to the seed compound were ignored unless the concentration deviated by ±0.1, as was usual for older testing methods. COMPARE analysis was conducted solely on five dose data for compounds **11** and **13** [38].

4. Conclusions

Novel ellipticines substituted at the 11-position are described and their activity evaluated against topoisomerase II and cell growth in the National Cancer Institute's 60 cell line screening platform. Two of the novel compounds (**13** and **16**) show limited promise as topoisomerase II inhibitors at high concentrations (>10 μM). On evaluation of anticancer effect at the NCI, compounds **11** and **13** show real promise as future leads. Benzylamide **11** and unsaturated ketone **13** appear to have different modes of action in their cellular effects with broad cytotoxicity seen for compound **13** but some selectivity of cellular response seen for compound **11**. COMPARE analysis identified a potential target for compound **11** in Aurora kinase due to correlation of 0.6 with the known inhibitor SCH1473759. This will be investigated further in the future by synthesis of a series of ellipticine 11-amides to probe if this activity can be tuned further.

Author Contributions: F.M.C. conceived and designed the experiments and wrote the manuscript; C.M.M. and E.O.S. performed the experiments, characterized the synthetic products and analysed the data.

Acknowledgments: The authors would like to acknowledge the Irish Research Council and the Higher Education Authority of Ireland under the PRTLI4 programme for funding. In addition, the authors would like to recognize the contribution from National Cancer Institute (NCI) screening program.

Abbreviations

The following abbreviations are used in this manuscript:

AKT	Protein Kinase B
CK2	Casein Kinase 2
GI50	Growth Inhibition 50%
LC50	Lethal concentration 50%
NCI	National Cancer Institute
NSC	numeric identifier for substances submitted to the National Cancer Institute (NCI)
Topo	Topoisomerase
SAR	Structure Activity Relationship

References

1. Hanahan, D.; Weinberg, R.A. Hallmarks of cancer: the next generation. *Cell* **2011**, *144*, 646–674. [CrossRef] [PubMed]
2. Goodwin, S.; Smith, A.F.; Horning, E.C. Alkaloids of Ochrosia elliptica Labill. *J. Am. Chem. Soc.* **1959**, *81*, 1903–1908. [CrossRef]
3. Miller, C.M.; McCarthy, F.O. Isolation, biological activity and synthesis of the natural product ellipticine and related pyridocarbazoles. *R. Soc. Chem. Adv.* **2012**, *2*, 8883–8918. [CrossRef]
4. O'Sullivan, E.C.; Miller, C.M.; Deane, F.M.; McCarthy, F.O. *Emerging Targets in the Bioactivity of Ellipticines and Derivatives. Studies in Natural Products Chemistry*; Elsevier: Amsterdam, The Netherlands, 2013; pp. 189–232.
5. Paoletti, C.; Le Pecq, J.B.; Dat-Xuong, N.; Juret, P.; Garnier, H.; Amiel, J.L.; Rouesse, J. Antitumor activity, pharmacology, and toxicity of ellipticines, ellipticinium, and 9-hydroxy derivatives: preliminary clinical trials of 2-methyl-9-hydroxy ellipticinium (NSC 264-137). *Recent Results Cancer Res.* **1980**, *74*, 107–123. [PubMed]
6. Ohashi, M.; Oki, T. Ellipticine and related anticancer agents. *Expert Opin. Ther. Pat.* **1996**, *6*, 1285–1294. [CrossRef]
7. Rouesse, J.; Spielmann, M.; Turpin, F.; Le Chevalier, T.; Azab, M.; Mondesir, J.M. Phase II study of elliptinium acetate salvage treatment of advanced breast cancer. *Eur. J. Cancer* **1993**, *6*, 856–859. [CrossRef]
8. Monnot, M.; Mauffret, O.; Simon, V.; Lescot, E.; Psaume, B.; Saucier, J.M.; Charra, M.; Belehradek, J., Jr.; Fermandjian, S. DNA-drug recognition and effects on topoisomerase II-mediated cytotoxicity. A three-mode binding model for ellipticine derivatives. *J. Biol. Chem.* **1991**, *266*, 1820–1829.
9. Froelich-Ammon, S.J.; Patchan, M.W.; Osheroff, N.; Thompson, R.B. Topoisomerase II binds to ellipticine in the absence or presence of DNA. Characterization of enzyme-drug interactions by fluorescence spectroscopy. *J. Biol. Chem.* **1995**, *270*, 14998–15004. [CrossRef]
10. Fossé, P.; René, B.; Charra, M.; Paoletti, C.; Saucier, J.M. Stimulation of topoisomerase II-mediated DNA cleavage by ellipticine derivatives: structure-activity relationship. *Mol. Pharmacol.* **1992**, *42*, 590–595.
11. Poljakova, J.; Eckschlager, T.; Hrabeta, J.; Hrebackova, J.; Smutny, S.; Frei, E.; Martinek, V.; Kizek, R.; Stiborova, M. The mechanism of cytotoxicity and DNA adduct formation by the anticancer drug ellipticine in human neuroblastoma cells. *Biochem. Pharmacol.* **2009**, *77*, 1466–1479. [CrossRef]
12. Vendôme, J.; Letard, S.; Martin, F.; Svinarchuk, F.; Dubreuil, P.; Auclair, C.; Le Bret, M. Molecular modelling of wild-type and D816V c-kit inhibition based on ATP-competitive binding of ellipticine derivatives to tyrosine kinases. *J. Med. Chem.* **2005**, *48*, 6194–6201. [CrossRef] [PubMed]
13. Prudent, R.; Vassal-Stermann, E.; Nguyen, C.-H.; Pillet, C.; Martinez, A.; Prunier, C.; Barette, C.; Soleilhac, E.; Filhol, O.; Beghin, A. Pharmacological inhibition of LIM kinase stabilizes microtubules and inhibits neoplastic growth. *Cancer Res.* **2012**, *72*, 4429–4439. [CrossRef] [PubMed]
14. Lu, C.; Wang, W.; El-Deiry, W.S. Non-genotoxic anti-neoplastic effects of ellipticine derivative NSC176327 in p53-deficient human colon carcinoma cells involve stimulation of p73. *Cancer Biol. Ther.* **2008**, *7*, 2039–2046. [CrossRef] [PubMed]
15. Andrews, W.J.; Panova, T.; Normand, C.; Gadal, O.; Tikhonova, I.G.; Panov, K.I. Old drug, new target: ellipticines selectively inhibit RNA polymerase I transcription. *J. Biol. Chem.* **2013**, *288*, 4567–4582. [CrossRef] [PubMed]

16. Brown, R.V.; Wang, T.; Chappeta, V.R.; Wu, G.; Onel, B.; Chawla, R.; Quijada, H.; Camp, S.M.; Chiang, E.T.; Lassiter, Q.R.; et al. The Consequences of Overlapping G-Quadruplexes and i-Motifs in the Platelet-Derived Growth Factor Receptor β Core Promoter Nuclease Hypersensitive Element Can Explain the Unexpected Effects of Mutations and Provide Opportunities for Selective Targeting of Both Structures by Small Molecules To Downregulate Gene Expression. *J. Am. Chem. Soc.* **2017**, *139*, 7456–7475. [PubMed]
17. Miller, C.M.; O'Sullivan, E.C.; Devine, K.J.; McCarthy, F.O. Synthesis and biological evaluation of novel isoellipticine derivatives and salts. *Org. Biomol. Chem.* **2012**, *10*, 7912–7921. [CrossRef]
18. Deane, F.M.; O'Sullivan, E.C.; Maguire, A.R.; Gilbert, J.; Sakoff, J.A.; McCluskey, A.; McCarthy, F.O. Synthesis and evaluation of novel ellipticines as potential anti-cancer agents. *Org. Biomol. Chem.* **2013**, *11*, 1334–1344. [CrossRef]
19. Russell, E.G.; O'Sullivan, E.C.; Miller, C.M.; Stanicka, J.; McCarthy, F.O.; Cotter, T.G. Ellipticine derivative induces potent cytostatic effect in acute myeloid leukaemia cells. *Investig. New Drugs* **2014**, *32*, 1113–1122. [CrossRef]
20. Russell, E.G.; Guo, J.; O'Sullivan, E.C.; O'Driscoll, C.M.; McCarthy, F.O.; Cotter, T.G. 7-formyl-10-methylisoellipticine, a novel ellipticine derivative, induces mitochondrial reactive oxygen species (ROS) and shows anti-leukaemic activity in mice. *Investig. New Drugs* **2016**, *34*, 15–23. [CrossRef]
21. Kutney, J.P.; Noda, M.; Lewis, N.G.; Monteiro, B.; Mostowicz, D.; Worth, B.R. Dihydropyridines in synthesis and biosynthesis. V. Synthesis of pyridocarbazole alkaloids: Olivacine and (±)-guantambuine. *Can. J. Chem.* **1982**, *60*, 2426–2430.
22. Mosher, C.W.; Crews, O.P.; Acton, E.M.; Goodman, L. Preparation and antitumor activity of olivacine and some new analogs. *J. Med. Chem.* **1966**, *9*, 237–241. [CrossRef] [PubMed]
23. Schmidt, U.; Theumer, G.; Jäger, A.; Kataeva, O.; Wan, B.; Franzblau, S.G.; Knölker, H.-J. Synthesis and Activity against Mycobacterium tuberculosis of Olivacine and Oxygenated Derivatives. *Molecules* **2018**, *23*, 1402. [CrossRef] [PubMed]
24. Awada, A.; Giacchetti, S.; Gerard, B.; Eftekhary, P.; Lucas, C.; de Valeriola, D.; Poullain, M.G.; Soudon, J.; Dosquet, C.; Brillanceau, M.-H. Clinical phase I and pharmacokinetic study of S 16020, a new olivacine derivative: report on three infusion schedules. *Ann. Oncol.* **2002**, *13*, 1925–1934. [CrossRef] [PubMed]
25. Thompson, D.; Miller, C.M.; McCarthy, F.O. Computer Simulations Reveal a Novel Nucleotide-type Binding Orientation for Ellipticine-based Anticancer c-kit Kinase Inhibitors. *Biochemistry* **2008**, *47*, 10333–10344. [CrossRef] [PubMed]
26. Gribble, G.W.; Saulnier, M.G.; Obaza-Nutaitis, J.A.; Ketcha, D.M. A versatile and efficient construction of the 6H-pyrido[4,3-b]carbazole ring system. Syntheses of the antitumor alkaloids ellipticine, 9-methoxyellipticine, and olivacine, and their analogs. *J. Org. Chem.* **1992**, *57*, 5891–5899. [CrossRef]
27. Saulnier, M.G.; Gribble, G.W. An efficient synthesis of ellipticine. *J. Org. Chem.* **1982**, *47*, 2810–2812. [CrossRef]
28. Saulnier, M.G.; Gribble, G.W. Efficient construction of the 10H-pyrido[3,4-b]carbazole ring system. Syntheses of isoellipticine and 7-methoxyisoellipticine. *J. Org. Chem.* **1983**, *48*, 2690–2695. [CrossRef]
29. Gribble, G.W.; Fletcher, G.L.; Ketcha, D.M.; Rajopadhye, M. Metalated heterocycles in the synthesis of ellipticine analogs. A new route to the 10H-pyrido[2,3-b]carbazole ring system. *J. Org. Chem.* **1989**, *54*, 3264–3269. [CrossRef]
30. Modi, S.P.; Carey, J.J.; Archer, S. Synthesis of 5-methyl-6h-pyrido[4,3-b]carbazole-11-methanol. *Tetrahedron Lett.* **1990**, *31*, 5845–5848. [CrossRef]
31. Modi, S.P.; Michael, M.A.; Archer, S.; Carey, J.J. An efficient synthesis of C-11 substituted 6H-pyrido[4,3-b] carbazoles. *Tetrahedron* **1991**, *47*, 6539–6548. [CrossRef]
32. Plug, J.P.M.; Koomen, G.-J.; Pandit, U.K. An Expedient Synthesis of 9-Hydroxyellipticine. *Synthesis* **1992**, *1992*, 1221–1222. [CrossRef]
33. Domcke, S.; Sinha, R.; Levine, D.A.; Sander, C.; Schultz, N. Evaluating cell lines as tumour models by comparison of genomic profiles. *Nat. Commun.* **2013**, *4*, 2126. [CrossRef] [PubMed]
34. Yu, T.; Tagat, J.R.; Kerekes, A.D.; Doll, R.J.; Zhang, Y.; Xiao, Y.; Esposite, S.; Belanger, D.B.; Curran, P.J.; Mandal, A.K.; et al. Discovery of a Potent, Injectable Inhibitor of Aurora Kinases Based on the Imidazo-[1,2-a]-Pyrazine Core. *ACS Med. Chem. Lett.* **2010**, *1*, 214–218. [CrossRef] [PubMed]
35. Pang, B.; Qiao, X.; Janssen, L.; Velds, A.; Groothuis, T.; Kerkhoven, R.; Nieuwland, M.; Ovaa, H.; Rottenberg, S.; van Tellingen, O.; et al. Drug-induced histone eviction from open chromatin contributes to the chemotherapeutic effects of doxorubicin. *Nat. Commun.* **2013**, *4*, 1908. [CrossRef] [PubMed]

36. National Cancer Institute. Developmental Therapeutics Program. NCI-60 Human Tumour Cell Lines Screen. Available online: https://dtp.cancer.gov/discovery_development/nci-60/default.htm (accessed on 14 May 2019).

37. Shoemaker, R.H. The NCI60 human tumour cell line anticancer drug screen. *Nat. Rev. Cancer* **2006**, *6*, 813–823. [CrossRef]

38. Paull, K.D.; Shoemaker, R.H.; Hodes, L.; Monks, A.; Scudiero, D.A.; Rubinstein, L.; Plowman, J.; Boyd, M.R. Display and Analysis of Patterns of Differential Activity of Drugs Against Human Tumor Cell Lines: Development of Mean Graph and COMPARE Algorithm. *J. Natl. Cancer Inst.* **1989**, *81*, 1088–1092. [CrossRef]

2

Design and Synthesis of Indoleamine 2,3-Dioxygenase 1 Inhibitors and Evaluation of their Use as Anti-Tumor Agents

Hui Wen †, Yuke Liu †, Shufang Wang, Ting Wang, Gang Zhang, Xiaoguang Chen, Yan Li, Huaqing Cui, Fangfang Lai * and Li Sheng *

State Key Laboratory of Bioactive Substances and Function of Natural Medicine, Institute of Materia Medica, Peking Union Medical College and Chinese Academy of Medical Sciences, Beijing 100050, China; wenhui@imm.ac.cn (H.W.); liuyuke@imm.ac.cn (Y.L.); wangshufang@imm.ac.cn (S.W.); wangtingdlf@imm.ac.cn (T.W.); gzhang@imm.ac.cn (G.Z.); chxg@imm.ac.cn (X.C.); yanli@imm.ac.cn (Y.L.); hcui@imm.ac.cn (H.C.)

* Correspondence: laifangfang@imm.ac.cn (F.L.); shengli@imm.ac.cn (L.S.);

† These two authors contributed equally to this paper.

Academic Editor: Qiao-Hong Chen

Abstract: Indoleamine 2,3-dioxygenase (IDO) 1 is the key enzyme for regulating tryptophan metabolism and is an important target for interrupting tumor immune escape. In this study, we designed four series of compounds as potential IDO1 inhibitors by attaching various fragments or ligands to indole or phenylimidazole scaffolds to improve binding to IDO1. The compounds were synthesized and their inhibitory activities against IDO1 and tryptophan 2,3-dioxygenase were evaluated. The cytotoxicities of the compounds against two tumor cell lines were also determined. Two compounds with a phenylimidazole scaffold (DX-03-12 and DX-03-13) showed potent IDO1 inhibition with IC_{50} values of 0.3–0.5 μM. These two IDO1 inhibitors showed low cell cytotoxicity, which indicated that they may exert their anti-tumor effect via immune modulation. Compound DX-03-12 was investigated further by determining the in vivo pharmacokinetic profile and anti-tumor efficacy. The pharmacokinetic study revealed that DX-03-12 had satisfactory properties in mice, with rapid absorption, moderate plasma clearance (~36% of hepatic blood flow), acceptable half-life (~4.6 h), and high oral bioavailability (~96%). Daily oral administration of 60 mg/kg of compound DX-03-12 decreased tumor growth by 72.2% after 19 days in a mouse melanoma cell B16-F10 xenograft model compared with the untreated control. Moreover, there was no obvious weight loss in DX-03-12-treated mice. In conclusion, compound DX-03-12 is a potent lead compound for developing IDO1 inhibitors and anti-tumor agents.

Keywords: indoleamine 2,3-dioxygenase; inhibitor; anti-tumor; immune modulation; tryptophan metabolism

1. Introduction

Tryptophan metabolism is an important pathway for cancer immunotherapy [1–3]. The accumulation of tryptophan can activate T cells, and a decrease in tryptophan concentration affects the regular function of T cells and interferes with the differentiation of naïve T cells. The accumulation of tryptophan metabolites, such as L-kynurenine and other downstream kynurenines (3-hydroxykynurenine and 3-hydroxyanthranilic acid), is toxic to T cells and induces T cell apoptosis. Thus, increasing tryptophan degradation inhibits the immune response [4–6].

Indoleamine 2,3-dioxygenase (IDO; E.C. 1.12.11.17) 1 is a monomeric 41 kDa enzyme that contains heme and converts L-tryptophan to *N*-formylkynurenine in non-hepatic tissues [7]. Tryptophan 2,3-dioxygenase (TDO; E.C. 1.13.11.11) also catalyzes the degradation of L-tryptophan to *N*-formylkynurenine [8]. However, these two enzymes are genetically distinct and have low sequence homology [8].

IDO1 is an important enzyme in tryptophan metabolism and contributes to creating peripheral immune tolerance by degrading L-tryptophan, which suppresses the function of T cells, and by producing *N*-formylkynurenine, which inhibits T cells [8]. In addition, IDO1 can also trigger other activators of anti-tumor immunity. Notably, IDO1 is overexpressed in a range of cancer tissues [4–6]. Thus, blocking the activity of IDO1 is a potential strategy for tumor immunotherapy.

The crystal structures of recombinant human IDO1 have been resolved [9,10], and biochemical studies have revealed that the heme iron in the active site of IDO1 binding and forms adducts with exogenous ligands including O_2^-, NO, CO, H_2S, and CN^- [9,11–14]. IDO1 tolerates various substrates, whereas TDO has strict substrate specificity. This difference can be used to develop selective IDO1 inhibitors [8].

During the development of anti-tumor drugs, potent IDO1 inhibitors were discovered, and intensive efforts have been made to develop potent IDO1/TDO inhibitors with various structural scaffolds. Some typical examples of IDO1/TDO inhibitors are shown in Figure 1 [1,15–21]. The indole and phenylimidazole scaffolds have produced several potent IDO1 inhibitors. For example, IDO1 inhibitors indoximod (pathway IC_{50} = 450 nM) and PF-0684003 (IDO1 IC_{50} = 410 nM) are indole derivatives [13], and GDC-0919 (IDO1 IC_{50} = 13 nM) and AMCL-17g (IDO1 IC_{50} = 77 nM) are phenylimidazole derivatives [20].

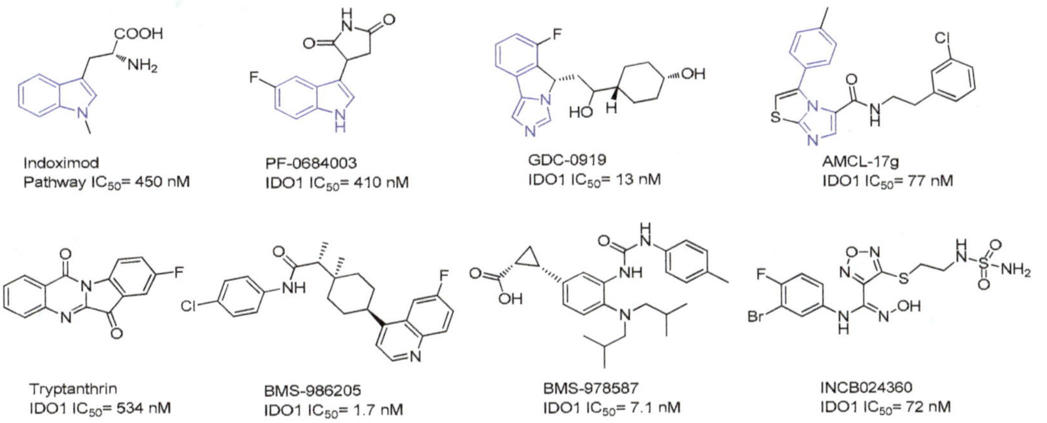

Figure 1. Reported IDO1 inhibitors. Indoximod and PF-0684003 have an indole scaffold and GDC-0919 and AMCL-17g have a phenylimidazole scaffold.

In this study, in the early stages of searching for new IDO1 inhibitors, we used indole and phenylimidazole as the core scaffolds. Four series of compounds were designed with different strategies. The compounds were synthesized and the IDO1/TDO inhibitory activities were determined. The in vivo pharmacokinetic profile and anti-tumor efficacy of a potent IDO1 inhibitor were evaluated to explore its potential as an anti-tumor agent.

2. Results and Discussion

2.1. Design Strategy for the Four Compound Series

Four series of compounds were designed (Figure 2) to explore the structure–activity relationship (SAR). The SAR information was used for further optimization. Indole is derived from tryptophan and phenylimidazole is an IDO1 inhibitor [18]. Thus, tryptophan and phenylimidazole fit into the active site of IDO1, and they were selected as the core scaffolds for designing the inhibitors. As we mentioned in the introduction, several exogenous ligands including hydroxylamine, O_2^-, NO, CO, H_2S, and CN^- were able to bind with the heme iron in the active site of IDO1 [9,11–14]. We attached various fragments and ligands to these scaffolds to strengthen the binding to the active site of IDO1.

In series 1, several ligands, such as hydroxylamine and SO, that interact strongly with heme iron were linked to the double bond of the indole scaffold. We hoped to observe a synergistic effect between the ligand and the indole ring in the IDO1 binding. Series 2 was based on compound PF-0684003 (Figure 1), which is an IDO1 inhibitor developed by Pfizer. The structure of PF-0684003 co-crystalized with IDO1 revealed that there was no interaction between PF-0684003 and the heme iron, which is usually observed between other IDO1 inhibitors and IDO1 [13]. Thus, several potential heme binding ligands, such as hydroxylamine and SO, were added to the structure of PF-0684003 to enhance the inhibitory activity.

Phenylimidazole is a weak IDO1 inhibitor. Crystal structures have revealed that the imidazole ring binds with the heme iron [18,19]. Thus, in series 3 and 4, we used phenylimidazole as the scaffold, and we attached fragments to either the imidazole ring (series 3) or the phenyl ring (series 4). These fragments were intended to improve the binding in the active site of IDO1 through various interactions, such as hydrogen bonds and π–π interactions.

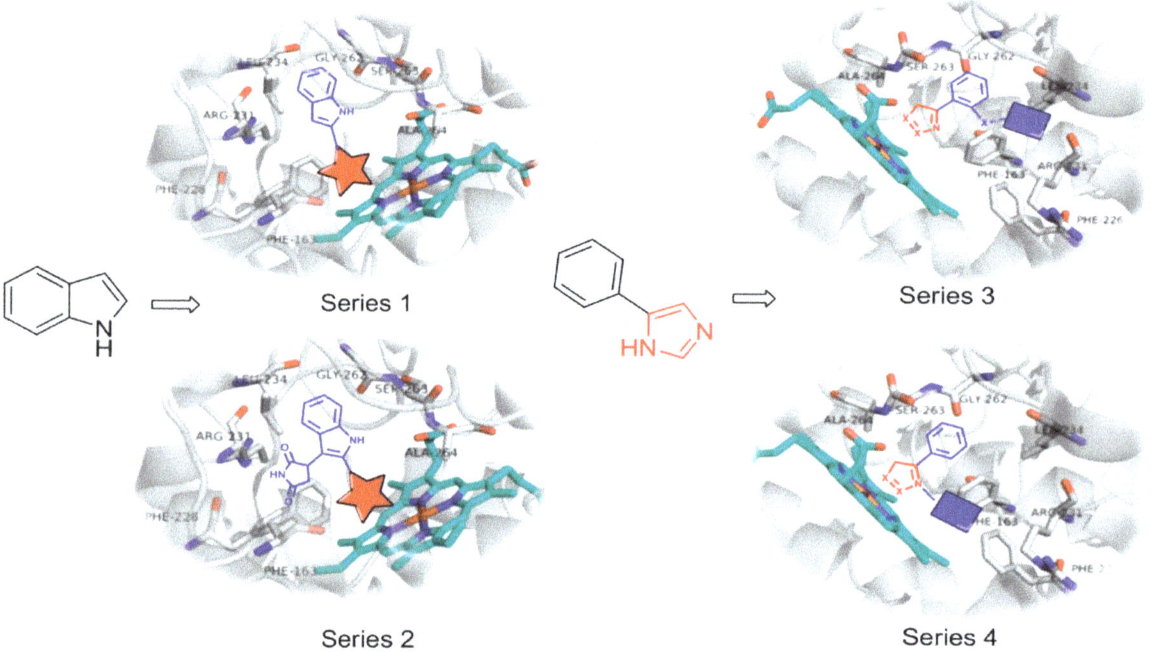

Figure 2. Design strategies of the four series of inhibitors. Because the parent compounds of series 1 and 2, indole and PF-0684003, respectively, do not interact with the heme iron, various heme binding ligands were attached to the indole scaffold. The imidazole ring interacts with the heme iron, and thus various fragments were attached to the phenyl ring in series 3 and the imidazole ring in series 4 to strengthen the binding to the active site of IDO1.

2.2. Synthesis of Selected Compounds

Although the compounds were classified into four series for examining the SAR, the structural diversity meant that they required a variety of synthetic routes. We describe representative synthetic schemes for four compounds. Syntheses for all the compounds are included in the Experimental section.

Scheme 1 shows the synthesis of DX-02-05. In the presence of a Lewis acid, ethyl 5-fluoro-1*H*-indole-2-carboxylate underwent a condensation reaction with 1*H*-pyrrole-2,5-dione to yield compound DX-02-03. Alcohol **1** was obtained by reducing DX-02-03, and then **1** was directly oxidized with MnO_2 to produce aldehyde **2**. Aldehyde **2** was condensed with hydroxylamine hydrochloride to obtain compound DX-02-04. Finally, the double bond in DX-02-04 was reduced with $NaBH_3CN$ to obtain compound DX-02-05.

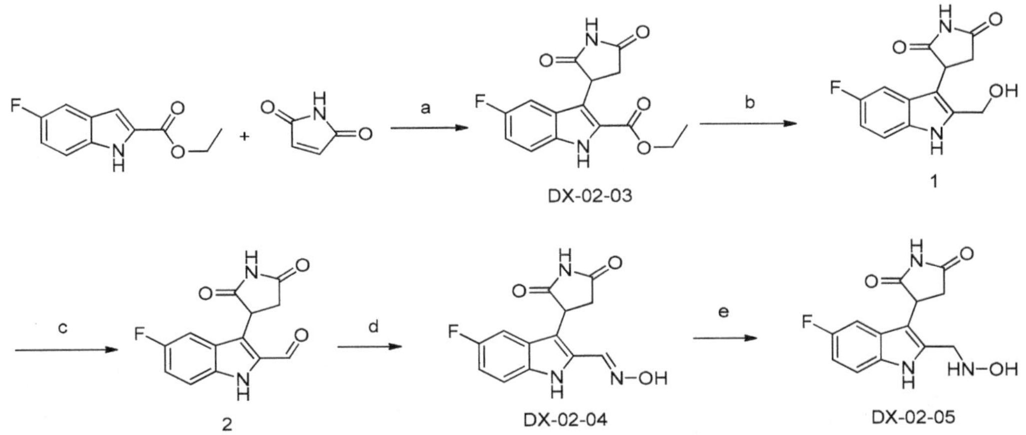

Scheme 1. Synthesis of DX-02-05. (a) BF_3-Et_2O, $ClCH_2CH_2Cl$, yield = 55%; (b) $LiAlH_4$, CH_3OH, yield = 86%; (c) MnO_2, dry dichloromethane, yield = 91%; (d) hydroxylamine hydrochloride, DIPEA, CH_3OH, yield = 66%; (e) $NaBH_3CN$, 12 N HCl, CH_3OH, yield = 43%.

Scheme 2 shows the synthesis of DX-02-07. Sulfur substitution of 5-fluoroindolin-2-one was performed with P_2S_5 to produce compound **3**. Under basic conditions, compound **4** was obtained through an SN_2 substitution reaction with CH_3I. A condensation reaction between **4** and 1*H*-pyrrole-2,5-dione was performed at 120 °C to obtain sulfide DX-02-06, which was oxidized to racemic sulfoxide DX-02-07.

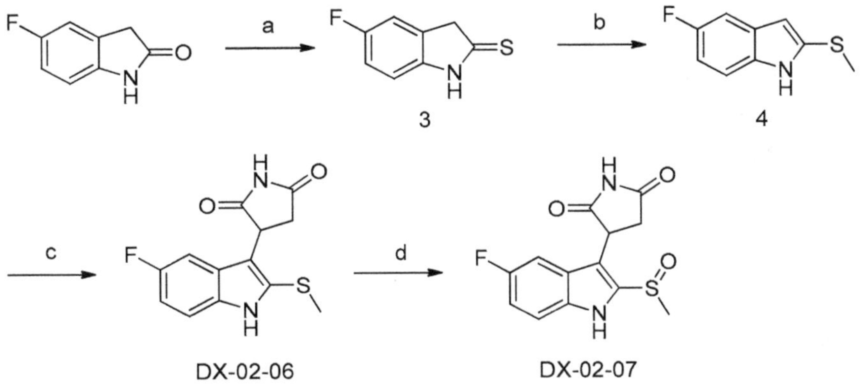

Scheme 2. Synthesis of DX-02-07. (a) P_2S_5, $NaHCO_3$, dry tetrahydrofuran, yield = 75%; (b) CH_3I, K_2CO_3, acetone, yield = 83%; (c) 1*H*-pyrrole-2,5-dione, CH_3CO_2H, yield = 61%; (d) m-CPBA, dry dichloromethane, yield = 35%.

Scheme 3 shows the synthesis of DX-03-12. First, the imidazole starting material was protected with trityl chloride to avoid various side reactions. Compound **6** was obtained by the Suzuki–Miyaura reaction with a boronic acid [22]. The methyl group was removed by BBr_3 to expose the hydroxyl group in compound **7**. Compound **8** was prepared in parallel by melting 3-chloropropylamine and isobenzofuran-1,3-dione together. Compounds **7** and **8** were subjected to an SN_2 nucleophilic reaction to obtain compound **9** under strong basic conditions. This step had a low yield, which was explained by the high steric hindrance of the large molecules and the weak nucleophilicity of compound **7**. The amine protecting group was removed with hydrazine hydrate to obtain compound **10**. Compound **10** was reacted with trifluoromethanesulfonylchloride under basic conditions to give compound **11**. Finally, DX-03-12 was obtained by removing the protecting group on the imidazole with acetic acid.

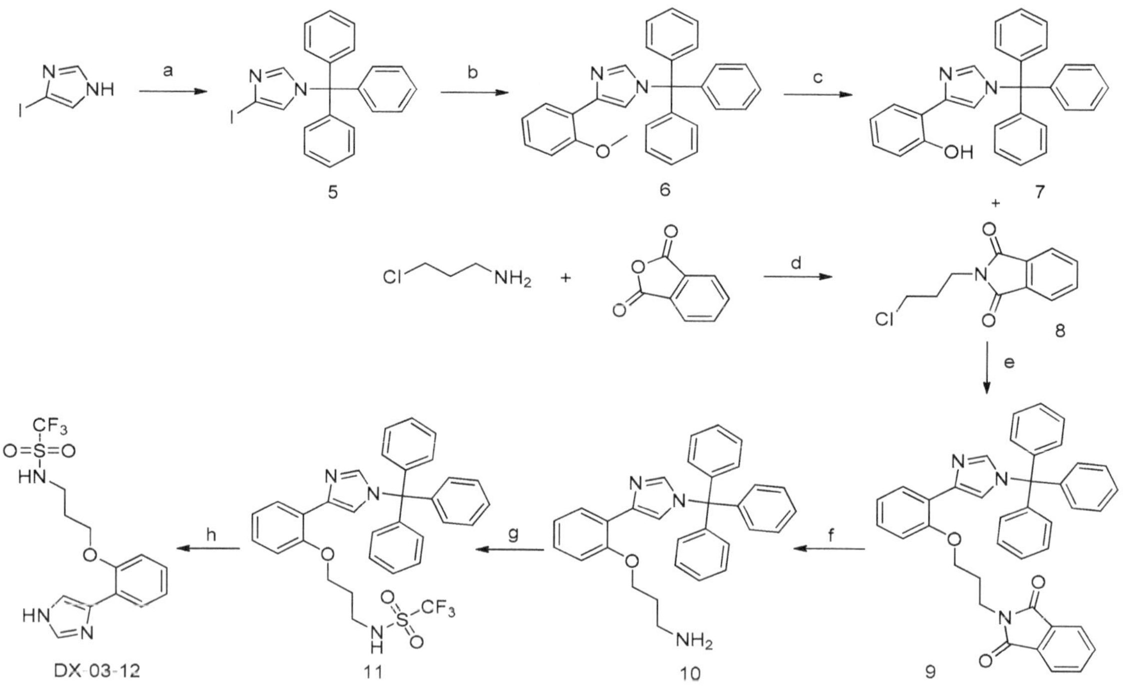

Scheme 3. Synthesis of DX-03-12. (a) Trityl Chloride, DIPEA, dry DMF, yield = 78%; (b) (2-methoxyphenyl)boronic acid, K_3PO_4, 14% $Pd(PPh_3)_4$, DMF, inert atmosphere, yield = 63%; (c) BBr_3, inert atmosphere, dry dichloromethane, yield = 65%; (d) solvent-free melt, yield = 55%; (e) KOH, dry DMF, yield = 71%; (f) hydrazine hydrate, CH_3OH; (g) trifluoromethanesulfonylchloride, DIPEA, dry dichloromethane, yield = 67%; (h) AcOH, CH_3OH, yield = 86%.

Scheme 4 shows the synthesis of DX-04-02. 2-Iodoimidazole was substituted with trifluoromethylbenzyl bromide to give compound **12**. Compound **12** underwent a Suzuki–Miyaura coupling reaction with (5-chloro-2-methoxyphenyl)boronic acid to obtain DX-04-01. Finally, the methyl group was removed with BBr_3 to obtain DX-04-02.

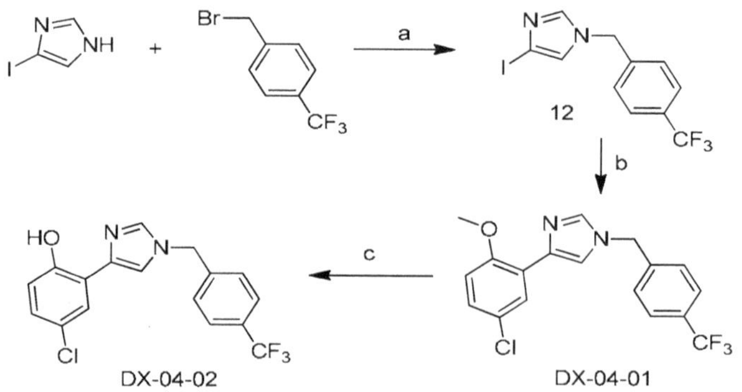

Scheme 4. Synthesis of DX-04-02. (a) DIPEA, dry DMF; (b) (5-chloro-2-methoxyphenyl)boronic acid, K_3PO_4, $Pd(PPh_3)_4$, DMF, inert atmosphere, yield = 72%; (c) BBr_3, inert atmosphere, yield = 53%.

2.3. *In Vitro Biological Evaluation*

We prepared the four series of compounds using the synthetic schemes in Section 2.2. Twelve commercially available compounds were purchased (see Section 3.1). In total, we screened 50 compounds in vitro for their IDO1 and TDO inhibitory activities and cell cytotoxicities against tumor cell lines H460 and MCF7 (Table 1). NLG919 was the reported potent IDO1/TDO inhibitor, and Taxol are known commercial anti-cancer drug. They were used as the reference compounds in this study.

Table 1. In vitro IDO1/TDO inhibitory activities and cell cytotoxicities of series 1.

Compound	Structure	IDO[a] IC_{50} or %	TDO [a] IC_{50} or %	H460 [a] IC_{50} or %	MCF7 [a] IC_{50} or %
DX-01-01	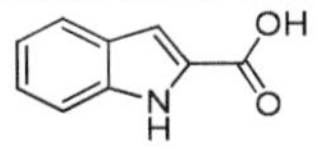	9.7%	8.9%	NA	NA
DX-01-02	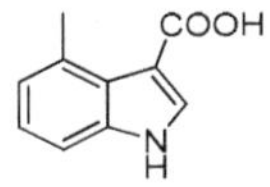	2.4%	10.0%	39.2%	43.1 μM
DX-01-03	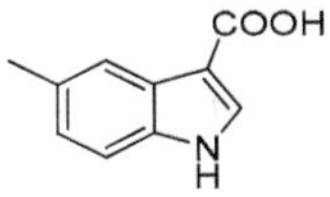	10.3%	10.1%	26.3%	37.6%
DX-01-04	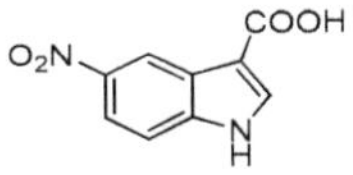	3.3%	6.0%	15.1%	24.3%
DX-01-05	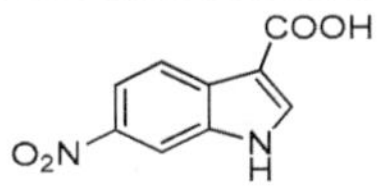	10.2%	10.5%	5.9%	29.7%
DX-01-06	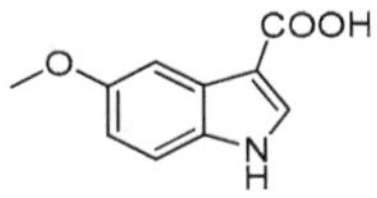	6.2%	8.4%	11.2%	25.7%
DX-01-07	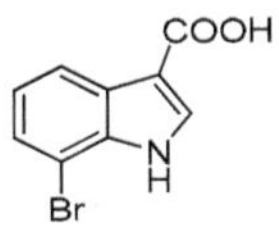	7.4%	16.9%	22.2%	34.6%
DX-01-08	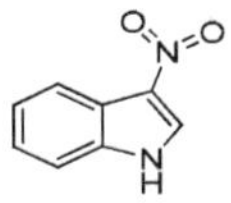	10.9%	3.2%	NA	NA
DX-01-09	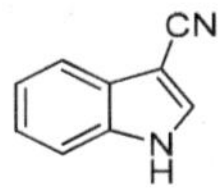	2.6%	7.8%	NA	NA
DX-01-10	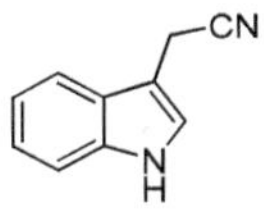	2.1%	8.9%	NA	NA
DX-01-11	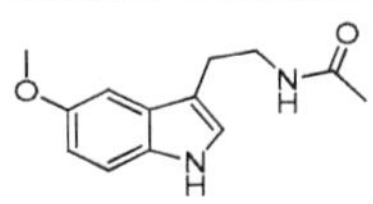	-	3.8%	NA	NA
DX-01-12	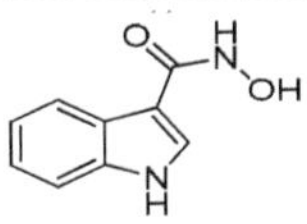	47.1%	33.9%	NA	NA
DX-01-13	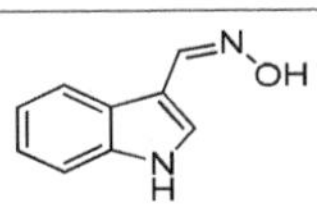	19.7%	8.1%	23.1%	10.1%
DX-01-14	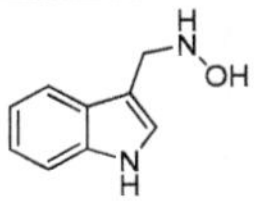	11.1 μM	38.2%	NA	NA

Table 1. *Cont.*

Compound	Structure	IDO[a] IC50 or %	TDO [a] IC50 or %	H460 [a] IC50 or %	MCF7 [a] IC50 or %
DX-01-15	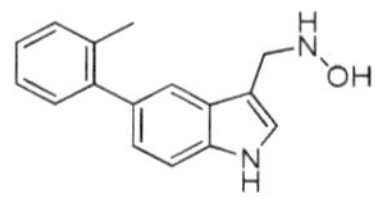	21.3 μM	35.4%	NA	NA
DX-01-16	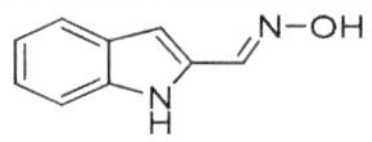	23.2 μM	19.7%	44.5%	20.9%
DX-01-17	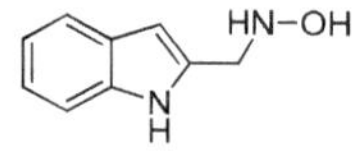	17.7 μM	42.2%	NA	NA
DX-01-18	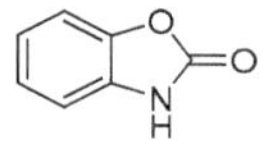	5.4%	-	NA	NA
DX-01-19	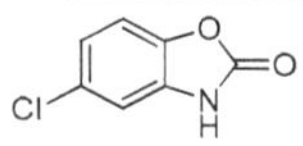	-	7.8%	NA	NA
DX-01-20	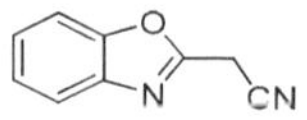	15.7%	3.8%	NA	NA
DX-01-21	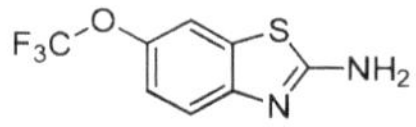	9.7%	9.2%	NA	NA
DX-01-22	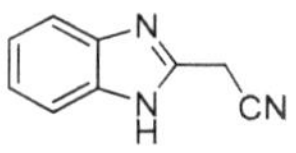	13.2%	4.5%	NA	NA
NLG919		0.064 μM	0.085 μM	NA	NA
Taxol		NA	NA	6 nM	15 nM

[a] When the calculated IC_{50} of a compound is >50 μM, we show the inhibition rate (%) at 50 μM. -: no detectable inhibition. NA: not tested.

The IDO1 and TDO inhibitory activities of the 22 compounds in series 1 were measured (Table 1). The series 1 compounds contained heme binding fragments including CO, NO, CN, H_2S, imidazole, and hydroxylamine; however, the inhibition data showed that most compounds in series 1 exhibited marginal IDO1/TDO inhibition. However, four compounds (DX-01-14, DX-01-15, DX-01-16, and DX-01-17) containing hydroxylamine had moderate IDO1 inhibitory activities. The most active IDO1 inhibitor in series 1 was compound DX-01-14 with an IC_{50} of 11.1 μM. In addition, cell cytotoxicity screening showed that most of the compounds were not toxic to mammalian cancer cell lines.

Generally speaking, these molecules have a rather low molecular weight, and the rather small moiety causes them hard to bind tightly inside the active center of IDO1. Thus, a poor SAR was observed for this series of compounds. Interestingly, for these four active compounds, they all contain the fragment of hydroxylamine. This may suggest that hydroxylamine is the ideal ligand to attach to the double bond of the indole scaffold, while still maintaining the binding with the heme iron.

Series 2 included seven compounds, which were all PF-0684003 derivatives (Table 2). However, the in vitro IDO1/TDO inhibitory activities of all these PF-0684003 derivatives were lower than that of the parent compound, and none were IDO1/TDO inhibitors. The cytotoxicity study demonstrated that these PF-0684003 derivatives were not toxic to cancer cell lines.

Table 2. In vitro IDO1/TDO inhibitory activities and cell cytotoxicities of series 2.

Compound	Structure	IDO [a] IC_{50} or %	TDO [a] IC_{50} or %	H460 [a] IC_{50} or %	MCF7 [a] IC_{50} or %
DX-02-01	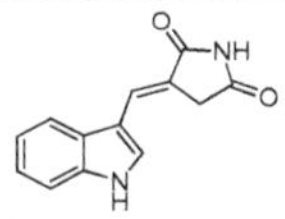	6.3%	-	NA	NA
DX-02-02	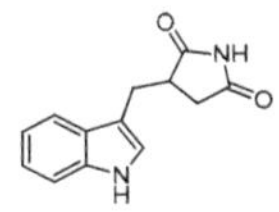	7.2%	2.3%	NA	NA
DX-02-03	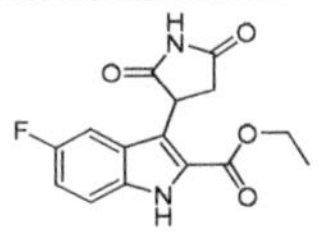	21.6%	15.4%	21.7%	22.1%
DX-02-04	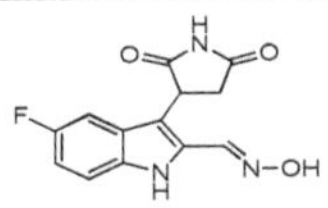	40.2%	14.5%	NA	NA
DX-02-05	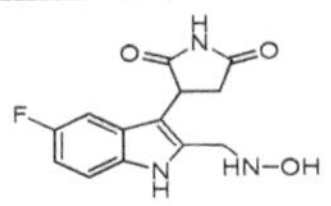	12.5%	16.3%	NA	NA
DX-02-06	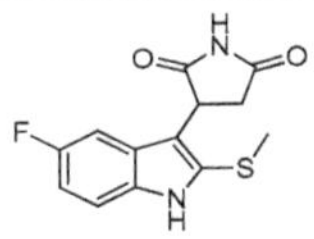	22.6%	19.6%	30.1%	19.9%
DX-02-07	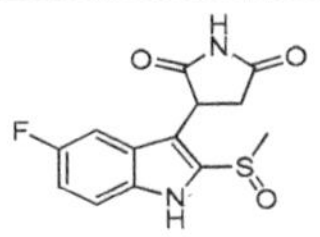	20.1%	13.9%	15.2%	11.0%
NLG919		0.064 μM	0.085 μM	NA	NA
Taxol		NA	NA	6 nM	15 nM

[a] When the calculated IC_{50} of a compound is >50 μM, we show the inhibition rate (%) at 50 μM. -: no detectable inhibition. NA: not tested.

The structure of PF-0684003 co-crystallized with IDO1 shows that PF-0684003 binds tightly in the active site of IDO1 but does not interact with the heme iron [18]. In the present study, the addition of the heme binding ligands [14] (SO and hydroxylamine in DX-02-07 and DX-02-05, respectively) to the double bond of the indole ring abrogated the IDO1 inhibition, similar to the optimization reported in a previous study.

Series 3 contains 13 phenylimidazole derivatives (Table 3). Compounds DX-03-01 to DX-03-10 showed marginal IDO1/TDO inhibition and weak cell cytotoxicities. However, compounds DX-03-11, DX-03-12, and DX-03-13 are potent IDO1 inhibitors with IC_{50} values of 0.3–2.4 μM. Interestingly, these three compounds show marginal TDO inhibition activity, and thus are IDO1/TDO selective inhibitors. In addition, these compounds are not toxic to mammalian cancer cell lines.

Compound DX-03-01 is a known compound [18], which binds to the active site in IDO1. The imidazole ring interacts with the heme iron, and the hydroxyl group binds to the nearby Ser167 in the active site [7]. However, the substitution of the hydroxyl group with hydroxylamine (DX-03-01 to DX-03-10) did not produce IDO1 inhibitors with higher activity. In DX-03-10 to DX-03-13, the hydroxyl group was used to attach an alkyl chain bearing terminal groups used in other reported IDO1 inhibitors [17,19]. The terminal fragments, such as sulfamide and urea, are important to maintain the binding [17,19].

Table 3. In vitro IDO1/TDO inhibitory activities and cell cytotoxicity of series 3.

Compound	Structure	IDO [a] IC_{50} or %	TDO [a] IC_{50} or %	H460 [a] IC_{50} or %	MCF7 [a] IC_{50} or %
DX-03-01	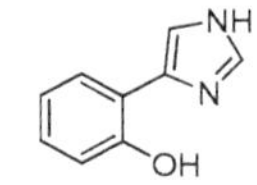	26.3%	10.3%	NA	NA
DX-03-02	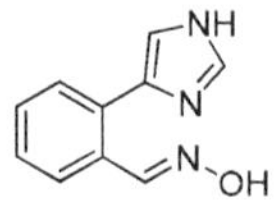	24.2%	13.9%	NA	NA
DX-03-03	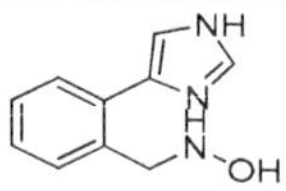	19.4%	11.1%	5.0%	22.2%
DX-03-04	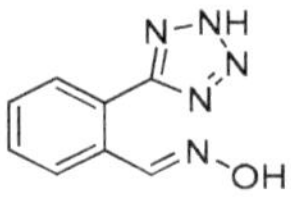	11.9%	20.3%	12.7%	34.7%
DX-03-05	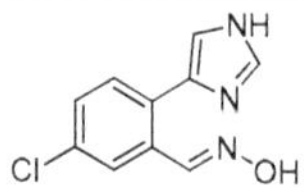	31.3%	12.1%	NA	NA
DX-03-06	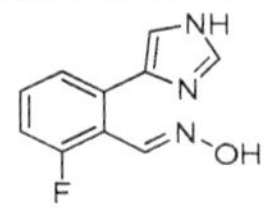	25.6%	12.9%	NA	NA
DX-03-07	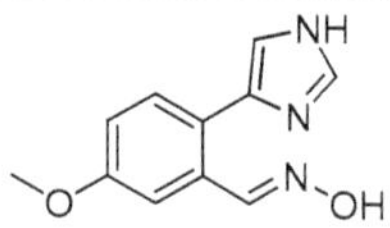	33.5%	15.1%	NA	NA
DX-03-08	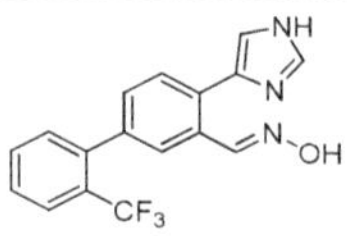	15.6%	11.1%	NA	NA
DX-03-09	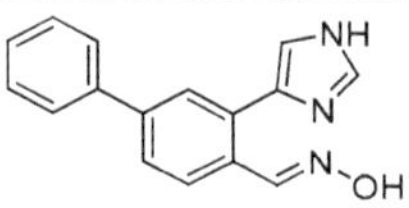	5.3%	6.4%	40.5%	37.7%
DX-03-10	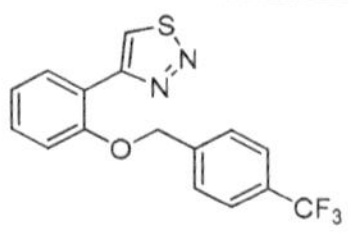	13.2%	21.5%	7.6%	24.7%
DX-03-11	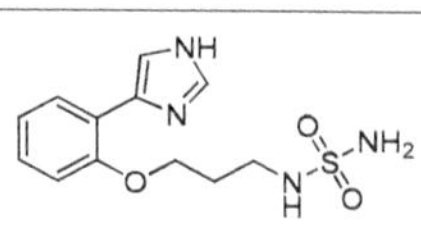	2.4 μM	38.2%	NA	NA
DX-03-12	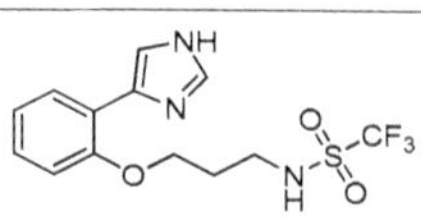	0.3 μM	36.4%	19.3%	6.6%
DX-03-13	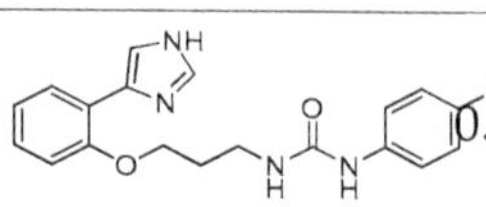	0.5 μM	38.9%	13.79	21.39
NLG919		0.064 μM	0.085 μM	NA	NA
Taxol		NA	NA	6 nM	15 nM

[a] When the calculated IC_{50} of a compound is >50 μM, we show the inhibition rate (%) at 50 μM. -: no detectable inhibition. NA: not tested.

Series 4 contains eight phenylimidazole derivatives (Table 4). Most compounds in this series showed marginal IDO1 inhibition, but compound DX-04-05 showed moderate IDO1 inhibition. However, compound DX-04-06, in which the hydroxyl group was methylated, showed decreased IDO1 inhibition. Most compounds in this series were toxic to the cancer cell lines H460 and MCF7 with an IC_{50} of around 10^{-5} M, which indicates the compounds also interrupt the function of other targets in the cells.

Table 4. In vitro IDO1/TDO inhibitory activities and cell cytotoxicities of series 4.

Compound	Structure	IDO [a] IC_{50} or %	TDO [a] IC_{50} or %	H460 [a] IC_{50} or %	MCF7 [a] IC_{50} or %
DX-04-01	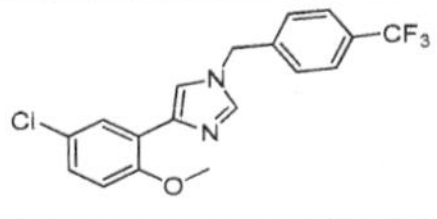	46.2%	26.5%	11.96 μM	8.53μM
DX-04-02	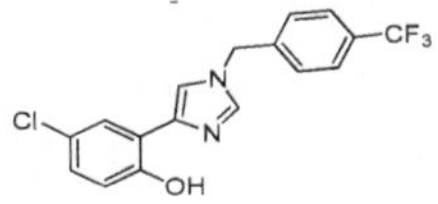	9.7%	18.0%	7.69 μM	35.72 μM
DX-04-03	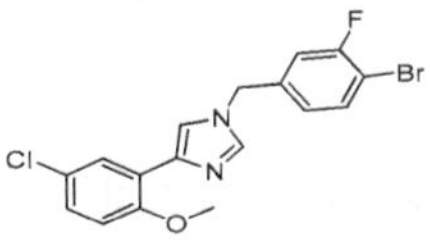	8.7%	17.3%	11.48 μM	15.44 μM
DX-04-04	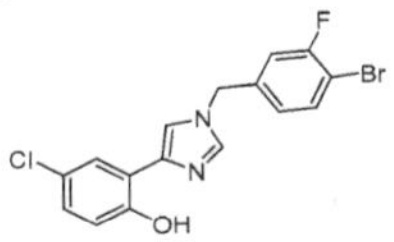	11.9%	23.8%	5.49 μM	20.95 μM
DX-04-05	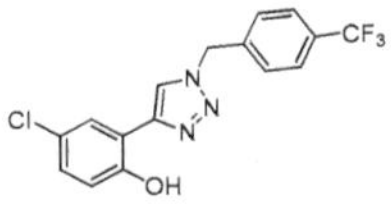	23 μM	22.4%	22.89 μM	42.55 μM
DX-04-06	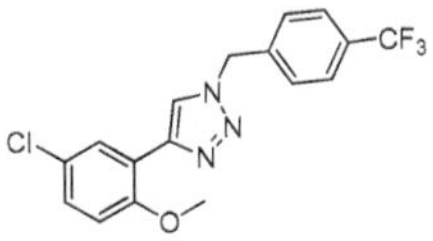	13.5%	23.6%	48.37 μM	49.34 μM
DX-04-07	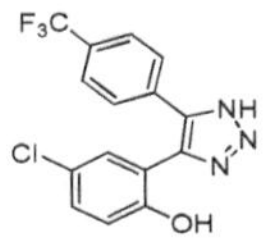	38.2%	21.4%	27.4 μM	12.28 μM
DX-04-08	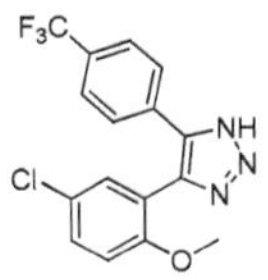	21.2%	11.2%	7.5%	24.9%
NLG919		0.064 μM	0.085 μM	NA	NA
Taxol		NA	NA	6 nM	15 nM

[a] When the calculated IC_{50} of a compound is >50 μM, we show the inhibition rate (%) at 50 μM. -: no detectable inhibition. NA: not tested.

In series 4, the design strategy was to attach fragments to the imidazole ring instead of the phenyl ring in series 3. However, this strategy does not maintain the IDO1 inhibitory activity. In addition, the free hydroxyl group in series 4 appears to be important for forming a hydrogen bond with an amino acid residue, such as Ser167 [7], in the active site; methylating this hydroxyl group decreased IDO1 inhibition (DX-04-05 versus DX-04-06).

In summary, based on the SAR study, compounds DX-03-12 and DX-03-13 showed potent IDO1 inhibition activity, and compound DX-03-13 has some structure similarity as previous published patent (WO2011/056652Al) [23]. Thus, the most potent IDO1 inhibitor DX-03-12 was used as the lead compound for further study.

2.4. Pharmacokinetic Study of DX-03-12

The in vivo pharmacokinetic properties of compound DX-03-12 were evaluated in male ICR mice. DX-03-12 was administered orally either as a bolus at a dose of 30 mg/kg or intravenously at a dose of 3 mg/kg. The plasma concentration-time profiles are shown in Figure 3. The pharmacokinetic parameters were determined by non-compartmental analysis (Table 5). After intravenous administration (3 mg/kg), compound DX-03-12 showed a moderate clearance of 33.3 mL/min/kg, which was approximately 36% of mouse hepatic blood flow (90 mL/min/kg). The volume of distribution in the steady state was 10 L/kg, suggesting that there was an extensive distribution of compound DX-03-12 in tissues. Compound DX-03-12 was rapidly absorbed after oral administration of 30 mg/kg. The plasma concentration was quantifiable at the first sampling time point (5 min) and remained detectable at 24 h. The maximum plasma concentration of compound DX-03-12 of 2963 ng/mL was observed 1 h post-dose. Compound DX-03-12 was eliminated relatively slowly with a half-life of 4.6 h. The oral bioavailability of compound DX-03-12 was calculated to be 96%.

The pharmacokinetic study revealed that compound DX-03-12 showed rapid absorption and almost complete oral bioavailability in mice. After oral administration of 30 mg/kg in mice, it exhibited a long half-life (4.6 h) due to moderate plasma clearance. The pharmacokinetic properties of compound DX-03-12 in mice indicate that it has the potential to be a once-a-day drug.

Table 5. Pharmacokinetic parameters of DX-03-12 after a single oral or intravenous dose in male ICR mice.

Parameters	Units	PO 30 mg/kg	iv 3 mg/kg
$t_{1/2\beta}$	h	4.61	3.49
T_{max}	h	1	0.033
C_{max}	ng/mL	2963	2138
$AUC_{(0\text{-}t)}$	h*ng/mL	12,902	1346
$AUC_{(0\text{-}\infty)}$	h*ng/mL	13,094	1500
V_{ss}	L/kg	-	10.1
Cl	mL/min/kg	-	33.3
F%		96	-

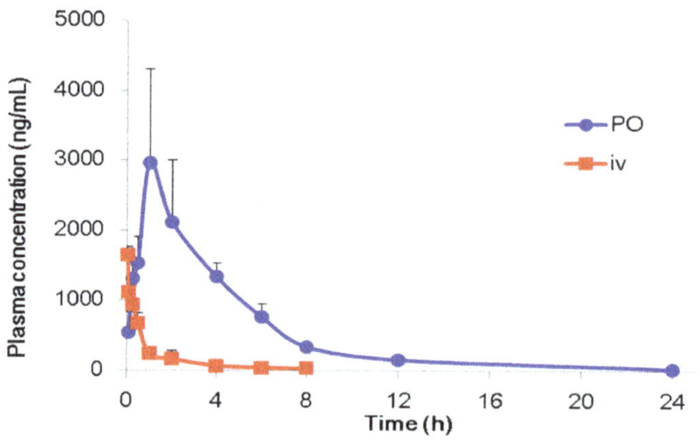

Figure 3. Mean plasma concentration-time profile in male ICR mice after administration of a single oral (30 mg/kg) or intravenous (3 mg/kg) dose of compound DX-03-12. PO stands for per os, which means oral administration of drug; iv stands for intravenous administration of drug.

2.5. In Vivo Anti-Tumor Efficacy Study of Compound DX-03-12

To determine whether the compound was effective against tumors in vivo, the anti-tumor effect of DX-03-12 was evaluated in a B16F10 subcutaneous xenograft model in syngeneic mice (Figure 4). Oral and intraperitoneal (i.p.) administration (30 or 60 mg/kg/day) of DX-03-12 significantly decreased the growth of melanoma B16F10 xenograft tumors in a dose-dependent manner. DX-03-12 oral treatment resulted in a 72.2% decrease in tumor weight and i.p. treatment resulted in a 72.3% decrease at a dose of 60 mg/kg compared with the control tumor after 19 days treatment. DX-03-12 had no obvious effect on the body weight of the mice and the peripheral white blood cells, which indicated that DX-03-12 had low toxicity in mice. In this study, the classic first line anti-cancer drug cyclophosphamide (CTX) was used as the reference drug.

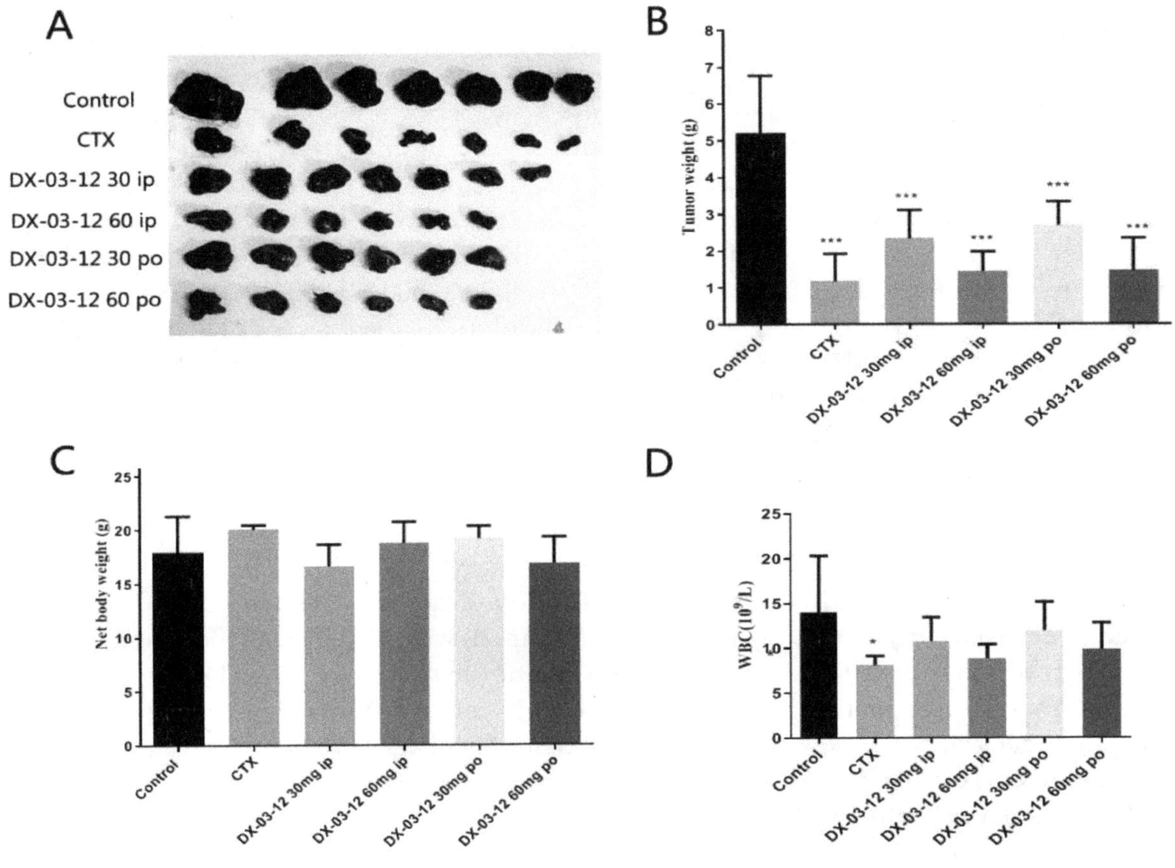

Figure 4. In vivo anti-tumor activity of DX-03-12 in B16F10 xenograft mice. (**A**,**B**) Tumors from each group after 19 days of treatment. Mice bearing B16F10 xenografts were dosed orally or i.p. with vehicle (0.5% methylcellulose), CTX (Cyclophosphamide, orally, 60 mg/kg twice a week), DX-03-12 (i.p., 30 mg/kg/day), DX-03-12 (i.p., 60 mg/kg/day), DX-03-12 (orally, 30 mg/kg/day), or DX-03-12 (orally, 60 mg/kg/day). Results are expressed as the mean ± SD (n = 5–7 for each group). * $p < 0.05$ and *** $p < 0.001$ versus vehicle. (**C**) The body weight from each group after the treatment. There is no obvious body weight difference among all of the groups. (**D**) The white blood cells detected in the blood of all groups of animals. There is also no obvious WBC difference among all of the groups.

3. Experiment Section

3.1. Chemistry

Reagents and solvents were obtained from commercial suppliers and used as received. ^{1}H-NMR spectra were obtained on an NMR spectrometer (Mercury, Varian, San Diego, CA, USA; 400 MHz). Electrospray ionization (ESI) mass spectra and high-resolution mass spectroscopy (HRMS) were performed with a liquid chromatograph/mass selective detector time-of-flight mass spectrometer

(LC/MSD TOF, Agilent Technologies, Santa Clara, CA, USA). silica gel column chromatography was performed with silica gel 60G (Qingdao Haiyang Chemical, Qingdao, China). Purity was determined using HPLC, LC/MS and NMR spectroscopy. All of the synthesized compounds have the purity over than 95%.

Several commercial available compounds were purchased from Beijing innochem Co. Ltd. (Beijing, China). They are DX-01-01, DX-01-08, DX-01-09, DX-01-10, DX-01-11, DX-01-12, DX-01-18, DX-01-19, DX-01-20, DX-01-21, DX-01-22, DX-03-01.

3.1.1. Preparation of (*R/S*) 3-(5-fluoro-2-((hydroxyamino)methyl)-1*H*-indol-3-yl)pyrrolidine-2,5-dione (DX-02-05)

Preparation of (*R/S*) Ethyl 3-(2,5-dioxopyrrolidin-3-yl)-5-fluoro-1*H*-indole-2-carboxylate (DX-02-03)

Ethyl 5-fluoro-1*H*-indole-2-carboxylate (2 g, 9.7 mmol) and 1*H*-pyrrole-2,5-dione (1.40 g, 14.4 mmol) were added to dry 1,2-dichloroethane (50 mL), and 46.5% BF_3-Et_2O (3.54 g, 11.6 mmol) was added to reaction mixture at 20 °C. After the reaction mixture was stirred at 90 °C, until the starting material disappeared in thin layer chromatography (TLC), the reaction mixture was distilled in vacuo, and dichloromethane (50 mL) was added to the mixture. The organic extract was washed twice with saturated aqueous $NaHCO_3$ and NaCl (20 mL) respectively, and the organic extract was dried over Na_2SO_4. After solvent was removed under vacuum, the product was purified as a white solid by silica gel column chromatography, 1.62 g, yield 55%. ^{1}H-NMR (400 MHz, DMSO-d_6): δ = 12.00 (s, 1H, NH-indolyl), 11.31 (s, 1H, NH), 7.49–7.45 (m, 2H, H-indolyl), 7.18 (td, *J* = 9.2, 2.6 Hz, 1H, H-indolyl), 4.82 (dd, *J* = 9.6, 6.6 Hz, 1H, CH), 4.33–4.27 (m, 2H, CH_2), 3.08 (dd, *J* = 17.7, 9.6 Hz, 1H, C<u>H'</u>H"), 2.70 (dd, *J* = 17.7, 6.6 Hz, 1H, CH'<u>H"</u>), 1.30 (t, *J* = 7.1 Hz, 3H, CH_3). ^{13}C-NMR (101 MHz, CD_3OD): δ =182.17, 180.15, 162.66, 160.66, 134.24, 129.01, 126.54, 119.11, 115.66, 114.82, 104.78, 62.19, 39.68, 39.37, 14.63. HRMS (ESI): *m/z* $[M + H]^+$ calculated for $C_{15}H_{14}O_4N_2F$: 305.09321; found: 305.09290.

Preparation of (*R/S*) 3-(5-fluoro-2-(hydroxymethyl)-1*H*-indol-3-yl) pyrrolidine-2,5-dione (**1**)

Ethyl 3-(2,5-dioxopyrrolidin-3-yl)-5-fluoro-1*H*-indole-2-carboxylate (DX-02-03, 1.3 g, 4.3 mmol) were added to dry CH_3OH (20 mL), $LiAlH_4$ (0.13 g, 4.3 mmol) was added to reaction mixture gradually at 20 °C. The reaction mixture was stirred at 20 °C until the starting material disappeared in TLC. The reaction mixture was distilled in vacuo, and ethyl acetate (50 mL) was added to the mixture. The organic extract was washed twice with saturated aqueous NaCl (20 mL), and the organic extract was dried over Na_2SO_4. After solvent was removed under vacuum, the product was purified as a white solid by silica gel column chromatography, 0.97 g, yield 86%. ^{1}H-NMR (400 MHz, CD_3OD): δ = 7.30 (dd, *J* = 8.8, 4.4 Hz, 1H, H-phenyl), 6.93 (dd, *J* = 9.9, 2.4 Hz, 1H, H-phenyl), 6.89–6.83 (m, 1H, H-phenyl), 4.72 (d, *J* = 1.3 Hz, 2H, CH_2), 4.46 (dd, *J* = 9.7, 5.6 Hz, 1H, CH), 3.20 (dd, *J* = 18.4, 9.7 Hz, 1H, C<u>H'</u>H"), 2.81 (dd, *J* = 18.4, 5.6 Hz, 1H, CH'<u>H"</u>). ^{13}C-NMR (101 MHz, CD_3OD): δ = 182.67, 180.16, 160.22, 157.85, 139.57, 133.85, 127.82, 113.46, 110.70, 103.45, 56.67, 39.93, 39.00. HRMS (ESI): *m/z* $[M + H]^+$ calculated for $C_{13}H_{12}N_2O_3F$: 263.08265; found: 263.08160.

Preparation of (*R/S*) 3-(2,5-dioxopyrrolidin-3-yl)-5-fluoro-1*H*-indole-2-carbaldehyde (**2**)

3-(5-Fluoro-2-(hydroxymethyl)-1*H*-indol-3-yl)pyrrolidine-2,5-dione (**1**, 0.8 g, 3.1 mmol) was added to dry dichloridemethane (20 mL), MnO_2 (0.36 g, 4.1 mmol) was added to reaction mixture gradually at 20 °C. The reaction mixture was stirred at 20 °C until the starting material disappeared in TLC. The reaction mixture was filtered, the solvent was removed under vacuum, and the product was purified as a white solid by silica gel column chromatography, 0.73g, yield 91%. ^{1}H-NMR (400 MHz, CD_3OD): δ = 10.00 (s, 1H, CHO), 7.50 (dd, *J* = 9.1, 4.3 Hz, 1H, H-phenyl), 7.27 (dd, *J* = 9.5, 2.3 Hz, 1H, H-phenyl), 7.19 (td, *J* = 9.1, 2.4 Hz, 1H, H-phenyl), 4.91 (dd, *J* = 9.7, 6.0 Hz, 1H, CH), 3.29–3.21 (m, 1H, C<u>H'</u>H"), 2.84 (dd, *J* = 18.1, 6.0 Hz, 1H, CH'<u>H"</u>). ^{13}C-NMR (101 MHz, CD_3OD): δ = 183.66,

181.23, 179.66, 160.59, 158.30, 135.75, 135.36, 127.61, 117.26, 115.66, 105.59, 39.77, 39.35. HRMS (ESI): *m/z* $[M + H]^+$ calculated for $C_{13}H_{10}N_2O_3F$: 261.06700; found: 261.06638.

Preparation of (*R/S*) (*E*)-3-(2,5-dioxopyrrolidin-3-yl)-5-fluoro-1*H*-indole-2-carbaldehyde oxime (DX-02-04)

3-(2,5-Dioxopyrrolidin-3-yl)-5-fluoro-1*H*-indole-2-carbaldehyde (0.5 g, 1.92 mmol) was added to dry CH_3OH (30 mL), then *N,N*-Diisopropylethylamine (0.5 g, 3.84 mmol) and hydroxylamine hydro -chloride (0.13 g, 1.92 mmol) were added respectively at 20 °C. The reaction mixture was stirred at 60 °C until the starting material disappeared in TLC. After solvent was removed under vacuum, the product was purified as a white solid by silica gel column chromatography, 0.35 g, yield 66%. ^{1}H-NMR (400 MHz, CD_3OD): δ = 8.22 (s, 1H, =CH), 7.32 (dd, *J* = 8.8, 4.4 Hz, 1H, H-indolyl), 7.06–6.86 (m, 2H, H-indolyl), 4.63 (dd, *J* = 9.7, 5.9 Hz, 1H, CH), 3.19 (dd, *J* = 18.3, 9.7 Hz, 1H, $\underline{CH'}$H"), 2.81 (dd, *J* = 18.7, 6.2 Hz, 1H, CH'$\underline{H"}$). ^{13}C-NMR (101 MHz, CD_3OD): δ =181.92, 179.89, 160.31, 157.98, 141.03, 136.51, 134.81, 132.30, 113.78, 112.58, 103.95, 39.83, 38.66. HRMS (ESI): *m/z* $[M + H]^+$ calculated for $C_{13}H_{11}N_3O_3F$: 276.07790; found: 276.07718.

Preparation of (*R/S*) 3-(5-fluoro-2-((hydroxyamino)methyl)-1*H*-indol-3-yl) pyrrolidine-2,5-dione (DX-02-05)

3-(2,5-Dioxopyrrolidin-3-yl)-5-fluoro-1*H*-indole-2-carbaldehyde oxime (DX-02-04, 0.3 g, 1.1 mmol) was added to CH_3OH (20 mL), then $NaBH_3CN$ (0.07 g, 1.1 mmol) was added at 20 °C. 12N HCl was added to reaction mixture continuously to keep acidic. The reaction mixture was stirred at 20 °C until the starting material disappeared in TLC. After solvent was removed under vacuum, the product was purified as a white solid by silica gel column chromatography, 0.13 g, yield 43%. ^{1}H-NMR (400 MHz, CD_3OD): δ = 7.30 (dd, *J* = 8.8, 4.5 Hz, 1H, H-indolyl), 6.93–6.88 (m, 1H, H-indolyl), 6.88–6.82 (m, 1H, H-indolyl), 4.50 (dd, *J* = 9.7, 5.5 Hz, 1H, CH), 4.12 (d, *J* = 3.6 Hz, 2H, $\underline{CH_2}$NH), 3.21 (dd, *J* = 18.5, 9.7 Hz, 1H, $\underline{CH'}$H"), 2.85 (dd, *J* = 18.5, 5.5 Hz, 1H, CH'$\underline{H"}$). ^{13}C-NMR (101 MHz, CD_3OD): δ = 160.27, 157.92, 135.20, 130.85, 130.02, 113.00, 110.85, 110.54, 104.55, 104.31, 50.48, 38.34, 30.37. HRMS (ESI): *m/z* $[M + H]^+$ calculated for $C_{13}H_{13}N_3O_3F$: 278.09355; found: 278.09291.

3.1.2. Preparation of (*R/S*) 3-(5-fluoro-2-(methylsulfinyl)-1*H*-indol-3-yl)pyrrolidine-2,5-dione (DX-02-07)

Preparation of 5-fluoroindoline-2-thione (**3**)

5-fluoroindolin-2-one (2 g, 13 mmol) and P_2S_5 (2.92 g, 13 mmol) were added to dry tetrahydrofuran (30 mL). After the reaction mixture was stirred at room temperature for 1 h. Until the starting material disappeared in thin layer chromatography (TLC), the $NaHCO_3$ (3.43 g, 39 mmol) was added gradually. After stirring at room temperature for 1 h, the reaction mixture was distilled in vacuo, dichloromethane (50 mL) was added to the mixture. The organic extract was washed twice with saturated aqueous NaCl (20 mL), and the organic extract was dried over Na_2SO_4. After solvent was removed under vacuum, the product was obtained as yellow crystals by re-crystallization using ethanol, 1.62 g, yield 75%. ^{1}H-NMR (400 MHz, $CDCl_3$): δ = 10.14 (s, 1H, NH), 7.05–6.95 (m, 1H, H-phenyl), 6.94–6.89 (m, 1H, H-phenyl), 4.08 (s, 1H, CH_2). ^{13}C-NMR (101 MHz, $CDCl_3$)): δ = 203.39, 159.10, 140.24, 132.15, 114.87, 112.47, 110.47, 49.15. HRMS (ESI): *m/z* $[M + H]^+$ calculated for C_8H_7NFS: 168.02777; found: 168.02773.

Preparation of 5-fluoro-2-(methylthio)-1*H*-indole (**4**)

5-fluoroindoline-2-thione (**3**, 1 g, 6 mmol), CH_3I (0.99 g, 7 mmol) and K_2CO_3 (0.97 g, 7 mmol) were added to acetone (30 mL), and the reaction mixture was stirred at room temperature until the starting material disappeared in TLC. The reaction mixture was distilled in vacuo, ethyl acetate (50 mL) was added to the mixture. The organic extract was washed twice with saturated aqueous NaCl (20 mL), and the organic extract was dried over Na_2SO_4. After solvent was removed under vacuum, the product was purified as a white solid by silica gel column chromatography, 0.90 g, yield 83%. ^{1}H-NMR (400 MHz, $CDCl_3$): δ = 8.04 (s, 1H, NH), 7.23–7.13 (m, 2H, H-indolyl), 6.91 (s, 1H, H-indolyl), 6.49 (s, 1H, H-indolyl), 2.52 (s, 3H, CH_3). ^{13}C-NMR (101 MHz, $CDCl_3$): δ = 159.18, 156.85, 133.57, 129.02, 110.94, 110.47, 105.31, 104.73, 18.86. HRMS (ESI): *m/z* $[M + H]^+$ calculated for C_9H_9NFS: 182.04342; found: 182.04425.

Preparation of (*R/S*) 3-(5-fluoro-2-(methylthio)-1*H*-indol-3-yl)pyrrolidine-2,5-dione (DX-02-06)

5-Fluoro-2-(methylthio)-1*H*-indole (**4**, 0.5 g, 2.7 mmol) and 1*H*-pyrrole-2,5-dione (0.54 g, 5.4 mmol) were added to dry CH_3CO_2H (30 mL), and the reaction mixture was stirred at 120 °C until the starting material disappeared in TLC. The reaction mixture was distilled in vacuo, ethyl acetate (100 mL) was added to the mixture. The organic extract was washed twice with saturated aqueous NaCl (30 mL), and the organic extract was dried over Na_2SO_4. After solvent was removed under vacuum, the product was purified as a white solid by silica gel column chromatography, 0.47 g, yield 61%. ^{1}H-NMR (400MHz, CD_3OD): δ = 7.28 (dd, *J* = 8.9, 4.5 Hz, 1H, H-phenyl), 7.00 (dd, *J* = 9.7, 2.4 Hz, 1H, H-phenyl), 6.91 (td, *J* = 9.2, 2.5 Hz, 1H, H-phenyl), 4.56 (dd, *J* = 9.8, 5.6 Hz, 1H, CH), 3.22 (dd, *J* = 18.3, 9.8 Hz, 1H, $C\underline{H}'H''$), 2.77 (dd, *J* = 18.3, 5.6 Hz, 1H, $CH'\underline{H''}$), 2.41 (s, 3H, CH_3). ^{13}C-NMR (101 MHz, CD_3OD): δ = 182.38, 180.11, 160.26, 135.05, 132.13, 127.67, 116.34, 113.18, 111.70, 103.25, 40.35, 39.10, 19.59. HRMS (ESI): *m/z* $[M + H]^+$ calculated for $C_{13}H_{12}O_2N_2FS$: 279.05980; found: 279.05930.

Preparation of (*R/S*) 3-(5-fluoro-2-(methylsulfinyl)-1*H*-indol-3-yl)pyrrolidine-2,5-dione (DX-02-07)

3-(5-Fluoro-2-(methylthio)-1*H*-indol-3-yl)pyrrolidine-2,5-dione (DX-02-06, 0.2 g, 0.7 mmol) was added to dry dichloridemethane (20 mL), and 3-Chloroperoxybenzoic acid (0.15 g, 0.9 mmol) was added gradually at 0 °C. The reaction mixture was stirred at 0 °C until the starting material disappeared in TLC, and $Na_2S_2O_3$ (0.11 g, 0.7 mmol) was added to the mixture. After reaction mixture was stirred for 20 min, the reaction mixture was washed twice with saturated aqueous NaCl (20 mL), and the organic extract was dried over Na_2SO_4. After solvent was removed under vacuum, the product was purified as a white solid by silica gel column chromatography, 0.074 g, yield 35%. ^{1}H-NMR (400MHz, DMSO-d_6): δ = 12.28 (s, 1H, NH), 11.51 (s, 1H, NH), 7.51–7.48 (m, 1H, H-phenyl), 7.19–7.13 (m, 2H, H-phenyl), 4.61 (ddd, *J* = 26.8, 9.7, 5.8 Hz, 1H, CH), 3.18 (ddd, *J* = 18.0, 9.7, 2.3 Hz, 1H, $C\underline{H}'H''$), 2.98 (d, *J* = 16.7 Hz, 3H, CH_3), 2.76 (ddd, *J* = 41.8, 18.1, 5.8 Hz, 1H, $CH'\underline{H''}$). ^{13}C-NMR (101 MHz, DMSO-d_6): δ = 179.74, 177.94, 158.72, 138.29, 134.14, 125.83, 114.50, 113.93, 113.53, 104.46, 41.67, 38.62, 38.11. HRMS (ESI): *m/z* $[M + H]^+$ calculated for $C_{13}H_{12}O_3N_2FS$: 295.05472; found: 295.05508.

3.1.3. Preparation of *N*-(3-(2-(1*H*-imidazol-5-yl)phenoxy)propyl)-1,1,1-trifluoromethane sulfonamide (DX-03-12)

Preparation of 4-iodo-1-trityl-1*H*-imidazole (**5**)

4-Iodo-1*H*-imidazole (5 g, 25.8 mmol) and *N,N*-diisopropylethylamine (6.65 g, 51.5 mmol) were added to dry dimethylformamide (30 mL), and (chloromethanetriyl)tribenzene (7.89 g, 28.4 mmol) was added to reaction mixture gradually at 20 °C. After the reaction mixture was stirred at 20 °C until the starting material disappeared in thin layer chromatography (TLC), the reaction mixture was distilled in vacuo, ethyl acetate (200 mL) was added to the mixture. The organic extract was washed twice with saturated aqueous NaCl (40 mL), and the organic extract was dried over Na_2SO_4. After solvent was removed under vacuum, the product was purified as a white solid by silica gel column chromatography, 8.77 g, yield 78%. ^{1}H-NMR (400 MHz, $CDCl_3$): δ = 7.38–7.33 (m, 10H, H-phenyl, H-imidazolyl), 7.13–7.09 (m, 6H, H-phenyl), 6.92 (d, *J* = 1.4 Hz, 1H, H-imidazolyl). ^{13}C-NMR (101 MHz, $CDCl_3$): δ = 141.83, 140.56, 129.72 (6C), 128.29 (3C), 128.18 (6C), 127.91, 126.89 (3C), 75.84. HRMS (ESI): *m/z* $[M + H]^+$ calculated for $C_{22}H_{18}N_2I$: 437.05092; found: 437.04934.

Preparation of 4-(2-methoxyphenyl)-1-trityl-1*H*-imidazole (**6**)

4-Iodo-1-trityl-1*H*-imidazole (**5**, 2 g, 4.58 mmol), (5-chloro-2-methoxyphenyl)boronic acid (0.852 g, 4.58 mmol), K_3PO_4 (2.9 g, 13.7 mmol), $Pd(PPh_3)_4$ (0.74 g, 0.64 mmol) were added to dry dimethylformamide (30 mL). The reaction mixture was stirred at 100 °C under inert atmosphere, until the starting material disappeared in TLC. The reaction mixture was distilled in vacuo, and ethyl acetate (100 mL) was added to the mixture. The organic extract was washed twice with saturated aqueous NaCl (20 mL), and the organic extract was dried over Na_2SO_4. After solvent was removed under vacuum, the product was purified as a white solid by silica gel column chromatography, 1.2 g, yield 63%. ^{1}H-NMR (400 MHz, $CDCl_3$): δ = 7.51–7.32 (m, 12H, H-phenyl, H-imidazolyl), 7.15–7.04 (m, 8H, H-phenyl, H-imidazolyl), 6.94 (d, *J* = 8.1 Hz, 1H, H-phenyl), 3.99 (s, 3H, CH_3). HRMS (ESI): *m/z* $[M + H]^+$ calculated for $C_{29}H_{25}N_2O$: 417.19614; found: 417.19647.

Preparation of 2-(1-trityl-1*H*-imidazol-4-yl)phenol (**7**)

4-(2-Methoxyphenyl)-1-trityl-1*H*-imidazole (**6**, 1.0 g, 2.4 mmol) was added to dry dichloridemethane (20 mL), BBr_3 (0.71 g, 2.9 mmol) was added to reaction mixture gradually at −70 °C. The reaction mixture was stirred under inert atmosphere until the starting material disappeared in TLC. The reaction mixture was diluted with dichloridemethane (50 mL), and was washed twice with saturated aqueous NaCl (20 mL), then the organic extract was dried over Na_2SO_4. After solvent was removed under vacuum, the product was purified as a white solid by silica gel column chromatography, 0.63 g, yield 65%. ^{1}H-NMR (400 MHz, DMSO-d_6): δ = 11.19 (s, 1H, OH), 7.49–7.36 (m, 2H, H-phenyl), 7.33–7.10 (m, 16H, H-phenyl, H-imidazolyl), 6.84–6.70 (m, 2H, H-phenyl), 6.45 (s, 1H, H-phenyl). ^{13}C-NMR (101 MHz, DMSO-d_6): δ = 147.24, 141.47, 137.70, 136.55, 128.71 (6C), 127.80 (6C), 127.56, 127.24 (3C), 126.99 (3C), 126.10, 118.39, 117.87, 115.68, 74.61. HRMS (ESI): *m/z* $[M + H]^+$ calculated for $C_{28}H_{23}N_2O$: 403.18049; found: 403.18134.

Preparation of 2-(3-chloropropyl)isoindoline-1,3-dione (**8**)

3-Chloropropan-1-amine (3.77 g, 40.5 mmol) and isobenzofuran-1,3-dione (2 g, 13.5 mmol) were mixed without solvent, and the reaction mixture was stirred at 140 °C (molten condition), until the starting material disappeared in TLC. The reaction mixture was distilled in vacuo, ethyl acetate (100 mL) was added to the mixture. The organic extract was washed twice with saturated aqueous NaCl (20 mL), and the organic extract was dried over Na_2SO_4. After solvent was removed under vacuum, the product was purified as a white solid by silica gel column chromatography, 1.66 g, yield 55%. ^{1}H-NMR (400 MHz, DMSO-d_6): δ = 7.85–7.78 (m, 4H, H-phenyl), 3.73–3.62 (m, 4H, CH_2, CH_2), 2.08–2.01(m, 2H, CH_2). ^{13}C-NMR (101 MHz, DMSO-d_6): δ = 167.38 (2C), 133.75 (2C), 131.19 (2C), 122.43 (2C), 42.31, 34.60, 30.39. HRMS (ESI): *m/z* $[M + H]^+$ calculated for $C_{11}H_{11}ClNO_2$: 224.04728; found: 224.04683.

Preparation of 2-(3-(2-(1-trityl-1*H*-imidazol-5-yl)phenoxy)propyl)isoindoline-1,3-dione (**9**)

2-(1-Trityl-1*H*-imidazol-4-yl)phenol (**7**, 0.5 g, 1.2 mmol) and KOH (0.14 g, 2.5 mmol) were added to dry dimethylformamide (20 mL), after the reaction mixture was stirred at 20 °C for 15 min, 2-(3-chloropropyl)isoindoline-1,3-dione (**8**, 0.294 g, 1.32 mmol) was added to reaction mixture at 20 °C. After the reaction mixture was stirred at 60 °C until the starting material disappeared in thin layer chromatography (TLC), the reaction mixture was distilled in vacuo, ethyl acetate (100 mL) was added to the mixture. The organic extract was washed twice with saturated aqueous NaCl (20 mL), and the organic extract was dried over Na_2SO_4. After solvent was removed under vacuum, the product was purified as a white solid by silica gel column chromatography, 0.5 g, yield 71%. ^{1}H-NMR (400 MHz, DMSO-d_6): δ = 8.08 (dd, *J* = 7.7, 1.6 Hz, 1H, H-phenyl), 7.88–7.81 (m, 4H, H-phenyl, H-imidazolyl), 7.44–7.35 (m, 10H, H-phenyl), 7.17–7.13 (m, 7H, H-phenyl, H-imidazolyl), 7.12–7.08 (m, 1H, H-phenyl), 6.97 (t, *J* = 7.5 Hz, 1H, H-phenyl), 6.92 (d, *J* = 8.2 Hz, 1H, H-phenyl), 3.93 (t, *J* = 6.4 Hz, 2H, CH_2), 3.43 (t, *J* = 6.5 Hz, 2H, CH_2), 1.82–1.69 (m, 2H, CH_2). ^{13}C-NMR (101 MHz, DMSO-d_6): δ = 167.25, 154.09,

141.77, 137.17, 134.72, 133.82, 131.11, 128.71 (6C), 128.65 (3C), 127.69, 127.66 (6C), 127.46, 127.36 (3C), 126.71, 125.92, 122.47, 121.86, 121.01, 120.60, 119.93, 111.33, 74.14, 64.42, 33.61, 27.54. HRMS (ESI): *m/z* $[M + H]^+$ calculated for $C_{39}H_{32}N_3O_3$: 590.24382; found: 590.24541.

Preparation of 3-(2-(1-trityl-1*H*-imidazol-4-yl)phenoxy)propan-1-amine (**10**)

2-(3-(2-(1-Trityl-1*H*-imidazol-4-yl)phenoxy)propyl)isoindoline-1,3-dione (**9**, 0.4 g, 0.68 mmol) and 35% hydrazine hydrate (0.12 g, 1.35 mmol) were added to CH_3OH, and the reaction mixture was stirred at 50 °C under inert atmosphere. After the starting material disappeared in thin layer chromatography (TLC), the reaction mixture was distilled in vacuo, ethyl acetate (100 mL) was added to the mixture. The organic extract was washed twice with saturated aqueous $NaHCO_3$ and NaCl (20 mL) respectively, and the organic extract was dried over Na_2SO_4. After solvent was removed under vacuum, the unpurified product was added to the next step directly.

Preparation of 1,1,1-trifluoro-*N*-(3-(2-(1-trityl-1*H*-imidazol-4-yl)phenoxy)propyl) Methane Sulfonamide (**11**)

3-(2-(1-Trityl-1*H*-imidazol-4-yl)phenoxy)propan-1-amine (crude **10**, 0.3 g, 0.65 mmol) and *N,N*-diisopropylethylamine (0.168 g, 1.3 mmol) were added to dry dichloridemethane (20 mL), and trifluoromethanesulfonylchloride (0.12 g, 0.71 mmol) was added to reaction mixture gradually at 20 °C. After the starting material disappeared in thin layer chromatography (TLC), the reaction mixture was distilled in vacuo, the reaction mixture was diluted with dichloridemethane (50 mL), and the organic extract was washed twice with saturated aqueous NaCl (20 mL), and the organic extract was dried over Na_2SO_4. After solvent was removed under vacuum, the product **11** was purified as a white solid by silica gel column chromatography, 0.257 g, yield 67%. ^{1}H-NMR (400 MHz, $CDCl_3$): δ = 7.80 (s, 1H, NH), 7.43–7.32 (m, 10H, H-phenyl, H-imidazolyl), 7.23–7.16 (m, 8H, H-phenyl, H-imidazol), 7.07 (d, *J* = 1.5 Hz, 1H, H-phenyl), 6.97–6.86 (m, 2H, H-phenyl), 4.16 (t, *J* = 5.2 Hz, 2H, CH_2), 3.57–3.46 (m, 2H, CH_2), 2.19–2.06 (m, 2H, CH_2). ^{13}C-NMR (101 MHz, $CDCl_3$): δ= 154.95, 142.08, 139.92, 138.22, 129.77 (6C), 128.56 (3C), 128.36, 128.15 (3C), 128.09 (6C), 121.68, 120.87, 119.04, 118.47, 111.86, 75.75, 67.83, 43.24, 29.80. HRMS (ESI): *m/z* $[M + H]^+$ calculated for $C_{32}H_{29}N_3O_3F_3S$: 592.18762; found: 592.18616.

Preparation of *N*-(3-(2-(1*H*-imidazol-5-yl)phenoxy)propyl)-1,1,1-trifluoromethane Sulfonamide (DX-03-12)

1,1,1-Trifluoro-*N*-(3-(2-(1-trityl-1*H*-imidazol-4-yl)phenoxy)propyl)methanesulfonamide (**11**, 0.2 g, 0.34 mmol) and AcOH (0.5 mL) were added to CH_3OH (10 mL), and the reaction mixture was stirred at 20 °C. After the starting material disappeared in thin layer chromatography (TLC), the reaction mixture was distilled in vacuo, the product was purified as a white solid by silica gel column chromatography, 0.101 g, yield 86%. ^{1}H-NMR (400 MHz, DMSO-d_6): δ =7.99 (d, *J* = 7.4 Hz, 1H, H-phenyl), 7.72 (s, 1H, H-imidazolyl), 7.49 (s, 1H, H-imidazolyl), 7.18 (t, *J* = 7.8 Hz, 1H, H-phenyl), 7.03 (d, *J* = 8.1 Hz, 1H, H-phenyl), 6.98 (t, *J* = 7.5 Hz, 1H, H-phenyl), 4.15 (t, *J* = 6.0 Hz, 2H, CH_2), 3.40 (t, *J* = 6.8 Hz, 2H, CH_2), 2.06–2.09 (m, 2H, CH_2). ^{13}C-NMR (101 MHz, DMSO-d_6): δ = 154.86, 135.47, 134.49, 127.46, 127.25, 124.99, 122.69, 120.97, 118.57, 112.34, 65.09, 41.39, 30.14. HRMS (ESI): *m/z* $[M + H]^+$ calculated for $C_{13}H_{15}O_3N_3F_3S$: 350.07807; found: 350.07782.

3.1.4. Preparation of 4-chloro-2-(1-(4-(trifluoromethyl)benzyl)-1*H*-imidazol-4-yl) Phenol (DX-04-02)

Preparation of 4-iodo-1-(4-(trifluoromethyl)benzyl)-1*H*-imidazole (**12**)

4-Iodo-1*H*-imidazole (1 g, 5.2 mmol) and *N,N*-diisopropylethylamine (1.34 g, 10.4 mmol) were added to dry dimethylformamide (20 mL), and 1-(bromomethyl)-4-(trifluoromethyl)benzene (1.48 g, 6.2 mmol) was added to reaction mixture at 20 °C. After the reaction mixture was stirred at 20 °C until the starting material disappeared in thin layer chromatography (TLC), the reaction mixture was distilled in vacuo, dichloromethane (50 mL) was added to the mixture. The organic extract was washed twice with saturated aqueous $NaHCO_3$ and NaCl (20 mL) respectively, and the organic extract was dried over Na_2SO_4. After solvent was removed under vacuum, the unpurified product was added to the next step directly.

Preparation of 4-(5-chloro-2-methoxyphenyl)-1-(4-(trifluoromethyl)benzyl)-1*H*-imidazole (DX-04-01)

4-Iodo-1-(4-(trifluoromethyl)benzyl)-1*H*-imidazole (crude **12**, 0.5 g, 1.4 mmol), (5-chloro-2-methoxyphenyl)boronic acid (0.27 g, 1.4 mmol), K_3PO_4 (0.9 g, 4.3 mmol), $Pd(PPh_3)_4$ (0.23 g, 0.2 mmol) were added to dry dimethylformamide (10 mL). The reaction mixture was stirred at 100 °C under inert atmosphere, until the starting material disappeared in TLC. The reaction mixture was distilled in vacuo, ethyl acetate (50 mL) was added to the mixture. The organic extract was washed twice with saturated aqueous NaCl (20 mL), and the organic extract was dried over Na_2SO_4. After solvent was removed under vacuum, DX-04-01 was purified as a white solid by silica gel column chromatography, 0.37 g, yield 72%. ^{1}H-NMR (400 MHz, CD_3OD): δ = 7.94 (d, *J* = 2.5 Hz, 1H, H-phenyl), 7.81 (s, 1H, H-imidazolyl), 7.65–7.63 (m, 3H, H-imidazolyl, H-phenyl), 7.40 (d, *J* = 8.0 Hz, 2H, H-phenyl), 7.15 (dd, *J* = 8.7, 2.5 Hz, 1H, H-phenyl), 6.96 (d, *J* = 8.8 Hz, 1H, H-phenyl), 5.34 (s, 2H, CH_2), 3.86 (s, 3H, CH_3). ^{13}C-NMR (101 MHz, CD_3OD): δ = 156.09, 142.76, 138.77, 137.13, 131.46, 129.05 (2C), 128.22, 127.44, 126.92 (2C), 124.85, 124.18, 121.78, 113.52, 112.48, 56.17, 51.22. HRMS (ESI): *m/z* $[M + H]^+$ calculated for$C_{18}H_{15}ON_2ClF_3$: 367.08195; found: 367.08374.

Preparation of 4-chloro-2-(1-(4-(trifluoromethyl)benzyl)-1*H*-imidazol-4-yl)phenol (DX-04-02)

4-(5-Chloro-2-methoxyphenyl)-1-(4-(trifluoromethyl)benzyl)-1*H*-imidazole (DX-04-01, 0.3 g, 0.82 mmol) was added to dry dichloridemethane (20 mL), BBr_3 (0.24 g, 0.98 mmol) was added to reaction mixture gradually at −70 °C. The reaction mixture was stirred under inert atmosphere until the starting material disappeared in TLC. The reaction mixture was diluted with dichloridemethane (50 mL), and was washed twice with saturated aqueous NaCl (20 mL), then the organic extract was dried over Na_2SO_4. After solvent was removed under vacuum, DX-04-02 was purified as a white solid by silica gel column chromatography, 0.15 g, yield 53%. ^{1}H-NMR (400 MHz, CD_3OD): δ = 7.85 (s, 1H, H-imidazolyl), 7.70–7.65 (m, 3H, H-imidazolyl, H-phenyl), 7.63 (d, *J* = 2.6 Hz, 1H, H-phenyl), 7.45 (d, *J* = 8.1 Hz, 2H, H-phenyl), 7.02 (dd, *J* = 8.7, 2.6 Hz, 1H, H-phenyl), 6.80 (d, *J* = 8.7 Hz, 1H, H-phenyl), 5.37 (s, 2H, CH_2). ^{13}C-NMR (101 MHz, CD_3OD): δ = 155.21, 142.66, 140.49, 137.67, 129.87, 129.60, 129.12 (2C), 128.42, 126.89 (2C), 126.06, 125.01, 121.01, 118.79, 118.28, 51.17. HRMS (ESI): *m/z* $[M + H]^+$ calculated for$C_{17}H_{13}ON_2ClF_3$: 353.06630; found: 353.06635.

3.1.5. Preparation of 4-methyl-1*H*-indole-3-carboxylic Acid (DX-01-02)

Methyl 4-methyl-1*H*-indole-3-carboxylate (200 mg, 1.06 mmol) used hydrolysis reaction (2 N NaOH water solution) to afford DX-01-02 (white solid, 151 mg, yield 82%). ^{1}H-NMR (400 MHz, CD_3OD): δ = 8.18 (dd, *J* = 3.9, 1.9 Hz, 1H, H-indolyl), 7.30 (d, *J* = 8.0 Hz, 1H, H-indolyl), 7.17 (t, *J* = 7.7 Hz, 1H, H-indolyl), 7.01 (dd, *J* = 7.3, 0.7 Hz, 1H, H-indolyl), 2.77 (s, 3H, CH_3). ^{13}C-NMR (101 MHz, CD_3OD): δ = 139.17, 133.89, 126.39, 125.96, 125.68, 120.61, 117.71, 112.19, 111.02, 23.30. HRMS (ESI): *m/z* $[M + H]^+$ calculated for $C_{10}H_{10}NO_2$: 176.07061; found: 176.07129.

3.1.6. Preparation of 5-methyl-1*H*-indole-3-carboxylic Acid (DX-01-03)

Methyl 5-methyl-1*H*-indole-3-carboxylate (200 mg, 1.06 mmol) used hydrolysis reaction (2 N NaOH water solution) to afford DX-01-03 (white solid, 150 mg, yield 81%). ^{1}H-NMR (400 MHz, CD_3OD): δ = 8.15 (d, *J* = 1.8 Hz, 1H, H-indolyl), 8.07 (s, 1H, H-indolyl), 7.39 (d, *J* = 8.3 Hz, 1H, H-indolyl), 7.15 (dd, *J* = 8.3, 1.1 Hz, 1H, H-indolyl), 2.46 (s, 3H, CH_3). ^{13}C-NMR (101 MHz, CD_3OD): δ = 137.41, 134.35, 127.80, 127.00, 122.51, 120.09, 117.20, 113.08, 110.78, 21.77. HRMS (ESI): *m/z* $[M + H]^+$ calculated for $C_{10}H_{10}NO_2$: 176.07061; found: 176.07094.

3.1.7. Preparation of 5-nitro-1*H*-indole-3-carboxylic Acid (DX-01-04)

Methyl 5-nitro-1*H*-indole-3-carboxylate (200 mg, 0.91 mmol) used hydrolysis reaction (2 N NaOH water solution) to afford DX-01-04 (white solid, 172 mg, yield 92%). ^{1}H-NMR (400 MHz, CD_3OD): δ = 8.99 (d, *J* = 2.2 Hz, 1H, H-indolyl), 8.14 (s, 1H, H-indolyl), 8.12 (dd, *J* = 9.0, 2.3 Hz, 1H, H-indolyl), 7.58 (d, *J* = 9.0 Hz, 1H, H-indolyl). ^{13}C-NMR (101 MHz, CD_3OD): δ = 167.81, 144.32, 141.16, 136.51, 127.01, 118.93, 118.80, 113.45, 111.10, 49.00. HRMS (ESI): *m/z* $[M + H]^+$ calculated for $C_9H_7N_2O_4$: 207.04003; found: 207.03940.

3.1.8. Preparation of 6-nitro-1*H*-indole-3-carboxylic Acid (DX-01-05)

Methyl 6-nitro-1*H*-indole-3-carboxylate (200 mg, 0.91 mmol) used hydrolysis reaction (2 N NaOH water solution) to afford DX-01-05 (white solid, 168 mg, yield 90%). ^{1}H-NMR (400 MHz, CD_3OD): δ = 8.38 (d, *J* = 1.5 Hz, 1H, H-indolyl), 8.22 (s, 1H, H-indolyl), 8.18 (d, *J* = 8.9 Hz, 1H, H-indolyl), 8.05 (dd, *J* = 8.8, 1.7 Hz, 1H, H-indolyl). ^{13}C-NMR (101 MHz, CD_3OD): δ = 167.87, 144.97, 138.31, 136.78, 132.29, 122.19, 117.33, 109.89, 109.69. HRMS (ESI): *m/z* $[M + H]^+$ calculated for $C_9H_7N_2O_4$: 207.04003; found: 207.03949.

3.1.9. Preparation of 5-methoxy-1*H*-indole-3-carboxylic Acid (DX-01-06)

Methyl 5-methoxy-1*H*-indole-3-carboxylate (200 mg, 0.97 mmol) used hydrolysis reaction (2 N NaOH water solution) to afford DX-01-06 (white solid, 140 mg, yield 75%). ^{1}H-NMR (400 MHz, CD_3OD): δ = 7.88 (s, 1H, H-indolyl), 7.57 (d, *J* = 2.4 Hz, 1H, H-indolyl), 7.31 (d, *J* = 8.8 Hz, 1H, H-indolyl), 6.83 (dd, *J* = 8.8, 2.5 Hz, 1H, H-indolyl), 3.83 (s, 3H, CH_3). ^{13}C-NMR (101 MHz, CD_3OD): δ = 156.99, 133.58, 128.36, 115.37, 114.23, 113.88, 113.61, 104.51, 103.64, 56.06. HRMS (ESI): *m/z* $[M + H]^+$ calculated for $C_{10}H_{10}NO_3$: 192.06552; found: 192.06645.

3.1.10. Preparation of 7-bromo-1*H*-indole-3-carboxylic Acid (DX-01-07)

Methyl 7-bromo-1*H*-indole-3-carboxylate (200 mg, 0.79 mmol) used hydrolysis reaction (2 N NaOH water solution) to afford DX-01-07 (white solid, 160 mg, yield 85%). ^{1}H-NMR (400 MHz, CD_3OD): δ = 8.06 (dd, *J* = 8.0, 0.9 Hz, 1H, H-indolyl), 7.98 (s, 1H, H-indolyl), 7.36 (dd, *J* = 7.6, 0.7 Hz, 1H, H-indolyl), 7.08 (t, *J* = 7.8 Hz, 1H, H-indolyl). ^{13}C-NMR (101 MHz, CD_3OD): δ = 168.56, 138.29, 134.03, 129.07, 126.24, 123.59, 121.46, 117.02, 106.02. HRMS (ESI): *m/z* $[M + H]^+$ calculated for $C_9H_7NO_2Br$: 239.96547; found: 239.96452.

3.1.11. Preparation of (*E*) 1*H*-indole-3-carbaldehyde Oxime (DX-01-13)

1*H*-indole-3-carbaldehyde (200 mg, 1.38 mmol) following the similar procedure described for the preparation of DX-02-04 afforded DX-01-13 (white solid, 158 mg, yield 72%). ^{1}H-NMR (400 MHz, DMSO-d_6): δ = 11.56 (s, 1H, OH), 11.17 (s, 1H, NH), 8.26 (s, 1H, =CH), 8.22 (d, *J* = 1.3 Hz, 1H, H-indolyl), 7.97 (d, *J* = 7.9 Hz, 1H, H-indolyl), 7.44 (d, *J* = 8.1 Hz, 1H, H-indolyl), 7.16 (t, *J* = 7.5 Hz, 2H, H-indolyl). ^{13}C-NMR (101 MHz, CD_3OD): δ = 146.89, 138.66, 132.19, 127.98, 123.30, 121.40, 118.79, 112.59, 107.56. HRMS (ESI): *m/z* $[M + H]^+$ calculated for $C_9H_9ON_2$: 161.07094; found: 161.07076.

3.1.12. Preparation of *N*-((1*H*-indol-3-yl)methyl)hydroxylamine (DX-01-14)

DX-01-13 (100 mg, 0.62 mmol) following the similar procedure described for the preparation of DX-02-05 afforded DX-01-14 (white solid, 70 mg, yield 69%). ^{1}H-NMR (400 MHz, DMSO-d_6): δ = 10.87 (s, 1H, NH-indolyl), 7.58 (d, *J* = 7.8 Hz, 1H, H-indolyl), 7.34 (d, *J* = 8.1 Hz, 1H, H-indolyl), 7.29 (br, 1H, NH), 7.24 (s, 1H, H-indolyl), 7.06 (t, *J* = 8.0 Hz, 1H, H-indolyl), 6.99–6.95 (m, 1H, H-indolyl), 5.66 (br, 1H, OH), 4.04 (s, 2H, CH_2). ^{13}C-NMR (101 MHz, CD_3OD): δ = 138.02, 128.61, 125.94, 122.58, 120.11, 119.41, 112.28, 110.24, 55.80. HRMS (ESI): *m/z* $[M + H]^+$ calculated for $C_9H_{11}ON_2$: 163.08659; found: 163.08611.

3.1.13. Preparation of *N*-((5-(o-tolyl)-1*H*-indol-3-yl)methyl)hydroxylamine (DX-01-15)

5-Bromo-1*H*-indole-3-carbaldehyde (300 mg, 1.34 mmol) and o-tolylboronic acid (183 mg, 1.34 mmol) following the similar procedure described for the preparation of DX-03-12 and DX-02-05 afforded DX-01-15 (white solid, 145 mg, yield 43% from 5-bromo-1*H*-indole-3-carbaldehyde). ^{1}H-NMR (400 MHz, CD_3OD): δ = 7.57–7.39 (m, 3H, H-phenyl, H-indolyl), 7.26–7.04 (m, 5H, H-phenyl, H-indolyl), 5.13 (s, 2H, CH_2), 2.24 (s, 3H, CH_3). ^{13}C-NMR (101 MHz, CD_3OD): δ = 144.63, 137.29, 136.60, 135.38, 131.19, 131.12, 128.56, 127.79, 126.62, 125.69, 124.87, 119.47, 112.33, 107.61, 62.12, 29.31. HRMS (ESI): *m/z* $[M + H]^+$ calculated for $C_{16}H_{17}N_2O$: 253.13354; found: 253.13471.

3.1.14. Preparation of (*E*)-1*H*-indole-2-carbaldehyde Oxime (DX-01-16)

1*H*-indole-2-carbaldehyde (200 mg, 1.38 mmol) following the similar procedure described for the preparation of DX-02-04 afforded DX-01-16 (white solid, 117 mg, yield 53%). ^{1}H-NMR (400 MHz, DMSO-d_6): δ = 11.29 (s, 1H, OH), 11.17 (s, 1H, NH), 8.14 (s, 1H, =CH), 7.52 (d, *J* = 8.0 Hz, 1H, H-indolyl), 7.37 (d, *J* = 8.2 Hz, 1H, H-indolyl), 7.12 (t, *J* = 7.6 Hz, 1H, H-indolyl), 6.98 (t, *J* = 7.5 Hz, 1H, H-indolyl), 6.56 (s, 1H, H-indolyl). ^{13}C-NMR (101 MHz, CD_3OD): δ = 142.67, 138.93, 132.77, 129.48, 124.71, 122.20, 120.89, 112.84, 108.61. HRMS (ESI): *m/z* $[M + H]^+$ calculated for $C_9H_9ON_2$: 161.07094; found: 161.07077.

3.1.15. Preparation of *N*-((1*H*-indol-2-yl)methyl)hydroxylamine (DX-01-17)

DX-01-16 (60 mg, 0.37 mmol) following the similar procedure described for the preparation of DX-02-05 afforded DX-01-17 (white solid, 39 mg, yield 65%). ^{1}H-NMR (400 MHz, DMSO-d_6): δ = 10.88 (s, 1H, NH-indolyl), 7.46–7.39 (m, 2H, H-indolyl, NH), 7.32 (d, *J* = 8.3 Hz, 1H, H-indolyl), 7.03–6.97 (m, 1H, H-indolyl), 6.93 (t, *J* = 8.1 Hz, 1H), 6.28 (s, 1H, H-indolyl), 6.17 (br, 1H, OH), 4.00 (s, 2H, CH_2). ^{13}C-NMR (101 MHz, CD_3OD): δ = 137.98, 136.56, 122.09, 120.86, 120.84, 120.01, 111.84, 101.86, 51.98. HRMS (ESI): *m/z* $[M + H]^+$ calculated for $C_9H_{11}ON_2$: 163.08659; found: 163.08636.

3.1.16. Preparation of (*E*)-3-((1*H*-indol-3-yl)methylene)pyrrolidine-2,5-dione (DX-02-01)

1*H*-indole-3-carbaldehyde (500 mg, 3.45 mmol) and 1*H*-pyrrole-2,5-dione (401 mg, 4.14 mmol) following the similar procedure described for the preparation of DX-02-04 afforded DX-02-01 (white solid, 398 mg, yield 51% from 1*H*-indole-3-carbaldehyde). ^{1}H-NMR (400 MHz, DMSO-d_6): δ = 11.94 (s, 1H, NH-indolyl), 11.18 (s, 1H, NH), 7.81 (dd, *J* = 12.1, 5.1 Hz, 2H, H-indolyl, =CH), 7.70 (t, *J* = 2.1 Hz, 1H, H-indolyl), 7.54–7.41 (m, 1H, H-indolyl), 7.21–7.16 (m, 2H, H-indolyl), 3.52 (d, *J* = 2.2 Hz, 2H). HRMS (ESI): *m/z* $[M + H]^+$ calculated for $C_{13}H_{11}O_2N_2$: 227.08150; found: 227.08134.

3.1.17. Preparation of (*R/S*) 3-((1*H*-indol-3-yl)methyl)pyrrolidine-2,5-dione (DX-02-02)

DX-02-01 (200 mg, 3.45 mmol) following the similar procedure described for the preparation of DX-02-04 afforded DX-02-02 (white solid, 65 mg, yield 32%). ^{1}H-NMR (400 MHz, DMSO-d_6): δ = 11.06 (s, 1H, NH-indolyl), 10.91 (s, 1H, NH), 7.51 (d, *J* = 7.8 Hz, 1H, H-indolyl), 7.33 (d, *J* = 8.0 Hz, 1H, H-indolyl), 7.16 (s, 1H, H-indolyl), 7.06 (t, *J* = 7.5 Hz, 1H, H-indolyl), 6.97 (t, *J* = 7.5 Hz, 1H, H-indolyl), 3.20–3.12 (m, 1H, CH′H″), 2.95 (dd, *J* = 14.0, 8.5 Hz, 1H, CH′H″), 2.70–2.61 (m, 2H, H-pyrrolidine-2,5-dione), 2.34 (dd, *J* = 18.0, 3.5 Hz, 1H, H-pyrrolidine-2,5-dione). HRMS (ESI): *m/z* $[M + H]^+$ calculated for $C_{13}H_{13}N_2O_2$: 229.09715; found: 229.09663

3.1.18. Preparation of (*E*) 2-(1*H*-imidazol-4-yl)benzaldehyde Oxime (DX-03-02)

Compound **5** (400 mg, 0.92 mmol) and (2-formylphenyl)boronic acid (138 mg, 0.92 mmol) following the similar procedure described for the preparation of DX-03-12 and DX-02-04 afforded DX-03-02 (white solid, 98 mg, yield 57% from (2-formylphenyl)boronic acid). ^{1}H-NMR (400 MHz, CD_3OD): δ = 8.32 (s, 1H, =CH), 7.85–7.84 (m, 1H, H-phenyl), 7.79 (s, 1H, H-imidazolyl), 7.52 (d, *J* = 7.7 Hz, 1H, H-phenyl), 7.42–7.38 (m, 1H, H-phenyl), 7.34–7.30 (m, 1H, H-phenyl), 7.12 (s, 1H, H-imidazolyl).

^{13}C-NMR (100 MHz, DMSO-d_6): δ = 148.70, 136.36, 133.83, 130.10, 129.50, 129.27, 128.72, 128.34, 127.09, 126.20. HRMS (ESI): *m/z* $[M + H]^+$ calculated for $C_{10}H_{10}ON_3$: 188.08184; found: 188.08191.

3.1.19. Preparation of *N*-(2-(1*H*-imidazol-4-yl)benzyl)hydroxylamine (DX-03-03)

Compound DX-03-02 (50 mg, 0.27 mmol) following the similar procedure described for the preparation of DX-02-04 afforded DX-03-03 (white solid, 32 mg, yield 63%). ^{1}H-NMR (400 MHz, CD_3OD): δ = 7.75 (s, 1H, H-imidazolyl), 7.53 (d, *J* = 1.7 Hz, 1H, H-phenyl), 7.47–7.44 (m, 1H, H-phenyl), 7.35–7.27 (m, 3H, H-imidazolyl, H-phenyl), 4.04 (s, 2H). HRMS (ESI): *m/z* $[M + H]^+$ calculated for $C_{10}H_{12}ON_3$: 190.09749; found: 190.09737.

3.1.20. Preparation of (*E*) 2-(2*H*-tetrazol-5-yl)benzaldehyde Oxime (DX-03-04)

2-(2H-tetrazol-5-yl)benzaldehyde (200 mg, 1.15 mmol) following the similar procedure described for the preparation of DX-03-12 and DX-02-04 afforded DX-03-04 (white solid, 78 mg, yield 36% from 2-(2*H*-tetrazol-5-yl)benzaldehyde). ^{1}H-NMR (400 MHz, DMSO-d_6): δ = 11.23 (s, 1H, OH), 11.07 (s, 1H, H-tetrazolyl), 8.29 (s, 1H, =CH), 7.73–7.56 (m, 4H, H-phenyl). ^{13}C-NMR (101 MHz, DMSO-d_6): δ = 156.17, 137.81, 132.14, 130.64, 129.27, 127.64, 116.84, 110.69. HRMS (ESI): *m/z* $[M + H]^+$ calculated for $C_8H_8N_5O$: 190.07234; found: 190.07158.

3.1.21. Preparation of (*E*) 5-chloro-2-(1*H*-imidazol-4-yl)benzaldehyde Oxime (DX-03-05)

Compound **5** (300 mg, 0.69 mmol) and (4-chloro-2-formylphenyl)boronic acid (127 mg, 0.69 mmol) following the similar procedure described for the preparation of DX-03-12 and DX-02-04 afforded DX-03-05 (white solid, 70 mg, yield 46% from (4-chloro-2-formylphenyl)boronic acid). ^{1}H-NMR (400 MHz, DMSO-d_6): δ = 12.38 (s, 1H, OH), 11.32 (s, 1H, NH-imidazolyl), 8.77 (s, 1H, =CH), 7.80 (s, 1H, H-imidazolyl), 7.74 (s, 1H, H-imidazolyl), 7.63 (d, *J* = 2.4 Hz, 1H, H-phenyl), 7.44–7.42 (m, 2H, H-phenyl). ^{13}C-NMR (101 MHz, DMSO-d_6): δ = 147.77, 138.56, 136.60, 133.12, 131.72, 131.48, 131.05, 129.25, 125.42, 116.28. HRMS (ESI): *m/z* $[M + H]^+$ calculated for $C_{10}H_9ClN_3O$: 222.04287; found: 222.04330.

3.1.22. Preparation of (*E*) 2-fluoro-6-(1*H*-imidazol-4-yl)benzaldehyde Oxime (DX-03-06)

Compound **5** (300 mg, 0.69 mmol) and (3-fluoro-2-formylphenyl)boronic acid (116 mg, 0.69 mmol) following the similar procedure described for the preparation of DX-03-12 and DX-02-04 afforded DX-03-06 (white solid, 75 mg, yield 53% from (3-fluoro-2-formylphenyl)boronic acid). ^{1}H-NMR (400 MHz, DMSO-d_6): δ = 12.37 (s, 1H, OH), 11.24 (s, 1H, NH-imidazolyl), 8.37 (s, 1H, =CH), 7.76 (s, 1H, H-imidazolyl), 7.52 (s, 1H, H-imidazolyl), 7.36–7.13 (m, 3H, H-phenyl). ^{13}C-NMR (101 MHz, DMSO-d_6): δ = 161.48, 159.00, 144.68, 136.29, 130.27, 124.36, 122.95, 117.89, 116.35, 113.98. HRMS (ESI): *m/z* $[M + H]^+$ calculated for $C_{10}H_9FN_3O$: 206.07242; found: 206.07250.

3.1.23. Preparation of (*E*) 2-(1*H*-imidazol-4-yl)-5-methoxybenzaldehyde Oxime (DX-03-07)

Compound **5** (300 mg, 0.69 mmol) and (2-formyl-4-methoxyphenyl)boronic acid (124 mg, 0.69 mmol) following the similar procedure described for the preparation of DX-03-12 and DX-02-04 afforded DX-03-07 (white solid, 113 mg, yield 76% from (2-formyl-4-methoxyphenyl)boronic acid). ^{1}H-NMR (400 MHz, CD_3OD): δ = 8.73 (s, 1H, H-imidazolyl), 7.78 (s, 1H, H-imidazolyl), 7.52–7.38 (m, 3H, H-phenyl), 7.15 (s, 1H, H-phenyl), 7.10–6.96 (m, 4H, H-phenyl), 3.85 (s, 3H, CH_3). ^{13}C-NMR (101 MHz, CD_3OD): δ = 141.55, 137.87, 133.07, 132.61, 121.44, 118.60, 117.79, 116.37, 113.90, 110.95, 55.90. HRMS (ESI): *m/z* $[M + H]^+$ calculated for $C_{11}H_{12}N_3O_2$: 218.09240; found: 218.09206.

3.1.24. Preparation of (*E*) 4-(1*H*-imidazol-4-yl)-2′-(trifluoromethyl)-[1,1′-biphenyl]-3-carbaldehyde Oxime (DX-03-08)

Compound **5** (300 mg, 0.69 mmol) and (3-formyl-2′-(trifluoromethyl)-[1,1′-biphenyl]-4-yl) boronic acid (202 mg, 0.69 mmol) following the similar procedure described for the preparation of DX-03-12 and DX-02-04 afforded DX-03-08 (white solid, 82mg, yield 36% from (3-formyl-2′-(trifluoromethyl)-[1,1′-biphenyl]-4-yl)boronic acid). ^{1}H-NMR (400 MHz, DMSO-d_6): δ = 12.38 (s, 1H, OH), 11.14 (s, 1H, NH-imidazolyl), 8.85(s, 1H, H-imidazolyl), 7.86–7.79 (m, 2H, H-imidazolyl, H-phenyl), 7.73–7.63 (m, 4H, H-phenyl), 7.46 (br, 2H, H-phenyl), 7.33 (s, 1H, H-phenyl). ^{13}C-NMR (101 MHz, DMSO-d_6): δ = 148.54, 140.58, 137.83, 136.56, 132.89, 132.57, 130.11, 129.84, 129.53, 128.94, 128.64, 126.58, 126.32, 126.23, 126.04, 123.22, 116.04. HRMS (ESI): *m/z* [M + H]$^+$ calculated for $C_{17}H_{13}F_3N_3O$: 332.10052; found: 332.10123.

3.1.25. Preparation of (*E*) 3-(1*H*-imidazol-4-yl)-[1,1′-biphenyl]-4-carbaldehyde Oxime (DX-03-09)

Compound **5** (300 mg, 0.69 mmol) and (4-formyl-[1,1′-biphenyl]-3-yl)boronic acid (156 mg, 0.69 mmol) following the similar procedure described for the preparation of DX-03-12 and DX-02-04 afforded DX-03-09 (white solid, 81 mg, yield 45% from (4-formyl-[1,1′-biphenyl]-3-yl)boronic acid). ^{1}H-NMR (400 MHz, DMSO-d_6): δ = 11.01 (s, 1H, OH), 10.34 (s, 1H, NH-imidazolyl), 8.55 (s, 1H, =CH), 8.39 (s, 1H, H-imidazolyl), 8.12 (s, 1H, H-imidazolyl), 7.58 (br, 1H, H-phenyl), 7.48–7.22 (m, 2H, H-phenyl), 7.11–7.02 (m, 2H, H-phenyl), 6.87–6,81 (m, 2H, H-phenyl), 6.50 (s, 1H, H-phenyl). HRMS (ESI): *m/z* [M + H]$^+$ calculated for $C_{16}H_{14}N_3O$: 264.11314; found: 264.11346.

3.1.26. Preparation of 4-(2-((4-(trifluoromethyl)benzyl)oxy)phenyl)-1,2,3-thiadiazole (DX-03-10)

2-(1,2,3-Thiadiazol-4-yl)phenol (100 mg, 0.56 mmol) and 1-(bromomethyl)-4-(trifluoromethyl)benzene (134 mg, 0.56 mmol) following the similar procedure described for the preparation of **12** afforded DX-03-10 (white solid, 128 mg, yield 68%). ^{1}H-NMR (400 MHz, DMSO-d_6): δ = 9.39 (s, 1H, H-thiadiazolyl), 8.26 (d, *J* = 7.5 Hz, 1H, H-phenyl), 7.76 (d, *J* = 8.2 Hz, 2H, H-phenyl), 7.70 (d, *J* = 8.5 Hz, 2H, H-phenyl), 7.48–7.43 (m, 1H, H-phenyl), 7.31 (d, *J* = 7.7 Hz, 1H, H-phenyl), 7.17 (t, *J* = 7.5 Hz, 1H, H-phenyl), 5.44 (s, 2H, CH_2). HRMS (ESI): *m/z* [M + H]$^+$ calculated for $C_{16}H_{12}F_3N_2OS$: 337.06169; found: 337.06116.

3.1.27. Preparation of *N*-(3-(2-(1*H*-imidazol-5-yl)phenoxy)propyl)-aminesulfonamide (DX-03-11)

Compound **9** (200 mg, 0.34 mmol) following the similar procedure described for the preparation of DX-03-12 afforded DX-03-11 (white solid, 45 mg, yield 45% from compound **9**). ^{1}H-NMR (400 MHz, CD_3OD): δ = 8.67 (s, 1H, NH-imidazolyl), 8.08 (s, 1H, H-imidazolyl), 7.83 (s, 1H, H-imidazolyl), 7.69 (d, *J* = 7.7 Hz, 1H, H-phenyl), 7.40 (t, *J* = 7.1 Hz, 1H, H-phenyl), 7.16 (d, *J* = 8.2 Hz, 1H, H-phenyl), 7.08 (t, *J* = 7.4 Hz, 1H, H-phenyl), 4.20 (t, *J* = 6.0 Hz, 2H, CH_2), 3.44 (t, *J* = 6.9 Hz, 2H, CH_2), 2.11–2.03 (m, 2H, CH_2). HRMS (ESI): *m/z* [M + H]$^+$ calculated for $C_{12}H_{17}O_3N_4S$: 297.10159; found: 297.10115.

3.1.28. Preparation of 1-(3-(2-(1*H*-imidazol-5-yl)phenoxy)propyl)-3-(4-(trifluoromethyl) phenyl)urea (DX-03-13)

Compound **9** (200 mg, 0.34 mmol) following the similar procedure described for the preparation of DX-03-12 afforded DX-03-13 (white solid, 77 mg, yield 56% from compound **9**). ^{1}H-NMR (400 MHz, DMSO-d_6): δ = 12.24 (s, 1H, NH-imidazolyl), 8.90 (s, 1H, H-imidazolyl), 8.01 (d, *J* = 7.4 Hz, 1H, H-phenyl), 7.75 (s, 1H, H-imidazolyl), 7.61–7.54 (m, 5H, H-phenyl), 7.21–7.15 (m, 1H, H-phenyl), 7.06 (d, *J* = 7.8 Hz, 1H, H-phenyl), 7.02–6.94 (m, 1H, H-phenyl), 6.48 (t, *J* = 5.7 Hz, 1H, H-phenyl), 4.14 (t, *J* = 6.1 Hz, 2H, CH_2), 3.38–3.32 (m, 2H, CH_2), 2.08–1.97 (m, 2H, CH_2). ^{13}C-NMR (101 MHz, DMSO-d_6): δ = 155.42, 155.08, 144.71, 135.42, 129.17, 127.38, 127.13, 126.38 (2C), 123.78, 122.81, 121.53, 121.21, 120.86, 117.71 (2C), 112.33, 65.82, 36.89, 29.98. HRMS (ESI): *m/z* [M + H]$^+$ calculated for $C_{20}H_{20}O_2N_4F_3$: 405.15329; found: 405.15302.

3.1.29. Preparation of 1-(3-bromo-4-fluorobenzyl)-4-(5-chloro-2-methoxyphenyl)-1*H*-imidazole (DX-04-03)

2-Bromo-4-(bromomethyl)-1-fluorobenzene (500 mg, 1.88 mmol) following the similar procedure described for the preparation of DX-04-02 afforded DX-04-03 (white solid, 480 mg, yield 65% from 2-bromo-4-(bromomethyl)-1-fluorobenzene). ^{1}H-NMR (400 MHz, CD_3OD): δ = 7.95 (d, *J* = 2.7 Hz, 1H, H-phenyl), 7.78 (d, *J* = 1.3 Hz, 1H, H-imidazolyl), 7.64 (d, *J* = 1.3 Hz, 1H, H-imidazolyl), 7.57 (dd, *J* = 6.5, 2.2 Hz, 1H, H-phenyl), 7.30–7.24 (m, 1H, H-phenyl), 7.20 (d, *J* = 8.5 Hz, 1H, H-phenyl), 7.16 (dd, *J* = 8.8, 2.7 Hz, 1H, H-phenyl), 6.98 (d, *J* = 8.8 Hz, 1H, H-phenyl), 5.22 (s, 2H, CH_2), 3.88 (s, 3H, CH_3). ^{13}C-NMR (101 MHz, CD_3OD): δ = 161.35, 158.96, 156.10, 138.33, 137.40, 133.91, 129.70, 128.04, 127.36, 126.81, 125.19, 121.53, 117.84, 113.47, 110.01, 56.13, 50.30. HRMS (ESI): *m/z* $[M + H]^+$ calculated for $C_{17}H_{14}ON_2BrClF$: 394.99566; found: 394.99728.

3.1.30. Preparation of 2-(1-(3-bromo-4-fluorobenzyl)-1*H*-imidazol-4-yl)-4-chlorophenol (DX-04-04)

DX-04-03 (200 mg, 0.51 mmol) following the similar procedure described for the preparation of DX-04-02 afforded DX-04-04 (white solid, 116 mg, yield 60%). ^{1}H-NMR (400 MHz, DMSO-d_6): δ = 9.12 (s, 1H, H-imidazolyl), 8.40 (s, 1H, H-imidazolyl), 8.01 (s, 1H, H-imidazolyl), 7.89 (dd, *J* = 6.5, 1.7 Hz, 1H, H-phenyl), 7.56–7.49 (m, 1H, H-phenyl), 7.45 (t, *J* = 8.6 Hz, 1H, H-phenyl), 7.34 (dd, *J* = 8.8, 2.5 Hz, 1H, H-phenyl), 7.00 (d, *J* = 8.8 Hz, 1H, H-phenyl), 5.42 (s, 2H, CH_2). ^{13}C-NMR (101 MHz, CD_3OD): δ = 161.85, 159.35, 154.93, 136.62, 134.79, 130.61, 130.34, 126.90, 125.53, 119.70, 118.77, 118.32, 118.09, 117.92, 110.27, 51.71. HRMS (ESI): *m/z* $[M + H]^+$ calculated for $C_{16}H_{12}ON_2BrClF$: 380.98001; found: 380.98065.

3.1.31. Preparation of 4-chloro-2-(1-(4-(trifluoromethyl)benzyl)-1*H*-1,2,3-triazol-4-yl)phenol (DX-04-05)

DX-04-06 (300 mg, 0.81 mmol) following the similar procedure described for the preparation of DX-04-02 afforded DX-04-05 (white solid, 176 mg, yield 61%). ^{1}H-NMR (400 MHz, DMSO-d_6): δ = 10.49 (s, 1H, OH), 7.85 (s, 1H, H-triazolyl), 7.64 (d, *J* = 8.1 Hz, 2H, H-phenyl), 7.34 (dd, *J* = 8.8, 2.7 Hz, 1H, H-phenyl), 7.20 (d, *J* = 8.1 Hz, 2H, H-phenyl), 7.16 (d, *J* = 2.7 Hz, 1H, H-phenyl), 6.98 (d, *J* = 8.8 Hz, 1H, H-phenyl), 5.62 (s, 2H, CH_2). ^{13}C-NMR (101 MHz, CD_3OD): δ = 155.39, 140.99, 136.49, 134.75, 132.46, 131.76, 131.11, 129.36 (2C), 126.49 (2C), 125.38, 124.09, 118.30, 116.15, 53.27. HRMS (ESI): *m/z* $[M + H]^+$ calculated for $C_{16}H_{12}ON_3ClF_3$: 354.06155; found: 354.06015.

3.1.32. Preparation of 4-(5-chloro-2-methoxyphenyl)-1-(4-(trifluoromethyl)benzyl)-1*H*-1,2,3-triazole (DX-04-06)

4-chloro-2-ethynyl-1-methoxybenzene (500 mg, 3.01 mmol) and 1-(bromomethyl)-4-(trifluoromethyl)benzene (717 mg, 3.01 mmol) following the similar procedure described for the preparation of DX-04-02 afforded DX-04-06 (white solid, 675 mg, yield 61% from 4-chloro-2-ethynyl-1-methoxybenzene). ^{1}H-NMR (400 MHz, CD_3OD): δ = 7.71 (s, 1H, H-triazolyl), 7.50 (d, *J* = 8.1 Hz, 2H, H-phenyl), 7.40 (dd, *J* = 8.9, 2.7 Hz, 1H, H-phenyl), 7.14 (d, *J* = 8.1 Hz, 2H, H-phenyl), 7.09 (d, *J* = 2.6 Hz, 1H, H-phenyl), 7.03 (d, *J* = 8.9 Hz, 1H, H-phenyl), 5.55 (s, 2H, CH_2), 3.64 (s, 3H, CH_3). ^{13}C-NMR (101 MHz, CD_3OD): δ = 154.74, 143.61, 131.20, 130.91, 129.93 (2C), 129.81, 129.39, 127.59, 127.02 (2C), 125.98, 125.64, 118.63, 117.43, 55.31, 55.04. HRMS (ESI): *m/z* $[M + H]^+$ calculated for $C_{17}H_{14}ON_3ClF_3$: 368.07720; found: 368.07599.

3.1.33. Preparation of 4-chloro-2-(5-(4-(trifluoromethyl)phenyl)-1*H*-1,2,3-triazol-4-yl)phenol (DX-04-07)

DX-04-08 (200 mg, 0.57 mmol) following the similar procedure described for the preparation of DX-04-02 afforded DX-04-07 (white solid, 144 mg, yield 75%). ^{1}H-NMR (400 MHz, DMSO-d_6): δ = 15.28 (s, 1H, H-triazolyl), 9.91 (s, 1H, NH-triazolyl), 7.75–7.68 (m, 4H, H-phenyl), 7.37 (br, 2H, H-phenyl), 6.94 (s, 1H, H-phenyl). ^{13}C-NMR (101 MHz, CD_3OD): δ = 155.58, 142.95, 137.77, 136.14, 131.62, 131.27,

130.86, 128.63 (2C), 126.43 (2C), 125.31, 124.28, 119.14, 118.53. HRMS (ESI): *m/z* $[M + H]^+$ calculated for $C_{15}H_{10}ON_3ClF_3$: 340.04590; found: 340.04453.

3.1.34. Preparation of 4-(5-chloro-2-methoxyphenyl)-5-(4-(trifluoromethyl)phenyl)-1*H*-1,2,3-triazole (DX-04-08)

4-chloro-2-ethynyl-1-methoxybenzene (300 mg, 1.81 mmol) and 1-iodo-4-(trifluoromethyl)benzene (491 mg, 1.81 mmol) following the similar procedure described for the preparation of DX-04-02 afforded DX-04-08 (white solid, 338 mg, yield 53% from 4-chloro-2-ethynyl-1-methoxybenzene). ^{1}H-NMR (400 MHz, DMSO-d_6): $\delta = 15.41$ (s, 1H, NH-triazolyl), 7.74 (d, $J = 8.1$ Hz, 2H, H-phenyl), 7.68–7.59 (m, 2H, H-phenyl), 7.54 (d, $J = 8.9$ Hz, 1H, H-phenyl), 7.48 (d, $J = 2.7$ Hz, 1H, H-phenyl), 7.15 (s, 1H, H-phenyl), 3.42 (s, 3H, CH_3). ^{13}C-NMR (101 MHz, CD_3OD): $\delta = 157.20$, 136.42, 131.71, 131.59, 131.14, 129.65, 128.37 (2C), 126.96, 126.75, 126.40 (2C), 124.27, 121.57, 114.17, 55.99. HRMS (ESI): *m/z* $[M + H]^+$ calculated for $C_{16}H_{12}ON_3ClF_3$: 354.06155; found: 354.06079.

3.2. Pharmacological Method

3.2.1. Enzyme-Based IDO1s or TDOs Activity Assay

The compounds on IDO1 or TDO activity were determined as follows [16,24,25]: A standard reaction mixture (100 μL) containing 100 mM potassium phosphate buffer (pH 6.5), 40 mM ascorbic acid (neutralized with NaOH), 200 μg/mL catalase, 20 μM methylene blue and 0.05 μM rhIDO1 or rhTDO was added to the solution containing the substrate L-tryptophan and the test sample at a determined concentration. The reaction was carried out at 37 °C for 45 min and stopped by adding 20 μL of 30% (*w/v*) trichloroacetic acid. After heating at 65 °C for 15 min, 100 μL of 2% (*w/v*) p-dimethylaminobenzaldehyde in acetic acid was added to each well. The yellow pigment derived from kynurenine was measured at 492 nm using a SYNERGY-H1 microplate reader (Biotek Instruments, Inc., Winooski, VT, USA). IC_{50} was analyzed using the GraphPad Prism 8.0 software (GraphPad Software, San Diego, CA, USA).

3.2.2. Cell Culture

B16-F10 mouse melanoma cells, NCI-H460 human lung cancer cell line and MCF7 were obtained from American Type Culture Collection (ATCC). All the cell lines were cultured with Dulbecco' modified Eagle's medium (DMEM) (Invitrogen Corporation, Waltham, MA, USA) supplemented with 10% fetal bovine serum (FBS) (Hyclone, Waltham, MA, USA) and 1% penicillin streptomycin (Invitrogen) at 37 °C in 5% CO_2.

3.2.3. Cell Viability Assay

The in vitro inhibitory effects of the compounds were measured by MTT assay [26]. Briefly, different kinds of cells were plated in 96-well plates at a density of 2000/well. After attachment for overnight at 37 °C, the cells were treated with the compounds at various concentrations. After 72 h culture, the MTT reagent was added to each well, and plates were incubated for another 4 h at 37 °C. Then, the blue-purple crystal formamidine was dissolved in DMSO after discarding the supernatant. Samples were measured using microplate reader at a wavelength of 570 nm (Biotek Instruments, Inc., Winooski, VT, USA). IC_{50} values were calculated with GraphPad Prism 8.0 software.

3.2.4. Mice

C57BL/6 mice were obtained from Beijing Vital River Laboratory Animal Technology Co., Ltd. (Beijing Vital River Laboratory Animal Technology Co., Ltd, Beijing, China). Studies involving mice were approved by the Experimental Animal Management and Welfare Committee at the Institute of Materia Medica, Peking Union Medical College.

3.2.5. Pharmacokinetic Studies

The animal Care and Welfare Committee of Institute of Materia Medica, Chinese Academy of Medical Sciences approved all animal care, housing, and laboratory procedures. Male ICR mice were used in the single dose pharmacokinetic studies. Compound DX-03-12 was prepared as 3 mg/mL suspension with 0.5% CMC (containing 0.3% Tween 80) for oral use and was formulated as 3 mg/mL solution with 5% DMSO in saline for intravenous injection. Twenty mice were divided into two groups, 10 in each group. After fasting 12 h with free access to water, mice were treated with a 3 mg/kg i.v. or 30 mg/kg oral dose of compound DX-03-12. Blood samples (50 μL) were collected at 5, 15, 30 min, 1, 2, 4, 6, 8, 12 and 24 h after oral administration and 2, 5, 15, 30 min, 1, 2, 4, 6, 8, 12 and 24 h after intravenous injection. After centrifugation, the plasma samples (15 μL) were precipitated by five volumes of acetonitrile. The supernatant were analyzed by liquid chromatography/tandem mass spectrometry (Agilent Technologies, Santa Clara, CA, USA) with a Zobax C18 column (50 mm × 2.1 mm, 3.5 μm). Compound detection was performed with the mass spectrometer in MRM (multiple reaction monitoring, Agilent Technologies, Santa Clara, CA, USA) negative ionization mode. The selected reaction monitoring transitions were *m/z* 348.5→160 for compound DX-03-12. The pharmacokinetic parameters were calculated with WinNonlin software V6.3 using non-compartmental analysis (Pharsight Corporation, Mountain View, CA, USA).

3.2.6. In Vivo Studies

The mouse melanoma cells B16F10 were cultured and harvested in saline. At day 0 of the experiment, 1×10^6 cells were injected subcutaneously into mice, and treatment was initiated at day 1 following the mice enrolled randomly in control and experimental groups [27]. For control group, 0.5% CMCNa was orally administered every day. Compound DX-03-12 was dissolved in 0.5% CMC for oral treatment or dissolved in saline for intraperitoneal treatment. When the mice were sacrificed, the tumors were stripped and weighted. The tumor growth inhibition (TGI) was calculated as TGI = $(1 - \text{tumor weight}_{\text{treatment}}/\text{tumor weight}_{\text{vehicle}}) \times 100\%$. The statistical analysis was performed with GraphPad Prism 8.0 software and the significance level was evaluated with a one-way ANOVA model.

4. Conclusions

We designed four series of IDO1 inhibitors using indole and phenylimidazole as the scaffolds. The design strategies were based on the mechanism of IDO1, focusing on the interaction between the inhibitor and the heme iron. The four series of compounds were synthesized and their IDO1 and TDO inhibition was evaluated. Most compounds showed marginal IDO1 inhibition, but eight compounds showed moderate IDO1 inhibition. In particular, DX-03-12 and DX-03-13 showed IDO1 inhibition with IC_{50}s of 0.3 and 0.5 μM and low cell cytotoxicities against two cancer cell lines. A pharmacokinetic study showed that DX-03-12 had satisfactory properties, with rapid absorption, moderate plasma clearance, acceptable half-life, and high oral bioavailability. The in vivo anti-tumor efficacy in a B16F10 subcutaneous xenograft mouse model showed that DX-03-12 orally administered at a dose of 60 mg/kg inhibited tumor growth by 72.2% compared with the control tumors. In summary, IDO1 inhibitor DX-03-12 exhibits promising drug like properties, good pharmacokinetic properties, low cellular toxicity, and impressive in vivo anti-tumor efficacy.

Author Contributions: L.S., F.L., and H.C. conceived and designed the experiments; H.W., Y.L. (Yuke Liu), S.W., T.W., and G.Z. performed the experiments, analyzed the data; Y.L. (Yan Li), and X.C. checked the data; L.S., F.L., and H.C. wrote the paper. Please contact L.S. for pharmacokinetic study, F.L. for pharmacology study and H.C. for medicinal chemistry.

Acknowledgments: We would like to express our appreciation to Jie Li of Beijing Chao-Yang Hospital for the clinical issue discussion.

References

1. Weng, T.; Qiu, X.; Wang, J.; Li, Z.; Bian, J. Recent discovery of indoleamine-2,3-dioxygenase 1 inhibitors targeting cancer immunotherapy. *Eur. J. Med. Chem.* **2018**, *143*, 656–669. [CrossRef] [PubMed]
2. Muller, A.J.; DuHadaway, J.B.; Donover, P.S.; Sutanto-Ward, E.; Prendergast, G.C. Inhibition of indoleamine 2,3-dioxygenase, an immunoregulatory target of the cancer suppression gene Bin1, potentiates cancer chemotherapy. *Nat. Med.* **2005**, *11*, 312–319. [CrossRef] [PubMed]
3. Platten, M.; Nollen, E.A.A.; Rohrig, U.F.; Fallarino, F.; Opitz, C.A. Tryptophan metabolism as a common therapeutic target in cancer, neurodegeneration and beyond. *Nat. Rev. Drug Discov* **2019**, *18*, 379–401. [CrossRef] [PubMed]
4. Cervenka, I.; Agudelo, L.; Ruas, J. Kynurenines: Tryptophan's metabolites in exercise, inflammation, and mental health. *Science* **2017**, *357*. [CrossRef] [PubMed]
5. Abdulla, A.-B.B. Kynurenine Pathway of Tryptophan Metabolism: Regulatory and Functional Aspects. *Int. J. Tryptophan. Res.* **2017**, *10*. [CrossRef]
6. Zhai, L.; Spranger, S.; Binder, D.C.; Gritsina, G.; Lauing, K.L.; Giles, F.J.; Wainwright, D.A. Molecular Pathways: Targeting IDO1 and Other Tryptophan Dioxygenases for Cancer Immunotherapy. *Clin. Cancer Res.* **2015**, *21*, 5427–5433. [CrossRef] [PubMed]
7. Chauhan, N.; Basran, J.; Efimov, I.; Svistunenko, D.A.; Seward, H.E.; Moody, P.C.; Raven, E.L. The role of serine 167 in human indoleamine 2,3-dioxygenase: A comparison with tryptophan 2,3-dioxygenase. *Biochemistry* **2008**, *47*, 4761–4769. [CrossRef] [PubMed]
8. Batabyal, D.; Yeh, S.R. Human tryptophan dioxygenase: A comparison to indoleamine 2,3-dioxygenase. *J. Am. Chem. Soc.* **2007**, *129*, 15690–15701. [CrossRef]
9. Sugimoto, H.; Oda, S.; Otsuki, T.; Hino, T.; Yoshida, T.; Shiro, Y. Crystal structure of human indoleamine 2,3-dioxygenase: Catalytic mechanism of O2 incorporation by a heme-containing dioxygenase. *Proc. Natl. Acad. Sci. USA* **2006**, *103*, 2611–2616. [CrossRef]
10. Rohrig, U.F.; Zoete, V.; Michielin, O. The Binding Mode of *N*-Hydroxyamidines to Indoleamine 2,3-Dioxygenase 1 (IDO1). *Biochemistry* **2017**, *56*, 4323–4325. [CrossRef]
11. Samelson-Jones, B.J.; Yeh, S.R. Interactions between nitric oxide and indoleamine 2,3-dioxygenase. *Biochemistry* **2006**, *45*, 8527–8538. [CrossRef] [PubMed]
12. Yanagisawa, S.; Sugimoto, H.; Shiro, Y.; Ogura, T. A specific interaction of L-tryptophan with CO of CO-bound indoleamine 2,3-dioxygenase identified by resonance Raman spectroscopy. *Biochemistry* **2010**, *49*, 10081–10088. [CrossRef] [PubMed]
13. Crosignani, S.; Bingham, P.; Bottemanne, P.; Cannelle, H.; Cauwenberghs, S.; Cordonnier, M.; Dalvie, D.; Deroose, F.; Feng, J.L.; Gomes, B.; et al. Discovery of a Novel and Selective Indoleamine 2,3-Dioxygenase (IDO-1) Inhibitor 3-(5-Fluoro-1*H*-indol-3-yl)pyrrolidine-2,5-dione (EOS200271/PF-06840003) and Its Characterization as a Potential Clinical Candidate. *J. Med. Chem.* **2017**, *60*, 9617–9629. [CrossRef] [PubMed]
14. Yang, D.; Li, T.; Li, Y.; Zhang, S.; Li, W.; Liang, H.; Xing, Z.; Du, L.; He, J.; Kuang, C.; et al. H_2S suppresses indoleamine 2, 3-dioxygenase 1 and exhibits immunotherapeutic efficacy in murine hepatocellular carcinoma. *J. Exp. Clin. Cancer Res.* **2019**, *38*, 88. [CrossRef] [PubMed]
15. Pham, K.N.; Yeh, S.R. Mapping the Binding Trajectory of a Suicide Inhibitor in Human Indoleamine 2,3-Dioxygenase 1. *J. Am. Chem. Soc.* **2018**, *140*, 14538–14541. [CrossRef] [PubMed]
16. Yang, S.; Li, X.; Hu, F.; Li, Y.; Yang, Y.; Yan, J.; Kuang, C.; Yang, Q. Discovery of tryptanthrin derivatives as potent inhibitors of indoleamine 2,3-dioxygenase with therapeutic activity in Lewis lung cancer (LLC) tumor-bearing mice. *J. Med. Chem.* **2013**, *56*, 8321–8331. [CrossRef] [PubMed]
17. Yue, E.W.; Douty, B.; Wayland, B.; Bower, M.; Liu, X.; Leffet, L.; Wang, Q.; Bowman, K.J.; Hansbury, M.J.; Liu, C.; et al. Discovery of potent competitive inhibitors of indoleamine 2,3-dioxygenase with in vivo pharmacodynamic activity and efficacy in a mouse melanoma model. *J. Med. Chem.* **2009**, *52*, 7364–7367. [CrossRef] [PubMed]

18. Kumar, S.; Jaller, D.; Patel, B.; LaLonde, J.M.; DuHadaway, J.B.; Malachowski, W.P.; Prendergast, G.C.; Muller, A.J. Structure based development of phenylimidazole-derived inhibitors of indoleamine 2,3-dioxygenase. *J. Med. Chem.* **2008**, *51*, 4968–4977. [CrossRef]
19. Rohrig, U.F.; Majjigapu, S.R.; Grosdidier, A.; Bron, S.; Stroobant, V.; Pilotte, L.; Colau, D.; Vogel, P.; Van den Eynde, B.J.; Zoete, V.; et al. Rational design of 4-aryl-1,2,3-triazoles for indoleamine 2,3-dioxygenase 1 inhibition. *J. Med. Chem.* **2012**, *55*, 5270–5290. [CrossRef]
20. Tojo, S.; Kohno, T.; Tanaka, T.; Kamioka, S.; Ota, Y.; Ishii, T.; Kamimoto, K.; Asano, S.; Isobe, Y. Crystal Structures and Structure-Activity Relationships of Imidazothiazole Derivatives as IDO1 Inhibitors. *ACS Med. Chem. Lett.* **2014**, *5*, 1119–1123. [CrossRef]
21. Zhu, M.M.T.; Dancsok, A.R.; Nielsen, T.O. Indoleamine Dioxygenase Inhibitors: Clinical Rationale and Current Development. *Curr. Oncol. Rep.* **2019**, *21*, 2. [CrossRef]
22. Yan, N.; He, Y.; Wen, H.; Lai, F.; Yin, D.; Cui, H. A Suzuki-Miyaura method for labelling proliferating cells containing incorporated BrdU. *Analyst* **2018**, *143*, 1224–1233. [CrossRef] [PubMed]
23. Mautino, M.; Kumar, S.; Jaipuri, F.; Kesharwani, T.; Zhang, X. Imidazole Derivatives as IDO inhibitors. WO2011056652A1, 12 May 2011.
24. Austin, C.J.; Mizdrak, J.; Matin, A.; Sirijovski, N.; Kosim-Satyaputra, P.; Willows, R.D.; Roberts, T.H.; Truscott, R.J.; Polekhina, G.; Parker, M.W.; et al. Optimised expression and purification of recombinant human indoleamine 2,3-dioxygenase. *Protein Expr. Purif.* **2004**, *37*, 392–398. [CrossRef] [PubMed]
25. Littlejohn, T.K.; Takikawa, O.; Skylas, D.; Jamie, J.F.; Walker, M.J.; Truscott, R.J. Expression and purification of recombinant human indoleamine 2, 3-dioxygenase. *Protein Expr. Purif.* **2000**, *19*, 22–29. [CrossRef]
26. Lai, F.; Shen, Z.; Wen, H.; Chen, J.; Zhang, X.; Lin, P.; Yin, D.; Cui, H.; Chen, X. A Morphological identification cell cytotoxicity assay using cytoplasm-localized fluorescent probe (CLFP) to distinguish living and dead cells. *Biochem. Biophys. Res. Commun.* **2017**, *482*, 257–263. [CrossRef] [PubMed]
27. He, Y.; Wen, J.; Cui, Q.; Lai, F.; Yin, D.; Cui, H. Quantitative Evaluation of in Vivo Target Efficacy of Anti-tumor Agents via an Immunofluorescence and EdU Labeling Strategy. *Front. Pharmacol.* **2018**, *9*, 812. [CrossRef] [PubMed]

3

Glycoconjugation of Betulin Derivatives Using Copper-Catalyzed 1,3-Dipolar Azido-Alkyne Cycloaddition Reaction and a Preliminary Assay of Cytotoxicity of the Obtained Compounds

Mirosława Grymel [1,2,*], Gabriela Pastuch-Gawołek [1,2], Anna Lalik [2,3], Mateusz Zawojak [1], Seweryn Boczek [1], Monika Krawczyk [1,2] and Karol Erfurt [4]

1 Department of Organic Chemistry, Bioorganic Chemistry and Biotechnology, Silesian University of Technology, B. Krzywoustego 4, 44-100 Gliwice, Poland; gabriela.pastuch@polsl.pl (G.P.-G.); mateuszzawojak@wp.pl (M.Z.); seweryn.boczek16@gmail.com (S.B.); monika.krawczyk@polsl.pl (M.K.)

2 Biotechnology Center, Silesian University of Technology, B. Krzywoustego 8, 44-100 Gliwice, Poland; anna.lalik@polsl.pl

3 Department of Systems Biology and Engineering, Silesian University of Technology, Akademicka 16, 44-100 Gliwice, Poland

4 Department of Chemical Organic Technology and Petrochemistry, Silesian University of Technology, B. Krzywoustego 4, 44-100 Gliwice, Poland; karol.erfurt@polsl.pl

* Correspondence: miroslawa.grymel@polsl.pl;

Academic Editors: José Antonio Lupiáñez, Amalia Pérez-Jiménez and Eva E. Rufino-Palomares

Abstract: Pentacyclic lupane-type triterpenoids, such as betulin and its synthetic derivatives, display a broad spectrum of biological activity. However, one of the major drawbacks of these compounds as potential therapeutic agents is their high hydrophobicity and low bioavailability. On the other hand, the presence of easily transformable functional groups in the parent structure makes betulin have a high synthetic potential and the ability to form different derivatives. In this context, research on the synthesis of new betulin derivatives as conjugates of naturally occurring triterpenoid with a monosaccharide via a linker containing a heteroaromatic 1,2,3-triazole ring was presented. It has been shown that copper-catalyzed 1,3-dipolar azide-alkyne cycloaddition reaction (CuAAC) provides an easy and effective way to synthesize new molecular hybrids based on natural products. The chemical structures of the obtained betulin glycoconjugates were confirmed by spectroscopic analysis. Cytotoxicity of the obtained compounds was evaluated on a human breast adenocarcinoma cell line (MCF-7) and colorectal carcinoma cell line (HCT 116). The obtained results show that despite the fact that the obtained betulin glycoconjugates do not show interesting antitumor activity, the idea of adding a sugar unit to the betulin backbone may, after some modifications, turn out to be correct and allow for the targeted transport of betulin glycoconjugates into the tumor cells.

Keywords: betulin glycoconjugates; click chemistry; 1,3-dipolar cycloaddition; anticancer activity

---

1. Introduction

For several decades, natural products (*NPs*) have been widely researched in terms of searching for potential therapeutic agents. One important class of natural plant products is pentacyclic lupane-type triterpenoids, among them betulin (*BN*). In recent years, due to a strong biological activity and low toxicity, the great interest of scientists has been focused on its naturally occurring bioactive skeleton, as evidenced by numerous new semi-synthetic derivatives reported every year. Betulin (*BN*, 3-lup-20(29)-ene-3,28-diol) is cheap, easily accessible from natural resources, and can be readily extracted from the bark of several species of trees, especially from the white birch (*Betula pubescens*) [1,2]. *BN* possesses a broad spectrum of biological activity confirmed by its anticancer [3–13], antibacterial [14,15], anti-HIV [14,16], anti-inflammatory [17–19], antiviral [20,21], antimalarial activity [17,19], and hepatoprotective properties [9,22,23].

One of the major drawbacks of betulin and analogs as potential therapeutic agents is its poor hydrophilicity, poor solubility in aqueous media like blood serum and polar solvents used for bioassays, and low bioavailability. However, due to the presence of easily transformable functional groups (including C3OH, C28OH) in the parent structure, betulin has a high synthetic potential and the ability to form numerous semisynthetic derivatives. Thus, the parent structure of betulin, being a biologically attractive scaffold with a high safety profile, makes it possible to carry out a variety of structural modifications to improve its pharmacokinetic properties. In some cases [5,6,9,12,24–26], the transformations gave compounds with a higher bioavailability and higher biological activity than the parent compound (Figure 1).

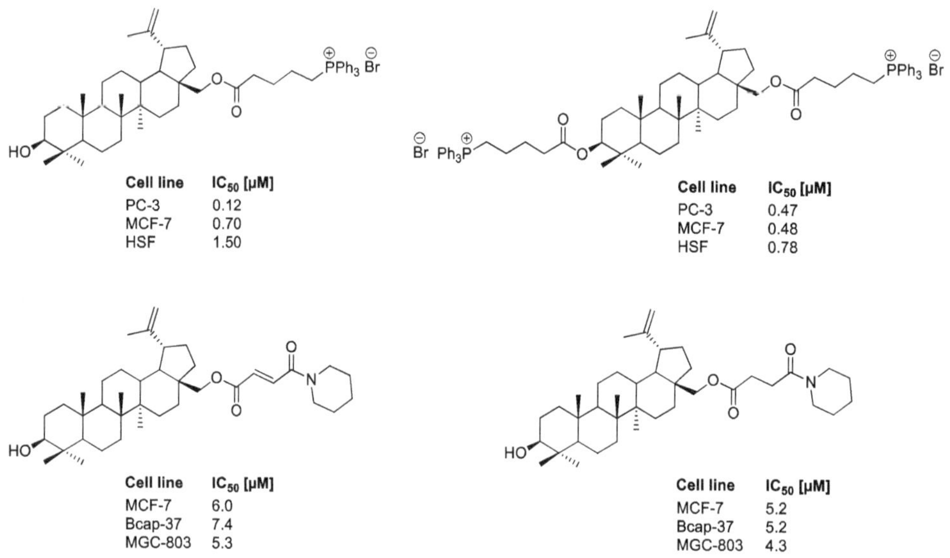

Figure 1. Antitumor activities of betulin derivatives against human breast carcinoma (MCF-7 and Bcap-37), human gastric carcinoma (MGC-803), human prostate carcinoma (PC-3), and human skin fibroblast (HSF) cell lines [12,27].

One of the strategies to improve the pharmacokinetic properties of betulin is its link to the 1,2,3-triazole ring, which is an important five-membered heterocyclic scaffold due to the extensive biological activities. This framework can be obtained through the copper-catalyzed azide-alkyne cycloaddition (CuAAC). In addition, the 1,2,3-triazole ring can be successfully used for conjugation in mild conditions and with high yields, with two or more molecules of interest. Due to the stability of triazoles in typical physiological conditions, they act as ideal linkers and could improve the hydrophilic property of the parent skeleton of NPs via the ability to create hydrogen bonding. The 1,2,3-triazole moiety mimics the naturally occurring amide bonds, and at the same time, it is more stable [28–31]. This methodology allows the functionalization of *BN* at position C3, C28, and C30, with different substrate (Scheme 1). Although the triazole derivatives of betulin have been widely researched, no structures have been found so far that would demonstrate cytotoxicity at a level that would allow them to be used as drugs [32].

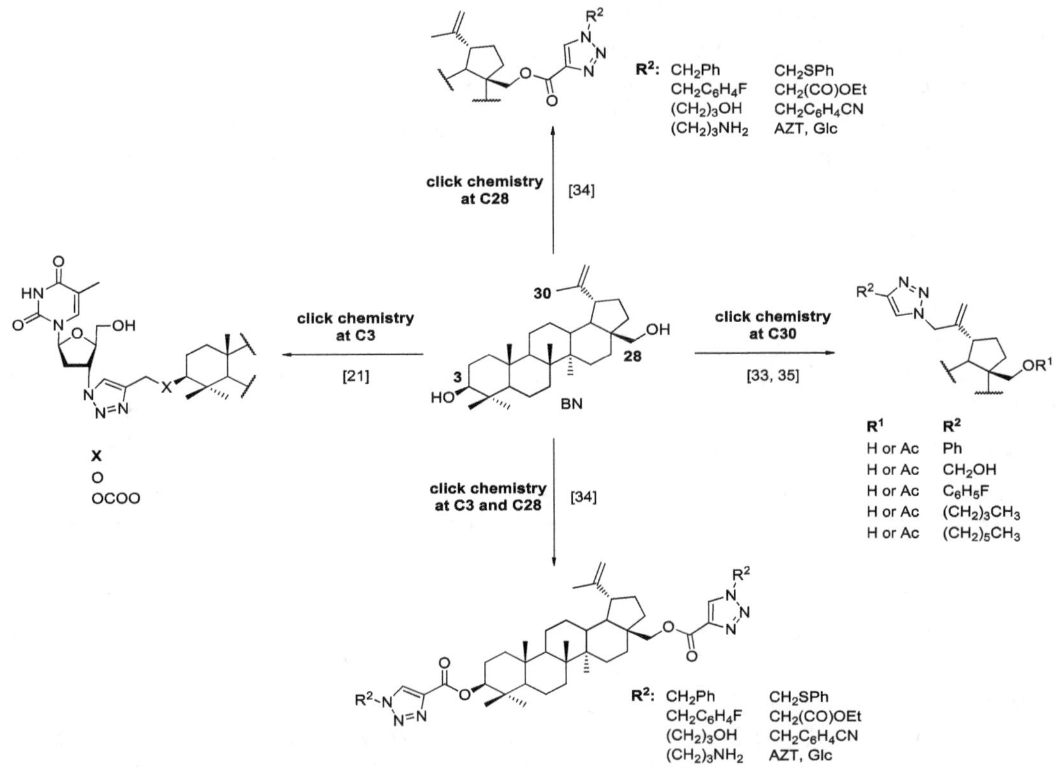

Scheme 1. Functionalization of betulin at the C3, C28, and C30 position via CuAAC [33–35].

The motivation for our research was the successes in the synthesis of molecular hybrids presented in Figure 2, obtained with the use of a natural biologically active compound, where the introduction of a triazole ring and a sugar unit into the parent structure of quinoline resulted in the improvement of pharmacological properties of the obtained glycoconjugates [36–39].

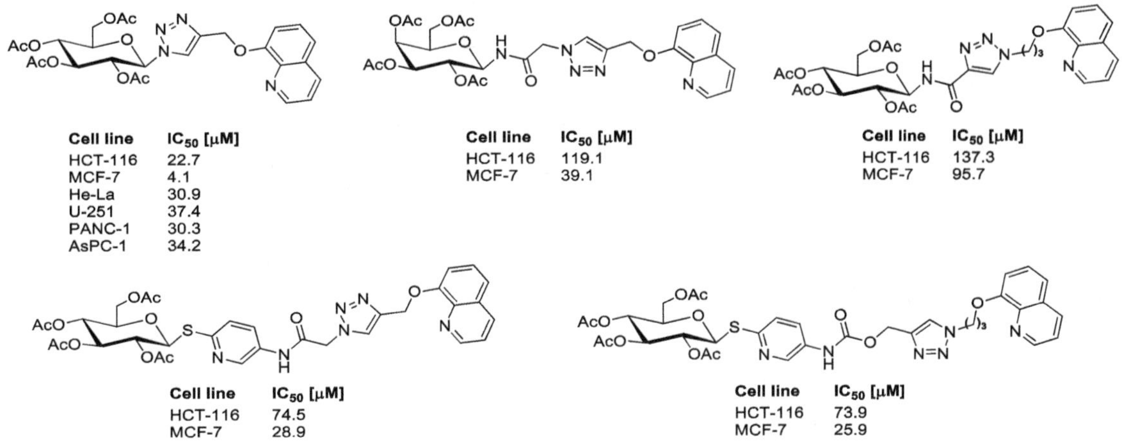

Figure 2. Selected quinoline glycoconjugates with anticancer activity.

The presence of a sugar unit in the hybrid molecules improves their pharmacokinetic properties, including solubility and intermembrane transport, as well as the selectivity in targeting drugs for a specific purpose. Sugar moieties are known to influence the pharmacokinetic properties of the respective compounds, such as absorption, distribution, and metabolism [40]. Since it is generally accepted that glycosides are more water soluble than the respective aglycones, glycosidation of triterpenes should increase hydrosolubility and improve the pharmacological properties. Furthermore, it is known that cancerous cells need a more significant sugar contribution than normal cells [41]. It is related to the specific metabolism of glucose by cancer cells as well as with their often-increased proliferation compared to healthy cells. This phenomenon is known as the Warburg effect and arises from mitochondrial metabolic changes. It consists in the fact that cancer cells produce their energy through glycolysis followed by lactic acid fermentation, characteristic of hypoxic conditions, and its level is much higher (more than 100 times) than in healthy cells, for which the main source of energy is mitochondrial oxidative phosphorylation [42]. An increased glycolysis process in cancer cells is associated with overexpression of GLUT transporters (special transmembrane proteins that facilitate concentration-dependent glucose uptake inside the cell) [43]. Consequently, this difference could be exploited to support the absorption of the therapeutic agent by the tumoral site, which allows for controlled drug delivery.

Our research group decided to focus on the synthesis of the new betulin glycoconjugates via click chemistry reaction. We designed semi-synthetic betulin derivatives as a combination of naturally occurring triterpenoid (BN) with proven broad biological activity, with a monosaccharide through a linker containing a heteroaromatic 1,2,3-triazole ring. The choice of the sugar unit for glycoconjugation was determined by the willingness to increase the selectivity of potential drugs by using the overexpression of GLUT transporters in some types of cancers. These transporters also recognize other sugars, such as galactose, mannose, and glucosamine [44]. It was decided to attach either D-glucose or D-galactose units due to the common occurrence of these sugars in nature. These sugars were supposed to perform the function of a drug carrier across the cell membrane by adapting to the structure of the GLUT transporter [43]. The configuration at the anomeric center of the sugar also seems important from the point of view of matching with the transporter. The results of research on the structural requirements for binding variously substituted sugars to the sugar transporters indicate that the β-configuration is preferred for binding to the GLUT transporters [45,46]. In order to obtain a library of compounds intended for the initial assessment of biological cytotoxicity, we tested two strategies for conjugating the sugar unit with the parent skeleton of betulin, both based on the 1,3-dipolar azido-alkyne cycloaddition reaction (Scheme 2).

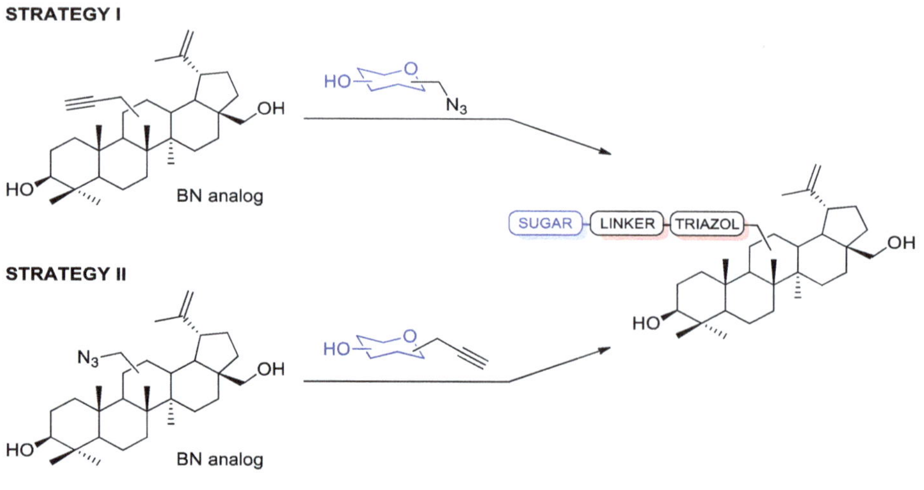

Scheme 2. Strategies for the synthesis of betulin glycoconjugates.

Strategy I involves the introduction of a propargyl moiety into the betulin structure at position C28 (monosubstituted betulin analogs) or C3 and C28 (disubstituted betulin analogs), followed by the synthesis of glycoconjugates containing the 1,2,3-triazole ring, resulting from combining propargyl betulin derivatives and appropriate sugar derivatives containing an azide moiety. *Strategy II*, on the other hand, consists of adding an appropriate linker ($O(CO)CH_2N_3$) to the betulin backbone one at position C28 or at two positions, C3 and C28, and the synthesis of glycoconjugates via click chemistry with the use of betulin azides and propargyl sugar derivatives. The linker that connects the betulin scaffold to the sugar unit is an important element that may influence the potential biological activity of the discussed betulin glycoconjugates. In this study, we report the synthesis of several glycoconjugates, having a linker containing a 1,2,3-triazole moiety and an additional ether (*O*-glycosidic bond), ester, or amide moiety (Figure 3). The triazole ring seems to be an ideal linker component as it improves water solubility, thus allowing in vivo administration; it is analogous to an amide function for its electronic properties but simultaneously is resistant to hydrolysis, it is sufficiently stable in biological systems, and finally, it is rigid enough, which allows avoidance of internal interaction between the two linked moieties. On the other hand, the presence of a glycosidic, amide, or ester linkage gives a chance for the hydrolysis of the glycoconjugate into its biologically active components after the compound enters the cell under the action of hydrolytic enzymes. The cytotoxicity of the obtained compounds was evaluated on a human breast adenocarcinoma cell line (MCF-7) and colorectal carcinoma cell line (HCT 116).

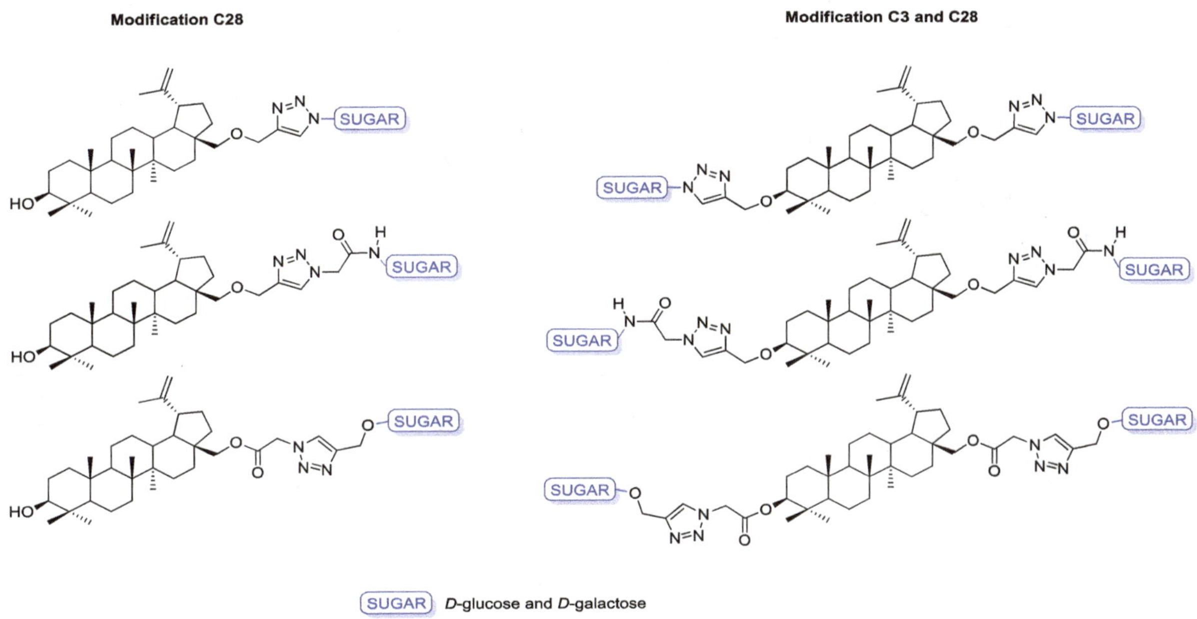

Figure 3. General structure of the betulin glycoconjugates.

2. Results and Discussion

2.1. Synthesis of Betulin Analogs

The introduction of a propargyl moiety into the betulin molecule was based on the procedure described by Khan et al. for betulinic acid [47]. It was assumed that both mono- and dipropargyl derivatives of betulin could be formed due to the presence in the substrate of the primary OH group at the C28 position and the secondary OH group at the C3 position. The propargylated betulin was prepared as shown in Scheme 3. Crystalline betulin was reacted with propargyl bromide in alkaline medium (NaH) in tetrahydrofuran. In the search for the optimal procedure, a number of modifications were made, by selecting the proportions of reagents, reaction time, and temperature. It was found that it is advantageous to use the reagents in a molar ratio (BN/NaH/HC≡CCH_2Br, 1:4:3.2) at ambient temperature for 24 h.

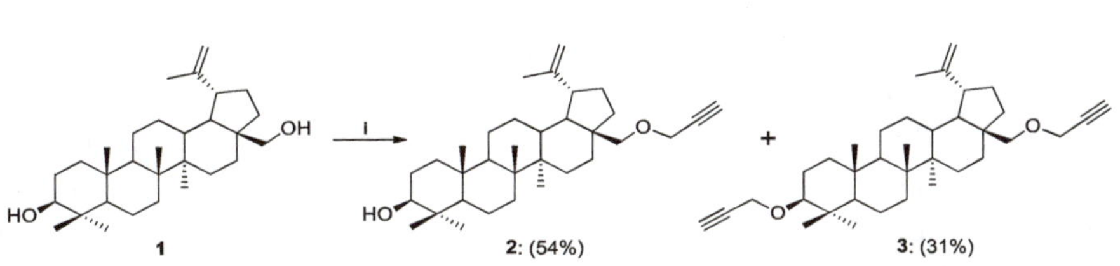

Scheme 3. Synthesis of propargyl derivatives of betulin **2** and **3**. Reagents and Conditions: (**i**) propargyl bromide, NaH, THF, r.t., 24 h.

The synthesis of 28-*O*-chloroacetylbetulin **4** and 3,28-*O,O′*-di(chloroacetyl)betulin **5** was performed by modifying the procedure described by Komissarova et al. in 2017 [48]. Chloroacetic chloride was added dropwise to the betulin solution in THF, while triethylamine (Et_3N) was replaced with *N,N*-diisopropylethylamine (DIPEA) and 4-(dimethylamino)pyridine (DMAP). We found that the application of twice the excess of chloroacetic chloride to BN results in the formation of only 3,28-*O,O′*-di(chloroacetyl)betulin **5** with a high yield (95%, Scheme 4). On the other hand, when the reagents were used in a molar ratio ($Cl(CO)CH_2Cl$/DIPEA/DMAP, 1.2:1.5:0.1), a modification of the betulin skeleton was observed at both the C28 and C3 positions. The maximum yield with which a monosubstituted product **4** can be obtained is 34%. Replacement of the chlorine anion in betulin analogs **4** and **5** by azide moiety was performed at an elevated temperature (90 °C) using NaN_3 and DMF as a solvent. 28-*O*-Azidoacetylbetulin **6** and 3,28-*O,O′*-di(azidoacetyl)betulin **7** were purified by column chromatography to give pure compounds with 64% and 72% yields, respectively (Scheme 4, Table 1).

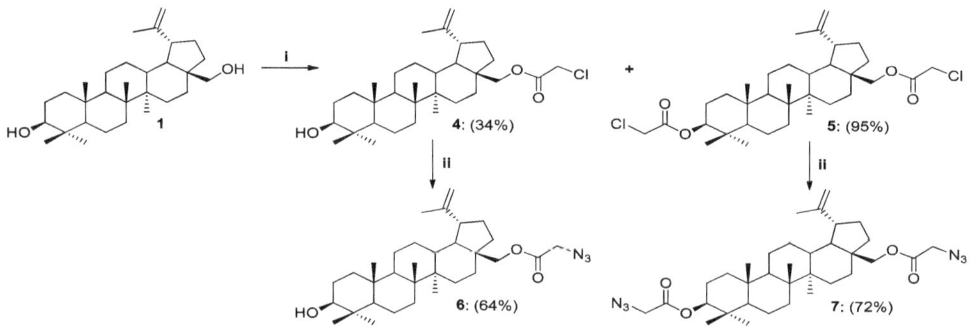

Scheme 4. Synthesis of betulin derivatives **4**–**7**. Reagents and Conditions: (**i**) $Cl(CO)CH_2Cl$, DIPEA, DMAP, THF, r.t., 24 h; (**ii**) NaN_3, DMF, 90 °C, 3 h.

Table 1. Synthesis of betulin derivatives **2**–**7**.

Entry	Substrate				Product			
	No.	**Solvent**	**Temp., °C**	**Time, h**	**No.**	**R (C3)**	**R¹ (C28)**	**Yield, %**
1	1	THF	r.t.	24	2	OH	OCH2C≡CH	54
					3	OCH2C≡CH	OCH2C≡CH	31
2	1	THF	r.t.	24	4	OH	O(CO)CH2Cl	34
3	1	THF	r.t.	24	5	O(CO)CH2Cl	O(CO)CH2Cl	95
4	4	DMF	90	3	6	OH	O(CO)CH2N3	64
5	5	DMF	90	3	7	O(CO)CH2N3	O(CO)CH2N3	72

2.2. *Synthesis of Sugar Derivatives*

Sugar derivatives substituted at the anomeric position were the second necessary structural element for the synthesis of betulin glycoconjugates. The synthetic route to the corresponding derivatives of D-glucose and D-galactose **9**–**14** is shown in Scheme 5. As mentioned before, the choice of such sugar moieties is dictated by the frequency of their natural occurrence as well as their importance for cell metabolism. All sugar derivatives were prepared according to known procedures involving the acetylation of free sugars **8a** or **8b** and conversion of per-*O*-acetylated derivatives **9a** or **9b** into the corresponding glycosyl bromides **11a** or **11b [49,50]**. The glycosyl bromides were used for further reactions leading to obtain 2,3,4,6-tetra-*O*-acetyl-β-glycosyl azides **12a** and **12b [36]**. D-Glucose derivative **10a**, in which the alkynyl moiety was introduced by the formation of an *O*-glycosidic linkage, was prepared by reacting per-*O*-acetylated D-glucose **9a** with propargyl alcohol in the presence of $BF_3{\cdot}Et_2O$ as a Lewis acid catalyst [51]. Sugar derivatives **13a** and **13b** containing an amide moiety at the sugar anomeric position were obtained in a two-step procedure. First, glycosyl azides **12a** and **12b** were converted to the corresponding 1-aminosugars through a hydrogenation reaction in a Parr apparatus using palladium hydroxide deposited on activated charcoal and then such obtained intermediates were reacted with chloroacetyl chloride in the presence of TEA, which neutralized the formed hydrogen chloride. Finally, the terminal chlorine atom in compounds **13a** and **13b** was exchanged with an azide group, which made it possible to obtain sugar derivatives **14a** and **14b** as a result of the reaction with sodium azide in anhydrous DMF [37].

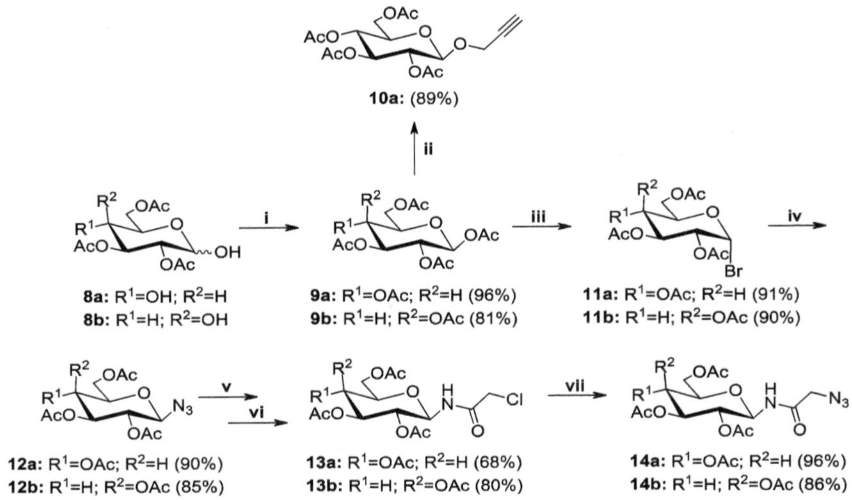

Scheme 5. Synthesis of sugar derivatives **9–14**. Reagents and Conditions: (**i**) CH_3COONa, Ac_2O, b.p., 1 h; (**ii**) propargyl alcohol, $BF_3 \cdot Et_2O$, DCM, 0 °C→r.t, 2 h; (**iii**) CH_3COOH, 33% HBr/AcOH, r.t., 1 h; (**iv**) NaN_3, TBASH, $CHCl_3/NaHCO_3$, r.t., 2 h; (**v**) 20% $Pd(OH)_2/C$, THF:EtOH (2:1, *v*/*v*), H_2, 1.5 bar, 2 h; (**vi**) chloroacetyl chloride, TEA, DCM, r.t., 1 h; (**vii**) NaN_3, DMF, r.t., 24 h.

2.3. *Modifications of the Natural Betulin Skeleton via Click Chemistry*

The copper-catalyzed azide-alkyne cycloaddition reaction (CuAAC) is widely used to modify natural bioactive compounds, and its main advantage is the ability to synthesize new molecular hybrids with high yields under mild conditions. In the course of our research, we developed a methodology for the synthesis of new previously unknown betulin derivatives, consisting of joining the triterpenoid skeleton with a monosaccharide through an appropriate linker containing a heteroaromatic 1,2,3-triazole ring. Glycoconjugation of betulin derivatives was based on the click chemistry reaction (CuAAC) using propargylbetulin derivatives **2**, **3** and protected D-glucose **12a**, **14a** or D-galactose **12b**, **14b** derivatives containing an azide group (Strategy I, Schemes 6 and 7) or propargyl *O*-glycoside derivative of *per-O*-acetylated-D-glucose **10a** with appropriate betulin azides **6**, **7** (Strategy II, Scheme 8). Building blocks designed in this way make it possible to obtain a whole range of betulin glycoconjugates, containing in the linker structure different combinations of an *O*-glycosidic linkage, an ester bond, an *O*-methylene 1,2,3-triazole linker, and an amide moiety.

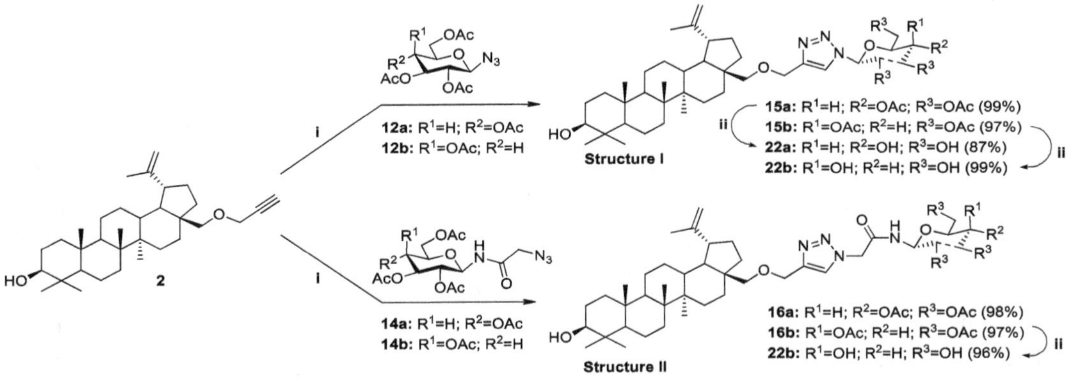

Scheme 6. Synthesis of glycoconjugates type I and II according to Strategy I. Reagents and Conditions: (**i**) $CuSO_4 \cdot 5H_2O$, NaAsc, *i*-PrOH/H_2O (1:1, *v*/*v*), r.t., 24 h; (**ii**) 1. NaOMe, MeOH, r.t., 0.5 h; 2. *Amberlyst*-15.

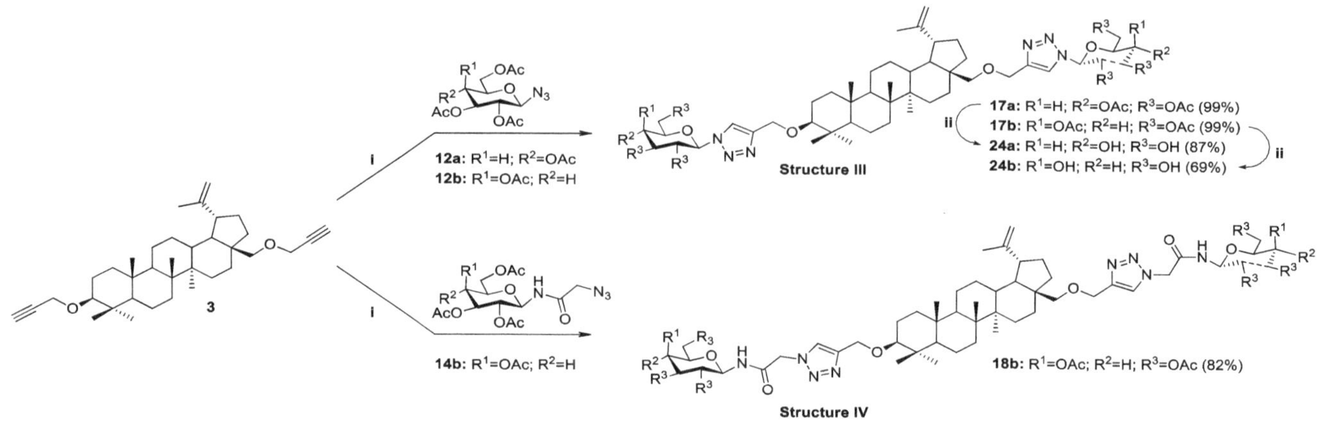

Scheme 7. Synthesis of glycoconjugates type **III** and **IV** according to Strategy I. Reagents and Conditions: (**i**) $CuSO_4{\cdot}5H_2O$, NaAsc, i-PrOH/H_2O (1:1, *v/v*), r.t., 24 h; (**ii**) 1. NaOMe, MeOH, r.t., 0.5 h: 2. *Amberlyst-15*.

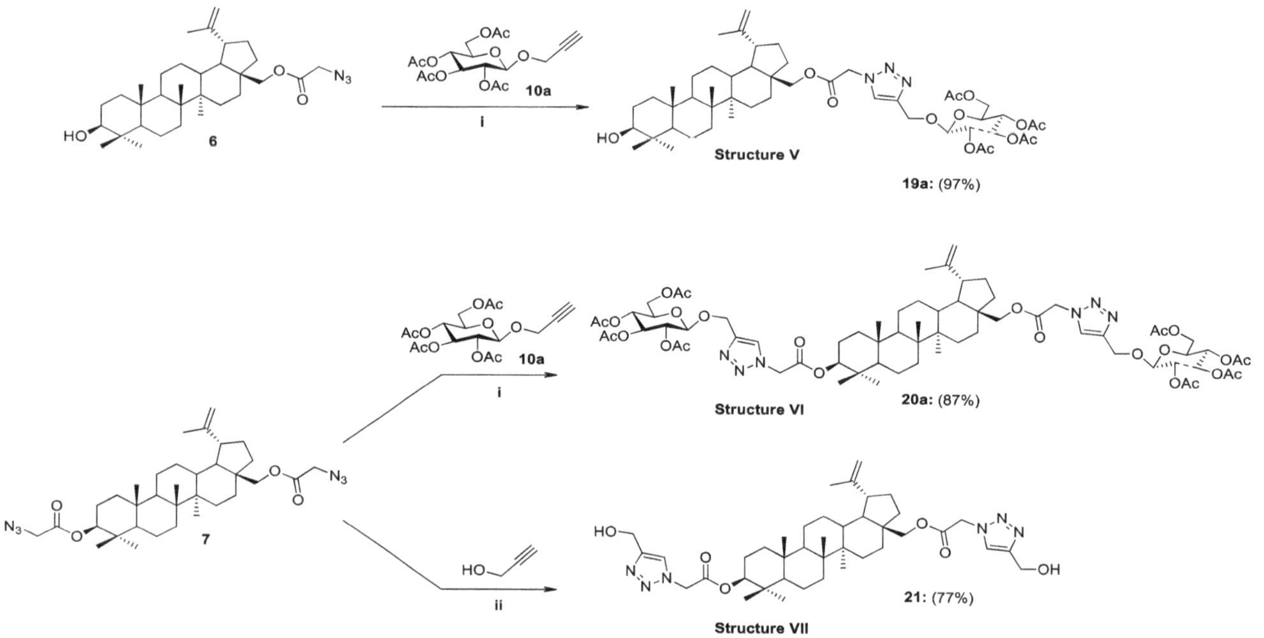

Scheme 8. Synthesis of glycoconjugates type **V–VII** according to Strategy II. Reagents and Conditions: (**i**) $CuSO_4{\cdot}5H_2O$, NaAsc, *i*-PrOH/THF/H_2O, r.t., 24 h, mol. ratio **6**/**10a**/$CuSO_4{\cdot}5H_2O$/NaAsc, 1:1:0.5:1.1; **7**/**10a**/$CuSO_4{\cdot}5H_2O$/NaAsc, 1:2:1.1:0.6; (**ii**) propargyl alcohol, $CuSO_4{\cdot}5H_2O$, NaAsc, *i*-PrOH/THF/H_2O (1.6:1:1.1, *v/v/v*), r.t., 24 h, mol ratio **7**/C_3H_4O /$CuSO_4{\cdot}5H_2O$/NaAsc, 1:3:1.2:2.2.

The general procedure of glycoconjugation of betulin derivatives involves mixing of 28-*O*-propargylbetulin **2** or 3,28-*O,O′*-di(propargyl)betulin **3** with the appropriate monosugar derivative (D-glucose or D-galactose) in the water-alcohol solvent system (*i*-PrOH/H_2O). In the case of 28-*O*-azidoacetylbetulin **6** and 3,28-*O,O′*-di(azidoacetyl)betulin **7**, due to the too low solubility of the substrates in the *i*-PrOH/H_2O solvent system, it was necessary to use an additional solvent (THF). In each case, the reaction was carried out under an argon atmosphere at room temperature for 24 h, using $CuSO_4{\cdot}5H_2O$ as a catalyst and sodium ascorbate (NaAsc) as an agent reducing Cu(II) to Cu(I).

As a result of the described reactions, five new monosubstituted betulin derivatives (**15a**, **15b**, **16a**, **16b**, and **19a**) modified at position C28, as well as four new disubstituted betulin derivatives (**17a**, **17b**, **18b**, and **20a**), modified at positions C3 and C28 were isolated by column chromatography in very good yields (97–99% and 82–99%, respectively, Table 2).

Table 2. Summary synthesis of betulin glycoconjugates **15–24**.

Entry	Substrate				Product		
	Analog BN	No.	Sugar	R^1, R^2, R^3	No.	Linker	Yield, %
STRATEGY I							
1	2	12a	Glc	OAc	15a	28-OCH2Triaz	99
2	2	12b	Gal	OAc	15b	28-OCH2Triaz	97
3	2	14a	Glc	OAc	16a	28-OCH2TriazCH2(CO)NH	98
4	2	14b	Gal	OAc	16b	28-OCH2TriazCH2(CO)NH	97
5	3	12a	Glc	OAc	17a	3,28-di-OCH2Triaz	99
6	3	12b	Gal	OAc	17b	3,28-di-OCH2Triaz	99
7	3	14b	Gal	OAc	18b	3,28-di-OCH2TriazCH2(CO)NH	82
STRATEGY II							
8	6	10a	Glc	OAc	19a	28-O(CO)CH2TriazCH2O	97
9	7	10a	Glc	OAc	20a	3,28-di-O(CO)CH2TriazCH2O	87
10	7	–	–	–	21	3,28-di-O(CO)CH2TriazOH	77
DEPROTECTION							
11	15a	–	Glc	OH	22a	28-OCH2Triaz	87
12	15b	–	Gal	OH	22b	28-OCH2Triaz	99
13	16b	–	Gal	OH	23b	28-OCH2TriazCH2(CO)NH	96
14	17a	–	Glc	OH	24a	3,28-di-OCH2Triaz	87
15	17b	–	Gal	OH	24b	3,28-di-OCH2Triaz	69

It has been considered that the use of an acyl protected sugar moiety may not be sufficient to achieve the desired hydrophilicity of the novel BN analogs. In order to compare the properties of glycoconjugates and assess the effect of acyl group presence, for the five per-*O*-acetylated glycoconjugates BN (**15a, 15b, 16a, 16b, 17b**), the deprotection of the sugar unit was performed by applying a standard Zemplén procedure [52], under mild conditions using 1 M methanolic solution of sodium methoxide in methanol. The reaction was carried out at room temperature for 120 min. The final step was to neutralize the reaction mixture with the use of *Amberlyst-15* ion exchange resin, after which the mixture was filtered to give betulin glycoconjugates (**22a, 22b, 23b, 24a**) in high yield (87-99%), except compound **24b** (69%), as shown in Table 2.

Our proposed concept of adding a linker to the scaffold of betulin is based on introducing a chloroacetyl moiety into its structure and then converting the obtained analogs into azidoacetyl derivatives. In the case of the analog **21**, in the final stage, the azide moiety was coupled with propargyl alcohol using the click chemistry reaction. As a result, a 3,28-disubstituted betulin **21** modified with a linker containing a 1,2,3-triazole ring substituted in the C4 position with a hydroxymethyl group was obtained in a yield of 77% (Scheme 8). The motivation to obtain a 3,28-*O,O′*-di(2-(4-(hydroxymethyl-*1H*-1,2,3-triazol-1-yl)acetyl)betulin **21** was the desire to check whether the addition of a sugar unit is necessary to improve the biological properties of BN or whether the introduction of the linker containing the 1,2,3-triazole ring alone would be sufficient. The structures of all synthesized compounds were confirmed by nuclear magnetic resonance (^{1}H-, ^{13}C-NMR, gHSQC), infrared spectroscopy (FT-IR), and high-resolution mass spectrometry (HRMS).

2.4. Cytotoxicity Studies

The obtained betulin glycoconjugates were screened to determine their cytotoxicity. The research was conducted on two cell lines: HCT 116 (colorectal carcinoma cell line) and MCF-7 (human breast adenocarcinoma cell line). In these lines, overexpression of the glucose and galactose transporters was observed [53–55]. The aim of the research was to initially estimate the influence of the modifications of the parent betulin backbone by adding a sugar unit/units, as well as to examine the influence of the structure of linker connecting betulin with sugar on the cytotoxicity of the tested compounds.

In the first stage, betulin glycoconjugates in which the hydroxyl groups of the sugar unit were protected with acetyl groups were selected for research. The choice of the type of hydroxyl group protection was dictated by the sensitivity of acetyl groups to the action of hydrolytic enzymes and the fact that these groups provide glycoconjugates with increased hydrophobicity, which should facilitate passive transport into the cell. The proliferation of tumor cells (HCT 116, MCF-7) treated with tested compounds (**15a**, **15b**, **16a**, **17a**, **17b**, **19a**) at 50- and 25-μM concentrations were determined after 24 and 48 h of incubation with the Cell Counting Kit-8 (CCK-8) based on the water-soluble tetrazole salt of WST-8. The CCK-8 kit, selected for the determination of viability and cytotoxicity, is less toxic and has higher sensitivity than other tetrazole salt-based tests, such as MTT or MTS [56]. The effect of these compounds was compared with the effect of betulin **1** doses, as shown in Figure 4.

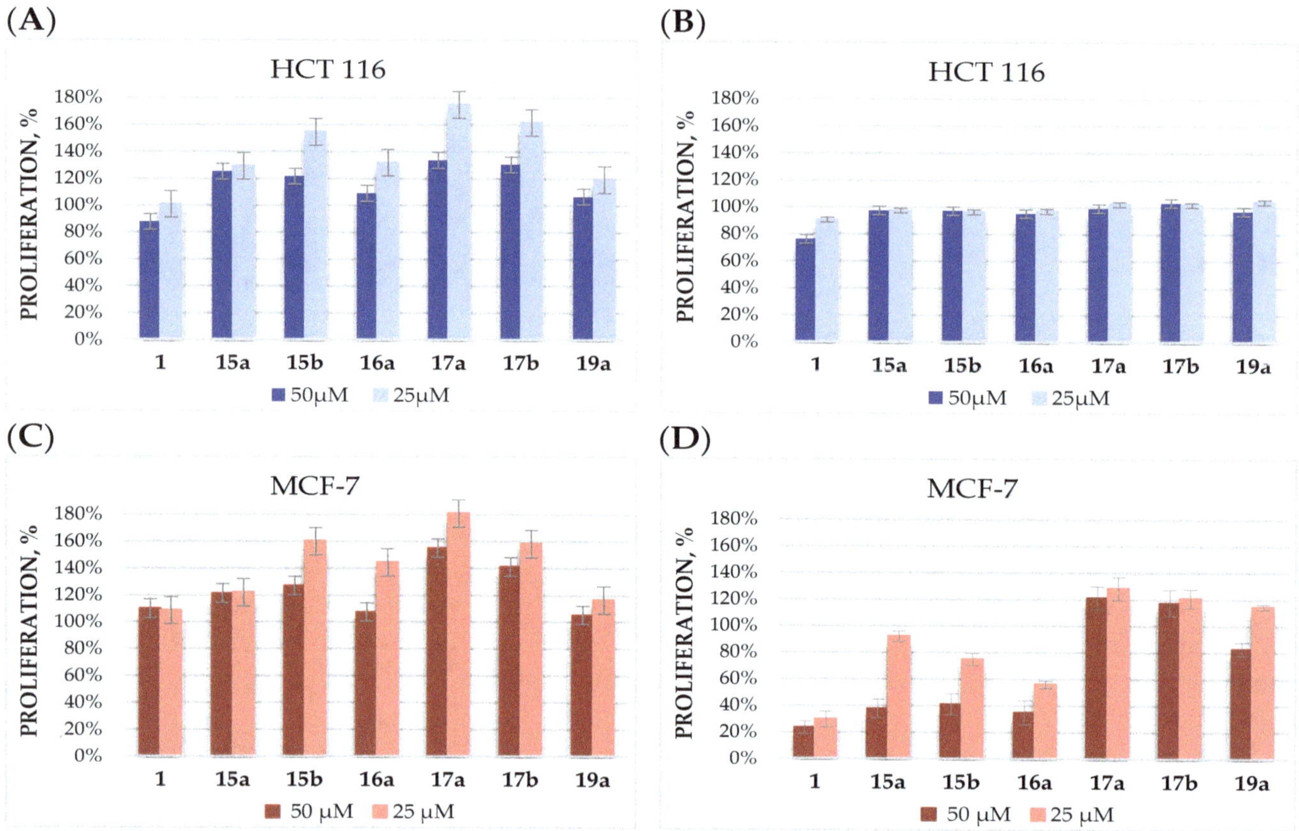

Figure 4. The dependence of HCT 116 and MCF-7 cell proliferation on the concentration of the betulin glycoconjugates, after 24 (**A,C**) or 48 h (**B,D**) of incubation.

Unfortunately, in the case of the HCT 116 cell line, it was found that the designed betulin glycoconjugates, both at 24 and 48 h, did not inhibit the proliferation of tumor cells. Additionally, it was observed that in some cases, the tested compounds even stimulate tumor cells to grow faster. It is especially visible after 24 h for analogs **15b**, **17a**, and **17b** (Figure 4A). Our hypothesis explaining this fact is based on the assumption that these derivatives are able to enter cancer cells, where they are degraded by hydrolytic enzymes with the release of sugar molecules, which is an additional source of energy allowing the proliferation growth. In the case of the MCF-7 cell line, after 24 h of incubation with the tested glycoconjugates, a similar effect was observed as for the HCT 116 cell line. However, after 48 h, a concentration-dependent cytotoxic effect of the glycoconjugates **15a**, **15b**, and **16a** was observed (Figure 4D). These glycoconjugates, given to cells at the 50-μM concentration, showed cytotoxicity comparable to that of betulin. In glycoconjugates **15a**, **15b**, and **16a**, the betulin skeleton was modified at position C28 by adding a sugar unit via an *O*-methylene-1,2,3-triazole linker or the same linker extended with an *N*-methyleneamide group. Presumably, the protection of the sugar hydroxyl groups improved the passive transport of the glycoconjugates inside the cell, where they released betulin under the action of hydrolytic enzymes. In the case of the disubstituted analogs BN **17a** and **17b**, modified at both the C3 and C28 positions, such a beneficial effect was not observed, which may be related to the prolonged effect of the release of as many as two glucose molecules (per each unit of betulin), which are the source of energy for increased proliferation. Quite unexpectedly, for the monosubstituted glycoconjugate **19a**, no significant cytotoxic activity was observed on tumor cells. Perhaps, the ester bond connecting the betulin backbone with the sugar unit is too labile and some part of the compound undergoes hydrolysis even before it penetrates the cell.

In order to check whether the introduction of the sugar unit increases the affinity of the obtained molecules for GLUT transporters, the acetyl protections in the sugar fragment of the obtained glycoconjugates were removed, and then cytotoxicity tests of the obtained compounds were carried out on the same cell lines (HCT 116, MCF-7). The cytotoxicity of the disubstituted BN derivative **21**, in which a linker contains only the 1,2,3-triazole system, without a sugar unit, was also tested. This study was designed to check the influence of the presence of the 1,2,3-triazole ring on the activity of the betulin derivative.

When the research was carried out on the HCT 116 cell line, both after 24 h and after 48 h, no significant effect of inhibition of tumor cell proliferation by the tested glycoconjugates was observed (**22a**, **22b**, **23b**, **24a**, **24b**). Interestingly, derivative **21** after 48 h shows slightly higher cytotoxicity compared to the activity of the parent BN backbone (Figure 5B). In the case of the MCF-7 cell line, after 24 h of incubation, the effect caused by the glycoconjugates (**22a**, **22b**, **23b**, **24a**) is only slightly better than that observed with BN. However, already after 48 h of incubation, the significantly higher cytotoxic activity of BN was observed compared to glycoconjugates. Surprisingly, as was in the case with the HCT 116 cell line, BN derivative **21** without a sugar unit, but only with an attached linker with the 1,2,3-triazole system, proved to be the most active. After 48 h of incubation, only 20% cell proliferation for this compound was observed as shown in Figure 5D.

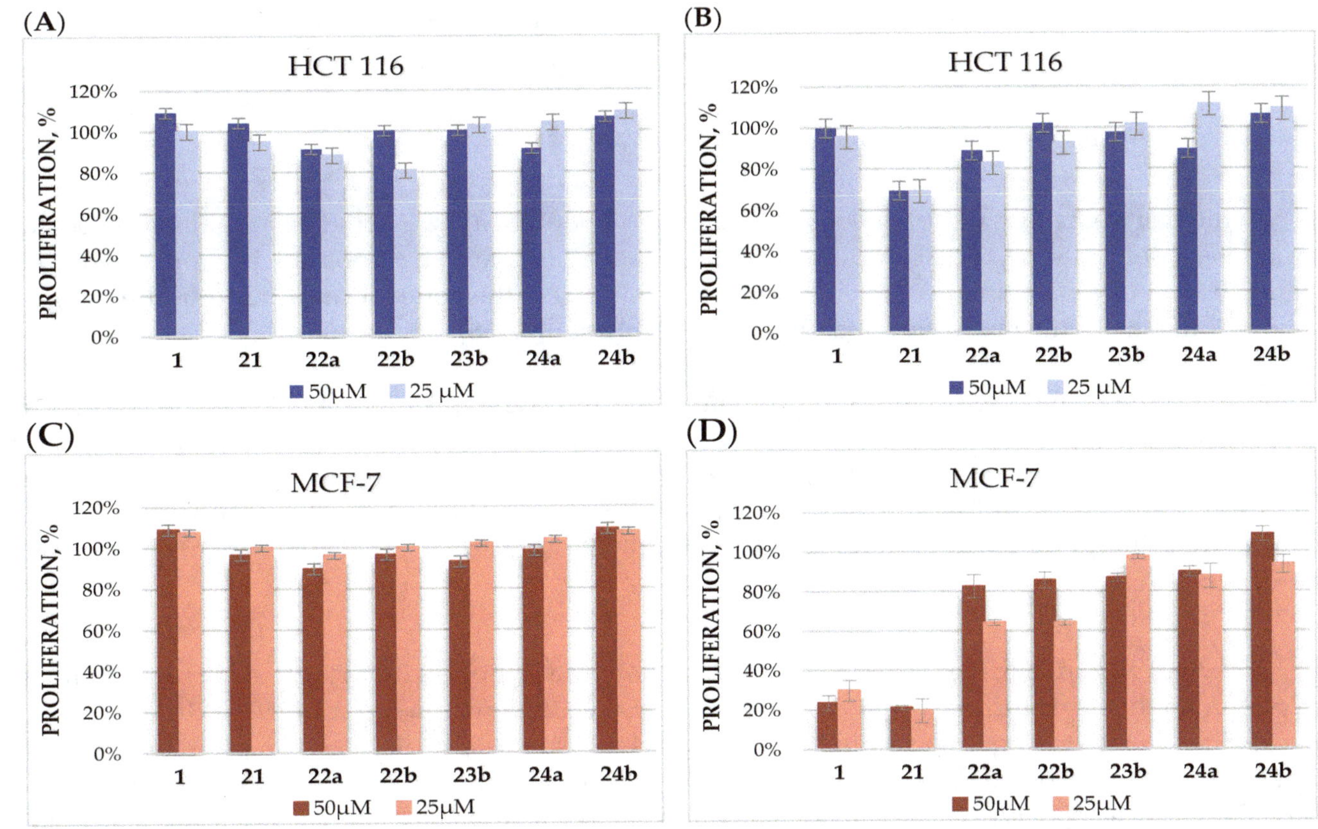

Figure 5. The dependence of HCT 116 and MCF-7 cell proliferation on the concentration of the betulin glycoconjugates, after 24 (**A**,**C**) or 48 h (**B**,**D**) of incubation.

In the course of further studies, for betulin **1** and its derivatives **15a**, **15b**, **16a,** and **21**, the ability to inhibit the proliferation of MCF-7 cells in a wider spectrum of concentrations was carried out in order to determine their IC_{50} value. The same compounds were also tested against NHDF cell line (normal human dermal fibroblast-neonatal cells), to assess the safety of their uses. Assays were performed in the concentration range of 50–6.25 μM for both tested cell lines. Unfortunately, it turned out that glycoconjugates **15a**, **15b**, and **16a** are equally cytotoxic in relation to healthy cells and to the tested tumor lines (Table 3). Additionally, the most active of betulin derivative **21**, even at the lowest tested dose, is extremely cytotoxic and allows the proliferation of both cell lines to be kept at only 20%. The cytotoxicity of compound **21** significantly exceeds that of betulin, which may suggest that further modification of this compound is necessary to improve its selectivity.

Table 3. Summary of cytotoxicity of BN and the betulin glycoconjugates.

Compound	Activity IC_{50} [μM] [a,b]	
	MCF-7	NHDF
1	12.40 ± 0.14	11.60 ± 0.22
15a	65.28 ± 0.68	60.62 ± 0. 64
15b	47.70 ± 0.72	47.61 ± 0.86
16a	29.77 ± 0.52	29.82 ± 0.45

[a] Cytotoxicity was evaluated using the CCK-8 assay; [b] Incubation time 48 h.

2.5. Cytotoxic Activity Predicted Lipophilicity

In medicinal chemistry, the aqueous solubility and lipophilicity of a drug are important molecular parameters determining the absorption and the bioavailability. The lipophilicity is indicated by the logarithm of a partition coefficient (logP), which reflects the concentration ratio of the drug at equilibrium partitioning between octanol and water phases [57,58].

Betulin **1**, which is the subject of our research, is characterized by a highly limited solubility in polar solvents. This property may result from the complex structure, the presence of five fused aliphatic rings, and the isopropenyl moiety. The only polar fragments of the molecule are the two hydroxyl groups at C3 and C28. In this study, in order to determine the effect of various substituents on the value of the logP coefficient for several betulin derivatives, we used the prediction base *MolInspirations* to evaluate in silico the parameter (Table 4).

As we expected, adding a sugar moiety decreases the lipophilicity (<logP) of betulin analogs. Moreover, in the case of triazole derivatives of betulin modified with a sugar unit, the difference was revealed when the structures containing a per-*O*-acetylated sugar unit **15–20** and an unprotected sugar unit **22–24** were compared. The linker type is also crucial. For compounds bearing a substituent of the OCH_2TriazGlc/Gal type at C3 and C28 position, the logP values are higher than for compounds bearing substituents with an ester moiety in the same position. On the other hand, the lowest values of the coefficient have derivatives in which an amide group is present in the linker structure. Only betulin glycoconjugates **23** and **24** have logP values smaller than 5 (Figure 6).

Table 4. LogP of BN and betulin analogs **2–24**.

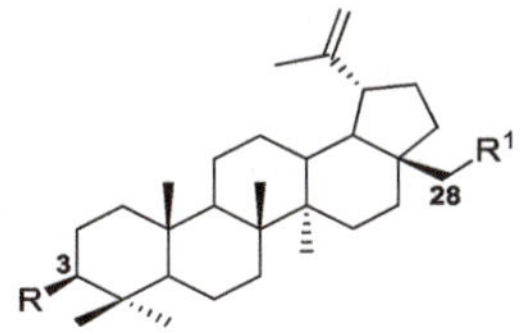

No.	R (C3)	R[1] (C28)	logP
1	OH	OH	7.16
2	OH	OCH2C≡CH	7.94
3	OCH2C≡CH	OCH2C≡CH	8.54
4	OH	O(CO)CH2Cl	8.23
5	O(CO)CH2Cl	O(CO)CH2Cl	8.86
6	OH	O(CO)CH2N3	8.31
7	O(CO)CH2N3	O(CO)CH2N3	8.94
15a	OH	OCH2TriazGlc(OAc)	7.59
16a	OH	OCH2TriazCH2(CO)NHGlc(OAc)	6.69
17a	OCH2TriazGlc(OAc)	OCH2TriazGlc(OAc)	8.01
18b	OCH2TriazCH2(CO)NHGal(OAc)	OCH2TriazCH2(CO)NHGal(OAc)	6.22
19a	OH	O(CO)CH2TriazCH2OGlc(OAc)	7.45
20a	O(CO)CH2TriazCH2OGlc(OAc)	O(CO)CH2TriazCH2OGlc(OAc)	7.74
21	O(CO)CH2TriazOH	O(CO)CH2TriazOH	6.38
22a	OH	OCH2TriazGlc(OH)	5.21
23b	OH	OCH2TriazCH2(CO)NHGal(OH)	4.31
24a	OCH2TriazGlc(OH)	OCH2TriazGlc(OH)	3.25

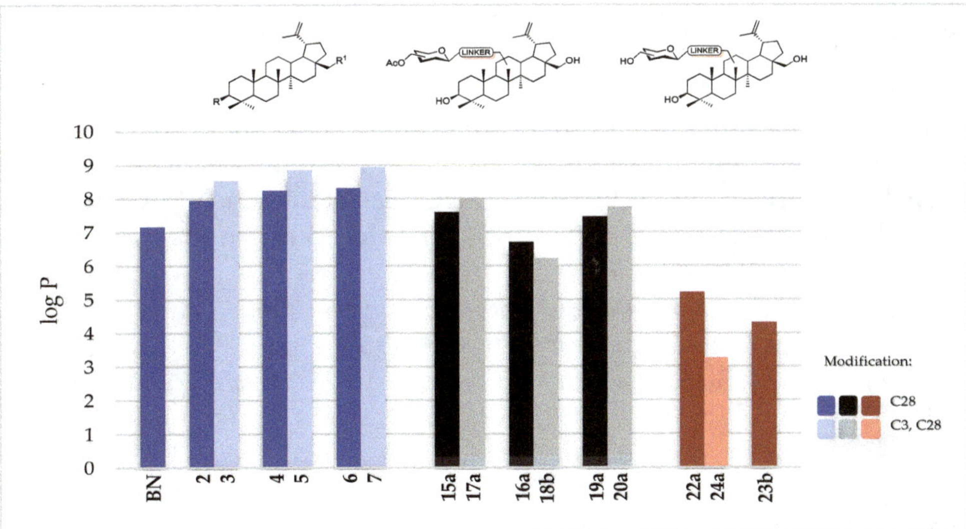

Figure 6. LogP of BN and betulin analogs **2–24**.

3. Materials and Methods

3.1. General Information

NMR spectra were recorded on a Varian spectrometer at operating frequencies of 600 or 400 and 150 or 100 MHz, respectively, using TMS as the resonance shift standard and NMR solvents ($CDCl_3$, CD_3OD or DMSO-d_6), which was purchased from ACROS Organics (Geel, Belgium). All chemical shifts (δ) are reported in ppm and coupling constants (*J*) in Hz. The following abbreviations were used to explain the observed multiplicities: s: singlet, d: doublet, dd: doublet of doublets, ddd: doublet of doublet of doublets, t: triplet, dd~t: doublet of doublets resembling a triplet (with similar values of coupling constants), m: multiplet, br: broad. IR-spectra were measured on an FTIR spectrophotometer

(ATR method). High-resolution mass spectrometry (HRMS) analyses were performed on a Waters LCT Premier XE system using the electrospray-ionization (ESI) technique. Optical rotations were measured with a JASCO P-2000 polarimeter using a sodium lamp (589.3 nm) at room temperature. Melting points were determined using a Boethius M HMK hot-stage apparatus. Reactions were monitored by TLC on precoated plates of silica gel 60 F254 (Merck Millipore). TLC plates were inspected under UV light (λ = 254 nm) or charring after spraying with 10% solution of sulfuric acid in ethanol. Crude products were purified using column chromatography performed on Silica Gel 60 (70–230 mesh, Fluka).

Cell viability was measured using a Cell Counting Kit-8 (Bimake) according to the manufacturer's protocol. The absorbance on the CKK-8 assay was measured spectrophotometrically at the 450-nm wavelength using a plate reader (Epoch, BioTek, USA).

28-*O*-Chloroacetylbetulin **4** and 3,28-*O,O'*-di(2-chloroacetyl)betulin **5** [48], 1,2,3,4,6-penta-*O*-acetyl-β-D-glucopyranose **9a**, 1,2,3,4,6-penta-*O*-acetyl-β-D-galactopyranose **9b** [53], propargyl 2,3,4,6-tetra-*O*-acetyl-β-D-glucopyranoside **10a** [55], 2,3,4,6-tetra-*O*-acetyl-α-D-glucopyranosyl bromide **11a**, 2,3,4,6-tetra-*O*-acetyl-α-D-galactopyranosyl bromide **11b** [54], 2,3,4,6-tetra-*O*-acetyl-β-D-glucopyranosyl azide **12a**, 2,3,4,6-tetra-*O*-acetyl-β-D-galactopyranosyl azide **12b** [36], 2,3,4,6-tetra-*O*-acetyl-*N*-(β-D-glucopyranosyl)chloroacetamide **13a**, 2,3,4,6-tetra-*O*-acetyl-*N*-(β-D-galacto-pyranosyl)chloroacetamide **13b**, 2,3,4,6-tetra-*O*-acetyl-*N*-(β-D-glucopyranosyl)azidoacetamide **14a**, and 2,3,4,6-tetra-*O*-acetyl-*N*-(β-D-galactopyranosyl)azidoacetamide **14b** [37] were prepared according to the respective published procedures. All used chemicals were purchased from Sigma-Aldrich, Fluka, Avantor, and ACROS Organics and were used without purification.

3.2. Chemistry

3.2.1. Procedure for the Synthesis of Betulin Analogs

Procedure for the Synthesis of 28-*O*-propargylbetulin **2** and 3,28-*O,O'*-di(propargyl)betulin **3**

Betulin **1** (0.226 mmol, 100.0 mg) and sodium hydride (NaH, 0.904 mmol, 21.7 mg) were dissolved in dry THF (1.3 mL) followed by addition of propargyl bromide (0.723 mmol, 0.062 mL). The heterogenous reaction mixture was left on the magnetic stirrer for 24 h at room temperature. The reaction progress was monitored on TLC in an eluents system DCM:AcOEt (10:1). Then, NH_4Cl (0.411 mmol, 22.0 mg, 5 mL H_2O) was added, extracted with Et_2O (5 × 4 mL), brine (5 mL) added, and dried over $MgSO_4$. After, this was followed by filtration and evaporation in vacuo. The crude products were purified using column chromatography (DCM:AcOEt, gradient: 50:1 to 10:1).

28-O-Propargylbetulin **2** was obtained as a white solid (58.8 mg, 54% yield); m.p.: 81—85 °C; $[\alpha]^{25}_D$ = +11.3 (c 0.5, $CHCl_3$); HRMS (ESI^+): calcd for $C_{33}H_{53}O_2$ ($[M + H]^+$): *m/z* 481.4046; found: *m/z* 481.4050; ^1H NMR (400 MHz, $CDCl_3$): δ_H 4.68 (s, br, 1H, H-29a), 4.58 (s, br, 1H, H-29b), 4.18 (dd, 1H, J_1 2.4 Hz, J_2 16.0 Hz, $OCH_aC\equiv$), 4.11 (dd, 1H, J_1 2.4 Hz, J_2 16.0 Hz, $OCH_bC\equiv$), 3.70 (d, 1H, *J* 9.2 Hz, H-28a), 3.21-3.15 (m, 2H, H-28b, H-3), 2.45-2.38 (m, 1H, H-19), 2.42 (dd~t, 1H, *J* 2.4 Hz, ≡CH), 2.1-0.60 (m, 25H, CH, CH_2), 1.68 (s, 3H, H-30), 1.05, 0.97 br, 0.83, 0.76 (all s, 3H each, H-23—H-27) ppm; ^{13}C NMR (150 MHz, $CDCl_3$) δ_C 150.64, 109.56, 80.51, 78.97, 74.01, 68.27, 58.61, 55.28, 50.42, 48.91, 47.99, 42.66, 40.98, 38.86, 38.69, 37.17, 34.69, 34.22, 29.90, 29.79, 27.99, 27.39, 27.14, 25.22, 20.87, 19.09, 18.29, 16.11, 15.98, 15.37, 14.83 ppm (Supplementary Materials, Table S1); IR (ATR) ν: 3350-3200, 2940, 2871, 1640, 1457, 1092, 882 cm^{-1}.

3,28-O,O'-Di(propargyl)betulin **3** was obtained as a yellow resin (36.5 mg, 31% yield); m.p.: resin; $[\alpha]^{25}_D$ = +31.9 (c 0.5, $CHCl_3$); HRMS (ESI^+): calcd for $C_{36}H_{55}O_2$ ($[M + H]^+$): *m/z* 519.4202; found: *m/z* 519.4202; ^1H NMR (600 MHz, $CDCl_3$): δ_H 4.68 (d, 1H, *J* 2.4 Hz, H-29a), 4.58 (dd, 1H, J_1 1.8 Hz, J_2 2.4 Hz, H-29b), 4.21-4.12 (m, 4H, 2x $CH_2C\equiv$), 3.70 (dd, 1H, J_1 1.2 Hz, J_2 8.4 Hz, H-28a), 3.16 (d, 1H, *J* 9.0 Hz, H-28b), 3.00 (dd, 1H, J_1 4.2 Hz, J_2 11.4 Hz, H-3), 2.44-2.39 (m, 1H, H-19), 2.41 i 2.36 (all dd~t, 1H each, *J* 2.4 Hz, ≡CH), 2.10-0.60 (m, 24H, CH, CH_2), 1.68 (s, 3H, H-30), 1.04, 0.98, 0.97, 0.83, 0.76 (all s, 3H each, H-23—H-27) ppm; ^{13}C NMR (150 MHz, $CDCl_3$) δ_C 150.64, 109.56, 85.86, 80.96, 80.50, 74.01, 73.41, 68.25, 58.62, 56.42, 55.87, 50.41, 48.92, 48.00, 47.02, 42.65, 41.03, 38.55, 37.12, 34.69, 34.24, 29.91, 29.71, 27.99,

27.12, 25.24, 20.91, 18.25, 19.11, 16.10, 16.00, 15.99, 14.79 ppm (Supplementary Materials, Table S1); IR (ATR) ν: 3314, 3261, 2952, 1610, 1453, 1377, 1085, 1068, 881 cm^{-1}.

Procedure for the Synthesis of 28-*O*-(2-azidoacetyl)betulin **6**

28-*O*-(2-Chloroacetyl)betulin **4** (0.193 mmol, 100.0 mg) was dissolved in DMF (1.93 mL) and sodium azide (0.963 mmol, 62.6 mg) was added. The heterogenous reaction mixture was stirred at 90 °C for 3 h. Then, H_2O (1 mL) and saturated $NaHCO_3$ solution (4 mL) was added. It was extracted with DCM (5 × 4 mL) and dried over $MgSO_4$. After that, this was followed by filtration and evaporation in vacuo. The crude product was purified using column chromatography (DCM:MeOH, gradient: 100:1 to 10:1).

28-O-(2-Azidoacetyl)betulin **6** was obtained as a white solid (65.0 mg, 64% yield); ^1H NMR (600 MHz, $CDCl_3$): δ_H 4.70 (d, 1H, *J* 1.8 Hz, H-29a), 4.60 (d, 1H, *J* 1.2 Hz, H-29b), 4.41 (dd, 1H, J_1 1.2 Hz, J_2 10.8 Hz, H-28a), 3.99 (d, 1H, *J* 11.4 Hz, H-28b), 3.89 (s, 2H, CH_2N_3), 3.18 (dd, 1H, J_1 4.8 Hz, J_2 11.4 Hz, H-3), 2.44 (td, 1H, J_1 5.8 Hz, J_2 10.9 Hz, H-19), 2.10–0.60 (m, 25H, CH, CH_2), 1.68 (s, 3H, H-30), 1.04, 0.98, 0.97, 0.83, 0.76 (all s, 3H each, H-23–H-27) ppm; ^{13}C NMR (150 MHz, $CDCl_3$) δ_C 168.65, 149.76, 109.92, 78.84, 64.31, 55.21, 50.41, 50.26, 48.72, 47.57, 46.33, 42.62, 40.79, 38.77, 38.62, 37.06, 34.39, 34.09, 29.59, 27.89, 27.30, 26.92, 25.09, 20.67, 19.04, 18.19, 16.00, 15.94, 15.27, 14.69 ppm (Supplementary Materials, Table S1).

Procedure for the Synthesis of 3,28-*O*,*O'*-di(2-azidoacetyl)betulin **7**

3,28-*O*,*O'*-Di(2-chloroacetyl)betulin **5** (0.168 mmol, 100.0 mg) was dissolved in 0.71 mL DMF and sodium azide (0.897 mmol, 58.3 mg) was added. The heterogenous reaction mixture was stirred at 90 °C for 3 h. Then, H_2O and saturated $NaHCO_3$ solution (4 mL) was added. It was extracted with DCM (4 × 4 mL) and dried over $MgSO_4$. After that, this was followed by filtration and evaporation in vacuo. The crude product was purified using column chromatography (DCM:MeOH, gradient: 100:1 to 10:1).

3,28-O,O'-Di(2-azidoacetyl)betulin **7** was obtained as a white solid (73.6 mg, 72% yield); ^1H NMR (600 MHz, $CDCl_3$): δ_H 4.70 (d, 1H, *J* 1.2 Hz, H-29a), 4.61–4.58 (m, 2H, H-29b, H-3), 4.42 (d, 1H, *J* 11.4 Hz, H-28a), 3.98 (d, 1H, *J* 10.8 Hz, H-28b), 3.89 and 3.85 (all s, 2H each, 2x CH_2N_3), 2.44 (td, 1H, J_1 5.7 Hz, J_2 10.8 Hz, H-19), 2.10–0.60 (m, 24H, CH, CH_2), 1.69 (s, 3H, H-30), 1.04, 0.98, 0.87, 0.866, 0.862 (all s, 3H each, H-23–H-27) ppm; ^{13}C NMR (150 MHz, $CDCl_3$) δ_C 168.75, 168.15, 149.84, 110.07, 83.21, 64.40, 55.36, 50.67, 50.52, 50.25, 48.80, 47.69, 46.43, 42.67, 40.91, 38.34, 37.89, 37.06, 34.49, 34.08, 29.67, 27.94, 27.00, 25.06, 23.68, 20.74, 19.05, 18.15, 16.54, 16.15, 16.04, 14.75 ppm (Supplementary Materials, Table S1); IR (ATR) ν: 2942, 2867, 1728, 1243, 1181, 1017, 979, 754 cm^{-1}.

3.2.2. General Procedure for the Synthesis of Betulin Glycoconjugates **15–16** according to Strategy I (Modification C28)

To a well-stirred 28-*O*-propargylbetulin **2** (0.208 mmol, 100.0 mg) and 2,3,4,6-tetra-*O*-acetyl-β-D-galactopyranosyl or 2,3,4,6-tetra-*O*-acetyl-β-D-glucopyranosyl azide **12a–b** (0.208 mmol, 77.7 mg) or **14a–b** (0.208 mmol, 89.5 mg) in *i*-PrOH (2 mL) were added $CuSO_4{\cdot}5H_2O$ (0.125 mmol, 31.2 mg) dissolved in H_2O (1 mL) and sodium ascorbate (0.229 mmol, 45.3 mg) dissolved in H_2O (1 mL) succesively. The reaction mixture was stirred under argon atmosphere for 24 h at room temperature. After completion of the reaction (was monitored by TLC), the reaction mixture was extracted with DCM (**15a–b**: 5 × 5 mL) or AcOEt (**16a–b**: 5 × 5 mL), then the mixture was dried over $MgSO_4$ and was concentrated in vacuo. The crude residue was separated/purified using column chromatography (**15a–b**: DCM:AcOEt, gradient: 20:1 to 1:1; **16a–b**: DCM:MeOH, gradient: 50:1 to 10:1).

Product **15a** *(28-OCH₂TriazGlcBN)* was obtained as a white solid (175.1 mg, 99% yield); m.p.: 108–109 °C; $[\alpha]^{25}{}_D = -21.8$ (c 0.5, $CHCl_3$); HRMS (ESI^+): calcd for $C_{47}H_{72}N_3O_{11}$ ($[M + H]^+$): *m/z* 854.5167; found: *m/z* 854.5165; ^1H NMR (600 MHz, $CDCl_3$): δ_H 7.75 (s, br, 1H, H-$5_{triaz.}$), 5.89 (d, 1H, *J*

9.0 Hz, H-1_{Glc}), 5.46 (dd~t, 1H, J_1 9.1 Hz, J_2 9.5 Hz, H-3_{Glc}), 5.42 (dd~t, 1H, J_1 9.0 Hz, J_2 9.5 Hz, H-2_{Glc}), 5.25 (dd~t, 1H, J_1 9.1 Hz, J_2 10.2 Hz, H-4_{Glc}), 4.67 (d, 1H, J 13.2 Hz, OCH_a), 4.66 (s, br, 1H, H-29a), 4.60 (d, 1H, J 12.6 Hz, OCH_b), 4.55 (dd, 1H, J_1 1.2 Hz, J_2 2.4 Hz, H-29b), 4.30 (dd, 1H, J_1 5.0 Hz, J_2 12.6 Hz, H-$6a_{Glc}$), 4.14 (dd, 1H, J_1 2.1 Hz, J_2 12.6 Hz, H-$6b_{Glc}$), 4.00 (ddd, 1H, J_1 2.1 Hz, J_2 5.0 Hz, J_3 10.2 Hz, H-5_{Glc}), 3.63 (d, 1H, J 8.4 Hz, H-28a), 3.19–3.17 (m, 2H, H-28a, H-3), 2.38 (td, 1H, J_1 5.8 Hz, J_2 11.1 Hz, H-19), 2.10–0.60 (m, 25H, CH, CH_2), 2.08, 2.07, 2.03, 1.88 (all s, 3H each, 4x CH_3CO), 1.66 (s, 3H, H-30), 1.02, 0.97, 0.96, 0.83, 0.76 (all s, 3H each, H-23–H-27) ppm; ^{13}C NMR (150 MHz, $CDCl_3$) δ_C 170.45, 169.90, 169.32, 168.87, 150.57, 146.62, 120.58, 109.60, 85.73, 78.95, 75.12, 72.73, 70.32, 68.94, 67.72, 64.95, 61.58, 55.31, 50.42, 48.85, 47.88, 47.26, 42.68, 40.92, 38.88, 38.73, 37.51, 37.17, 34.77, 34.26, 29.91, 29.85, 28.00, 27.42, 25.22, 20.85, 20.66, 20.53, 20.51, 20.20, 19.06, 18.32, 16.11, 16.03, 15.37, 14.79 ppm (Supplementary Materials, Table S2); IR (ATR) ν: 3400–3500, 2941, 1751, 1650, 1455, 1367, 1216, 1038, 731 cm^{-1}.

Product **15b** *(28-OCH_2TriazGalBN)* was obtained as a white solid (201.7 mg, 97% yield); m.p.: 117–118 °C; $[\alpha]^{25}_D = -9.4$ (c 0.5, $CHCl_3$); HRMS (ESI$^+$): calcd for $C_{47}H_{71}N_3O_{11}Na$ ([M + Na]$^+$): *m/z* 876.4986; found: *m/z* 876.4989; ^1H NMR (600 MHz, $CDCl_3$): δ_H 7.80 (s, br, 1H, H-$5_{triaz.}$), 5.84 (d, 1H, J 9.3 Hz, H-1_{Gal}), 5.58 (dd, 1H, J_1 9.3 Hz, J_2 10.2 Hz, H-2_{Gal}), 5.55 (dd, 1H, J_1 0.8 Hz, J_2 3.4 Hz, H-4_{Gal}), 5.25 (dd, 1H, J_1 3.4 Hz, J_2 10.2 Hz, H-3_{Gal}), 4.69–4.57 (m, 4H, OCH_2, H-29a, H-29b), 4.24–4.18 (m, 2H, H-$6a_{Gal}$, H-5_{Gal}), 4.13 (d, 1H, J_1 6.3 Hz, J_2 10.9 Hz, H-$6b_{Gal}$), 3.63 (d, 1H, J 8.2 Hz, H-28a), 3.21–3.17 (m, 2H, H-28a, H-3), 2.40 (td, 1H, J_1 6.0 Hz, J_2 11.1 Hz, H-19), 2.30–0.60 (m, 25H, CH, CH_2), 2.22, 2.04, 2.01, 1.90 (all s, 3H each, 4x CH_3CO), 1.66 (s, 3H, H-30), 1.02, 0.97, 0.96, 0.83, 0.76 (all s, 3H each, H-23–H-27). ppm; ^{13}C NMR (150 MHz, $CDCl_3$) δ_C 170.28, 169.95, 169.80, 169.04, 150.61, 146.46, 120.76, 109.60, 86.27, 78.96, 74.02, 70.89, 68.94, 67.85, 66.87, 64.91, 61.15, 55.30, 50.41, 48.84, 47.87, 47.26, 42.69, 40.93, 38.88, 38.72, 37.50, 37.17, 34.79, 34.25, 29.95, 29.86, 28.00, 27.42, 27.23, 25.22, 20.84, 20.66, 20.62, 20.49, 20.30, 19.06, 18.33, 16.11, 16.00, 15.37, 14.80 ppm (Supplementary Materials, Table S2); IR (ATR) ν: 3600–3200, 2930, 2868, 1749, 1650, 1456, 1370, 1214, 1042, 731 cm^{-1}.

Product **16a** *(28-OCH_2TriazCH_2(CO)NHGlcBN)* was obtained as a white solid (190.0 mg, 99% yield); m.p.: 127-129 °C; $[\alpha]^{25}_D = +11.4$ (c 0.5, $CHCl_3$); HRMS (ESI$^+$): calcd for $C_{49}H_{74}N_4O_{12}Na$ ([M + Na]$^+$): *m/z* 933.5201; found: *m/z* 933.5202; ^1H NMR (600 MHz, $CDCl_3$): δ_H 7.66 (s, br, 1H, H-$5_{triaz.}$), 6.99 (d, 1H, J 8.8 Hz, NH), 5.29 (dd~t, 1H, J 9.5 Hz, H-1_{Glc}), 5.21 (dd, 1H, J_1 8.9 Hz, J_2 9.4 Hz, H-$3_{Glc}{}^{a}$), 5.12 (d, 1H, J 16.6 Hz, $OCH_a{}^{b}$), 5.05 (dd, 1H, J_1 9.4 Hz, J_2 10.1 Hz, H-$4_{Glc}{}^{a}$), 5.04 (d, 1H, J 16.5 Hz, $OCH_b{}^{b}$), 4.90 (dd~t, 1H, J 9.6 Hz, H-$2_{Glc}{}^{a}$), 4.67 (s, br, 3H, H-29a, CH_2CO^{b}), 4.57 (dd, 1H, J_1 1.4 Hz, J_2 2.1 Hz, H-29b), 4.28 (dd, 1H, J_1 4.4 Hz, J_2 12.5 Hz, H-$6a_{Glc}$), 4.09 (dd, 1H, J_1 2.2 Hz, J_2 12.5 Hz, H-$6b_{Glc}$), 3.81 (ddd, 1H, J_1 2.2 Hz, J_2 4.4 Hz, J_3 10.1 Hz, H-5_{Glc}), 3.63 (d, 1H, J 9.1 Hz, H-28a), 3.22-2.18 (m, 2H, H-28b, H-3), 2.39 (td, 1H, J_1 5.8 Hz, J_2 10.8 Hz, H-19), 2.15–0.60 (m, 25H, CH, CH_2), 2.08, 2.03, 2.02, 2.01 (all s, 3H each, 4x CH_3CO), 1.67 (s, 3H, H-30), 0.97, 0.96, 0.956, 0.82, 0.77 (all s, 3H each, H-23–H-27) ppm; ^{13}C NMR (150 MHz, $CDCl_3$) δ_C 170.86, 170.57, 169.84, 169.49, 165.68, 150.53, 146.71, 123.76, 109.64, 78.99, 78.41, 73.80, 72.51, 70.32, 68.95, 68.01, 65.14, 61.56, 55.28, 52.59, 50.38, 48.83, 47.88, 47.23, 42.64, 40.88, 38.86 38.70, 37.49, 37.15, 34.73, 34.23, 29.86, 29.69, 28.01, 27.40, 27.16, 25.18, 20.83, 20.73, 20.56, 20.54, 19.08, 18.33, 16.12, 15.93, 15.41, 14.79 ppm (Supplementary Materials, Table S2); IR (ATR) ν: 3200–3400, 2937, 1749, 1650, 1450, 1367, 1223, 1037, 993, 907, 882, 753 cm^{-1}. [a,b] Reverse signal assignment is possible.

Product **16b** *(28-OCH_2TriazCH_2(CO)NHGalBN)* was obtained as a white solid (184.0 mg, 97% yield); m.p.: 117-120 °C; $[\alpha]^{25}_D = +14.3$ (c 0.5, $CHCl_3$); HRMS (ESI$^+$): calcd for $C_{49}H_{74}N_4O_{12}Na$ ([M + Na]$^+$): *m/z* 933.5201; found: *m/z* 933.5202; ^1H NMR (600 MHz, $CDCl_3$): δ_H 7.66 (s, br, 1H, H-$5_{triaz.}$), 6.93 (d, 1H, J 8.9 Hz, NH), 5.43 (dd, 1H, J_1 0.9 Hz, J_2 3.3 Hz, H-4_{Gal}), 5.19 (dd, 1H, J_1 8.9 Hz, J_2 9.2 Hz, H-1_{Gal}), 5.12 and 4.99 (qAB, 2H, J 3.3 Hz, CH_2CO), 5.11 (dd, 1H, J_1 3.3 Hz, J_2 10.3 Hz, H-3_{Gal}), 5.06 (dd, 1H, J_1 9.2 Hz, J_2 10.3 Hz, H-2_{Gal}), 4.68 (s, 2H, OCH_2), 4.67 and 4.57 (s, br, 1H each, H-29a, H-29b), 4.11 (dd, 1H, J_1 6.9 Hz, J_2 11.3 Hz, H-$6a_{Gal}$), 4.07 (dd, 1H, J_1 6.2 Hz, J_2 11.23 Hz, H-$6b_{Gal}$), 4.02 (m, 1H, H-5_{Gal}), 3.63 (d, 1H, J 8.9 Hz, H-28a), 3.22–3.18 (m, 2H, H-28b, H-3), 2.39 (td, 1H, J_1 5.9 Hz, J_2 10.8 Hz, H-19), 2.30–0.60 (m, 25H, CH, CH_2), 2.15, 2.04, 2.03, 1.98 (all s, 3H each, 4x CH_3CO), 1.67 (s, 3H, H-30), 0.97, 0.96, 0.957, 0.82, 0.77 (all s, 3H each, H-23–H-27) ppm; ^{13}C NMR (150 MHz, $CDCl_3$) δ_C 171.00, 170.37,

169.98, 169.73, 165.67, 150.53, 146.60, 123.86, 109.63, 78.98, 78.61, 72.56, 70.71, 68.98, 68.06, 67.08, 65.13, 61.08, 55.29, 52.55, 50.39, 48.84, 47.89, 47.24, 42.65, 40.89, 38.87, 38.71, 37.50, 37.16, 34.74, 34.24, 29.88, 29.86, 28.01, 27.39, 27.17, 25.19, 20.84, 20.67, 20.64, 20.60, 20.50, 19.08, 18.33, 16.12, 15.94, 15.40, 14.79 ppm (Supplementary Materials, Table S2); IR (ATR) ν: 3100–2800, 1749, 1650, 1368, 1222, 1084, 1046, 752 cm^{-1}.

3.2.3. General Procedure for the Synthesis of Betulin Glycoconjugates **17–18** according to Strategy I (Modification C3 and C28)

To a well-stirred 3,28-*O,O′*-di(2-propargyl)betulin **3** (0.193 mmol, 100.0 mg) and per-*O*-acetylated glucopyranosyl or galactopyranosyl azides **12a–b** (0.385 mmol, 143.9 mg) or **14a–b** (0.385 mmol, 165.9 mg) in *i*-PrOH (6.6 mL), $CuSO_4{\cdot}5H_2O$ (0.231 mmol, 57.8 mg) dissolved in H_2O (3.3 mL) and sodium ascorbate (0.424 mmol, 84.0 mg) dissolved in H_2O (3.3 mL) were added successively. The reaction mixture was stirred under argon atmosphere for 24 h at room temperature. After completion of the reaction (was monitored by TLC), the reaction mixture was extracted with (**17a–b**: DCM 5 × 5 mL; **18b**: AcOEt 5 × 5 mL), then the mixture was dried over $MgSO_4$ and was concentrated in vacuo. The crude residue was separated/purified using column chromatography (**17a–b**: DCM:AcOEt, gradient: 15:1 to 1:1; **18b**: DCM:MeOH, gradient: 40:1 to 10:1).

*Product **17a** (3,28-di(OCH$_2$TriazGlc)BN)* was obtained as a white solid (242.0 mg, 99% yield); m.p.: 126–127 °C; $[\alpha]^{25}{}_D = -6.1$ (c 0.5, $CHCl_3$); HRMS (ESI^+): calcd for $C_{64}H_{93}N_6O_{20}$ ($[M + H]^+$): *m/z* 1265.6445; found: *m/z* 1265.6426; ^{1}H NMR (600 MHz, $CDCl_3$): δ_H 7.75 and 7.74 (all s, 1H each, 2x H-5$_{triaz.}$), 5.90 and 5.89 (all d, 1H each, J_1 9.0 Hz and J_2 9.4 Hz, 2x H-1$_{Glc}$), 5.50-5.40 (m, 4H, 2x H-2$_{Glc}$, 2x H-3$_{Glc}$)), 5.24 and 5.25 19 (all dd, 1H each, J_1 9.4 Hz, J_2 10.1 Hz and J_1 9.2 Hz, J_2 10.1 Hz, 2x H-4$_{Glc}$), 4.78–4.54 (m, 3H, OCH_2, H-29b), 4.32–4.28 (m, 2H, 2x H-6a$_{Glc}$), 4.36-4.13 (m, 2H, 2x H-6b$_{Glc}$), 4.03-4.00 (m, 2H, 2x H-5$_{Glc}$), 3.62 (d, 1H, *J* 8.4 Hz, H-28a), 3.18 (d, 1H, *J* 9.0 Hz, H-28b), 2.95 (dd, 1H, J_1 4.2 Hz, J_2 12.0 Hz, H-3), 2.38 (td, 1H, J_1 5.7 Hz, J_2 11.0 Hz, H-19), 2.20-0.60 (m, 24H, CH, CH_2), 2.08, 2.07, 2.069, 2.031, 2.029, 1.88, 1.87 (all s, 3H each, 8x CH_3CO), 1.66 (s, 3H, H-30), 1.01, 0.95, 0.89, 0.84, 0.78 (all s, 3H each, H-23–H-27) ppm; ^{13}C NMR (150 MHz, $CDCl_3$) δ_C 170.46, 170.44, 169.91, 169.89, 169.32, 168.86, 168.79, 150.57, 147.26, 146.59, 120.58, 120.50, 109.61, 86.65, 85.69, 85.62, 75.08 75.04, 72.81 72.71, 70.31 70.18, 68.92, 67.71 67.70, 64.93, 62.88, 61.57, 55.68, 50.36, 48.82, 47.84, 47.25, 42.65, 40.94, 38.81, 38.52, 37.48, 37.11, 34.76, 34.24, 29.89, 29.83, 27.97, 27.18, 25.20, 22.83, 20.85, 20.66, 20.53, 20.51, 20.17, 19.05, 18.24, 16.25, 16.12, 16.02, 14.73 ppm (Supplementary Materials, Table S2); IR (ATR) ν: 2942, 1750, 1457, 1368, 1216, 1091, 1055, 1036, 913, 732 cm^{-1}.

*Product **17b** (3,28-di(OCH$_2$TriazGal)BN)* was obtained as a white solid (242.0 mg, 99% yield); m.p.: 122-123 °C; $[\alpha]^{25}{}_D = +4.9$ (c 0.5, $CHCl_3$); HRMS (ESI $^+$): calcd for $C_{64}H_{92}N_6O_{20}Na$ ($[M + Na]^+$): *m/z* 1287.6264; found: *m/z* 1287.6206; ^{1}H NMR (600 MHz, $CDCl_3$): δ_H 7.80 and 7.79 (all s, br, 1H each, 2x H-5$_{triaz.}$), 5.86 and 5.856 (all d, 1H each, *J* 9.4 Hz, 2x H-1$_{Gal}$), 5.61 and 5.58 (all dd, 1H each, J_1 9.4 Hz, J_2 10.2 Hz, 2x H-2$_{Gal}$), 5.56–5.54 (m, 2H, 2x H-4$_{Gal}$), 5.25 and 5.26 (all dd, 1H each, J_1 5.4 Hz, J_2 10.2 Hz, 2x H-3$_{Gal}$), 4.78–4.56 (m, 6H, 2x OCH_2, H-29a, H-29b), 4.26–4.23 (m, 2H, 2x H-5$_{Gal}$), 4.22–4.10 (m, 4H, 2x H-6a$_{Gal}$, 2x H-6b$_{Gal}$), 3.62 (d, 1H, *J* 8.8 Hz, H-28a), 3.20 (d, 1H, *J* 9.1 Hz, H-28b), 2.97 (dd, 1H, J_1 4.3 Hz, J_2 11.7 Hz, H-3), 2.40 (td, 1H, J_1 5.7 Hz, J_2 11.1 Hz, H-19), 2.23, 2.22, 2.044, 2.04, 2.013, 2.01, 1.90, 1.88 (all s, 3H each, 8x CH_3CO), 2.30–0.60 (m, 24H, CH, CH_2), 1.67 (s, 3H, H-30), 1.01, 0.95, 0.90, 0.84, 0.78 (all s, 3H each, H-23–H-27) ppm; ^{13}C NMR (150 MHz, $CDCl_3$) δ_C 170.31, 170.28, 169.95, 169.79, 169.03, 168.93, 150.59, 147.06, 146.42, 120.77, 120.66, 109.62, 86.63, 86.22, 86.17, 73.98, 70.94, 70.86, 68.91, 67.86, 67.74, 66.91, 64.88, 61.18, 55.68, 52.88, 50.36, 48.83, 47.86, 47.25, 42.66, 40.95, 38.82, 38.53, 37.48, 37.12, 34.78, 34.24, 29.94, 29.84, 27.96, 27.20, 22.87, 25.20, 20.86, 20.66, 20.63, 20.49, 20.29, 20.27, 19.05, 18.26, 16.26, 16.13, 16.00, 14.74 ppm (Supplementary Materials, Table S2); IR (ATR) ν: 2942, 1748, 1457, 1368, 1213, 1089, 1043, 921, 730 cm^{-1}.

*Product **18b** (3,28-di(OCH$_2$TriazCH$_2$(CO)NHGal)BN)* was obtained as a white solid (216.9 mg, 82% yield); m.p.: 142–145 °C; $[\alpha]^{25}{}_D = +4.9$ (c 0.5, $CHCl_3$); HRMS (ESI^+): calcd for $C_{68}H_{99}N_8O_{22}$ ($[M + H]^+$): *m/z* 1379.6900; found: *m/z* 1379.6533; ^{1}H NMR (600 MHz, $CDCl_3$): δ_H 7.66 and 7.64 (all s, 1H each, 2x H-$5_{triaz.}$), 6.86 and 6.85 (all d, 1H each, *J* 8.8 Hz, 2x NH), 5.45-5.40 (m, 2H, 2x H-4_{Gal}), 5.22-5.18 (m, 2H, 2x H-1_{Gal}), 5.14–4.98 (m, 8H, 2x H-2_{Gal}, 2x H-3_{Gal}, 2x CH_2), 4.84–4.57 (m, 6H, H-29a, H-29b, 2x CH_2), 4.14-4.07 (m, 4H, 2x H-$6a_{Gal}$, 2x H-$6b_{Gal}$), 4.06–4.01 (m, 2H, 2x H-5_{Gal}), 3.63 (d, 1H, *J* 8.9 Hz, H-28a), 3.22 (d, 1H, *J* 9.0 Hz, H-28b), 2.97 (dd, 1H, J_1 4.2 Hz, J_2 11.7 Hz, H-3), 2.39 (td, 1H, J_1 5.9 Hz, J_2 10.6 Hz, H-19), 2.30–0.60 (m, 24H, CH, CH_2), 2.15, 2.14, 2.04, 2.03, 2.02, 1.98, 1.977, 1.96 (all s, 3H each, 8x CH_3CO), 1.67 (s, 3H, H-30), 0.96, 0.95, 0.92, 0.83, 0.77 (all s, 3H each, H-23–H-27) ppm; ^{13}C NMR (150 MHz, $CDCl_3$) δ_C 171.03, 170.92, 170.34, 169.98, 169.71, 165.68, 165.55, 150.54, 147.49, 146.77, 123.75, 123.61, 109.65, 86.89, 78.75, 78.72, 72.59, 72.57, 70.67, 70.64, 69.01, 68.06, 68.00, 67.06, 65.21, 63.20, 61.11, 61.00, 55.69, 52.71, 52.65, 50.36, 48.85, 47.90, 47.25, 42.65, 40.93, 38.85, 38.52, 37.50, 37.14, 34.75, 34.24, 29.88, 29.69, 28.10, 27.17, 25.20, 22.86, 20.87, 20.67, 20.62, 20.60, 20.59, 20.50, 19.09, 18.26, 16.30, 16.15, 15.96, 14.76, ppm (Supplementary Materials, Table S2); IR (ATR) ν: 2950, 1748, 1620, 1510, 1450, 1368, 1218, 1084, 1045, 970, 890, 720 cm^{-1}.

3.2.4. Procedure for the Synthesis of Betulin Glycoconjugates **19a** according to Strategy II (Modification C28)

To a well-stirred 28-*O*-(2-azidoacetyl)betulin **6** (0.190 mmol, 100.0 mg) and *per-O*-acetylated glucopyranosyl propargyl **10a** (0.190 mmol, 73.5 mg) in *i*-PrOH (2 mL) and THF (1 mL), $CuSO_4{\cdot}5H_2O$ (0.114 mmol, 22.6 mg) dissolved in H_2O (1 mL) and sodium ascorbate (0.209 mmol, 52.2 mg) dissolved in H_2O (1 mL) were added successively. The reaction mixture was stirred under argon atmosphere for 24 h at room temperature. After completion of the reaction (was monitored by TLC), the reaction mixture was extracted with DCM (5 × 5 mL), then the mixture was dried over $MgSO_4$ and was concentrated in vacuo. The crude residue was separated/purified using column chromatography (DCM:MeOH, gradient: 50:1 to 10:1).

*Product **19a** (28-O(CO)CH_2TriazCH$_2$OGlcBN)* was obtained as a white solid (168.3 mg, 97% yield); m.p.: 99–101 °C; $[\alpha]^{25}{}_D = -15.6$ (c 0.5, $CHCl_3$); HRMS (ESI+): calcd for $C_{49}H_{73}N_3O_{13}Na$ ($[M + Na]^+$): m/z 934.5041; found: m/z 934.5045; ^1H NMR (600 MHz, $CDCl_3$): δ_H 7.69 (s, br, 1H, H-$5_{triaz.}$), 5.22-5.17 (m, 2H, H-1_{Glc}, H-3_{Glc}), 5.10 (dd~t, 1H, J_1 9.6 Hz, J_2 9.8 Hz, H-2_{Glc}), 5.02 (ddt, 1H, J_1 8.0 Hz, J_2 9.5 Hz, H-4Glc), 4.97 and 4.86 (qAB, 2H, CH_2), 4.68 (s, br, 2H, CH_2), 4.68 and 4.60 (all s, br, 1H each, H-29a, H-29b), 4.43 (d, 1H, *J* 10.9 Hz, H-28a), 4.26 (dd, 1H, J_1 4.7 Hz, J_2 12.3 Hz,H-$6a_{Glc}$), 4.17 (dd, 1H, J_1 2.1 Hz, J_2 12.3 Hz, H-$6b_{Glc}$), 3.97 (d, 1H, *J* 11.0 Hz, H-28b), 3.73 (ddd, 1H, J_1 2.1 Hz, J_2 4.7 Hz, J_3 9.5 Hz, H-5_{Glc}), 3.18 (dd, 1H, J_1 4.7 Hz, J_2 11.5 Hz, H-3), 2.41 (td, 1H, J_1 5.7 Hz, J_2 10.7 Hz, H-19), 2.20-0.60 (m, 25H, CH, CH_2), 2.10, 2.03, 2.004, 2.00 (all s, 3H each, 4x CH_3CO), 1.68 (s, 3H, H-30), 1.01, 0.98, 0.97, 0.82, 0.76 (all s, 3H each, H-23–H-27) ppm; ^{13}C NMR (150 MHz, $CDCl_3$) δ_C 170.65, 170.18, 169.45, 169.42, 166.55, 149.73, 124.28, 110.10, 78.94, 72.79, 71.94, 71.21, 68.36, 61.80, 50.86, 64.96, 62.93, 55.29, 50.85, 50.33, 48.80, 47.64, 46.45, 42.71, 40.88, 38.87, 38.71, 37.68, 37.15, 34.39, 34.18, 29.60, 29.44, 27.99, 27.01, 27.39, 25.16, 20.78, 20.74, 20.67, 20.60, 19.11, 18.28, 16.10, 16.01, 15.36, 14.78 ppm (Supplementary Materials, Table S2); IR (ATR) ν: 3400–3200, 2942, 1747, 1640, 1456, 1366, 1218, 1037, 982, 883, 769 cm^{-1}.

3.2.5. Procedure for the Synthesis of Betulin Glycoconjugates **20a** according to Strategy II (Modification C3 and C28)

To a well-stirred 3,28-*O,O'*-di(2-azidoacetyl)betulin **7** (0.164 mmol, 100.0 mg) and per-*O*-acetylated glucopyranosyl propargyl **10a** (0.329 mmol, 126.9 mg) in *i*-PrOH (4.2 mL) and THF (1.8 mL), $CuSO_4{\cdot}5H_2O$ (0.181 mmol, 45.1 mg) dissolved in H_2O (2.1 mL) and sodium ascorbate (0.099 mmol, 19.5 mg) dissolved in H_2O (2.1 mL) were added successively. The reaction mixture was stirred under argon atmosphere for 24 h at room temperature. After completion of the reaction (was monitored by TLC), the reaction mixture was extracted with DCM (5 × 5 mL), then the mixture was dried over MgSO4 and was concentrated in vacuo. The crude residue was separated/purified using column chromatography (DCM:MeOH, gradient: 30:1 to 10:1).

*Product **20a** (3,28-di(O(CO)CH_2TriazCH$_2$OGlc)BN)* was obtained as a white solid (198.0 mg, 87% yield); m.p.: 109–112 °C; $[\alpha]^{25}{}_D = -19.0$ (c 0.5, $CHCl_3$); HRMS (ESI+): calcd for $C_{68}H_{97}N_6O_{24}$ ([M +

H]$^+$): m/z 1381.6554; found: m/z 1381.6218; ^{1}H NMR (600 MHz, $CDCl_3$): δ_H 7.68 and 7.66 (all s, 1H each, 2x H-5$_{triaz.}$), 5.23-5.13 (m, 4H, 2x (H-1$_{Glc}$ H-3$_{Glc}$)), 5.12–5.06 (m, 2H, 2x H-2$_{Glc}$), 5.05-4.99 (m, 2H, 2x H-4$_{Glc}$), 4.99-4.83 (m, 4H, 2x CH_2), 4.69–4.66 (m, 5H, H-29a, 2x CH_2), 4.60 (s, br, 1H, H-29b), 4.43 (d, 1H, J 10.6 Hz, H-28a), 4.26 and 4.27 (all dd, 1H each, J_1 1.0 Hz, J_2 12.4 Hz, 2x H-6a$_{Glc}$), 4.19–4.14 (m, 2H, 2x H-6b$_{Glc}$), 3.96 (d, 1H, *J* 11.0 Hz, H-28b), 3.75–3.70 (m, 2H, 2x H-5$_{Glc}$), 4.56 (dd, 1H, J_1 5.2 Hz, J_2 10.1 Hz, H-3), 2.41 (td, 1H, J_1 5.7 Hz, J_2 10.7 Hz, H-19), 2.20–0.60 (m, 24H, CH, CH_2), 2.093, 2.09, 2.028, 2.025, 2.03, 2.00, 1.998, 1.994 (all s, 3H each, 8x CH_3CO), 1.68 (s, 3H, H-30), 1.01, 0.98, 0.97, 0.84, 0.77 (all s, 3H each, H-23–H-27) ppm; ^{13}C NMR (150 MHz, $CDCl_3$) δ_C 170.64, 170.16, 169.43, 166.56, 165.90, 160.42, 149.68, 144.65, 144.55, 124.25, 124.24, 110.16, 83.86, 68.37, 72.80, 71.94, 71.22, 68.37, 62.94, 61.81, 61.80, 55.30, 51.05, 50.83, 50.21, 48.77, 47.65, 46.45, 42.73, 40.89, 38.27, 37.90, 37.65, 37.03, 34.38, 34.05, 29.57, 29.43, 28.01, 27.00, 25.08, 23.61, 21.96, 20.77, 20.66, 20.65, 20.60, 19.10, 18.11, 16.39, 16.12, 16.00, 14.75 ppm (Supplementary Materials, Table S2); IR (ATR) ν: 2930, 1744, 1620, 1367, 1216, 1037, 979, 880, 752 cm^{-1}.

3.2.6. Procedure for the Synthesis of 3,28-*O*,*O*′-di(2-(4-(hydroxymethyl-1H-1,2,3-triazol-1-yl)acetyl)betulin **21**

To a well-stirred 3,28-*O*,*O*′-di(2-azidoacetyl)betulin **7** (0.663 mmol, 403.6 mg) in *i*-PrOH (7.6 mL) and THF (4.8 mL), propargyl alcohol (1.989 mmol, 111.5 mg, 0.116 mL) and $CuSO_4 \cdot 5H_2O$ (0.796 mmol, 198.6 mg) dissolved in H_2O (2.7 mL) and sodium ascorbate (1.458 mmol, 288.9 mg) dissolved in H_2O (2.7 mL) were added successively. The reaction mixture was stirred under argon atmosphere for 24 h at room temperature. After completion of the reaction (was monitored by TLC), the reaction mixture was extracted with DCM (9 × 30 mL), then mixture was dried over $MgSO_4$ and was concentrated in vacuo. The crude residue was separated/purified using column chromatography (DCM:MeOH, gradient: 20:1 to 5:1).

Product **21** *(3,28-di(O(CO)CH$_2$TriazCH$_2$OH)BN)* was obtained as a white solid (367.2 mg, 77% yield); m.p.: 105–108 °C; $[\alpha]^{25}_D$ = +4.7 (c 0.5, $CHCl_3$); HRMS (ESI$^+$): calcd for $C_{40}H_{61}N_6O_6$ ([M + H]$^+$): *m/z* 721.4653; found: *m/z* 721.4650; ^{1}H NMR (600 MHz, $CDCl_3$): δ_H 7.68 and 7.66 (all s, 1H each, 2x H-5$_{triaz.}$), 5.19 (d, 2H, *J* 1.0 Hz, O(CO)CH_2), 5.15 (d, 2H, *J* 0.6 Hz, O(CO)CH_2), 4.82 (br s, 4H, 2x $\underline{CH_2}$OH), 4.69 (d, 1H, *J* 1.6 Hz, H-29a), 4.60 (s, 1H, H-29b), 4.57–4.54 (m, 1H, H-3),4.42 (d, 1H, *J* 10.9 Hz, H-28a), 3.96 (d, 1H, *J* 10.9 Hz, H-28b), 2.41 (m, 3H, H-19, 2x $CH_2O\underline{H}$), 2.10–0.60 (m, 24H, CH, CH_2), 1.67 (s, 3H, H-30), 1.00, 0.96, 0.83, 0.828, 0.75 (all s, 3H each, H-23–H-27) ppm; ^{13}C NMR (150 MHz, $CDCl_3$) δ_C 165.97, 165.61, 149.96, 149.66, 148.09, 123.08 110.12, 83.85, 64.92, 56.50; 55.28, 55.23, 51.08; 50.86, 50.20, 48.75, 47.65, 46.43, 42.71, 40.88, 38.26, 37.88, 37.64, 37.02, 34.37, 34.04, 29.56, 29.43, 28.00, 26.98, 25.07, 23.58, 20.73, 19.09, 18.10, 16.36, 16.11, 16.00, 14.75 ppm (Supplementary Materials, Table S3); IR (ATR) ν: 3500–300, 2927, 2871, 1743, 1456, 1376, 1266, 1219, 1040, 1006, 977, 882, 805 cm^{-1}.

3.2.7. Procedure for the Deprotection of Betulin Glycoconjugates **15–17**

Glycoconjugates **15–17** (1.0 mmol) were dissolved in MeOH (**15a–b**: 16 mL, **16a–b**: 35 mL, **17a–b**: 30 mL). Then, 1M solution of MeONa in MeOH (**15a–b**: 0.2 mmol, 0.2 mL, **16a–b**: 0.4 mmol, 0.4 mL, **17a–b**: 0.15 mmol, 0.15 mL) was added. Reaction was carried out for 120 min at room temperature. The reaction progress was monitored on TLC. After the reaction was complete, the mixture was neutralized with *Amberlyst-15*, filtered, and the filtrate was evaporated in vacuo. The crude products were crystallized from methanol.

Product ***22a*** *(28-OCH$_2$TriazGlcBN)* was obtained as a white solid (69.9 mg, 87% yield); m.p.: 174–175 °C; $[\alpha]^{25}_D$ = +4.1 (c 0.5, MeOH); HRMS (ESI$^+$): calcd for $C_{39}H_{63}N_3O_7Na$ ([M + Na]$^+$): *m/z* 708.4564; found: *m/z* 708.4555; ^{1}H NMR (400 MHz, MeOD): δ_H 8.19 (s, br, 1H, H-5$_{triaz.}$), 5.62 (d, 1H, *J* 9.2 Hz, H-1$_{Glc}$), 4.68–4.55 (m, 4H, H-29a, H-29b, OCH_2), 3.91–3.86 (m, 2H, H-6a$_{Glc}$, H-5$_{Glc}$), 3.73 (dd, 1H, J_1 5.2 Hz, J_2 12.1 Hz, H-6b$_{Glc}$), 3.65 (d, 1H, *J* 8.9 Hz, H-28a), 3.61–3.49 (m, 3H, H-4$_{Glc}$, H-3$_{Glc}$, H-2$_{Glc}$), 3.23 (d, 1H, *J* 9.0 Hz, H-28b), 3.12 (dd, 1H, J_1 4.9 Hz, J_2 11.2 Hz, H-3), 2.43 (td, 1H, J_1 5.2 Hz, J_2 10.9 Hz, H-19), 2.05-0.60 (m, 25H, CH, CH_2), 1.67 (s, 3H, H-30), 1.00, 0.98, 0.95, 0.86, 0.76 (all s, 3H each, H-23–H-27) ppm; ^{13}C NMR (150 MHz, MeOD) δ_C 151.86, 146.36, 124.41, 110.25, 89.70, 81.18, 79.75, 78.60, 74.10, 71.00, 69.88, 65.31, 62.47, 56.90, 51.94, 50.24, 43.82, 42.21, 40.14, 38.99, 38.35, 35.83, 35.53, 31.05, 30.75, 28.68, 28.39, 28.12, 26.71, 22.06, 19.52, 18.40, 16.76, 16.68, 16.15, 15.33 ppm (Supplementary Materials, Table S3); IR (ATR) ν: 3600-3100, 2941, 2871, 1620, 1450, 1390, 1100, 1043, 1013, 880 cm^{-1}.

Product ***22b*** *(28-OCH$_2$TriazGalBN)* was obtained as a white solid (79.5 mg, 99% yield); m.p.: 218–220 °C; $[\alpha]^{25}_D$ = +9.1 (c 0.5, MeOH); HRMS (ESI $^+$): calcd for $C_{39}H_{63}N_3O_7Na$ ($[M + Na]^+$): *m/z* 708.4564; found: *m/z* 708.4553; ^{1}H NMR (400 MHz, MeOD): δ_H 8.21 (s, br, 1H, H-5$_{triaz.}$), 5.57 (d, 1H, *J* 9.2 Hz, H-1$_{Glc}$), 4.68-4.56 (m, 4H, OCH$_2$, H-29a, H-29b), 4.15 (dd~t, 1H, *J* 9.3 Hz, H-2$_{Gal}$), 4.00 (dd, 1H, J_1 0.9 Hz, J_2 3.3 Hz, H-4$_{Gal}$), 3.85–3.69 (m, 3H, 2H-6$_{Gal}$, H-5$_{Gal}$), 3.70 (dd, 1H, J_1 3.3 Hz, J_2 9.5 Hz, H-3$_{Gal}$), 3.64 (d, 1H, *J* 8.6 Hz, H-28a), 3.23 (d, 1H, *J* 8.8 Hz, H-28b), 3.12 (dd, 1H, J_1 5.0 Hz, J_2 11.1 Hz, H-3), 2.43 (td, 1H, J_1 5.9 Hz, J_2 10.9 Hz, H-19), 2.01-0.60 (m, 25H, CH, CH$_2$), 1.67 (s, 3H, H-30), 0.99, 0.98, 0.95, 0.86, 0.76 (all s, 3H each, H-23–H-27) ppm; ^{13}C NMR (150 MHz, MeOD) δ_C 151.87, 146.54, 123.87, 110.28, 90.28, 79.90, 79.71, 75.40, 71.50, 70.32, 69.67, 65.33, 62.30, 56.86, 51.90, 50.17, 43.79, 42.15, 39.99, 40.09, 38.95, 38.32, 35.82, 35.46, 30.99, 30.79, 28.65, 28.34, 28.09, 26.64, 22.02, 19.41, 19.50, 16.76, 16.62, 16.16, 15.28 ppm (Supplementary Materials, Table S3); IR (ATR) ν: 3600–3100, 2932, 2869, 1630, 1456, 1374, 1093, 1044, 880 cm^{-1}.

Product ***23b*** *(28-OCH$_2$TriazCH$_2$(CO)NHGalBN)* was obtained as a white solid (78.3 mg, 96% yield); m.p.: 187-190 °C; $[\alpha]^{25}_D$ = +6.9 (c 0.5, $CHCl_3$); HRMS (ESI $^+$): calcd for $C_{41}H_{67}N_4O_8$ ($[M + H]^+$): *m/z* 743.4959; found: *m/z* 743.4962; ^{1}H NMR (400 MHz, MeOD): 7.96 (s, br, 1H, H-5$_{triaz.}$), 7.46 (s, 1H, NH), 5.22 (q, 2H, *J* 16.4 Hz, CH$_2$N), 4.90 (d, 1H, *J* 8.8 Hz, H-1$_{Gal}$), 4.68 and 4.57 (s, br, 1H, H-29a, H-29b), 4.65 (s, 2H, OCH$_2$), 3.94 (d, 1H, *J* 2.8 Hz, H-4$_{Gal}$), 3.83–3.54 (m, 5H, H-28a, H-2$_{Gal}$, H-3$_{Gal}$, H-5$_{Gal}$, H-6a$_{Gal}$, H-6b$_{Gal}$), 3.39 (s, 2H, CH$_2$CO), 3.24 (d, 1H, *J* 9.2 Hz, H-28b), 3.18–3.14 (m, 1H, H-3), 2.39 (td, 1H, J_1 5.9 Hz, J_2 10.8 Hz, H-19), 2.05–0.60 (m, 25H, CH, CH$_2$), 1.68 (s, 3H, H-30), 0.99, 0.98, 0.96, 0.84, 0.76 (all s, 3H each, H-23–H-27) ppm; ^{13}C NMR (150 MHz, MeOD) δ_C 168.57, 151.91, 146.42, 126.86, 110.24, 81.77, 79.75, 78.48, 75.82, 71.51, 70.49, 69.49, 65.15, 56.90, 51.92, 50.23, 43.80, 42.18, 40.12, 40.01, 38.98, 38.35, 35.86, 35.52, 31.04, 30.78, 28.67, 28.36, 28.12, 26.67, 22.05, 19.53, 19.44, 16.77, 16.59, 16.17, 15.30 ppm (Supplementary Materials, Table S3); IR (ATR) ν: 3600–3000, 2942, 1698, 1374, 1228, 1083, 1045, 879 cm^{-1}.

Product ***24a*** *(3,28-di(OCH$_2$TriazGlc)BN)* was obtained as a white solid (63.9 mg, 87% yield); m.p.: 176–178 °C; $[\alpha]^{25}_D$ = +16.4 (c 0.5, MeOH); HRMS (ESI $^+$): calcd for $C_{48}H_{76}N_6O_{12}Na$ ($[M + Na]^+$): *m/z* 951.5419; found: *m/z* 951.5441; ^{1}H NMR (600 MHz, MeOD): δ_H 8.18 i 8.14 (all s, br, 1H each, 2x H-5$_{triaz.}$), 5.61 and 5.59 (all d, 1H each, *J* 8.7 Hz, 2x H-1$_{Glc}$), 4.74–4.50 (m, 6H, H-29a, H-29b, 2x OCH$_2$), 3.90–3.87 (m, 4H, 2x H-6a$_{Glc}$, 2x H-5$_{Glc}$), 3.74–3.48 (m, 9H, H-28a, 2x H-2$_{Glc}$, 2x H-3$_{Glc}$, 2x H-4$_{Glc}$, 2x H-6b$_{Glc}$), 3.23 (d, 1H, *J* 9.0 Hz, H-28b), 2.98 (dd, 1H, J_1 4.2 Hz, J_2 11.4 Hz, H-3), 2.43 (td, 1H, J_1 5.9 Hz, J_2 11.0 Hz, H-19), 2.00–0.65 (m, 25H, CH, CH$_2$), 1.68 (s, 3H, H-30), 0.99, 0.98, 0.92, 0.87, 0.75 (all s, 3H each, H-23–H-27) ppm; ^{13}C NMR (150 MHz, MeOD) δ_C 151.89, 146.99, 146.42, 124.33, 124.18, 110.24, 88.07, 89.65, 81.20, 78.64, 74.11, 71.00, 69.82, 65.36, 63.50, 62.49, 57.23, 51.93, 50.25, 43.85, 42.25, 39.85, 39.96, 39.00, 38.37, 35.84, 35.52, 31.07, 30.76, 28.67, 28.41, 28.40, 26.71, 22.10, 19.43, 18.40, 16.82, 16.79, 16.70, 15.32 ppm (Supplementary Materials, Table S3); IR (ATR) ν: 3600–3100, 2936, 1620, 1460, 1374, 1093, 1042, 896 cm^{-1}.

Product ***24b*** *(3,28-di(OCH$_2$TriazGal)BN)* was obtained as a white solid (50.7 mg, 69% yield); m.p.: 178–179 °C; $[\alpha]^{25}_D$ = +22.4 (c 0.5, MeOH); HRMS (ESI^+): calcd for $C_{48}H_{77}N_6O_{12}$ ($[M + H]^+$): *m/z* 929.5599; found: *m/z* 929.5621; ^{1}H NMR (600 MHz, MeOD): δ_H 8.21 and 8.18 (all s, br, 1H each, 2x H-5$_{triaz.}$), 5.57 and 5.56 (all d, 1H each, *J* 9.0 Hz, 2x H-1$_{Gal}$), 4.74-4.51 (m, 6H, 2x OCH$_2$, H-29a, H-29b), 4.15 and 4.14 (all dd~t, 2H each, *J* 9.4 Hz, 2x H-2$_{Gal}$), 3.99 (m, 2H, 2x H-4$_{Gal}$), 3.85-3.69 (m, 8H, 2x H-3$_{Gal,}$ 2x H-5$_{Gal}$, 2x H-6a$_{Gal}$, 2x H-6b$_{Gal}$), 3.64 (d, 1H, *J* 9.4 Hz, H-28a), 3.23 (d, 1H, *J* 9.0 Hz, H-28b), 2.98 (dd, 1H, J_1 4.3 Hz, J_2 11.8 Hz, H-3), 2.43 (td, 1H, J_1 5.9 Hz, J_2 10.7 Hz, H-19), 2.00–0.70 (m, 25H, CH, CH$_2$), 1.68 (s, 3H, H-30), 0.99, 0.98, 0.92, 0.87, 0.76 (all s, 3H each, H-23–H-27)ppm; ^{13}C NMR (150 MHz, MeOD) δ_C 151.89, 147.19, 146.56, 123.89, 123.64, 110.27, 90.27, 88.04, 80.04, 79.02, 75.44, 71.56, 71.55, 69.77, 65.38; 63.56, 62.50, 62.34, 57.22, 51.91, 50.22, 43.83, 42.22, 39.83, 39.97, 39.96, 38.34, 35.84, 35.48,

31.05, 30.78, 28.66, 28.37, 28.42, 26.68, 22.08, 19.42, 18.41, 16.83, 16.80, 16.66, 15.30 ppm (Supplementary Materials, Table S3); IR (ATR) ν: 3600–3100, 2925, 2869, 1650, 1456, 1374, 1219, 1090, 1045, 879 cm^{-1}.

3.3. Biological Assays

3.3.1. Cell Lines

HCT 116 and MCF-7 cells were purchased from the American Type Culture Collection. NHDF cells were purchased from Lonza. All cells were cultured under standard conditions at 37 °C in a humidified atmosphere at 5% CO_2 in DMEM/F12 medium (PAA) supplemented with 10% FBS (EURx).

3.3.2. CCK-8 Assay

A Cell Counting Kit-8 (CCK-8) from Bimake was used to assess cell viability. Briefly, cells were seeded in 96-well plates, with three duplicate wells in each group. Cells were treated with betulin or its derivatives and incubated for 24 or 48 h. Then, CCK-8 solution was added to each well and the plate was incubated for 2 h at 37 °C. Subsequently, the absorbance at 450 nm was measured using a microplate reader (Epoch, BioTek). Cell viability rate was calculated using *CalcuSyn software* (version 2.0, Biosoft, Cambridge, UK).

4. Conclusions

In conclusion, we designed and synthesized a library of novel glycoconjugates of natural pentacyclic triterpenoid (BN) by employing click chemistry. The CuAAC reactions are extensively employed in the conjugate synthesis of various organic compounds, owing to their versatility, high chemoselectivity, and mild conditions. In this study, we successfully prepared new mono- and disubstituted betulin derivatives containing a sugar unit attached via a linker inclusive of the 1,2,3-triazole ring at the C3 and C28 position of the parent skeleton of BN. We confirmed that the click chemistry approach in a simple, easy and inexpensive way leads to a wide range of products with high yield, purity, and selectivity.

The methodology developed by us extends the synthetic possibilities of modifying the betulin skeleton. Importantly, it enables the simple preparation of both mono-(modification C28) and disubstituted betulin derivatives (modification C3 and C28) with high yields. The construction of the linker connecting betulin to the sugar unit depends on the type of building blocks used. According to Strategy I, synthesis starts with the preparation of an alkyne betulin derivative, which is then clicked with a 1-azido sugar. The second option is to modify the betulin with an azide moiety and click it with propargyl *O*-glucoside.

Unfortunately, a preliminary cytotoxicity assay of the obtained betulin glycoconjugates showed that the addition of a sugar unit to the native betulin structure via a few selected linkers containing a 1,2,3-triazole ring is not a significant way for biological activity. Monosubstituted betulin glycoconjugates show comparable or slightly lower activity than that of betulin alone while betulin derivatives containing two sugar units protected with acetyl groups increase cell viability, which may result from the release of glucose from the tested glycoconjugates under physiological conditions. In turn, the observed lack of biological activity of deprotected betulin glycoconjugates may be due to the insufficient affinity of these compounds for glucose transporters.

3,28-*O*,*O*′-Di(2-(4-(hydroxymethyl-*1H*-1,2,3-triazol-1-yl)acetyl)betulin **21**, modified only by introducing a fragment containing the 1,2,3-triazole system without the sugar unit, turned out to be surprisingly active. Unfortunately, it also turned out to be very toxic. This indicates that modifying the betulin backbone by introducing a 1,2,3-triazole ring significantly improves its cytotoxicity. However, further work should be done on increasing the selectivity of the obtained connections.

The obtained results show that despite the fact that the obtained betulin glycoconjugates do not show interesting antitumor activity, the idea of adding a sugar unit to the betulin backbone may, after some modifications, turn out to be correct and allow for the targeted transport of biologically active compounds into the tumor cells. The position used in the sugar unit for conjugation with the betulin derivative appears to be crucial for maintaining its affinity for GLUT transporters. Based on literature reports [59,60], it can be assumed that the 6-OH group (the group least involved in binding to the GLUT transporter) is the most neutral position that can be modified in sugar, so as not to reduce its affinity to the transport protein on the surface of cancer cells. Due to the above, it seems advisable to undertake further research on the chemical modifications of betulin by attaching sugar through the functionalization of this position. Glycoconjugation of betulin with the use of sugar derivatives modified in the C-6 position will be carried out both with the use of 1,3-dipolar azide-alkyne cycloaddition, as well as by creating bonds that can be broken under the action of intracellular enzymes (ester, amide, or carbamate).

Author Contributions: Conceptualization and methodology, M.G. and G.P.-G.; synthesis and characterization of chemical compounds, M.Z., S.B. and M.K.; cytotoxicity tests, A.L.; mass spectra, K.E.; supervision, M.G. and G.P.-G.; analysis and interpretation of the results, M.G., G.P.-G., M.Z. and S.B.; writing-original draft preparation, M.G. and G.P.-G.; writing-review and editing, M.G. and G.P.-G. All authors have read and agreed to the published version of the manuscript.

References

1. Krasutsky, P.A. Birch bark research and development. *Nat. Prod. Rep.* **2006**, *23*, 919–942. [CrossRef] [PubMed]
2. Safe, S.; Kasiappan, R. Natural Products as Mechanism-based Anticancer Agents: Sp Transcription Factors as Targets. *Phytother. Res.* **2016**, *30*, 1723–1732. [CrossRef] [PubMed]
3. Hordyjewska, A.; Ostapiuk, A.; Horecka, A. Betulin and betulinic acid in cancer research. *J. Pre-Clin. Clin. Res.* **2018**, *12*, 72–75. [CrossRef]
4. Dutta, D.; Chakraborty, B.; Sarkar, A.; Chowdhury, C.; Das, P. A potent betulinic acid analogue ascertains an antagonistic mechanism between autophagy and proteasomal degradation pathway in HT-29 cells. *BMC Cancer* **2016**, *16*, 23. [CrossRef] [PubMed]
5. Boryczka, S.; Bębenek, E.; Wietrzyk, J.; Kempińska, K.; Jastrzębska, M.; Kusz, J.; Nowak, M. Synthesis, Structure and Cytotoxic Activity of New Acetylenic Derivatives of Betulin. *Molecules* **2013**, *18*, 4526–4543. [CrossRef]
6. Baratto, L.C.; Porsani, M.V.; Pimentel, I.C.; Netto, A.B.P.; Paschke, R.; Oliveira, B.H. Preparation of betulinic acid derivatives by chemical and biotransformation methods and determination of cytotoxicity against selected cancer cell lines. *Eur. J. Med. Chem.* **2013**, *68*, 121–131. [CrossRef]
7. Kommera, H.; Kaluđerović, G.N.; Kalbitz, J.; Dräger, B.; Paschke, R. Small structural changes of pentacyclic lupane type triterpenoid derivatives lead to significant differences in their anticancer properties. *Eur. J. Med. Chem.* **2010**, *45*, 3346–3353. [CrossRef]
8. Kommera, H.; Kaluđerović, G.N.; Dittrich, S.; Kalbitz, J.; Dräger, B.; Mueller, T.; Paschke, R. Carbamate derivatives of betulinic acid and betulin with selective cytotoxic activity. *Bioorg. Med. Chem. Lett.* **2010**, *20*, 3409–3412. [CrossRef]
9. Dangroo, N.A.; Singh, J.; Rath, S.K.; Gupta, N.; Qayum, A.; Singh, S.; Sangwan, P.L. A convergent synthesis of novel alkyne–azide cycloaddition congeners of betulinic acid as potent cytotoxic agent. *Steroids* **2017**, *123*, 1–12. [CrossRef]
10. Gauthier, C.; Legault, J.; Lebrun, M.; Dufour, P.; Pichette, A. Glycosidation of lupane-type triterpenoids as potent in vitro cytotoxic agents. *Bioorg. Med. Chem.* **2006**, *14*, 6713–6725. [CrossRef]

11. Drąg-Zalesińska, M.; Kulbacka, J.; Saczko, J.; Wysocka, T.; Zabel, M.; Surowiak, P.; Drag, M. Esters of betulin and betulinic acid with amino acids have improved water solubility and are selectively cytotoxic toward cancer cells. *Bioorg. Med. Chem. Lett.* **2009**, *19*, 4814–4817. [CrossRef] [PubMed]
12. Yang, S.-J.; Liu, M.-C.; Xiang, H.-M.; Zhao, Q.; Xue, W.; Yang, S. Synthesis and in vitro antitumor evaluation of betulin acid ester derivatives as novel apoptosis inducers. *Eur. J. Med. Chem.* **2015**, *102*, 249–255. [CrossRef] [PubMed]
13. Zhang, D.-M.; Xu, H.-G.; Wang, L.; Li, Y.-J.; Sun, P.; Wu, X.-M.; Wang, G.; Chen, W.-M.; Ye, W.-C. Betulinic Acid and its Derivatives as Potential Antitumor Agents. *Med. Res. Rev.* **2015**, *35*, 1127–1155. [CrossRef] [PubMed]
14. Zhao, H.; Liu, Z.; Liu, W.; Han, X.; Zhao, M. Betulin attenuates lung and liver injuries in sepsis. *Int. Immunopharmacol.* **2016**, *30*, 50–56. [CrossRef] [PubMed]
15. Moghaddam, M.G.; Ahmad, F.B.H.; Samzadeh-Kermani, A. Biological Activity of Betulinic Acid: A Review. *Pharmacol. Pharm.* **2012**, *3*, 119–123. [CrossRef]
16. Zhao, H.; Zheng, Q.; Hu, X.; Shen, H.; Li, F. Betulin attenuates kidney injury in septic rats through inhibiting TLR4/NF-κB signaling pathway. *Life Sci.* **2016**, *144*, 185–193. [CrossRef]
17. Fulda, S.; Kroemer, G. Targeting mitochondrial apoptosis by betulinic acid in human cancers. *Drug Discov. Today* **2009**, *14*, 885–890. [CrossRef]
18. Suman, P.; Patel, A.; Solano, L.; Jampana, G.; Gardner, Z.S.; Holt, C.M.; Jonnalagadda, S.C. Synthesis and cytotoxicity of Baylis-Hillman template derived betulinic acid-triazole conjugates. *Tetrahedron* **2017**, *73*, 4214–4226. [CrossRef]
19. Jonnalagadda, S.; Suman, P.; Morgan, D.; Seay, J. Recent Developments on the Synthesis and Applications of Betulin and Betulinic Acid Derivatives as Therapeutic Agents. *Bioact. Nat. Prod. (Part O)* **2017**, *53*, 45–84. [CrossRef]
20. Baltina, L.A.; Kazakova, O.B.; Nigmatullina, L.; Boreko, E.I.; Pavlova, N.; Nikolaeva, S.; Savinova, O.; Tolstikov, G. Lupane triterpenes and derivatives with antiviral activity. *Bioorg. Med. Chem. Lett.* **2003**, *13*, 3549–3552. [CrossRef]
21. Bori, I.D.; Hung, H.-Y.; Qian, K.; Chen, C.-H.; Morris-Natschke, S.L.; Lee, K.-H. Anti-AIDS agents 88. Anti-HIV conjugates of betulin and betulinic acid with AZT prepared via click chemistry. *Tetrahedron Lett.* **2012**, *53*, 1987–1989. [CrossRef]
22. Amiri, S.; Dastghaib, S.; Ahmadi, M.; Mehrbod, P.; Khadem, F.; Behrouj, H.; Aghanoori, M.-R.; Machaj, F.; Ghamsari, M.; Rosik, J.; et al. Betulin and its derivatives as novel compounds with different pharmacological effects. *Biotechnol. Adv.* **2020**, *38*, 107409. [CrossRef]
23. Zdzisińska, B. Właściwości lecznicze betuliny i kwasu betulinowego, składników ekstraktu z kory brzozy. *Farm. Przegl. Nauk.* **2010**, *3*, 33–39.
24. Grymel, M.; Zawojak, M.; Adamek, J. Triphenylphosphonium Analogues of Betulin and Betulinic Acid with Biological Activity: A Comprehensive Review. *J. Nat. Prod.* **2019**, *82*, 1719–1730. [CrossRef] [PubMed]
25. Pokorný, J.; Horka, V.; Sidova, V.; Urban, M. Synthesis and characterization of new conjugates of betulin diacetate and bis(triphenysilyl)betulin with substituted triazoles. *Mon. Für Chem.—Chem. Mon.* **2018**, *149*, 839–845. [CrossRef]
26. Bhunia, D.; Pallavi, P.M.C.; Bonam, S.R.; Reddy, S.A.; Verma, Y.K.; Halmuthur, S.K.M. Design, Synthesis, and Evaluation of Novel 1,2,3-Triazole-Tethered Glycolipids as Vaccine Adjuvants. *Arch. Pharm.* **2015**, *348*, 689–703. [CrossRef] [PubMed]
27. Ye, Y.; Zhang, T.; Yuan, H.; Li, D.; Lou, H.; Fan, P. Mitochondria-Targeted Lupane Triterpenoid Derivatives and Their Selective Apoptosis-Inducing Anticancer Mechanisms. *J. Med. Chem.* **2017**, *60*, 6353–6363. [CrossRef] [PubMed]
28. Dalvie, D.K.; Kalgutkar, A.S.; Khojasteh-Bakht, S.C.; Obach, R.S.; O'Donnell, J.P. Biotransformation Reactions of Five-Membered Aromatic Heterocyclic Rings. *Chem. Res. Toxicol.* **2002**, *15*, 269–299. [CrossRef]
29. Valverde, I.E.; Bauman, A.; Kluba, C.A.; Vomstein, S.; Walter, M.A.; Mindt, T.L. 1,2,3-Triazoles as Amide Bond Mimics: Triazole Scan Yields Protease-Resistant Peptidomimetics for Tumor Targeting. *Angew. Chem. Int. Ed.* **2013**, *52*, 8957–8960. [CrossRef]
30. Dheer, D.; Singh, V.; Shankar, R. Medicinal attributes of 1,2,3-triazoles: Current developments. *Bioorganic Chem.* **2017**, *71*, 30–54. [CrossRef]

31. Thirumurugan, P.; Matosiuk, D.; Jozwiak, K. Click Chemistry for Drug Development and Diverse Chemical–Biology Applications. *Chem. Rev.* **2013**, *113*, 4905–4979. [CrossRef] [PubMed]
32. Pokorný, L.B.A.M.U.J.; Borkova, L.; Urban, M. Click Reactions in Chemistry of Triterpenes—Advances Towards Development of Potential Therapeutics. *Curr. Med. Chem.* **2018**, *25*, 636–658. [CrossRef] [PubMed]
33. Antimonova, A.N.; Petrenko, N.I.; Shakirov, M.M.; Rybalova, T.V.; Frolova, T.S.; Shul'Ts, E.E.; Kukina, T.P.; Sinitsyna, O.I.; Tolstikov, G.A. Synthesis and study of mutagenic properties of lupane triterpenoids containing 1,2,3-triazole fragments in the C-30 position. *Chem. Nat. Compd.* **2013**, *49*, 657–664. [CrossRef]
34. Bębenek, E.; Jastrzębska, M.; Kadela-Tomanek, M.; Chrobak, E.; Orzechowska, B.; Zwolińska, K.; Latocha, M.; Mertas, A.; Czuba, Z.P.; Boryczka, S. Novel Triazole Hybrids of Betulin: Synthesis and Biological Activity Profile. *Molecules* **2017**, *22*, 1876. [CrossRef] [PubMed]
35. Shi, W.; Tang, N.; Yan, W. Synthesis and cytotoxicity of triterpenoids derived from betulin and betulinic acid via click chemistry. *J. Asian Nat. Prod. Res.* **2015**, *17*, 159–169. [CrossRef] [PubMed]
36. Krawczyk, M.; Pastuch-Gawołek, G.; Mrozek-Wilczkiewicz, A.; Kuczak, M.; Skonieczna, M.; Musiol, R. Synthesis of 8-hydroxyquinoline glycoconjugates and preliminary assay of their β1,4-GalT inhibitory and anti-cancer properties. *Bioorg. Chem.* **2019**, *84*, 326–338. [CrossRef] [PubMed]
37. Krawczyk, M.; Pastuch-Gawołek, G.; Pluta, A.; Erfurt, K.; Domiński, A.; Kurcok, P. 8-Hydroxyquinoline Glycoconjugates: Modifications in the Linker Structure and Their Effect on the Cytotoxicity of the Obtained Compounds. *Molecules* **2019**, *24*, 4181. [CrossRef]
38. Krawczyk, M.; Pastuch-Gawołek, G.; Hadasik, A.; Erfurt, K. 8-Hydroxyquinoline Glycoconjugates Containing Sulfur at the Sugar Anomeric Position—Synthesis and Preliminary Evaluation of Their Cytotoxicity. *Molecules* **2020**, *25*, 4174. [CrossRef]
39. Domiński, A.; Krawczyk, M.; Konieczny, T.; Kasprów, M.; Foryś, A.; Pastuch-Gawołek, G.; Kurcok, P. Biodegradable pH-responsive micelles loaded with 8-hydroxyquinoline glycoconjugates for Warburg effect based tumor targeting. *Eur. J. Pharm. Biopharm.* **2020**, *154*, 317–329. [CrossRef]
40. Křen, V.; Martinkova, L. Glycosides in Medicine: "The Role of Glycosidic Residue in Biological Activity". *Curr. Med. Chem.* **2001**, *8*, 1303–1328. [CrossRef]
41. A Smith, T. Facilitative glucose transporter expression in human cancer tissue. *Br. J. Biomed. Sci.* **1999**, *56*, 285–292. [PubMed]
42. Heiden, M.G.V.; Cantley, L.C.; Thompson, C.B. Understanding the Warburg Effect: The Metabolic Requirements of Cell Proliferation. *Science* **2009**, *324*, 1029–1033. [CrossRef] [PubMed]
43. Calvaresi, E.C.; Hergenrother, P.J. Glucose conjugation for the specific targeting and treatment of cancer. *Chem. Sci.* **2013**, *4*, 2319–2333. [CrossRef] [PubMed]
44. Zhao, F.-Q. Functional Properties and Genomics of Glucose Transporters. *Curr. Genom.* **2007**, *8*, 113–128. [CrossRef]
45. Barnett, J.E.G.; Holman, G.D.; Munday, K.A. Structural requirements for binding to the sugar-transport system of the human erythrocyte. *Biochem. J.* **1973**, *131*, 211–221. [CrossRef]
46. Ma, J.; Liu, H.; Xi, Z.; Hou, J.; Li, Y.; Niu, J.; Liu, T.; Bi, S.; Wang, X.; Wang, C.; et al. Protected and De-protected Platinum(IV) Glycoconjugates With GLUT1 and OCT2-Mediated Selective Cancer Targeting: Demonstrated Enhanced Transporter-Mediated Cytotoxic Properties in vitro and in vivo. *Front. Chem.* **2018**, *6*, 386. [CrossRef]
47. Khan, I.; Guru, S.K.; Rath, S.K.; Chinthakindi, P.K.; Singh, B.; Koul, S.; Bhushan, S.; Sangwan, P.L. A novel triazole derivative of betulinic acid induces extrinsic and intrinsic apoptosis in human leukemia HL-60 cells. *Eur. J. Med. Chem.* **2016**, *108*, 104–116. [CrossRef]
48. Komissarova, N.G.; Dubovitskii, S.N.; Shitikova, O.V.; Vyrypaev, E.M.; Spirikhin, L.V.; Eropkina, E.M.; Lobova, T.G.; Eropkin, M.; Yunusov, M.S. Synthesis of Conjugates of Lupane-Type Pentacyclic Triterpenoids with 2-Aminoethane- and N-Methyl-2-Aminoethanesulfonic Acids. Assessment of in vitro Toxicity. *Chem. Nat. Compd.* **2017**, *53*, 907–914. [CrossRef]
49. Yang, Q.-R.; Qiao, W.-H.; Zhang, S.-M.; Qu, J.-P.; Liu, D.-L. Synthesis and Characterization of a New Cationic Galactolipid with Carbamate for Gene Delivery. *Tenside Surfactants Deterg.* **2010**, *47*, 294–299. [CrossRef]
50. Rajaram, H.; Palanivelu, M.K.; Arumugam, T.V.; Rao, V.M.; Shaw, P.N.; McGeary, R.P.; Ross, B.P. 'Click' assembly of glycoclusters and discovery of a trehalose analogue that retards Aβ40 aggregation and inhibits Aβ40-induced neurotoxicity. *Bioorg. Med. Chem. Lett.* **2014**, *24*, 4523–4528. [CrossRef]

51. Lancuški, A.; Bossard, F.; Fort, S. Carbohydrate-Decorated PCL Fibers for Specific Protein Adhesion. *Biomacromolecules* **2013**, *14*, 1877–1884. [CrossRef] [PubMed]
52. Zemplén, G.; Pacsu, E. Über die Verseifung acetylierter Zucker und verwandter Substanzen. *Berichte Dtsch. Chem. Ges. (A B Ser.)* **1929**, *62*, 1613–1614. [CrossRef]
53. Brown, R.S.; Wahl, R.L. Overexpression of Glut-1 glucose transporter in human breast cancer. An im-munohistochemical study. *Cancer* **1993**, *72*, 2979–2985. [CrossRef]
54. Haber, R.S.; Rathan, A.; Weiser, K.R.; Pritsker, A.; Itzkowitz, S.H.; Bodian, C.; Slater, G.; Weiss, A.; Burstein, D.E. GLUT1 glucose transporter expression in colorectal carcinoma: A marker for poor progno-sis. *Cancer* **1998**, *83*, 34–40. [CrossRef]
55. Kumamoto, K.; Goto, Y.; Sekikawa, K.; Takenoshita, S.; Ishida, N.; Kawakita, M.; Kannagi, R. Increased expression of UDP-galactose transporter messenger RNA in human colon cancer tissues and its implica-tion in synthesis of Thomsen-Friedenreich antigen and sialyl Lewis A/X determinants. *Cancer Res.* **2001**, *61*, 4620–4627.
56. Lutter, A.-H.; Scholka, J.; Richter, H.; Anderer, U. Applying XTT, WST-1, and WST-8 to human chondrocytes: A comparison of membrane-impermeable tetrazolium salts in 2D and 3D cultures. *Clin. Hemorheol. Microcirc.* **2017**, *67*, 327–342. [CrossRef]
57. Van De Waterbeemd, H.; Smith, D.A.; Jones, B.C. Lipophilicity in PK design: Methyl, ethyl, futile. *J. Comput. Mol. Des.* **2001**, *15*, 273–286. [CrossRef]
58. Lombardo, F.; Obach, R.; Shalaeva, M.Y.; Gao, F. Prediction of Volume of Distribution Values in Hu-mans for Neutral and Basic Drugs Using Physicochemical Measurements and Plasma Protein Binding Data. *J. Med. Chem.* **2002**, *45*, 2867–2876. [CrossRef]
59. Deng, D.; Xu, C.; Sun, P.; Wu, J.; Yan, C.; Hu, M.; Yan, N. Crystal structure of the human glucose transporter GLUT1. *Nat. Cell Biol.* **2014**, *510*, 121–125. [CrossRef]
60. Fernández, C.; Nieto, O.; Rivas, E.; Montenegro, G.; Fontenla, J.A.; Fernández-Mayoralas, A. Synthesis and biological studies of glycosyl dopamine derivatives as potential antiparkinsonian agents. *Carbohydr. Res.* **2000**, *327*, 353–365. [CrossRef]

4

The Cytotoxic Effect of Newly Synthesized Ferrocenes against Cervical Carcinoma Cells Alone and in Combination with Radiotherapy

Hana Skoupilova [1], Vladimir Rak [2], Jiri Pinkas [3], Jindrich Karban [4] and Roman Hrstka [1,*]

1 Research Centre for Applied Molecular Oncology, Masaryk Memorial Cancer Institute, Zluty kopec 7, 656 53 Brno, Czech Republic; hana.skoupilova@med.muni.cz

2 Department of Radiation Oncology, Masaryk Memorial Cancer Institute, Zluty kopec 7, 656 53 Brno, Czech Republic; vladimir.rak@mou.cz

3 J. Heyrovský Institute of Physical Chemistry, Academy of Sciences of the Czech Republic, v. v. i., Dolejškova 2155/3, 182 23 Prague 8, Czech Republic; jiri.pinkas@jh-inst.cas.cz

4 Institute of Chemical Process Fundamentals, Academy of Sciences of the Czech Republic, v. v. i., Rozvojová 135, 165 02 Prague 6, Czech Republic; karban@icpf.cas.cz

* Correspondence: hrstka@mou.cz;

Abstract: Cervical cancer is one of the most common types of cancer in women, with approximately 500,000 new cases and 250,000 deaths every year. Radiotherapy combined with chemotherapy represents the treatment of choice for advanced cervical carcinomas. The role of the chemotherapy is to increase the sensitivity of the cancer cells to irradiation. Cisplatin, the most commonly used drug for this purpose, has its limitations. Thus, we used a family of ferrocene derivatives (in addition, one new species was prepared using standard Schlenk techniques) and studied their effects on cervical cancer cells alone and in combination with irradiation. We applied colorimetric assay to determine the cytotoxicity of the compounds; flow cytometry to analyze the production of reactive oxygen species (ROS), cell cycle, and mitochondrial membrane potential (MMP); immunochemistry to study protein expression; and colony forming assay to evaluate changes in radiosensitivity. Treatment with ferrocenes exhibited significant cytotoxicity against cervical cancer cells, associated with increasing ROS production and MMP changes, suggesting the induction of apoptosis. The combined activity of ferrocenes and ionizing radiation highlighted ferrocenes as potential radiosensitizing drugs, while their higher single-agent toxicity in comparison with routinely used cisplatin could also be promising. Our results demonstrate antitumor activity of several tested ferrocenes both alone and in combination with radiotherapy.

Keywords: ferrocenes; chemotherapy; cytotoxic effect; radiotherapy; radiosensitization; irradiation; cell death

---

1. Introduction

Worldwide, cervical carcinoma is the second most common malignancy specific to women. It was estimated that in 2012, more than half a million women were diagnosed with cervical cancer around the world, and approximately quarter of a million died [1,2].

Fortunately, the incidence of cervical cancer is steadily declining in most developed countries [3]. Two main reasons for this trend are effective screening and vaccination against the most common oncogenic human papilloma virus (HPV) strains which cause almost all cervical cancers [4]. Treatment of cervical cancer depends on the stage of disease and ranges from conization (simple removal of abnormal cervical epithelium) or trachelectomy (removal of the whole cervix) to hysterectomy and/or radiotherapy [5]. Radiotherapy is usually used in more advanced cases, either to remove remaining microscopic disease after surgery (adjuvant therapy) or as a main treatment when surgery cannot be performed (curative therapy).

Curative radiotherapy is often combined with chemotherapy to improve the treatment outcome [6]. The most commonly used chemotherapeutic drug in this case is cisplatin. Adding a weekly infusion of cisplatin to radiotherapy improves five-year overall survival by 6% and disease-free survival by 8% [6].

Although platinum substances are widely used, they can cause serious side effects, including renal, neural, and gastrointestinal toxicity, that limit their usefulness [7]. Thus, not only the advantages but also the disadvantages of cisplatin stimulated further research into other types of compounds containing metal in their structure. Besides platinum complexes, species containing iron, titanium, ruthenium, gold, or palladium have been synthesized and tested [8–14]. Among the most intensively studied substances exhibiting radiosensitization effects are ruthenium compounds [15–17] or gold nanoparticles [16], as demonstrated also by in vivo screenings [18–20]. Nevertheless, despite a great deal of research into iron-containing antitumor compounds, there have been only a few investigations into the potential radiosensitizing effects of these compounds in cancer cells [21,22].

This article is focused on the series of ferrocene derivatives of the general formula $[Fe(\eta^5\text{-}C_5H_4CH_2(p\text{-}C_6H_4)CH_2(N\text{-het}))_2]$ bearing either substituted or unsubstituted saturated five- and six-membered nitrogen-containing heterocycles (Figure 1). In vitro cytotoxicity analysis was performed on cell lines derived from cervical cancer. In the case of highly toxic ferrocenes, we focused especially on their mechanisms of action in terms of the disruption of cell metabolism and examination of cellular mechanisms leading to cell death. The combined effect of ferrocenes with ionizing radiation was also determined to test the possible use of these ferrocenes as potential radiosensitizing agents.

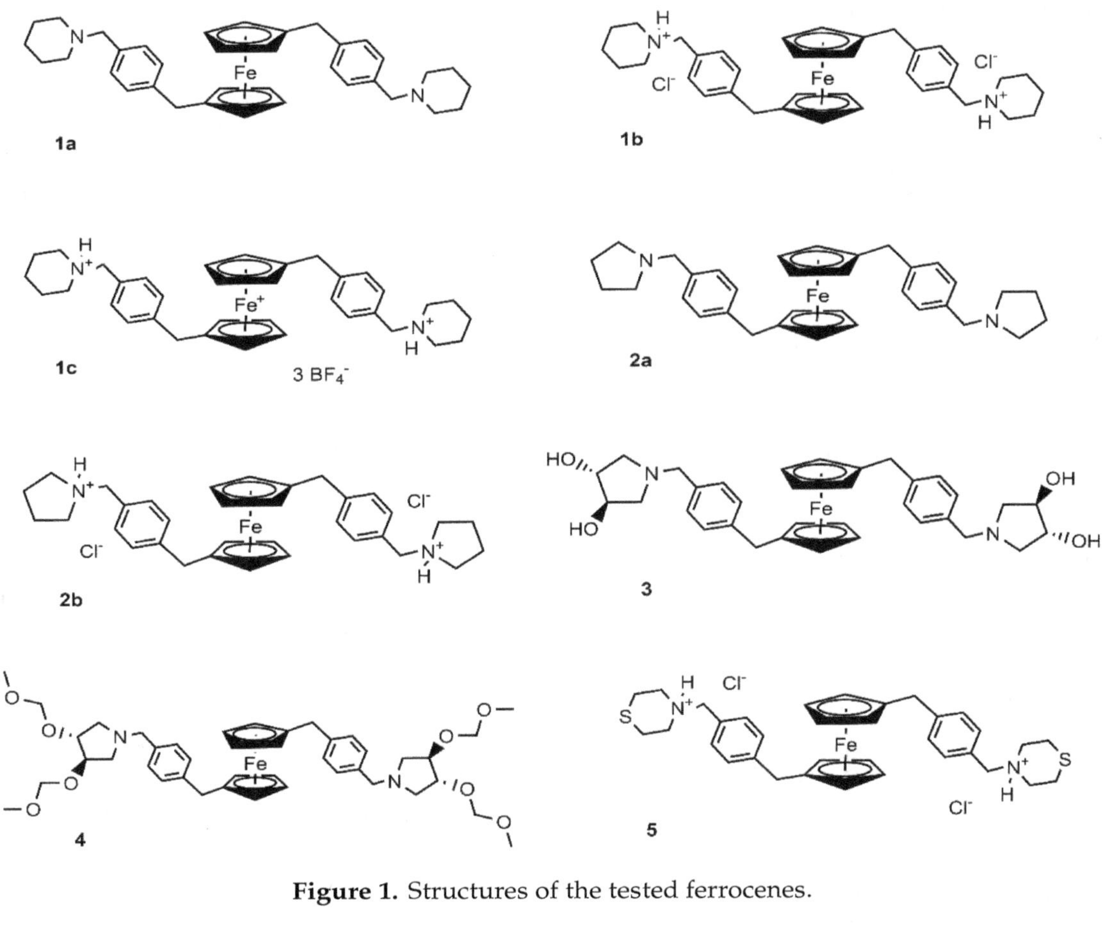

Figure 1. Structures of the tested ferrocenes.

2. Materials and Methods

2.1. Preparation and Characterization of Ferrocenes

Ferrocenes **1a**, **1b**, **2a**, **2b**, **3**, **4**, and **5** were prepared under argon atmosphere using standard Schlenk techniques, as was previously published [23]. Ferrocene **1c** was prepared from **1b** (155 mg, 244 μmol) and $AgBF_4$ (149 mg, 764 μmol) (Scheme 1). The substances were dried under vacuum for 1 h. The vacuum was replaced with argon and dry acetone (10 mL) was added, which caused an immediate color change from yellow to dark green. The mixture was then stirred for 2 days with light exclusion and then filtered. The filtrate was evaporated to dryness to obtain **1c** as a green solid substance with yield 200 mg (99%). M.p. 82 °C. ATR (Si); cm^{-1}: 3151 (sh, vw), 3115 (w), 2961 (w), 2932 (sh, vw), 2870 (vw), 1614 (vw), 1518 (w), 1462 (m), 1417 (m), 1367 (w), 1284 (w), 1226 (vw), 1054 (vs), 1035 (sh, s), 857 (m), 839 (sh, w), 764 (vw), 578 (w), 520 (m), 416 (w). Elemental analysis for **1c**—$C_{36}H_{46}B_3F_{12}FeN_2$ calculated C, 52.53; H, 5.63; N, 3.40%, found C, 51.41; H, 5.49; N, 3.35%. Its infrared spectrum (ATR) is characterized by the presence of a very strong and broad band at 1054 cm^{-1}, which could be assigned to stretching B–F vibration of the $[BF_4]^-$ anion.

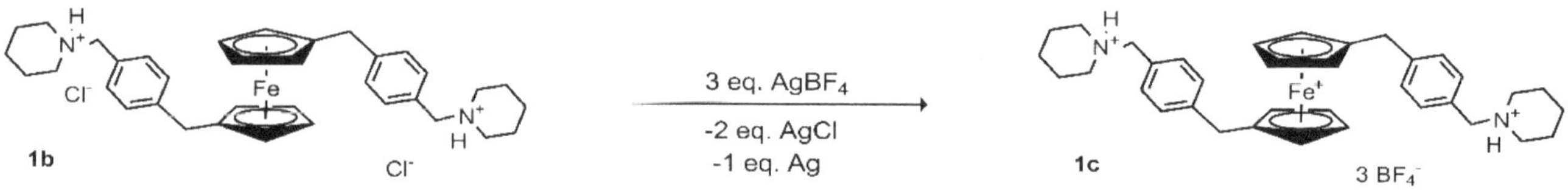

Scheme 1. Preparation of **1c**.

Ferrocene derivatives **1a**, **1b**, **2a**, **2b**, **3**, **4**, and **5** were characterized by elemental analysis, melting point, nuclear magnetic resonance (NMR), electrospray ionization mass spectrometry (ESI-MS), and X-ray diffraction analysis, as reported previously [23,24].

2.2. Cell Lines and Cultivation

Cervical cancer cell lines Ca Ski (ATCC® CRL-1550™), SiHa (ATCC® HTB-35™), and HeLa (ATCC® CCL-2™) were used. As nonmalignant controls we used the hTERT (human telomerase reverse transcriptase) immortalized retinal epithelium cell line RPE-1 (ATCC® CRL-4000™) and immortalized HEK 293 cells (ATCC® CRL-1573™) derived from human embryonic renal epithelium. All these cell lines were obtained from the American Type Culture Collection (ATCC, Manassas, Virginia, USA). Ca Ski and SiHa were maintained in high-glucose RPMI-1640 Medium (Sigma-Aldrich, St. Louis, USA) at 37 °C in a humidified atmosphere with 5% CO_2. HeLa and noncancerous cell lines HEK 293 and RPE-1 were maintained in high-glucose Dulbecco's modified Eagle's medium (DMEM) (Sigma-Aldrich, St. Louis, Missouri, USA) under the same conditions. Both media were supplemented with 10% fetal bovine serum (Gibco, Thermo Fisher Scientific, Waltham, Massachusetts, USA), 300 μg/mL L-glutamine (Sigma-Aldrich, St. Louis, Missouri, USA), and 100 μg/mL HyClone Penicillin–Streptomycin 100× solution (BioSera, Nuaille, France). The culture medium was changed during each cell passage. Cells were grown to 60–80% confluence prior to experimental treatments with ferrocenes at concentrations from 1 to 100 μM. Cells were mycoplasma-free throughout the duration of all experiments.

2.3. Cell Viability Assay

Due to their different sizes and growth rates, SiHa and Ca Ski cells were seeded at a density of 10,000 cells; HeLa, 8000 cells; HEK 293, 5000 cells; and RPE-1, 4000 cells per well in 96-well plates. The next day, the cells were exposed to the tested ferrocenes diluted in dimethyl sulfoxide (DMSO; Sigma-Aldrich, St. Louis, Missouri, USA) in concentrations from 0 to 100 μM (each in pentaplicate) for 24 h. Cell viability was measured using colorimetric MTT (3-(4,5-dimethylthiazol-2-yl)-2,5-diphenyltetrazolium bromide) assay as described previously [25]. All experiments were performed in three independent runs (twice, when cytotoxicity was over 100 μM). Data from cytotoxicity assays were measured using a Microplate Reader: Infinite® M1000 PRO (Tecan, Männedorf, Zürich, Switzerland) and analyzed using GraphPad Software (San Diego, California, USA) as IC_{50} values (concentrations of compounds that cause metabolic inhibition of 50% of cells).

2.4. Cell Cycle

The cell cycle was measured by a modified propidium iodide (PI) staining protocol as described previously [26,27]. Cells in 6-well plates were treated with 5 μM ferrocenes or cisplatin (positive control), and half of the wells were irradiated with 4 Gy (discussed in detail in Section 2.11); all samples were then incubated for 24 h. Afterwards, cells were trypsinized, washed with PBS (phosphate-buffered saline), and centrifuged at 1000 rpm for 5 min. Pellets were washed and resuspended in 0.5 mL of PBS. Cells were then fixed in 70% EtOH for at least 4 h at 4 °C. After fixation, the cells were centrifuged at 1000 rpm for 5 min and washed in PBS again. Subsequently, the cells were stained in 1 mL of staining solution: 0.1% Triton X-100, 10 μg/mL PI (both Sigma-Aldrich, St. Louis, USA), and 100 μg/mL DNase-free RNase A (Invitrogen, Carlsbad, California, USA) for 10 min at 37 °C. The DNA content was measured using a flow cytometer (Navios, Beckman Coulter, USA).

2.5. Reactive Oxygen Species (ROS) Production

SiHa or HeLa cells were seeded at 8000 cells per well in dark 96-well plates and incubated under standard conditions for 24 h. The next day, the medium was changed with 100 μL of Hanks' balanced salt solution (HBSS) (0.137 M NaCl, 5.4 mM KCl, 0.25 mM Na_2HPO_4, 0.1 g glucose, 0.44 mM KH_2PO_4, 1.3 mM $CaCl_2$, 1.0 mM $MgSO_4$, 4.2 mM $NaHCO_3$). Cells were incubated for 1 h. The solution was subsequently aspirated, and 100 μL of HBSS with 5 μM concentration of general oxidative stress indicator 5-(and-6)-chloromethyl-2′,7′-dichlorodihydrofluorescein diacetate, acetyl ester (CM-H_2DCFDA; Invitrogen, Carlsbad, California, USA) was added. After 30 min the cells were washed twice and treated with 10 μM ferrocenes or 50 μM H_2O_2, serving as a positive control, or 10 mM N-acetylcysteine (NAC), serving as a negative control. ROS production was measured after 2, 4, and 6 h.

2.6. Mitochondrial Membrane Potential Changes

The changes in mitochondrial membrane potential were measured using a 1,1′,3,3′-Tetraethyl-5,5′,6,6′-tetrachloroimidacarbocyanine iodide dye—mitochondrial membrane potential probe (JC-1; Invitrogen, Carlsbad, California, USA) [28,29]. The cells were harvested with trypsin and seeded at a density of 0.15–0.2 million of cells per well in 12-well plates, then allowed to adhere overnight. The cells were exposed to ferrocenes in 5 μM concentration for 24 h. Since SiHa cells were more resistant, the conditions were modified to 40 μM concentration for 6 h. Treatment with valinomycin (Molecular probes, Eugene, Oregon, USA) in 50 μM concentration for 2 h served as a positive control. Cells were collected with a rubber scraper, washed with PBS, and centrifuged at 1000 rpm for 5 min. Pellets were washed, centrifuged, and resuspended in PBS with JC-1 probe in concentration 5 μg/mL. Mitochondrial potential changes were measured using a BD FACS Aria sorter (BD Biosciences, Franklin Lakes, New Jersey, USA).

2.7. Annexin V–Fluorescein Isothiocyanate (FITC)/PI Binding Assay

HeLa cells were incubated for 24 h at 37 °C in 6-well plates with 10 μM ferrocenes. SiHa cells were more resistant; thus, the conditions were modified to 20 μM concentrations. Cells were harvested by acutase, washed twice with PBS, centrifuged at 1000 rpm for 5 min, and then resuspended in Annexin V Binding buffer (10 mM HEPES/NaOH, pH 7.4; 14 mM NaCl; 2.5 mM $CaCl_2$) at a concentration of 1 million cells/mL. A volume of 100 μL of cell suspension was pipetted into the 1.5 mL tube and mixed with fluorescein isothiocyanate (FITC)-labeled Annexin V (BioLegend, San Diego, USA) and PI solutions. The cells were gently vortexed and incubated for 15 min at 22 °C in the dark. After incubation,

400 μL of Annexin V Binding buffer was added and samples were measured using a flow cytometer (Navios, Beckman Coulter, USA).

2.8. *Western Blot Analysis*

Hela and SiHa cell lines were treated with 2 μM concentration of selected ferrocenes, and half of them were subsequently irradiated with 4 Gy of ionizing radiation. All samples were then incubated for 24 h. Cells were washed twice with ice-cold PBS, scraped off with a rubber scraper, and then lysed in nonyl phenoxypolyethoxylethanol (NP-40) lysis buffer (150 mM NaCl, 50 mM TrisHCl pH 8.0, 5 mM NaF, 5 mM EDTA, 1% NP-40, 1:100 phosphatase inhibitor cocktail, and 1:100 protease inhibitor cocktail, both cocktails from Sigma-Aldrich, St. Louis, USA). The protein concentrations were measured via Bradford protein assay (Bio-Rad, Hercules, California, USA). A quantity of 20 μg of protein lysate per sample was applied and separated on 10% SDS polyacrylamide gel, then transferred onto nitrocellulose blotting membrane (Pall Life Sciences, New York, USA). The accuracy of sample loading was verified with Ponceau staining. Membranes were blocked in 5% milk with 0.1% Tween 20 in PBS and probed overnight with the following antibodies: anti β-actin monoclonal antibody (Sigma-Aldrich, St. Louis, Missouri, USA) served as a loading control, SQSTM1 p62 antibody (A-6) (Santa Cruz Biotechnology, Dallas, Texas, USA), and LC3B antibody (Novus Biologicals, Littleton, USA). Membranes were washed with PBS containing 0.1% Tween and incubated with secondary IgG antibodies SWAR-Px (Swine Anti-Rabbit Immunoglobulins- horseradish peroxidase, #P0217) and RAM-Px (Rabbit Anti-Mouse Immunoglobulins- horseradish peroxidase, #P0161) (Dako, Glostrup, Denmark) for 1 h. Positive signals were visualized with enhanced chemiluminescence reagent (ECL; Amersham Pharmacia Biotech, UK) using a G:BOX Chemi XX6 System (Syngene, Cambridge, United Kingdom). Ordinarily used chemicals were obtained from Sigma-Aldrich (St. Louis, Missouri, USA).

2.9. *Immunofluorescence Staining*

Cells were seeded on coverslips in 12-well plates. After 24 h of incubation at 37 °C with 5 μM concentration of ferrocenes **1b**, **2a**, and **3** and with 0.2 μM Bafilomycin A as a positive control, coverslips with adherent cells were washed with PBS solution and fixed with 4% formaldehyde. After permeabilization with 0.2% Triton-X100 (Sigma-Aldrich, St. Louis, Missouri, USA), cells were incubated with primary antibodies recognizing p62 and LC3B, respectively, for 1 h at 37 °C. The cells were then washed and incubated with fluorescent-dye-conjugated secondary antibodies (ab96899 for LC3B and ab96881 for p62; Abcam, Cambridge, United Kingdom) for 1 h at room temperature. In parallel, Hoechst staining was used to visualize nuclei. PBS was used for washing and Vectashield (Cole-Parmer, Vernon Hills, Illinois, USA) for mounting the coverslip. Cells were visualized on a Nuance Multispectral Tissue Imaging System FX (PerkinElmer, Waltham, Massachusetts, USA).

2.10. *Colony Forming Assay (CFA)*

The radiosensitizing properties of the selected compounds were tested in vitro according to the standardized protocol for colony forming assay [30]. Briefly, cells were trypsinized, centrifuged, and resuspended in fresh medium. The suspensions were then plated at a density of 250 cells per well in 12-well plates and left for 24 h in an incubator to adhere. The next day, selected ferrocenes were added in concentrations of 0.5 and 1.0 μM for HeLa cells and 1.0 and 2.0 μM for the more-resistant SiHa cells. Following 1–2 h of incubation, the cells were irradiated according to the protocol in Section 2.11. The cells were then further incubated under standard conditions for 14 days, and colonies were fixed with crystal violet staining/fixing solution—1% methanol (Penta, Chrudim, Czech Republic), 0.05% crystal violet (Merck Millipore, Burlington, Massachusetts, USA), and 3.7% formaldehyde (Sigma-Aldrich, St. Louis, USA) in PBS and manually counted. Surviving fractions (SF) were calculated by comparing the number of colonies in irradiated and nonirradiated (control) plates using a linear-quadratic model for cell death after irradiation. To obtain the final radiosensitizing effect, dose-modifying factors (DMF) were calculated as the ratios of surviving fractions in cells irradiated with and without tested ferrocenes at selected doses.

2.11. Ionizing Radiation

Orthovoltage X-ray irradiation was performed using an Xstrahl 200 radiotherapy system (Xstrahl, Surrey, England) as a single fraction of 2, 4, or 6 Gy with energy 200 kV with a half-value layer of 1 mm of Cu. The field size was 20 × 20 cm, the distance from source to irradiated wells was 50 cm, and the dose rate was 0.38 Gy/min. To obtain an adequate dose at a surface, wells were covered with a 1 cm thick bolus material. Control cells were taken from the incubator and handled similarly to treated cells, except during irradiation when they were placed outside the treatment room to avoid any exposure to ionizing radiation. All treatments were done at room temperature.

3. Results

3.1. Cytotoxic Activity

The cytotoxicity of ferrocenes was tested in vitro against cervical cancer cell lines CaSki, SiHa, and HeLa using MTT tests. Since nephrotoxicity remains the main side effect of cisplatin treatment, the toxicity of the selected (most active) complexes against noncancerous human embryonic kidney cells (HEK 293) was evaluated along with retinal epithelial cells (RPE-1). Table 1 shows the IC_{50} values for particular ferrocenes. According to the cytotoxicity results, the three most active substances—**1b**, **2a**, and **3**—were selected and used for further testing.

Table 1. Cytotoxic effects of the studied ferrocenes in micromolar concentrations after 24 h against selected cell lines.

Comp.	Ca Ski	SiHa	HeLa	RPE-1	HEK 293
Cisplatin	35.1 ± 8.7	26.6 ± 4.1	28.2 ± 5.9	46.8 ± 6.0	25.3 ± 8.6
1a	69.4 ± 8.6	17.1 ± 3.4	61.5 ± 2.9	82.8 ± 3.7	>100
1b	6.2 ± 2.1	9.9 ± 2.2	6.4 ± 1.6	5.1 ± 0.8	35.6 ± 6.2
1c	12.5 ± 0.6	18.2 ± 3.1	10.6 ± 2.5	11.0 ± 2.4	16.7 ± 2.0
2a	8.3 ± 2.3	14.1 ± 3.4	7.3 ± 1.2	4.7 ± 0.1	6.2 ± 1.6
2b	15.0 ± 1.0	30.2 ± 2.9	13.0 ± 0.6	8.2 ± 0.4	5.4 ± 0.6
3	7.6 ± 1.3	11.1 ± 1.5	6.5 ± 0.4	8.5 ± 1.1	9.5 ± 1.0
4	>100	>100	>100	>100	>100
5	>100	91.8 ± 9.4	7.7 ± 1.1	7.4 ± 2.0	3.0 ± 0.3

3.2. Effect of Selected Ferrocenes on Cell Cycle

To determine the effect of the tested ferrocenes on the cell cycle, PI assay was used. HeLa cells showed significant changes in cell cycle distribution, especially an increased proportion of cells in S phase and a corresponding decrease in G0/G1 phases (Figure 2). On the other hand, SiHa cells showed no significant changes in cell cycle distribution in response to the tested ferrocenes (data not shown). Importantly, the applied doses of irradiation in our experiment had no significant effect on cell cycle distribution except for increased accumulation of HeLa cells in the G2/M phase in response to **3**.

3.3. Analysis of Cell Death

Since MTT tests clearly confirmed the cytotoxicity of the selected compounds, closer examination of the specific mechanisms and pathways associated with cell death was performed.

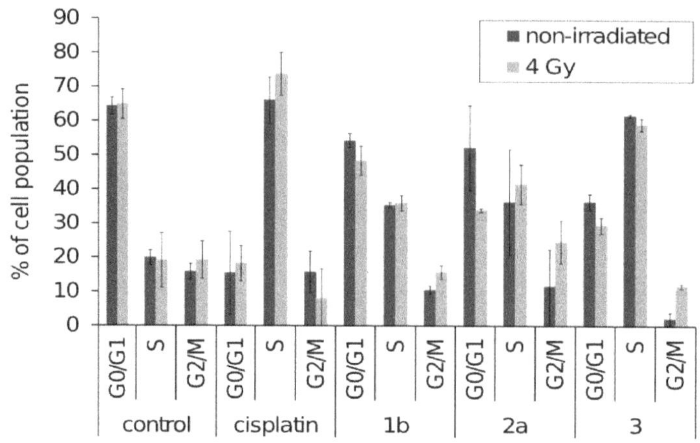

Figure 2. Cell cycle analysis of HeLa cells exposed for 24 h to 5 μM ferrocenes either with or without 4 Gy irradiation.

3.3.1. Effect of Selected Ferrocenes on ROS Production

A cell-membrane-permeable chloromethyl derivative of H_2DCFDA was used to determine the production of reactive oxygen species. An increased amount of ROS was measured after 2 h of treatment with selected ferrocenes in 10 μM concentration. Untreated cells and cells treated with hydrogen peroxide were used as controls. The relative fluorescence values are summarized in Figure 3.

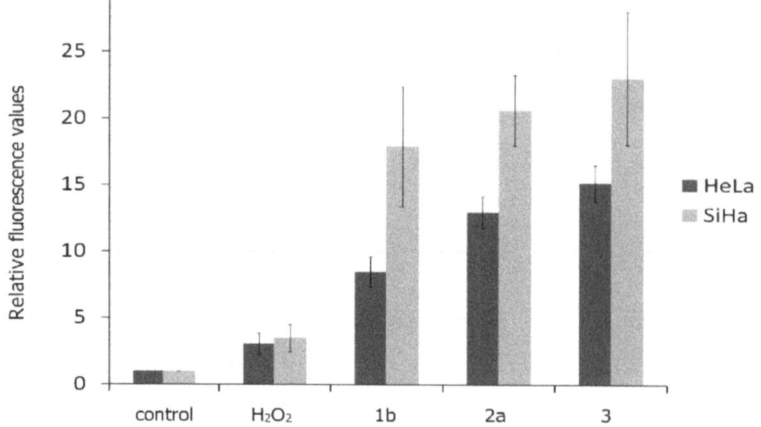

Figure 3. Reactive oxygen species (ROS) production in HeLa and SiHa cells after treatment with the most active ferrocenes. Untreated cells were used as a negative control, H_2O_2 was used as a positive control. Data were normalized to control untreated cells.

3.3.2. Effect of **1b**, **2a**, and **3** on Mitochondrial Membrane Potential

Increased levels of reactive oxygen species can be closely associated with mitochondrial metabolism [31–33]. Thus, the JC-1 probe, routinely used for measuring the state of mitochondrial membranes and their potential in a wide spectrum of cell types, was applied [34–37]. Increased mitochondrial potential in HeLa cells (by about 50% to 100%) was observed after treatment with 5 μM ferrocenes. SiHa cells were resistant under the same conditions, but increasing the concentration to 40 μM caused a similar change in mitochondrial potential (Figure 4).

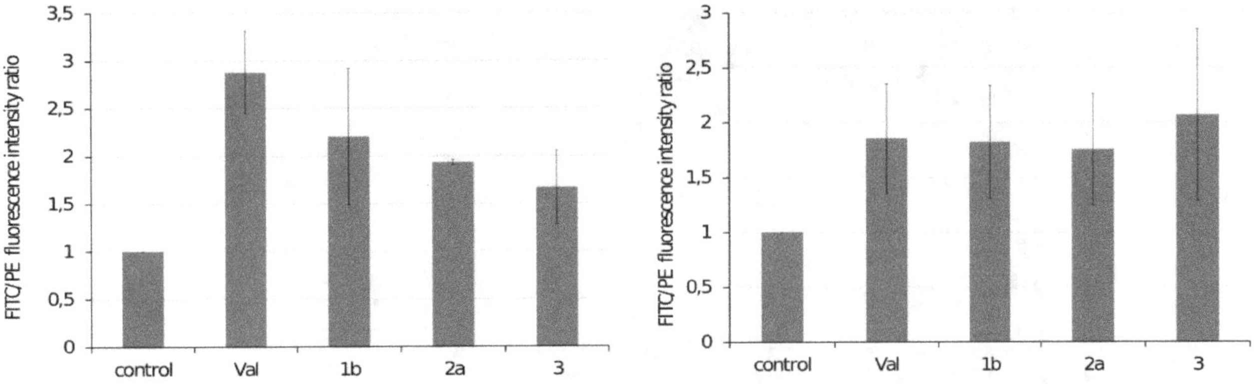

(a) (b)

Figure 4. Determination of mitochondrial membrane depolarization in (**a**) HeLa cells exposed to 5 μM ferrocenes for 24 h and (**b**) SiHa cells exposed to 40 μM ferrocenes for 6 h. Valinomycin (Val) was used as a positive control. Fluorescein isothiocyanate (FITC) and Phycoerythrin (PE) fluorescence intensity ratio were determined. Data are reported in relation to untreated cells (control).

3.3.3. Analysis of Apoptosis

Increased production of reactive oxygen radicals along with the disruption of the mitochondrial membrane may indicate the involvement of apoptosis as a possible mode of cell death. Annexin V labeling with FITC was used for cytometric measurement of the translocation of phosphatidylserine to the outer surface of the plasma membrane [38–40]. PI staining of DNA was used to detect the late phase of apoptosis. Treatment with active ferrocenes was associated with the induction of both early and late phases of apoptosis in either cell line. Necrotic cells were not observed in significant amounts (Figure 5).

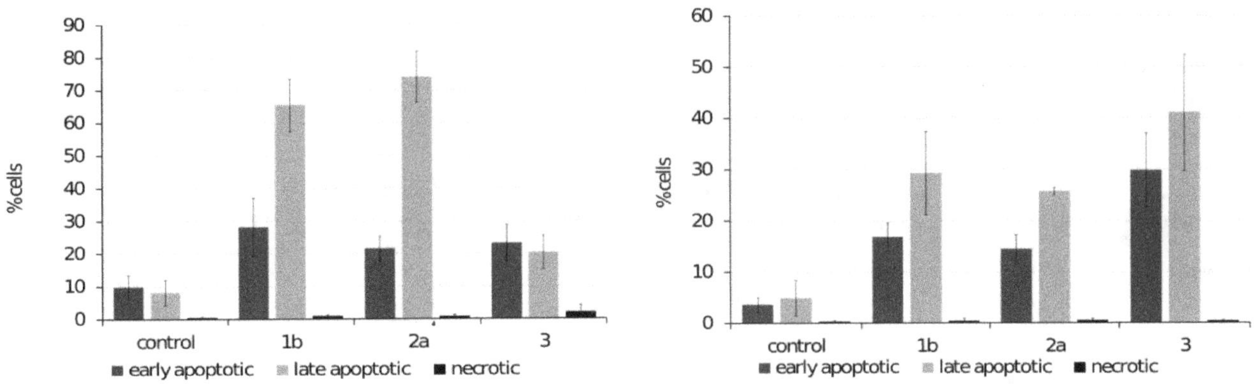

(a) (b)

Figure 5. Determination of apoptosis by flow cytometry in (**a**) HeLa cells treated with 10 μM ferrocenes and (**b**) SiHa cells treated with 20 μM ferrocenes.

3.4. Autophagy Detection

The production of ROS is not specific only to apoptotic cells. Autophagy can also be induced by higher levels of reactive oxygen species [41,42]. To elucidate whether autophagy is also elevated in response to treatment with ferrocenes, the levels of autophagy-associated proteins p62 and cleaved LC3B were determined by immunofluorescent staining in HeLa cells. Indeed, increased levels of both p62 and LC3B were observed in these cells exposed to particular ferrocenes (Figure 6). Clear elevation of the LC3B level was also confirmed by Western blot analysis in both cell lines exposed to particular ferrocenes (Figure 7). In parallel, we also analyzed the combined effect of irradiation on LC3B cleavage. Interestingly, a clear decrease in the LC3B level was observed, predominantly in SiHa cells.

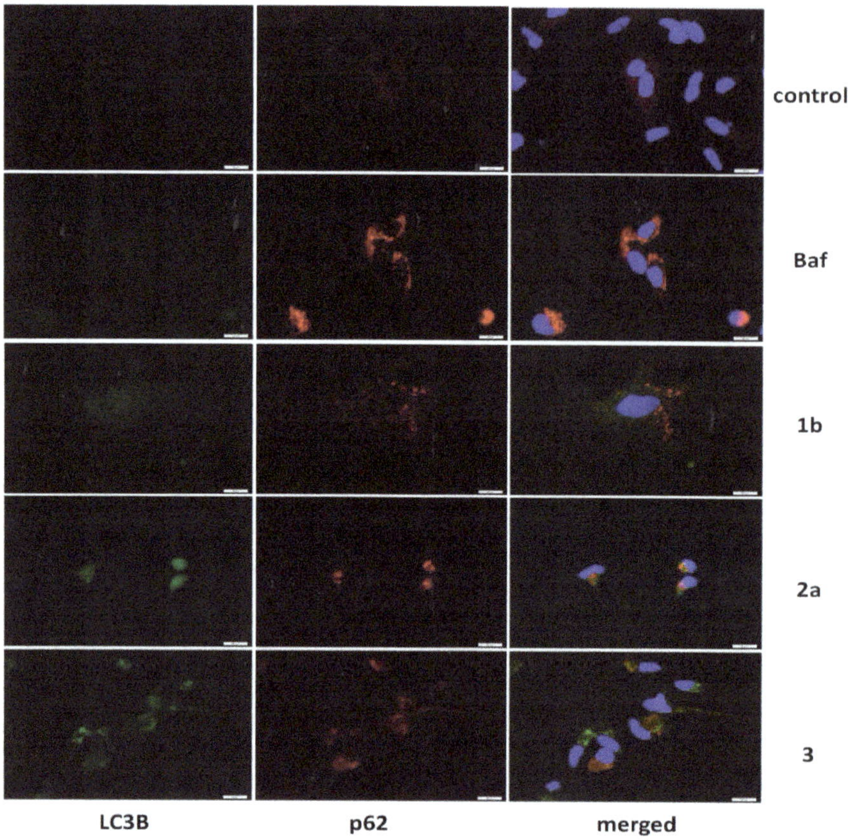

Figure 6. Detection of autophagy-related proteins in HeLa cells exposed to 5 μM ferrocenes for 24 h. Disruptor of autophagic flux Bafilomycin A (Baf) [43] was used as a positive control. Nuclei are stained with DAPI.

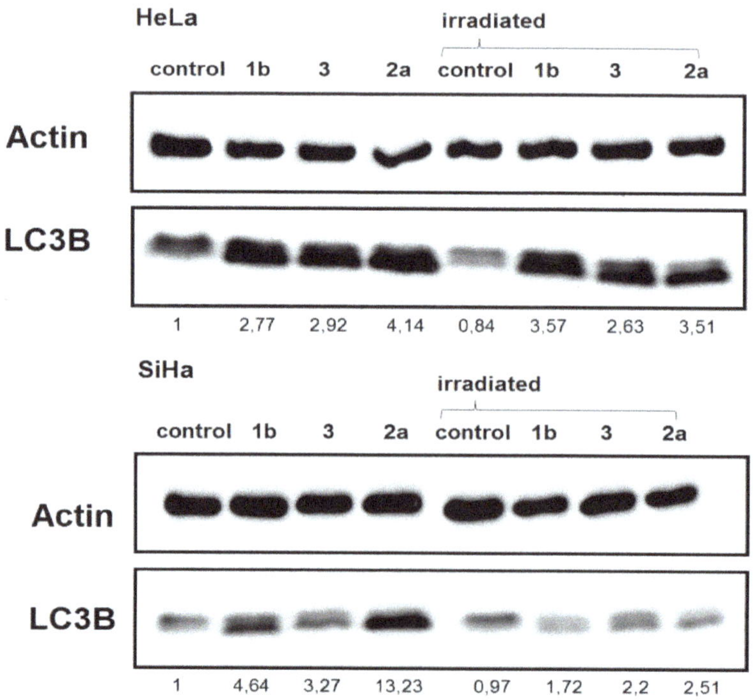

Figure 7. Detection of autophagy-associated protein LC3B in HeLa (upper part) and SiHa (lower part) cells. β-actin served as a loading control. Cells were treated with 2 μM concentrations of selected ferrocenes with or without a 4 Gy dose of irradiation.

3.5. Sensitivity to Ionizing Radiation

Radiotherapy is a standard treatment option in advanced cervical carcinomas. Colony forming assay was used to evaluate the potential radiosensitizing effect of the selected ferrocenes [30].

3.5.1. Determination of the Surviving Fraction

The surviving fraction (SF) calculated from CFA is the ratio of surviving colonies in the irradiated and nonirradiated plates. Figure 8 shows that ferrocene **1b** had a potent radiosensitizing effect on both cell lines. In the SiHa cell line, a similar, albeit smaller, effect was observed for **2a**.

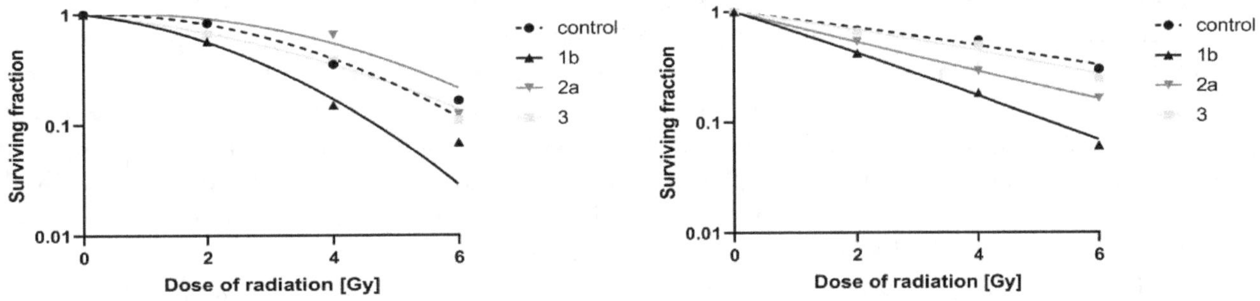

(a) (b)

Figure 8. Graphical interpretation of the surviving fraction (SF) for the combination of selected ferrocenes with different doses of irradiation in (**a**) HeLa cells exposed to 1 μM ferrocenes and (**b**) SiHa cells treated with 2 μM ferrocenes.

3.5.2. Evaluation of Dose-Modifying Factors

Dose-modifying factors (DMFs) assess the additive effect of a tested drug when used in combination with ionizing radiation. They are the ratios of doses needed to obtain the same surviving fractions in cells irradiated with and without the tested ferrocenes [44]. Values below 0.8 were considered as showing an antagonistic effect, values between 0.8 and 1.2 as showing no effect, and values above 1.2 as showing a synergistic effect (Table 2).

Table 2. Dose-modifying factors for the selected ferrocenes in HeLa and SiHa cells.

HeLa Cells				SiHa Cells			
Conc.	**1b**	**2a**	**3**	**Conc.**	**1b**	**2a**	**3**
0.5 μM	0.9 ± 0.08	1.0 ± 0.1	0.9 ± 0.08	1 μM	1.4 ± 0.19	1.3 ± 0.07	0.9 ± 0.08
1 μM	1.6 ± 0.13	0.9 ± 0.2	1.2 ± 0.08	2 μM	1.8 ± 0.5	1.4 ± 0.17	1.2 ± 0.08

4. Discussion

In recent articles, syntheses of some ferrocenes have been published [23,24]. Several of these compounds showed a clear cytotoxic effect that was equal or even greater when compared with cisplatin, which has become a mainstay of cancer therapy. We hypothesize that ferrocenes, similarly to cisplatin, may, in combination with ionizing radiation, show a synergistic cytotoxic effect. This radiosensitization effect could be particularly beneficial in the treatment of chemoresistant malignancies, e.g., cervical tumors that are generally perceived as resistant to cisplatin [45,46].

In previous studies, the mechanisms of transport of substituted ferrocenes were investigated using differential pulse voltammetry and inductively coupled plasma mass spectrometry. We identified membrane transferrin-receptor-mediated endocytosis of transferrin-bound ferrocene as the major mechanism of cellular uptake. Importantly, the rate of ferrocene accumulation in cancer cells is proportional to its cytotoxic effects [24,47]. To assess the exact mode of action of the studied ferrocenes, several methods were used. First, while no changes in cell cycle distribution were observed in SiHa cells, HeLa cells showed increased accumulation of cells in the S phase in response to treatment with all tested ferrocenes.

However, the increase in proportion of cells in the S phase predominantly after treatment with **1b** and **2a** was significantly lower when compared to that in cisplatin-treated cells. This could be of potential interest, since the doses of cisplatin used probably slow down DNA synthesis due to repairing its damage, which is associated with the accumulation of cells in the S phase [48], and cells in S phase are generally considered to be more radioresistant [49]. Thus, even though cisplatin is commonly used with radiotherapy, the effect of ionizing radiation in this combination is probably partly attenuated because cisplatin actually increases the proportion of cells in the S phase [50,51]. Therefore, treatment with ferrocenes resulting in the induction of cell cycle arrest in the S phase to a much lesser extent compared to cisplatin would be more effective, bringing greater benefit to these patients.

Second, a potent increase in reactive oxygen species was observed upon treatment with the selected ferrocenes. This can be explained by the basic chemical structure of the ferrocene core that is known as a catalyst in a Fenton reaction generating both hydroxyl radicals and higher oxidation states of the iron. Thus, in the presence of transition metals, H_2O_2, a product of mitochondrial oxidative respiration, is reduced inside the cells; this generates oxygen radicals responsible for damage to all macromolecules, including DNA, proteins, and membrane phospholipids that are damaged by the peroxidation of unsaturated fatty acids in exposed cells [52–54]. In recent years, several studies have confirmed potent induction of ROS by a range of organometallic complexes, including ferrocenes, in cancer cells [55–62]. These studies imply their possible utilization in cancer research and treatment. Our current results show a large increase in levels of reactive oxygen species after treatment with ferrocenes **1b**, **2a**, and **3**, which indicates their impact on the redox homeostasis in tumor cells.

Third, due to the aforementioned increase in ROS production, the effect of the tested compounds on mitochondrial function was also analyzed. Our experiments showed clear changes in mitochondrial membrane potential. These changes are generally considered to be an early step in apoptosis after treatment with different drugs [63,64]. Depolarization of the mitochondrial membrane leads to the release of cytochrome c from the mitochondria. This process triggers the formation of an apoptosome and the activation of caspases, launching the intrinsic apoptotic pathway [65]. Furthermore, early and late stages of apoptosis were both detected via Annexin V assay and DNA labeling by PI. These findings are in agreement with those of other studies showing that many different ferrocene-containing compounds, e.g., ferrocifens, Pt–ferrocene complexes [66,67], and ferrocenes combined with retinoids, are able to activate apoptotic cell death in cancer cells [68–70].

Elevated levels of ROS can also lead to the induction of autophagy as a defense mechanism that allows cell survival during stress conditions. An increase in autophagy-related proteins was observed, especially for cleaved-form LC3B. These changes were most prominent after treatment with ferrocenes **1b** and **2a**. It is well known that autophagy can play a dual role in response to drug treatment. On one hand, upregulation of autophagy could help in the formation of cancer cells resistant to chemotherapy [71]. On the other hand, excessive elevation of autophagy may assist in the induction of programmed cell death [72]. In our study, combination of ferrocenes with irradiation led to a decrease in the amount of LC3B protein. The decrease was most pronounced in response to ferrocene **2a**. It can therefore be assumed that autophagy induction helps cells to overcome exposure to ferrocenes. In line with these findings, combined treatment with ionizing radiation attenuates autophagy induction and results in significantly higher anti-tumor efficacy. This correlates with the CFA results, which showed decreased colony formation rates after combination of ferrocene **1b** and partially **2a** with radiotherapy when compared to radiotherapy alone. To quantify this interplay, the dose-modifying factor for each ferrocene was calculated. The most pronounced synergistic effect was observed for ferrocene **1b** (1.6× increased effectiveness of radiotherapy in HeLa and 1.8× in SiHa cell lines) and for ferrocene **2a** (1.4× for the SiHa cell line).

5. Conclusions

A series of ferrocenes based on the general formula $[Fe(\eta^5\text{-}C_5H_4CH_2(p\text{-}C_6H_4)CH_2(N\text{-het}))_2]$ bearing either substituted or unsubstituted saturated five- and six-membered nitrogen-containing heterocycles showed higher cytotoxic activity than cisplatin against cervical cancer cell lines. These ferrocenes were able to increase the production of reactive oxygen species and disrupt mitochondrial homeostasis. As a consequence of these processes, the onset of a cell death mechanism via apoptosis and the activation of autophagy were observed. Furthermore, two of these ferrocenes—**1b** and **2a**—showed increased cytotoxic effects when combined with irradiation. However, the precise relationship between ionizing radiation and ferrocene derivatives needs further investigation. On the other hand, to put this problem into perspective, precise knowledge of the interaction between ionizing radiation and cisplatin is also unknown, and this holds true for many other chemotherapeutic drugs as well.

The combination of ferrocene **1b** and, to a lesser degree, **2a** with irradiation resulted in greater efficacy than either treatment alone in cervical cancer cell lines. Thus, our results suggest that the selected ferrocenes could be used in combination with radiotherapy, representing promising candidates for further investigation. Alternatively, the addition of ferrocene compounds to standard chemoradiation with cisplatin could also be considered. However, care needs to be taken to evaluate the potential increase in toxicity, since the studied ferrocenes and cisplatin have partly overlapping effects, mainly in the production of reactive oxygen species.

Author Contributions: Conceptualization, H.S. and V.R.; methodology, H.S.; software, H.S. and V.R.; validation H.S. and V.R.; chemical synthesis, J.P. and J.K., formal analysis, H.S.; investigation, H.S.; writing—original draft preparation, H.S.; writing—review and editing, V.R. and H.R.; visualization, H.S.; supervision, R.H.; project administration, R.H.; funding acquisition, J.P., J.K. and R.H. All authors have read and agreed to the published version of the manuscript.

Acknowledgments: At this point we would like to thank L. Sommerova for help with flow cytometry analyses.

References

1. International Agency for Research on Cancer. Cancer Incidence in Five Continents Time Trends. Available online: http://ci5.iarc.fr/CI5plus/Default.aspx (accessed on 24 June 2018).
2. Chovanec, J.; Náležinská, M. Přehled diagnostiky a léčby karcinomu děložního hrdla. *Onkologie* **2014**, *8*, 269–274.
3. Ferlay, J.; Colombet, M.; Bray, F. Cancer Incidence in Five Continents, CI5plus: IARC CancerBase No. 9. Available online: http://ci5.iarc.fr (accessed on 18 October 2019).
4. Walboomers, J.M.; Jacobs, M.V.; Manos, M.M.; Bosch, F.X.; Kummer, J.A.; Shah, K.V.; Snijders, P.J.; Peto, J.; Meijer, C.J.; Munoz, N. Human papillomavirus is a necessary cause of invasive cervical cancer worldwide. *J. Pathol.* **1999**, *189*, 12–19. [CrossRef]
5. Marth, C.; Landoni, F.; Mahner, S.; McCormack, M.; Gonzalez-Martin, A.; Colombo, N. Cervical cancer: ESMO Clinical Practice Guidelines for diagnosis, treatment and follow-up. *Ann. Oncol. Off. J. Eur. Soc. Med. Oncol.* **2018**, *29*, 262. [CrossRef] [PubMed]
6. Vale, C.; Tierney, J.F.; Stewart, L.A.; Brady, M.; Dinshaw, K.; Jakobsen, A.; Parmar, M.K.; Thomas, G.; Trimble, T.; Alberts, D.S.; et al. Reducing uncertainties about the effects of chemoradiotherapy for cervical cancer: A systematic review and meta-analysis of individual patient data from 18 randomized trials. *J. Clin. Oncol.* **2008**, *26*, 5802–5812.
7. Galanski, M.; Jakupec, M.A.; Keppler, B.K. Update of the preclinical situation of anticancer platinum complexes: Novel design strategies and innovative analytical approaches. *Curr. Med. Chem.* **2005**, *12*, 2075–2094. [CrossRef] [PubMed]
8. Peter, S.; Aderibigbe, B.A. Ferrocene-Based Compounds with Antimalaria/Anticancer Activity. *Molecules* **2019**, *24*, 3604. [CrossRef] [PubMed]
9. Sirignano, E.; Saturnino, C.; Botta, A.; Sinicropi, M.S.; Caruso, A.; Pisano, A.; Lappano, R.; Maggiolini, M.; Longo, P. Synthesis, characterization and cytotoxic activity on breast cancer cells of new half-titanocene derivatives. *Bioorg. Med. Chem. Lett.* **2013**, *23*, 3458–3462. [CrossRef]

10. Saturnino, C.; Sirignano, E.; Botta, A.; Sinicropi, M.S.; Caruso, A.; Pisano, A.; Lappano, R.; Maggiolini, M.; Longo, P. New titanocene derivatives with high antiproliferative activity against breast cancer cells. *Bioorg. Med. Chem. Lett.* **2014**, *24*, 136–140. [CrossRef]
11. Saturnino, C.; Barone, I.; Iacopetta, D.; Mariconda, A.; Sinicropi, M.S.; Rosano, C.; Campana, A.; Catalano, S.; Longo, P.; Ando, S. N-heterocyclic carbene complexes of silver and gold as novel tools against breast cancer progression. *Future Med. Chem.* **2016**, *8*, 2213–2229. [CrossRef]
12. Iacopetta, D.; Mariconda, A.; Saturnino, C.; Caruso, A.; Palma, G.; Ceramella, J.; Muia, N.; Perri, M.; Sinicropi, M.S.; Caroleo, M.C.; et al. Novel Gold and Silver Carbene Complexes Exert Antitumor Effects Triggering the Reactive Oxygen Species Dependent Intrinsic Apoptotic Pathway. *Chem. Med. Chem.* **2017**, *12*, 2054–2065. [CrossRef]
13. Alessio, E.; Messori, L. The Deceptively Similar Ruthenium(III) Drug Candidates KP1019 and NAMI-A Have Different Actions. What Did We Learn in the Past 30 Years? *Met. Life Sci.* **2018**, *18*, 141.
14. Ari, F.; Cevatemre, B.; Armutak, E.I.; Aztopal, N.; Yilmaz, V.T.; Ulukaya, E. Apoptosis-inducing effect of a palladium(II) saccharinate complex of terpyridine on human breast cancer cells in vitro and in vivo. *Bioorg. Med. Chem.* **2014**, *22*, 4948–4954. [CrossRef]
15. Carter, R.; Westhorpe, A.; Romero, M.J.; Habtemariam, A.; Gallevo, C.R.; Bark, Y.; Menezes, N.; Sadler, P.J.; Sharma, R.A. Radiosensitisation of human colorectal cancer cells by ruthenium(II) arene anticancer complexes. *Sci. Rep.* **2016**, *6*, 20596. [CrossRef]
16. Mesbahi, A. A review on gold nanoparticles radiosensitization effect in radiation therapy of cancer. *Rep. Pract. Oncol. Radiother. J. Greatpoland Cancer Cent. Pozn. Pol. Soc. Radiat. Oncol.* **2010**, *15*, 176–180. [CrossRef]
17. Gill, M.R.; Menon, J.U.; Jarman, P.J.; Owen, J.; Skaripa-Koukelli, I.; Able, S.; Thomas, J.A.; Carlisle, R.; Vallis, K.A. (111)In-labelled polymeric nanoparticles incorporating a ruthenium-based radiosensitizer for EGFR-targeted combination therapy in oesophageal cancer cells. *Nanoscale* **2018**, *10*, 10596–10608. [CrossRef]
18. Hainfeld, J.F.; Slatkin, D.N.; Smilowitz, H.M. The use of gold nanoparticles to enhance radiotherapy in mice. *Phys. Med. Biol.* **2004**, *49*, 309–315. [CrossRef]
19. Chang, M.Y.; Shiau, A.L.; Chen, Y.H.; Chang, C.J.; Chen, H.H.; Wu, C.L. Increased apoptotic potential and dose-enhancing effect of gold nanoparticles in combination with single-dose clinical electron beams on tumor-bearing mice. *Cancer Sci.* **2008**, *99*, 1479–1484. [CrossRef]
20. Hainfeld, J.F.; Smilowitz, H.M.; O'Connor, M.J.; Dilmanian, F.A.; Slatkin, D.N. Gold nanoparticle imaging and radiotherapy of brain tumors in mice. *Nanomedicine* **2013**, *8*, 1601–1609. [CrossRef]
21. Teicher, B.A.; Jacobs, J.L.; Cathcart, K.N.; Abrams, M.J.; Vollano, J.F.; Picker, D.H. Some complexes of cobalt(III) and iron(III) are radiosensitizers of hypoxic EMT6 cells. *Radiat. Res.* **1987**, *109*, 36–46. [CrossRef]
22. Joy, A.M.; Goodgame, D.M.; Stratford, I.J. High efficiency of ferricenium salts as radiosensitizers of V79 cells in vitro and the KHT tumor in vivo. *Int. J. Radiat. Oncol. Biol. Phys.* **1989**, *16*, 1053–1056. [CrossRef]
23. Hodík, T.; Lamač, M.; Červenková Šťastná, L.; Cuřínová, P.; Karban, J.; Skoupilová, H.; Hrstka, R.; Císařová, I.; Gyepes, R.; Pinkas, J. Improving cytotoxic properties of ferrocenes by incorporation of saturated N-heterocycles. *J. Organomet. Chem.* **2017**, *846*, 141–151. [CrossRef]
24. Bartosik, M.; Koubkova, L.; Karban, J.; Cervenkova Stastna, L.; Hodik, T.; Lamac, M.; Pinkas, J.; Hrstka, R. Electrochemical analysis of a novel ferrocene derivative as a potential antitumor drug. *Analyst* **2015**, *140*, 5864–5867. [CrossRef]
25. Kvardova, V.; Hrstka, R.; Walerych, D.; Muller, P.; Matoulkova, E.; Hruskova, V.; Stelclova, D.; Sova, P.; Vojtesek, B. The new platinum(IV) derivative LA-12 shows stronger inhibitory effect on Hsp90 function compared to cisplatin. *Mol. Cancer* **2010**, *9*, 147. [CrossRef]
26. Darzynkiewicz, Z.; Halicka, H.D.; Zhao, H. Analysis of cellular DNA content by flow and laser scanning cytometry. *Adv. Exp. Med. Biol.* **2010**, *676*, 137–147.
27. Koubkova, L.; Vyzula, R.; Karban, J.; Pinkas, J.; Ondrouskova, E.; Vojtesek, B.; Hrstka, R. Evaluation of cytotoxic activity of titanocene difluorides and determination of their mechanism of action in ovarian cancer cells. *Investig. New Drugs* **2015**, *33*, 1123–1132. [CrossRef]
28. Matarrese, P.; Tinari, A.; Mormone, E.; Bianco, G.A.; Toscano, M.A.; Ascione, B.; Rabinovich, G.A.; Malorni, W. Galectin-1 sensitizes resting human T lymphocytes to Fas (CD95)-mediated cell death via mitochondrial hyperpolarization, budding, and fission. *J. Biol. Chem.* **2005**, *280*, 6969–6985. [CrossRef]

29. Ruan, Q.; Lesort, M.; MacDonald, M.E.; Johnson, G.V. Striatal cells from mutant huntingtin knock-in mice are selectively vulnerable to mitochondrial complex II inhibitor-induced cell death through a non-apoptotic pathway. *Hum. Mol. Genet.* **2004**, *13*, 669–681. [CrossRef]
30. Franken, N.A.; Rodermond, H.M.; Stap, J.; Haveman, J.; van Bree, C. Clonogenic assay of cells in vitro. *Nat. Protoc.* **2006**, *1*, 2315–2319. [CrossRef]
31. Starkov, A.A. The role of mitochondria in reactive oxygen species metabolism and signaling. *Ann. N. Y. Acad. Sci.* **2008**, *1147*, 37–52. [CrossRef]
32. Marchi, S.; Giorgi, C.; Suski, J.M.; Agnoletto, C.; Bononi, A.; Bonora, M.; De Marchi, E.; Missiroli, S.; Patergnani, S.; Poletti, F.; et al. Mitochondria-ros crosstalk in the control of cell death and aging. *J. Signal Transduct.* **2012**, *2012*, 329635. [CrossRef]
33. Di Meo, S.; Reed, T.T.; Venditti, P.; Victor, V.M. Role of ROS and RNS Sources in Physiological and Pathological Conditions. *Oxid. Med. Cell. Longev.* **2016**, *2016*, 1245049. [CrossRef]
34. Cossarizza, A.; Ceccarelli, D.; Masini, A. Functional heterogeneity of an isolated mitochondrial population revealed by cytofluorometric analysis at the single organelle level. *Exp. Cell Res.* **1996**, *222*, 84–94. [CrossRef]
35. Di Lisa, F.; Blank, P.S.; Colonna, R.; Gambassi, G.; Silverman, H.S.; Stern, M.D.; Hansford, R.G. Mitochondrial membrane potential in single living adult rat cardiac myocytes exposed to anoxia or metabolic inhibition. *J. Physiol.* **1995**, *486*, 1–13. [CrossRef]
36. Sick, T.J.; Perez-Pinzon, M.A. Optical methods for probing mitochondrial function in brain slices. *Methods* **1999**, *18*, 104–108. [CrossRef]
37. White, R.J.; Reynolds, I.J. Mitochondrial depolarization in glutamate-stimulated neurons: An early signal specific to excitotoxin exposure. *J. Neurosci.* **1996**, *16*, 5688–5697. [CrossRef]
38. Sekine, C.; Moriyama, Y.; Koyanagi, A.; Koyama, N.; Ogata, H.; Okumura, K.; Yagita, H. Differential regulation of splenic CD8- dendritic cells and marginal zone B cells by Notch ligands. *Int. Immunol.* **2009**, *21*, 295–301. [CrossRef]
39. Galski, H.; Oved-Gelber, T.; Simanovsky, M.; Lazarovici, P.; Gottesman, M.M.; Nagler, A. P-glycoprotein-dependent resistance of cancer cells toward the extrinsic TRAIL apoptosis signaling pathway. *Biochem. Pharm.* **2013**, *86*, 584–596. [CrossRef]
40. Seguier, S.; Tartour, E.; Guerin, C.; Couty, L.; Lemitre, M.; Lallement, L.; Folliguet, M.; El Naderi, S.; Terme, M.; Badoual, C.; et al. Inhibition of the differentiation of monocyte-derived dendritic cells by human gingival fibroblasts. *PLoS ONE* **2013**, *8*, e70937. [CrossRef]
41. Azad, M.B.; Chen, Y.; Gibson, S.B. Regulation of autophagy by reactive oxygen species (ROS): Implications for cancer progression and treatment. *Antioxid. Redox Signal.* **2009**, *11*, 777–790. [CrossRef]
42. Cordani, M.; Donadelli, M.; Strippoli, R.; Bazhin, A.V.; Sanchez-Alvarez, M. Interplay between ROS and Autophagy in Cancer and Aging: From Molecular Mechanisms to Novel Therapeutic Approaches. *Oxid. Med. Cell. Longev.* **2019**, *2019*, 8794612. [CrossRef]
43. Yamamoto, A.; Tagawa, Y.; Yoshimori, T.; Moriyama, Y.; Masaki, R.; Tashiro, Y. Bafilomycin A1 prevents maturation of autophagic vacuoles by inhibiting fusion between autophagosomes and lysosomes in rat hepatoma cell line, H-4-II-E cells. *Cell Struct. Funct.* **1998**, *23*, 33–42. [CrossRef] [PubMed]
44. Thames, H.D., Jr.; Rasmussen, S.L. A test for dose-modifying factors. *Radiat. Res.* **1978**, *76*, 308–324. [CrossRef] [PubMed]
45. Minagawa, Y.; Kigawa, J.; Itamochi, H.; Kanamori, Y.; Shimada, M.; Takahashi, M.; Terakawa, N. Cisplatin-resistant HeLa cells are resistant to apoptosis via p53-dependent and -independent pathways. *Jpn. J. Cancer Res.* **1999**, *90*, 1373–1379. [CrossRef] [PubMed]
46. Chen, J.; Solomides, C.; Parekh, H.; Simpkins, F.; Simpkins, H. Cisplatin resistance in human cervical, ovarian and lung cancer cells. *Cancer Chemother. Pharm.* **2015**, *75*, 1217–1227. [CrossRef]
47. Skoupilova, H.; Bartosik, M.; Sommerova, L.; Pinkas, J.; Vaculovic, T.; Kanicky, V.; Karban, J.; Hrstka, R. Ferrocenes as new anticancer drug candidates: Determination of the mechanism of action. *Eur. J. Pharm.* **2020**, *867*, 172825. [CrossRef]
48. Velma, V.; Dasari, S.R.; Tchounwou, P.B. Low Doses of Cisplatin Induce Gene Alterations, Cell Cycle Arrest, and Apoptosis in Human Promyelocytic Leukemia Cells. *Biomark. Insights* **2016**, *11*, 113–121. [CrossRef]
49. Pawlik, T.M.; Keyomarsi, K. Role of cell cycle in mediating sensitivity to radiotherapy. *Int. J. Radiat. Oncol. Biol. Phys.* **2004**, *59*, 928–942. [CrossRef] [PubMed]

50. Cruet-Hennequart, S.; Villalan, S.; Kaczmarczyk, A.; O'Meara, E.; Sokol, A.M.; Carty, M.P. Characterization of the effects of cisplatin and carboplatin on cell cycle progression and DNA damage response activation in DNA polymerase eta-deficient human cells. *Cell Cycle* **2009**, *8*, 3039–3050. [CrossRef]
51. Wagner, J.M.; Karnitz, L.M. Cisplatin-induced DNA damage activates replication checkpoint signaling components that differentially affect tumor cell survival. *Mol. Pharm.* **2009**, *76*, 208–214. [CrossRef]
52. Wang, Y.; Yin, W.; Ke, W.; Chen, W.; He, C.; Ge, Z. Multifunctional Polymeric Micelles with Amplified Fenton Reaction for Tumor Ablation. *Biomacromolecules* **2018**, *19*, 1990–1998. [CrossRef]
53. Liu, C.; Chen, W.; Qing, Z.; Zheng, J.; Xiao, Y.; Yang, S.; Wang, L.; Li, Y.; Yang, R. In Vivo Lighted Fluorescence via Fenton Reaction: Approach for Imaging of Hydrogen Peroxide in Living Systems. *Anal. Chem.* **2016**, *88*, 3998–4003. [CrossRef] [PubMed]
54. Halliwell, B.; Gutteridge, J.M. Role of free radicals and catalytic metal ions in human disease: An overview. *Methods Enzymol.* **1990**, *186*, 1–85. [PubMed]
55. Acevedo-Morantes, C.Y.; Meléndez, E.; Singh, S.P.; Ramírez-Vick, J.E. Cytotoxicity and Reactive Oxygen Species Generated by Ferrocenium and Ferrocene on MCF7 and MCF10A Cell Lines. *J. Cancer Sci. Ther.* **2012**, *4*, 271–275.
56. Gasser, G.; Ott, I.; Metzler-Nolte, N. Organometallic anticancer compounds. *J. Med. Chem.* **2011**, *54*, 3–25. [CrossRef]
57. Mooney, A.; Tiedt, R.; Maghoub, T.; O'Donovan, N.; Crown, J.; White, B.; Kenny, P.T. Structure–activity relationship and mode of action of N-(6-ferrocenyl-2-naphthoyl) dipeptide ethyl esters: Novel organometallic anticancer compounds. *J. Med. Chem.* **2012**, *55*, 5455–5466. [CrossRef] [PubMed]
58. Peng, X.; Gandhi, V. ROS-activated anticancer prodrugs: A new strategy for tumor-specific damage. *Ther. Deliv.* **2012**, *3*, 823–833. [CrossRef]
59. Podolski-Renić, A.; Bösze, S.; Dinić, J.; Kocsis, L.; Hudecz, F.; Csámpai, A.; Pešić, M. Ferrocene-Cinchona Hybrids with Triazolyl-chalcone Linker Act as Prooxidants and Sensitize Human Cancer Cell Lines to Paclitaxel. *Metallomics* **2017**, *9*, 1132–1141. [CrossRef]
60. Kovjazin, R.; Eldar, T.; Patya, M.; Vanichkin, A.; Lander, H.M.; Novogrodsky, A. Ferrocene-induced lymphocyte activation and anti-tumor activity is mediated by redox-sensitive signaling. *FASEB J. Off. Publ. Fed. Am. Soc. Exp. Biol.* **2003**, *17*, 467–469.
61. van Staveren, D.R.; Metzler-Nolte, N. Bioorganometallic chemistry of ferrocene. *Chem. Rev.* **2004**, *104*, 5931–5985. [CrossRef]
62. Santos, M.M.; Bastos, P.; Catela, I.; Zalewska, K.; Branco, L.C. Recent Advances of Metallocenes for Medicinal Chemistry. *Mini Rev. Med. Chem.* **2017**, *17*, 771–784. [CrossRef]
63. Satoh, T.; Enokido, Y.; Aoshima, H.; Uchiyama, Y.; Hatanaka, H. Changes in mitochondrial membrane potential during oxidative stress-induced apoptosis in PC12 cells. *J. Neurosci. Res.* **1997**, *50*, 413–420. [CrossRef]
64. Zhang, Y.H.; Wu, Y.L.; Tashiro, S.; Onodera, S.; Ikejima, T. Reactive oxygen species contribute to oridonin-induced apoptosis and autophagy in human cervical carcinoma HeLa cells. *Acta. Pharm. Sin.* **2011**, *32*, 1266–1275. [CrossRef] [PubMed]
65. Elena-Real, C.A.; Diaz-Quintana, A.; Gonzalez-Arzola, K.; Velazquez-Campoy, A.; Orzaez, M.; Lopez-Rivas, A.; Gil-Caballero, S.; De la Rosa, M.A.; Diaz-Moreno, I. Cytochrome c speeds up caspase cascade activation by blocking 14-3-3epsilon-dependent Apaf-1 inhibition. *Cell Death Dis.* **2018**, *9*, 365. [CrossRef]
66. Niioka, T.; Uno, T.; Yasui-Furukori, N.; Takahata, T.; Shimizu, M.; Sugawara, K.; Tateishi, T. Pharmacokinetics of low-dose nedaplatin and validation of AUC prediction in patients with non-small-cell lung carcinoma. *Cancer Chemother. Pharm.* **2007**, *59*, 575–580. [CrossRef]
67. Jaouen, G.; Vessieres, A.; Top, S. Ferrocifen type anti cancer drugs. *Chem. Soc. Rev.* **2015**, *44*, 8802–8817. [CrossRef]
68. Cortes, R.; Tarrado-Castellarnau, M.; Talancon, D.; Lopez, C.; Link, W.; Ruiz, D.; Centelles, J.J.; Quirante, J.; Cascante, M. A novel cyclometallated Pt(II)-ferrocene complex induces nuclear FOXO3a localization and apoptosis and synergizes with cisplatin to inhibit lung cancer cell proliferation. *Metallomics* **2014**, *6*, 622–633. [CrossRef]
69. Wlassoff, W.A.; Albright, C.D.; Sivashinski, M.S.; Ivanova, A.; Appelbaum, J.G.; Salganik, R.I. Hydrogen peroxide overproduced in breast cancer cells can serve as an anticancer prodrug generating apoptosis-stimulating hydroxyl radicals under the effect of tamoxifen-ferrocene conjugate. *J. Pharm. Pharm.* **2007**, *59*, 1549–1553. [CrossRef]

70. Ivanova, D.; Gronemeyer, H.; de Lera, A.R. Design and stereoselective synthesis of retinoids with ferrocene or N-butylcarbazole pharmacophores that induce post-differentiation apoptosis in acute promyelocytic leukemia cells. *Chem. Med. Chem.* **2011**, *6*, 1518–1529. [CrossRef]
71. Guo, J.Y.; Chen, H.Y.; Mathew, R.; Fan, J.; Strohecker, A.M.; Karsli-Uzunbas, G.; Kamphorst, J.J.; Chen, G.; Lemons, J.M.; Karantza, V.; et al. Activated Ras requires autophagy to maintain oxidative metabolism and tumorigenesis. *Genes Dev.* **2011**, *25*, 460–470. [CrossRef]
72. Yonekawa, T.; Thorburn, A. Autophagy and cell death. *Essays Biochem.* **2013**, *55*, 105–117.

5

Phenylpyrazalopyrimidines as Tyrosine Kinase Inhibitors: Synthesis, Antiproliferative Activity and Molecular Simulations

Bhupender S. Chhikara [1,2], Sajda Ashraf [3], Saghar Mozaffari [4], Nicole St. Jeans [2], Dindyal Mandal [2,4], Rakesh Kumar Tiwari [2,4], Zaheer Ul-Haq [3,*] and Keykavous Parang [2,4,*]

1. Department of Chemistry, Aditi Mahavidyalaya, University of Delhi, Bawana, Delhi 110039, India; bschhikara@gmail.com
2. Department of Biomedical and Pharmaceutical Sciences, College of Pharmacy, University of Rhode Island, Rhode Island, Kingston, RI 02881, USA; nicolestjean@ymail.com (N.S.J.); mandal@chapman.edu (D.M.); tiwari@chapman.edu (R.K.T.)
3. Dr. Panjwani Center for Molecular Medicine and Drug Research, ICCBS, University of Karachi, Karachi 75210, Pakistan; sajda.ashraf@yahoo.com
4. Center For Targeted Drug Delivery, Department of Biomedical and Pharmaceutical Sciences, Chapman University School of Pharmacy, Harry and Diane Rinker Health Science Campus, California, Irvine, CA 92618, USA; mozaf100@mail.chapman.edu

* Correspondence: zaheer.qasmi@iccs.edu (Z.U.-H.); parang@chapman.edu (K.P.);

Academic Editor: Qiao-Hong Chen

Abstract: *N*1-(α,β-Alkene)-substituted phenylpyrazolopyrimidine derivatives with acetyl and functionalized phenyl groups at α- and β-positions, respectively, were synthesized by the reaction of 3-phenylpyrazolopyrimidine (PhPP) with bromoacetone, followed by a chalcone reaction with differently substituted aromatic aldehydes. The Src kinase enzyme assay revealed modest inhibitory activity (half maximal inhibitory concentration, IC_{50} = 21.7–192.1 μM) by a number of PhPP derivatives. Antiproliferative activity of the compounds was evaluated on human leukemia (CCRF-CEM), human ovarian adenocarcinoma (SK-OV-3), breast carcinoma (MDA-MB-231), and colon adenocarcinoma (HT-29) cells in vitro. 4-Chlorophenyl carbo-enyl substituted 3-phenylpyrazolopyrimidine (**10**) inhibited the cell proliferation of HT-29 and SK-OV-3 by 90% and 79%, respectively, at a concentration of 50 μM after 96 h incubation. The compound showed modest inhibitory activity against c-Src (IC_{50} = 60.4 μM), Btk (IC_{50} = 90.5 μM), and Lck (IC_{50} = 110 μM), while it showed no activity against Abl1, Akt1, Alk, Braf, Cdk2, and PKCa. In combination with target selection and kinase profiling assay, extensive theoretical studies were carried out to explore the selectivity behavior of compound **10**. Specific interactions were also explored by examining the changing trends of interactions of tyrosine kinases with the phenylpyrazolopyrimidine derivative. The results showed good agreement with the experimental selectivity pattern among c-Src, Btk, and Lck.

Keywords: protein kinase; phenylpyrazolopyrimidine; antiproliferative activity; enzyme inhibition; molecular simulation

---

1. Introduction

Cancer cells show the overexpression of different protein tyrosine kinases (PTKs). These enzymes catalyze the phosphorylation of many protein substrates by the transfer of the γ-phosphate group from ATP to specific tyrosine residues. PTKs have critical roles in signal transduction pathways.

Src family kinases (SFKs) have nine different PTKs, including c-Src, c-Yes, Fyn, Lck, Lyn, Hck, Frk, Blk, and c-Fgr of which Src is the prototype [1]. SFKs have essential roles in the regulation of a wide variety of normal cellular signal transduction pathways, such as cell division, differentiation, growth factor signaling, survival, adhesion, migration, and invasion [2]. Src tyrosine kinase expression is frequently elevated in several tumors, including breast, colon, prostate, lung, ovary, and pancreas, when it is compared with the adjacent healthy tissues. Src kinase was shown to be the critical modulator of cancer cell metastasis and invasion [3].

In recent years, a number of small cell-permeable inhibitors of protein kinases were investigated for the treatment of different cancers [4]. Different small molecules that were actively investigated as kinase inhibitor include quinazolines [5], quinolinecarbonitriles [6], pyrazolopyrimidines [7,8], imidazo [1,5-a]pyrazines [9], Calixarene [10], benzotriazines [11,12], indoles [13], and ATP- phosphopeptide conjugates [14]. The research effort led to the generation of small molecules for the treatment of different malignancies. Imatinib, a 2-phenylaminopyrimidine, was approved for the treatment of chronic myelogenous leukemia (CML) and gastrointestinal stromal tumors (GISTs) [15]. Dasatinib (BMS-354825), a pyrimidinylthiazole derivative, was approved to use in patients with CML after imatinib treatment [16], and bosutinib (SKI-606), a 3-quinolinecarbonitrile analogue, is known to suppress migration and invasion of human breast cancer cells [17]. Ibrutinib (Figure 1) is a pyrazolopyrimidine-based [18] small-molecule kinase inhibitor that was approved for the treatment of B-cell cancers like mantle cell lymphoma, chronic lymphocytic leukemia, and Waldenström's macroglobulinemia [19,20].

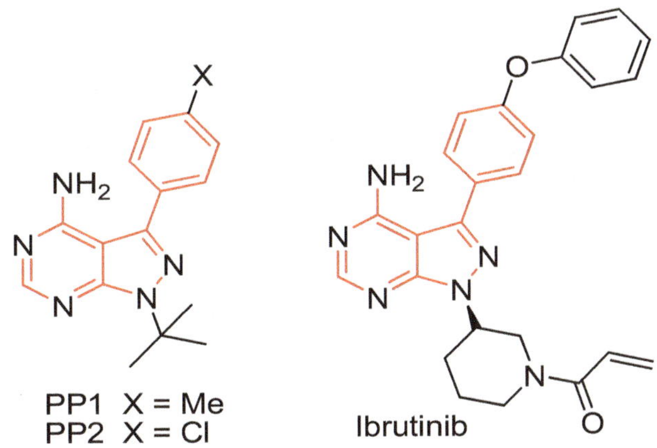

Figure 1. Chemical structures of 3-phenylpyrazolopyrimidine (PhPP) derivatives (PP1 and PP2) and Ibrutinib.

A number of crystallographic studies showed that adenosine 5′-(β,γ-imido)triphosphate (AMP-PNP), an ATP mimic, binds to the ATP-binding site of c-Src (Protein Data Bank (PDB) 2SRC) [21]. Furthermore, complexes of 3-phenylpyrazolopyrimidine (PhPP) derivatives (PP1 and PP2) (Figure 1) act as ATP-binding site inhibitors of Hck (PDB 1QCF) and Lck (PDB 1QPE) [22]. Indeed, the pyrazolopyrimidine core of PP1 and PP2 (Figure 1) mimics the adenine base of ATP in binding to the nucleotide-binding site. In another study [8], we showed that the 3-phenyl group interacts with a large hydrophobic pocket in the ATP-binding site, contributing significantly to Src kinase inhibitory activity. There is also another cavity formed from side chains of helix αC and helix αD that is normally occupied by a carbohydrate moiety followed by a triphosphate group of ATP. This cavity is mostly unfilled by the tert-butyl of 3-phenylpyrazolopyrimidines (PP1 and PP2). Furthermore, we investigated the variation of *N*1 substitution in 3-phenylpyrazolopyrimidines with different 1,2,3-triazoles containing hydrophobic residues to interact with amino acids of this cavity and contribute to the enhancement of Src kinase inhibitory potency [8]. The cysteine residue present in the cavity could be a potential target to bind with PhPP molecules irreversibly, leading to a potential increase in kinase inhibition.

Here, we describe the synthesis and evaluation of kinase inhibitory activity of *N*1-substituted PhPP with α-acetyl-β-phenyl-alkene groups (Figure 2). We hypothesized that this substitution at the *N*1 position of PhPP could contribute significantly to the kinase inhibition through generating specific interactions. We further extended our study to investigate the selectivity profile of one of the active compounds (**10**) with a panel of nine different kinases by applying MD and MMGBSA calculations. This study helped to reveal the inhibitory mechanism of PhPP derivatives based on their distinct structural characteristics required for its interaction with a specific kinase.

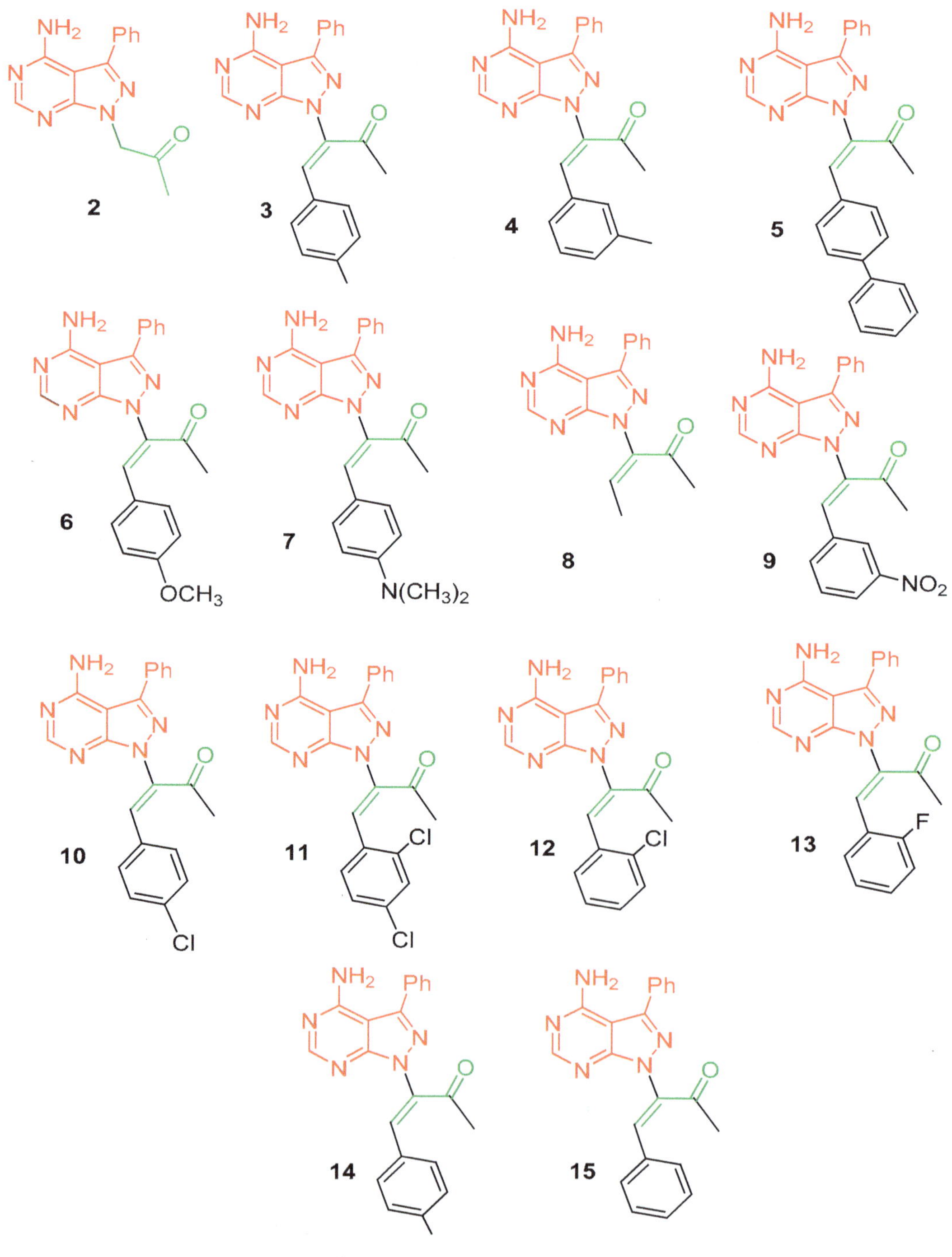

Figure 2. Chemical structures of *N*1-substituted PhPP with α-acetyl-β-phenyl-alkene groups (*E* and *Z* isomers).

2. Results and Discussion

2.1. Chemical Synthesis

The products were synthesized by following the chemical pathway shown in Scheme 1. The PhPP (**1**) was synthesized according to a reported procedure [23]. The N1 of **1** was substituted with bromoacetone in the presence of potassium carbonate as a base. Product **2** was confirmed by NMR, which showed the disappearance of the proton peak of NH at 8.07 ppm of **1** and appearance of the peak at 5.24 ppm and 2.21 ppm for CH_2 and CH_3, respectively, in ^1H NMR. Furthermore, ^{13}C NMR showed peaks at 201.34 ppm, 56.15 ppm, and 27.14 ppm representing the carbonyl group, CH_2, and CH_3, respectively, in product **2**.

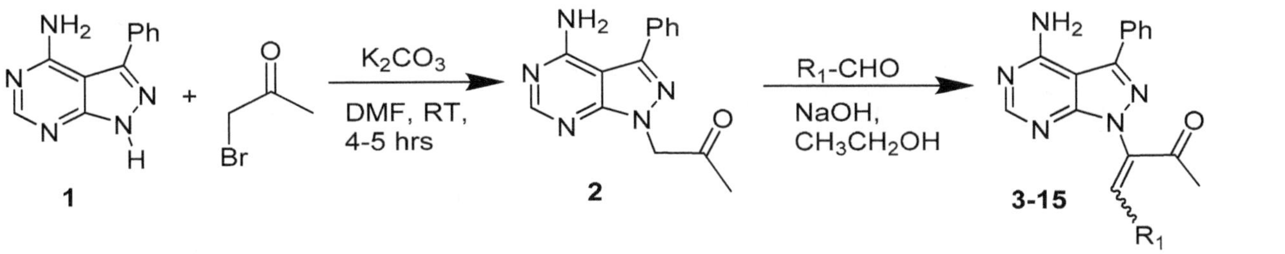

	R_1		
3	*p*-(CH_3)Ph-	**10**	*p*-(Cl)Ph-
4	*m*-(CH_3)Ph-	**11**	2,4-diCl-Ph-
5	4-(Ph)-Ph-	**12**	*o*-(Cl)Ph
6	4- (OCH_3)Ph-	**13**	*o*-(F)Ph-
7	*p*-($N(CH_3)_2$Ph-	**14**	p-(F)Ph-
8	-CH_3	**15**	Ph-
9	*m*-(NO_2)Ph-		

Scheme 1. Chemical synthesis of PhPP derivatives.

Next, the double bond group was introduced by the chalcone reaction. The anion of **2** generated by sodium hydroxide was reacted with different benzaldehydes at room temperature to give product **3**. The ratio of starting material and amount of solvent defined the formation of product and side products. A higher concentration (i.e., less amount of solvent ethanol) and the presence of higher equivalents of **2** than the aldehyde lead to a second internal Michael reaction where the anion of **2** reacts with product **3**, leading to the formation of side product as indicated by Electrospray Ionization Mass Spectrometry (ESI-MS) at 659 Da (data not shown). In an optimum condition, the aldehyde and reactant **2** should be present in more than 1.4:1 equivalent, and solvent ethanol should be present in approximately 20 mL for 26 mg (0.1 mmol) of **2**. Out of two possible products after the conjugation of **2** with 4-methylbenzaldehyde, only product **3** was observed, suggesting the reaction of the carbanion of methylene (CH_2) group between the carbonyl and nitrogen rather than that of methyl (CH_3). The formation of product **3** was confirmed by ESI-MS by the presence of a mass peak at 370 Da $[M + H]^+$. This was confirmed by ^1H NMR, which showed the absence of a peak at 5.24 ppm for CH_2 of **2,** while the three protons for CH_3 were present at 2.31 ppm. Correspondingly, in ^{13}C NMR, the peak at 56.15 ppm (assigned to CH_2) was absent in **3** while the peak at 26.13 ppm (assigned to CH_3 with slight upfield shift) was present. Furthermore, out of EZ possible isomers for the double bond, both the isomers were present as indicated by NOE NMR spectra, possibly by rotation introduced due to keto-enol tautomerism.

In the case of product **8**, the chalcone reaction was carried with precaution to avoid the formation of side products due to the presence of α-hydrogen in acetaldehyde. The anion of **2** was generated first with 1.1 equivalent of sodium hydroxide over extended time and added to the solution of acetaldehyde (1.2 equivalents). The reaction was quenched with acetic acid after 30 min. The product was confirmed by ESI-MS and NMR. The products were purified by HPLC and showed a purity of 95–99%.

2.2. Src-Kinase Assay

In vitro Src kinase assay for some of the compounds was conducted, as presented in Table 1. As results indicated, the compounds were moderately active against the Src kinase. Among all the tested compounds, compounds **6** and **4** were found to be the most potent with IC_{50} values of 21.7 and 24.7 μM, respectively. Compounds **3** and **7** exhibited IC_{50} values of 32.9 μM and 36.8, respectively. Compound **5** showed the lowest activity with an IC_{50} of 192.1 μM. Since the compounds showed only moderate Src kinase inhibitory activity, they were evaluated for antiproliferative activity first to find the lead compound for further kinase inhibitory assays.

Table 1. In vitro Src kinase inhibition assay for the selected compounds.

Compound No.	IC_{50} (μM) [a]
3	32.9
4	24.7
5	192.1
6	21.7
7	36.9
Staurosporine	0.6
PP2	0.5

[a] All experiments were repeated in triplicate. All the standard deviations were in the range of 6–13%.

2.3. Antiproliferative Activities

The effect of compounds on the cell proliferation of cancer cells was evaluated in vitro in a human leukemia cell line (CCRF-CEM) according to the previously reported procedures [24,25], breast adenocarcinoma (MDA-MB-231), ovarian adenocarcinoma (SK-OV-3), and colon adenocarcinoma (HT-29) cell lines up to 72 h. Doxorubicin (Dox) was used as a positive control as shown previously [26–29]. These cell lines were selected to determine the antiproliferative activity against diverse cancer cells. Compounds **10** and **11** consistently inhibited the cell proliferation 72–96 h in all cell lines. The percentage of cell proliferation was significantly reduced in HT-29 cells in the presence of **10** and **11** when compared with Dox and other compounds. Compound **10** was more effective in the order of HT-29 (90%) > CCRF-CEM, SK-OV-3 (79%) > MDA-MB-231 (60%), while Dox showed HT-29 (75%) > CCRF-CEM, SK-OV-3 (73%) > MDM-MB-231 (64%) after 96 h. Compounds **2**, **7**, **9**, and **12** were found to be inactive in reducing the cell proliferation in all the cell lines after 24–96 h while other compounds **3** and **13–15** exhibited comparable or slightly less antiproliferative activity (Figure 3A–D) than compounds **10** and **11** after 96 h. These data indicate that the presence of the chlorine group at the para position in compounds **10** and **11** were effective in improving the antiproliferative activities. However, the absence of phenyl and/or double bonds in compounds **2** and **8** significantly reduced the antiproliferative activities versus **10** and **11**. The presence of *p*-dimethylamino, *m*-nitro, and *o*-chlorine in **7**, **9**, and **12** were not productive while *o*-fluorine (**13**), *p*-fluorine (**14**), unsubstituted phenyl (**15**), and *p*-Cl (**10** and **11**) enhanced the antiproliferative activity. Compounds **5** and **6** with *p*-ph and *p*-methoxy exhibited antiproliferative activity against some of the cell lines, with **5** being more active in HT-29 and **6** in CCRF-CEM and SK-OV3 cells. However, their activity was generally less than compounds **3**, **10**, **11**, **13**, and **14**. Compounds **10** and **11** exhibited IC_{50} values of 25.5 μM and 34.3 μM, respectively, after 72 h incubation against SK-OV-3 cells (Figure 4).

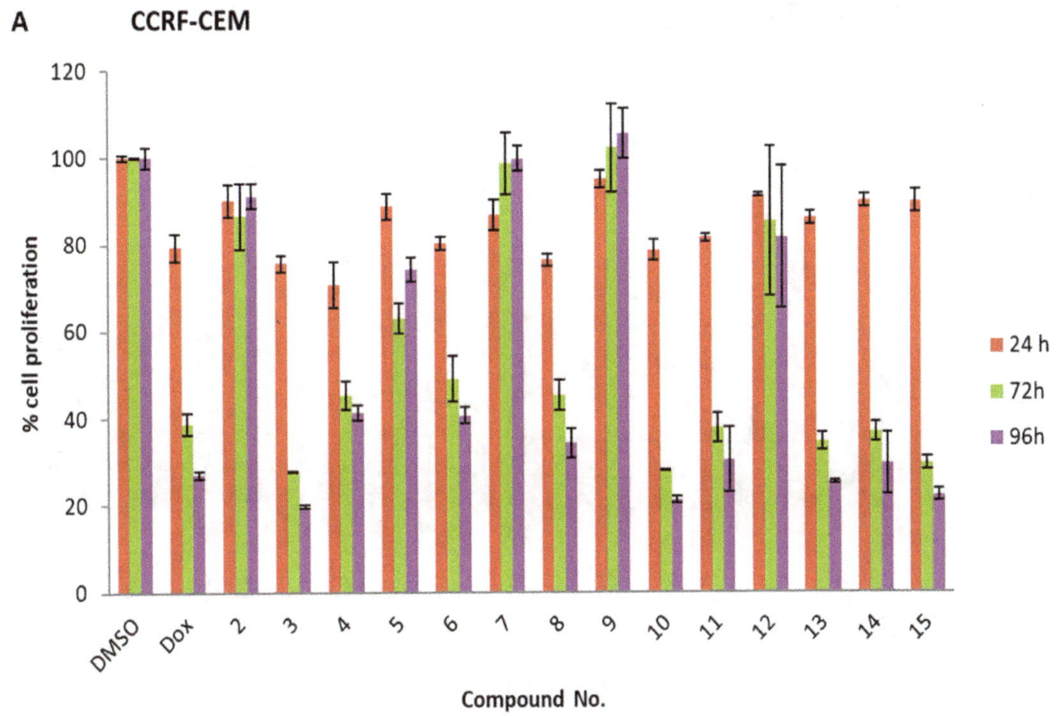

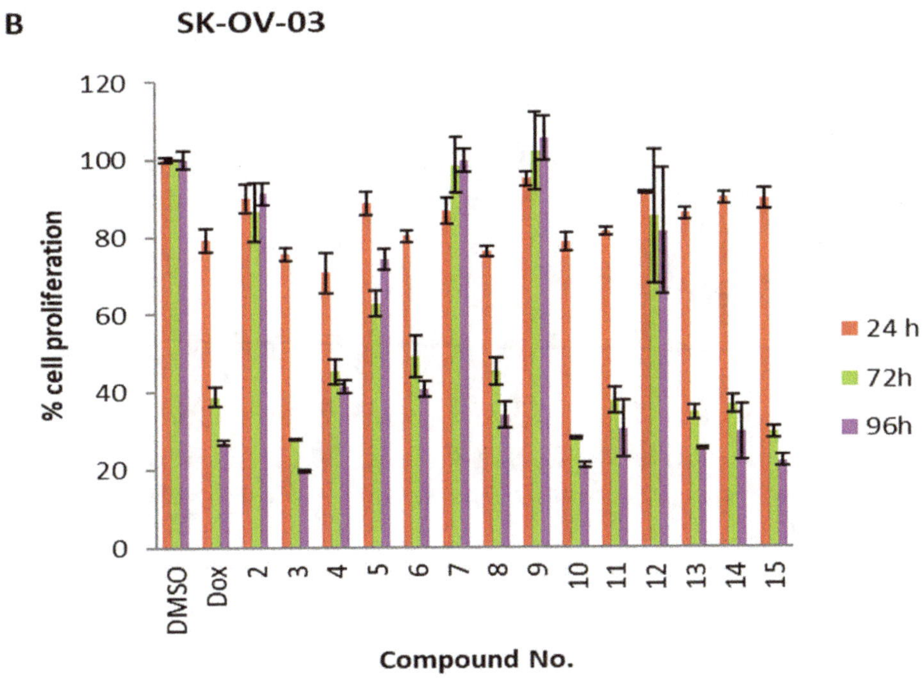

Figure 3. *Cont.*

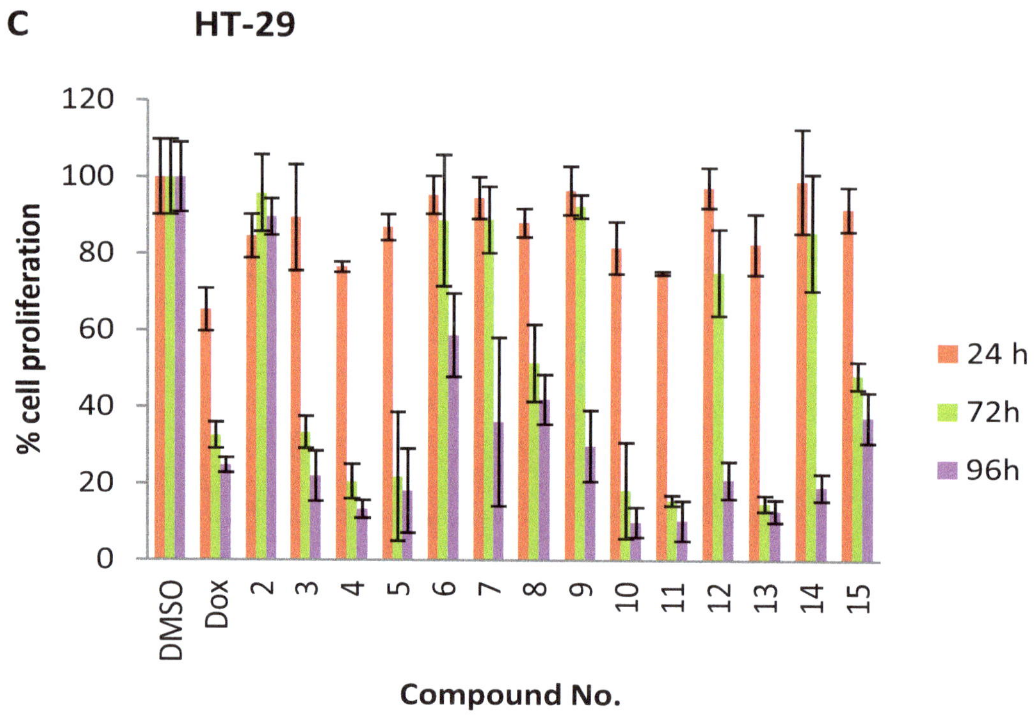

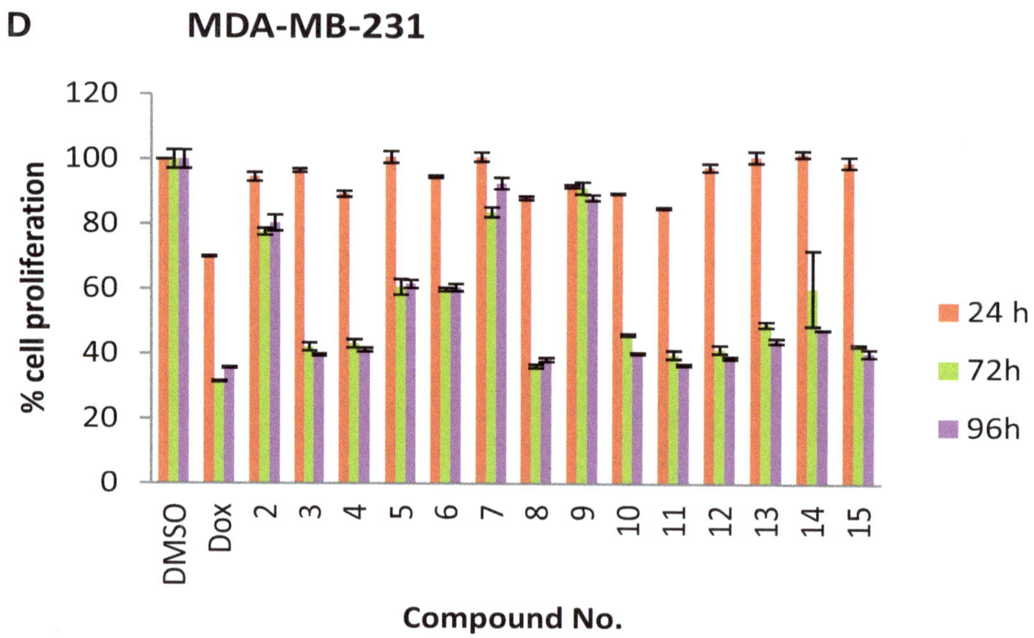

Figure 3. Antiproliferative activity of PhPP derivatives (50 μM) and doxorubicin (Dox) (1 μM) against CCRF-CEM (**A**), SK-OV-3 (**B**), HT-29 (**C**), and MDA-MB-231 (**D**) cell lines. All experiments were repeated in triplicate.

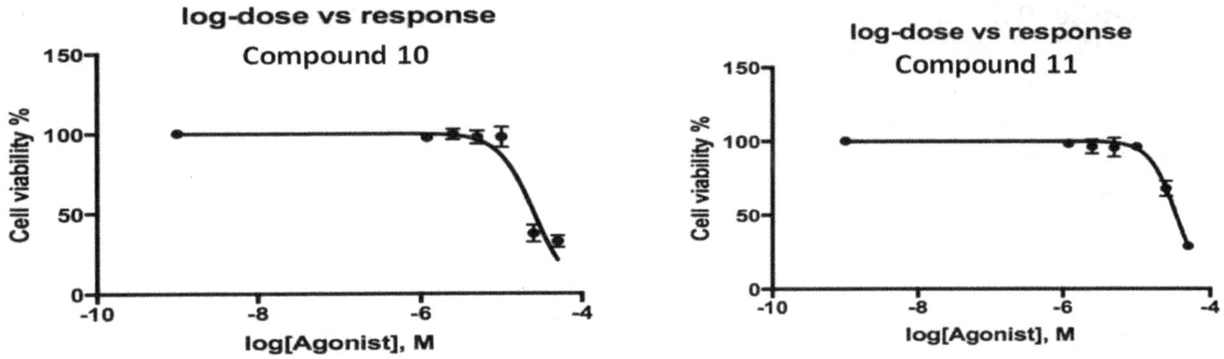

Figure 4. Dose-response curves of **10** (**left**) and **11** (**right**) after 72 h incubation against SK-OV-3 cells.

Compound **10** was selected for further evaluation against a panel of kinases to determine the mechanism of activity. The results are shown in Table 2 against Abl1, Akt1, Alk, Braf, Btk, Cdk2, cSrc, Lck, and PKCa enzymes. The data indicate modest activity against Btk, c-Src, and Lck while the compound was inactive or showed very low inhibition activity against other kinases.

Table 2. The activity of compound **10** against a panel of protein kinases.

Kinase	Compound 10 IC_{50} (μM)	Control Compound IC_{50} (μM)
Abl1	NA[a]	0.85 [b]
Akt1	>150	0.012 [b]
Alk	NA	0.01 [b]
Braf	NA	0.018 [c]
Btk	95.4	0.067 [b]
Cdk2/Cyclin A1	NA	0.0039 [b]
c-Src	64.1	0.0085 [b]
Lck	110	0.011 [b]
PKCa	NA	0.0016 [b]

[a] Not active (NA) indicates no inhibition or compound activity that could not be fit to an IC_{50} curve; [b] Staurosporine; [c] GW5074.

2.4. *Molecular Modeling*

To rationalize the activity of compound **10**, KEGG pathway and molecular dynamics simulation studies were utilized to explore the specific behavior of the *Z* configuration compound **10** against multiple kinases.

2.4.1. Target Identification

Conventional identification of drug targets is an expensive, time-consuming, and difficult process; only a few drug targets can be identified. In contrast, the computational method permits a great deal of analysis within a short period and brings a large number of potential drug targets from a pool of information [30]. In the present study, an integrated in silico approach was used to identify potential targets [31] for the active compound **10**. Initially, the disease search tool in the KEGG database was used against breast, ovarian, and colorectal cancer to extract the targets that may be involved in these diseases (Figures 5–7) [32]. KEGG uses the knowledge of gene function and linking this information with advanced order functional information by using systematic analysis. The schematic presentation of the KEGG pathway shows genes marked as light-blue color as a drug target and genes marked as pink as associated with the disease, whereas when the gene is linked with both a disease and a drug target, its color is split into light blue and pink. There were several target proteins involved in one pathway; therefore, protein-drug association servers Similarity Ensemble Approach (SEA, http://sea.bkslab.org/) [33], Search Tool for the Retrieval of Interacting Genes (STRING, http://string-db.org) [34], and Search Tool for Interacting Chemicals (STITCH, http://stitch.embl.de/) [35] were used. The STRING database was used to explain the molecular function, biological processes, cellular components, and pathways of the target proteins. The SEA relates target proteins based on set-wise chemical similarity among their compounds. A total of 14 potential targets (Btk, Itk, c-Src, EGFR, Akt1, Fyn, Lyn, Lck, PKC, Abl1, Hck, Cdk2, Braf, and Her2) were selected based on the data obtained from these servers that further proved the reliability of text mining and molecular docking.

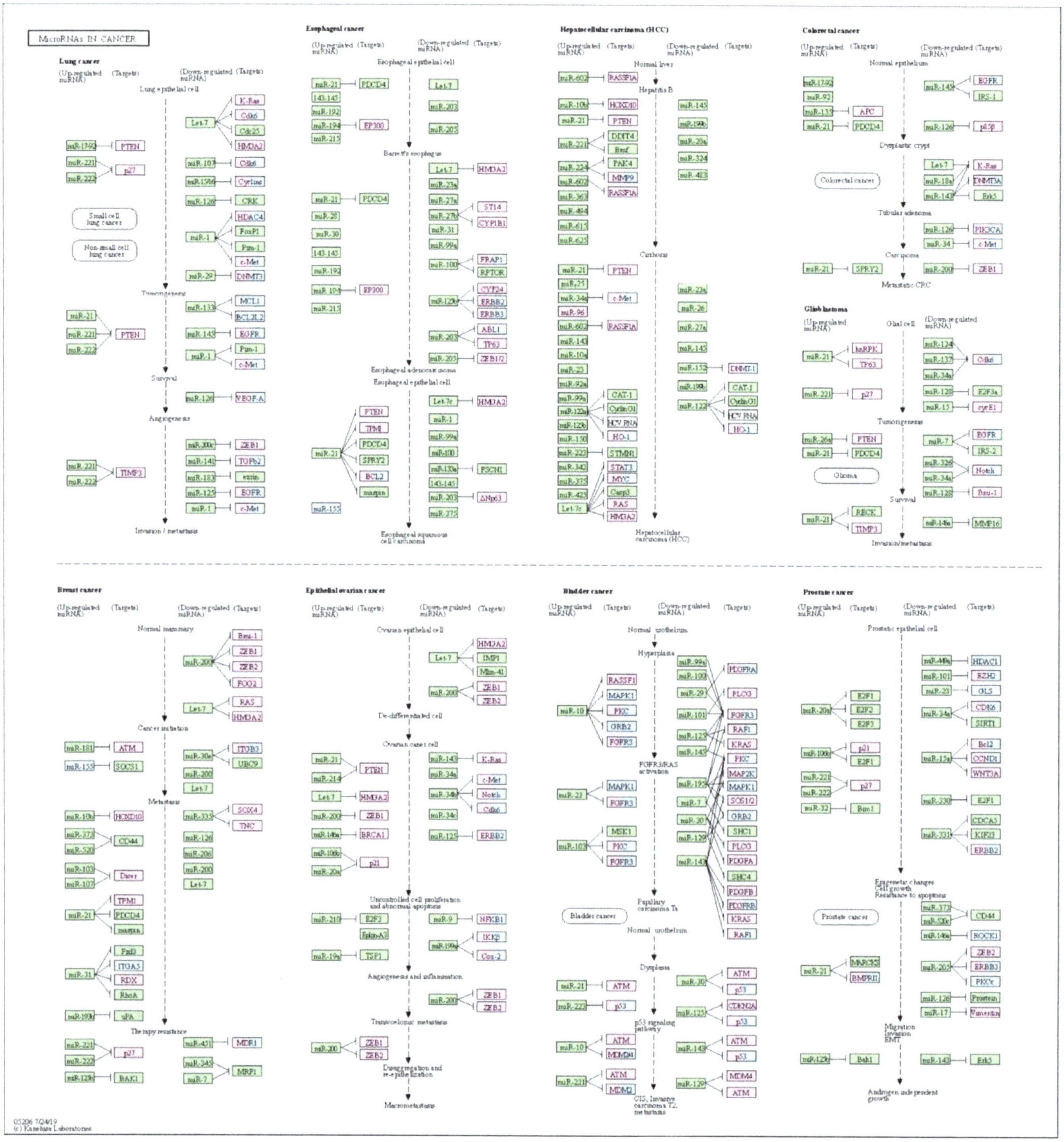

Figure 5. The KEGG pathway for ovarian cancer.

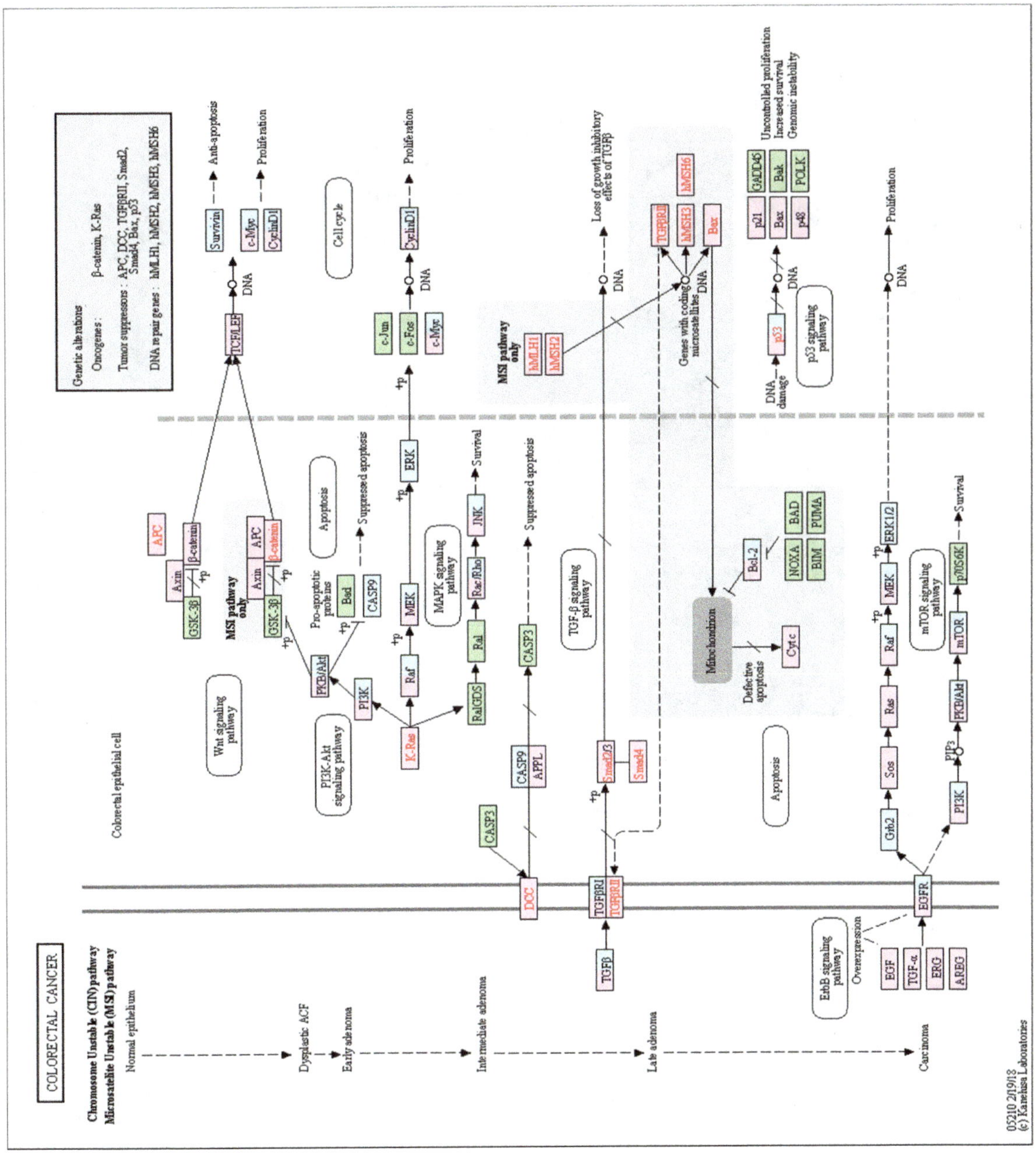

Figure 6. The KEGG pathway for colorectal cancer.

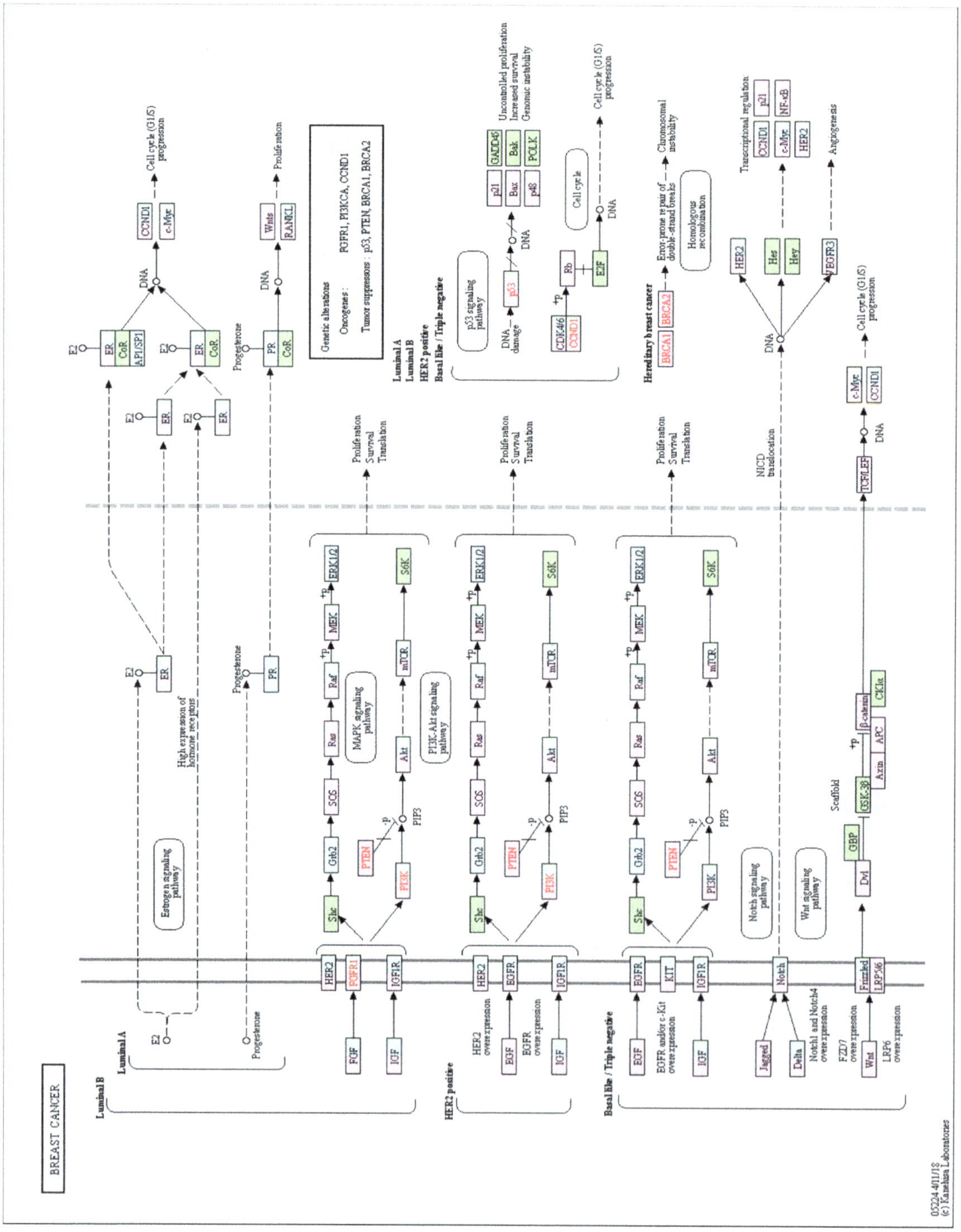

Figure 7. The KEGG pathway for breast cancer.

2.4.2. Docking Studies

The known compounds that were already reported as inhibitors of the target proteins, as well as nature and crucial active site residues, were specified in their accessible complexes, used as a positive control. Prior to docking, validation of the software and docking conditions was performed by retrieving the control compounds from their crystal complexes and then redocking by MOE against their relevant targets. The redocking results are presented in Table 3. After validation, docking of compound **10** was performed with all 14 targets, and their docking scores were compared with the control in order to select a target with the highest docking score. We observed that compound **10** presented good scores against Btk, Itk, c-Src, EGFR, Akt1, Fyn, Lyn, Lck, PKC, and Abl1 kinase as compared to Hck, Cdk2, Braf, and Her2. The docking scores of compound **10** are presented in Table 4.

Table 3. Predicted binding affinity (docking scores in kcal/mol) and root-mean-square deviation (RMSD) of control inhibitors against related proteins.

Target Proteins	Docking Score of Comp. 10	RMSD (Å)
c-Src	−8.3240	1.5
Btk	−7.6201	0.75
Itk	−8.1748	1.4
EGFR	−7.7890	1.56
Fyn	−7.5002	1.32
Lyn	−5.9252	1.23
Hck	−5.1107	0.9
Her2	−8.7522	0.54
Lck	−7.7834	0.45
PKC	−6.4224	0.82
Braf	−6.8762	1.52
Abl1	−6.7421	0.85
Akt1	−7.8654	0.74
Cdk2	−5.2409	0.95

Table 4. MM/PBSA derived binding free energies of complexes computed from the MD simulations.

	c-Src	PKC	Akt	Alk	Btk	CDK2	Lck	Abl1	Braf
VDWAALS	−40.343	−46.197	−35.635	−35.533	−46.946	−50.067	−34.248	−40.962	−31.802
EEL	−13.296	−19.577	−15.181	−3.935	−13.128	−29.554	−15.558	−18.300	−10.603
EPB/EGB	32.183	39.385	33.442	23.836	36.678	54.064	32.371	39.952	26.077
ESURF/ECAVITY/ ENPOLAR	−5.024	−5.873	−3.961	−4.54	−5.820	−6.421	−4.623	−5.313	−4.283
DELTA G binding (PB)	−20.633	−21.653	−15.645	−5.210	−15.683	−6.893	−18.093	−9.629	−20.433

2.4.3. Structure Architecture of Kinases

The structure of all protein kinase domains is composed of a small, typically β-stranded *N*-lobe linked with a small hinge region to a bigger α-helical *C*-lobe. In protein kinases, ATP binds to the cavity that lies between *N*- and C-terminal lobes creating the kinase activation site, where the adenine moiety of ATP is packed like a sandwich between hydrophobic residues, while it is associated with the hinge region by hydrophilic contact. Typical kinase elements include the G-loop (glycine-rich residues forming the active site roof), A-loop, or activation loop crucial for kinase activation and deactivation, C-helix responsible for the selectivity of the active site, and the hinge region that plays a vital role in inhibitor binding. The ATP-binding site categorized into five distinct regions: adenine region where the adenine moiety of ATP forms a hydrogen bond with the hinge, hydrophobic region-I corresponds to the entrance pocket, hydrophobic region-II also known as the selectivity pocket is determined by an extremely conserved DFG (aspartate-phenylalanine-glycine) motif, a hydrophilic region where the ATP sugar binds, and a solvent-exposed region for phosphate binding.

2.4.4. Molecular Dynamic Simulation

Although X-ray crystallography and molecular docking are powerful techniques for biological macromolecules, they are unable to examine the protein's flexibility and they provide a momentary binding mode. Therefore, MD simulation was used to investigate the ligand-protein interactions [36] and the conformational changes which occur in the structure of kinases with respect to motions. Based on the docking results, nine complexes were selected for further MD simulation to understand the binding mechanism of compound **10** and its stability against multiple kinases.

c-Src

The stereo view of the binding mode of Src (PDB ID: 2SRC) is depicted in Figure 8A. It was found that, initially, compound **10** was bound to the active site of Src kinase similar to a cognate ligand by making a hydrogen bond with the NH group of Met341 and CO group of Glu339, while these bonds were observed to undergo destabilization during the simulation. Comparatively, three new hydrogen bonds were formed, involving the side chain amino group of Lys295 (solvent accessible area) and the hydroxyl group of Ser345, which interact with the pyrazolopyrimidine scaffold located in the adenine region of Src kinase. The spatial position of the compound was found to be different from the observed dock pose because of major conformational changes during simulation.

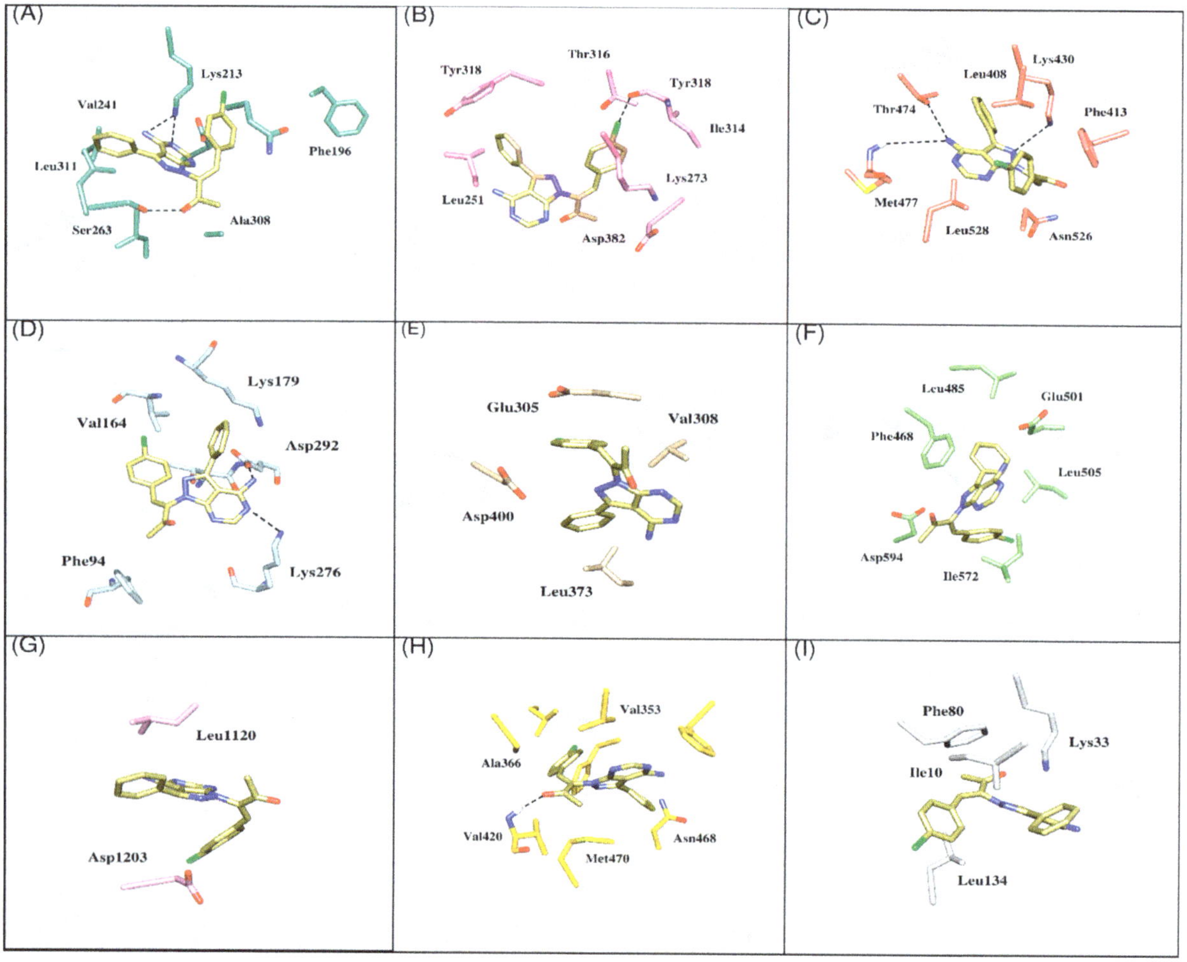

Figure 8. Binding mode of Z configuration of compound **10** (khaki) with the active site residues of (**A**) c-Src, (**B**) Lck, (**C**) Btk, (**D**) Akt, (**E**) Abl1, (**F**) Braf, (**G**) Alk, (**H**) PKC, and (**I**) Cdk2. Amino acid residues involved in crucial interactions are labeled.

The activation loop in the DFG-in conformation provides enough space to accommodate the ring of compound **10**, which may cause a collision with Phe405 of the DFG-out conformation. Moreover, distinct hydrophobic interactions were also observed with Leu273, and Val281 (hydrophobic region I) that maintain the binding mode of complexes. The MD results suggest that the non-flexible part of the compound might be the reason for its moderate activity as compared to the reference compound.

Lck

The binding elements responsible for the modest activity of Lck kinase are depicted in Figure 8B. Consistent with the results from other reported studies, compound **10** is well accommodated in the ATP site of Lck by forming multiple hydrophobic, π-stacking, π-cation, and Van der Waals interactions with Leu251, Ala271, Lys273, Thr316, Lys318, and Asp382. Due to the different conformation of the DFG motif, compound **10** slightly moves toward the adenine region with its core pyrimidine ring in the adenine region by forming a hydrophilic interaction with Met319. In the meantime, Phe385 of the DFG motif is involved in a weak hydrophobic interaction due to the far distance. The chloro-benzene ring engages the gatekeeper residue Thr316 via hydrophobic interaction, while the non-substituted benzene ring occupies the extended hydrophobic pocket, forming π-stacking and Van der Waals interactions with Leu251, Ala271, and Tyr318. The complex was further stabilized by the formation of a halogen bond between the backbone of the carbonyl oxygen of Ile314 and the fluorine of the compound **10**. In summary, a marked similarity of interaction was observed with the reference compound except for the hydrophilic interaction responsible for the inhibitory activity of Lck kinase.

Btk

The docked complex of BTK presented a number of hydrophilic and hydrophobic interactions with the active site residues Leu408, Val416, Lys430, Thr474, Glu475, Met477, Leu528, Asp539, and Phe540. The compound occupied the same position consistent with the reference compound. Molecular dynamics studies revealed that compound **10** binding to BTK, is stable and it was found to involve in hydrogen bond interactions with key residues of the glycine-rich P-loop like Leu408, Gly409, and Asp539. Transient hydrogen bond interactions were also detected with crucial active site residues Glu475 and Met477 of the hinge region, catalytic residue Lys430, and the DFG motif that is crucial for kinase activity, indicating that compound **10** probably has the appropriate interaction profile with BTK (Figure 8C).

Akt

According to the binding mode of the Akt complex [37], compound **10** adopts a Y-shape conformation, where the presence of residues Phe469 and Phe472 that are essential for the regulatory control of Akt1, make the pocket hydrophobic. Initially, the pyrimidine ring occupies the adenosine portion of the binding site, forming hydrogen bonding to the hinge region of the kinase through Ala230 (Figure 8D). During the simulation, this hydrogen bond is replaced by hydrophobic interactions, while the phenyl substituent presents a parallel aromatic interaction with Phe438. Moreover, residues Lys179, Leu181, and Val164 also stabilize the compound by making hydrophobic contact. In general, theoretical studies indicate that compound **10** stabilizes Akt via hydrophobic interactions; however, after losing its interactions with the hinge region, the gatekeeper residue and the DFG motif lead to its low kinase inhibitory properties.

Abl

The binding mode of the Abl1 complex (Figure 8E) showed that the compound is accommodated in the lipophilic channel slightly away from the hinge region. The bent conformation of the molecule does not allow its tight binding to the ATP site. This resultant compound is unable to mimic interaction with the adenine moiety of ATP. Only a few hydrophobic interactions were observed with Glu305, Val308, Leu473, and Asp400, but these interactions were also not found to be persistent throughout the md simulation. It is hypothesized that the absence of specific interactions of compound **10** with the residues of the hinge region and DFG motif could be the reason for its inactivity.

Braf

According to the docking calculations, compound **10** is involved in a number of hydrophilic and hydrophobic interactions with Braf kinase. However, after a short 50 ns production run, the simulated binding mode provided a different picture to understand the selectivity trend. During the simulation, these non-bonded interactions were weakened due to loop flipping of the motif from the DGF-in to the DGF-out conformation. However, in order to accommodate the core pyrimidine ring, the benzene ring was required to tilt out of the plane due to restricted space. As a result of this movement, intermolecular interactions broke, which penalized the binding affinity of compound **10** for Braf (Figure 8F).

Alk

The binding interactions of the Alk with compound **10** are depicted in Figure 8G. The complex obtained after simulation indicates that the compound partially aligned on the reference compound ceritinib, and it was unable to form any hydrophilic interaction with the active site residues, especially with the hinge region. A similar type of binding mode was observed in the case of PKC (Figure 8H) and Cdk2 (Figure 8I).

2.4.5. Binding Free Energy Calculations

MM/PBSA is considered as the best choice for predicting the binding affinities of a protein-ligand complex with implicit solvent at a low computational cost. It has the potential to recognize the true binding structure of the complex from docking. In the present study, MM/PBSA was used to re-rank the nine complexes after a short production run of 50 ns. The calculated binding free energy of all complexes is presented in Table 4 [38]. The binding position and atomic interaction between protein kinases and ligand are the main factors that play a role in measuring the binding affinity. The predicted binding poses of compound **10** significantly overlaid with the reported inhibitors of c-Src, Lck, Btk, and Akt, but partially aligned in the case of Braf and Alk. According to Table 4, the binding free energy computed for c-Src, Lck, and Akt complexes was −20.63, −15.64, and −18.09, respectively, which were more stable than ALK, CDK2, and Abl1 kinases, agreeing with the selectivity profile observed experimentally. In order to comprehend the effect of the individual energy term in the binding process, total binding free energy was decomposed into the Eele, Evdw, EGB, and ESURF energy components. The values of these components indicated that van der Waals (ΔGvdw) energy contributed significantly to the total binding free energy. The superior contribution of Van der Waals interaction (Table 4) was in agreement with the fact that compound **10** mainly stabilizes via hydrophobic interactions with the kinases.

3. Experimental Protocols

3.1. Materials and Methods

Bromoacetone was purchased from ChemService Inc. (West Chester, PA, USA). Anhydrous dichloromethane, anhydrous pyridine, *N*,*N*-dimethylformamide (DMF), and other chemicals and reagents were purchased from Sigma-Aldrich Chemical Co. (Milwaukee, WI, USA). The chemical structures of final products were characterized by nuclear magnetic resonance spectra (^{1}H NMR, ^{13}C NMR) determined on a Bruker (Billerica, MA, USA) NMR spectrometer (400 MHz) or a Varian (Silicon Valley, CA, USA) NMR spectrometer (500 MHz). ^{13}C NMR spectra were fully decoupled. Chemical shifts were reported in parts per millions (ppm) using deuterated solvent peak as the standard. The chemical structures of final products were confirmed by a high-resolution Biosystems QStar Elite (QStar Technologies, Denver, CO, USA) time-of-flight electrospray mass spectrometer. Details of procedures and spectroscopic data of the respective compounds are presented below. Final compounds were purified on a Phenomenex (Torrance, CA, USA) Prodigy 10 μm ODS reverse-phase column (2.1 cm × 25 cm) with a Hitachi (Tokyo, Japan) HPLC system using a gradient system of acetonitrile or methanol and water ($CH_3CN/CH_3OH/H_2O$, 0–100%, pH 7.0, 60 min). The purity of final products (>99%) was confirmed by analytical HPLC. The analytical HPLC was performed on the Hitachi analytical HPLC system using a C18 Shimadzu (Kyoto, Japan) Premier 3 μm column (150 cm × 4.6 mm) using two different isocratic systems, and a flow rate of 1 mL/min with UV detection at 265 nm.

3.2. *Synthesis*

3-Phenyl-1*H*-pyrazolo[3,4-*d*]pyrimidin-4-amine (**1**): Compound **1** was synthesized according to a previously reported procedure [23].

1-(4-Amino-3-phenyl-1*H*-pyrazolo[3,4-*d*]pyrimidin-1-yl)propan-2-one (**2**): Compound **1** (156 mg, 0.73 mmol) and potassium carbonate (200 mg, 1.4 mmol) were taken in dry DMF (10 mL). Bromoacetone (100 mg, 0.72 mmol) was diluted with dry DMF (5 mL) and was added dropwise to the reaction mixture at room temperature. The reaction mixture was stirred for 4 h at room temperature. After completion of the reaction, the solvent was removed under reduced pressure, added water (50 mL) and extracted with dichloromethane. The organic layer was filtered through filter paper and dried over Na_2SO_4 (anhydrous). The crude product was further purified on silica gel flash chromatography using dichloromethane and methanol (0–20%) as eluents. 160 mg, 81% yield. ^{1}H-NMR ($CDCl_3$, 500 MHz, δ ppm): 8.3 (s, 1H), 7.7 (d, J = 11 Hz, 2H), 7.5–7.5 (m, 3H), 5.2 (s, 2H), 2.2 (s, 3H).^{13}C NMR ($CDCl_3$, 125 MHz, δ ppm): 201.3, 158.1, 156.2, 155.2, 145.4, 132.8, 129.4, 129.3, 128.4, 98.4, 56.1, 27.1. HR-MS (ESI-TOF) (*m*/*z*): calculated for $C_{14}H_{13}N_5O + H^+$: 268.1193; found, 268.0852 $[M + H]^+$.

General Procedure for the Synthesis of Pyrazolopyrimidine Chalcones:

Compound **2** (26 mg, 0.1 mmol) was dissolved in ethanol (5 mL). Sodium hydroxide (5 mg, 20 μL of 250 mg/mL NaOH solution in water) was added to the compound **2** solution. The reaction mixture solution was stirred for 15 min. Then, a solution of *p*-methylbenzaldehyde (24 mg, 0.2 mmol) in ethanol (15 mL) was added to the reaction mixture. The reaction mixture was allowed to stir at room temperature for 5 h. On completion of the reaction, the reaction mixture was neutralized with dilute acetic acid in ethanol and purified over reverse phase HPLC using water and methanol as eluents to obtain pure product **3** (22 mg, 61% yield). A similar procedure was adopted for the synthesis of other pyrazolopyrimidine derivatives.

3-(4-Amino-3-phenyl-1*H*-pyrazolo[3,4-*d*]pyrimidin-1-yl)-4-*p*-tolylbut-3-en-2-one (**3**). (Yield: 61%). ^{1}H-NMR ($CDCl_3$, 500 MHz, δ ppm): 8.3 (s, 1H), 7.7 (s, 1H), 7.7 (d, J = 7 Hz, 2H), 7.6–7.5 (m, 3H), 7.0 (d, J = 8.2 Hz, 2H), 6.9 (d, J = 8.2 Hz, 2H), 2.3 (s, 3H), 2.9 (s, 3H). ^{13}C NMR ($CDCl_3$, 125 MHz, δ ppm): 194.3, 157.9, 156.9, 155.8, 146.8, 141.8, 140.5, 132.7, 131.8, 130.7, 129.6, 129.5, 129.4, 128.5, 26.1, 21.5. HR-MS (ESI-TOF) (*m*/*z*): calculated for $C_{22}H_{19}N_5O + H^+$: 370.1662; found, 370.1534 $[M + H]^+$.

3-(4-Amino-3-phenyl-1*H*-pyrazolo[3,4-d]pyrimidin-1-yl)-4-*m*-tolylbut-3-en-2-one (**4**). (Yield: 64%). ^{1}H-NMR ($CDCl_3$, 500 MHz, δ ppm): 8.3 (s, 1H), 7.9 (s, 1H), 7.7 (d, J = 7 Hz, 2H), 7.6–7.5 (m, 3H), 7.1–7.0 (m, 2H), 6.8 (s, 1H), 6.7 (d, J = 10 Hz, 1H), 2.3 (s, 3H), 2.2 (s, 3H). ^{13}C NMR ($CDCl_3$, 125 MHz, δ ppm): 194.3, 157.8, 155.1, 154.9, 146.8, 140.6, 133.9, 131.7, 131.5, 130.2, 129.5, 129.4,128.6, 128.4, 26.2, 21.3. HR-MS (ESI-TOF) (*m*/*z*): calculated for $C_{22}H_{19}N_5O + H^+$: 370.1662; found, 370.1454 $[M + H]^+$.

3-(4-Amino-3-phenyl-1*H*-pyrazolo[3,4-d]pyrimidin-1-yl)-4-*p*-biphenylbut-3-en-2-one (**5**). (Yield: 59%). ^{1}H-NMR ($CDCl_3$, 500 MHz, δ ppm): 8.0 (s, 1H), 7.9 (s, 1H), 7.7 (d, J = 8.2 Hz, 2H), 7.6–7.6 (m, 3H), 7.6–7.4 (m, 9H), 2.3 (s, 3H). ^{13}C NMR ($CDCl_3$, 125 MHz, δ ppm): 191.9, 147.2, 135.2, 131.1, 130.3, 129.9, 129.9, 129.8, 129.4, 129.0, 128.7, 128.5, 128.5, 127.7, 127.3, 127.3, 127.2, 127.1, 127.0, 126.1, 22.5. HR-MS (ESI-TOF) (*m*/*z*): calculated for $C_{27}H_{21}N_5O + H^+$: 432.1819; found, 432.1616 $[M + H]^+$.

3-(4-Amino-3-phenyl-1*H*-pyrazolo[3,4-d]pyrimidin-1-yl)-4-(4-methoxyphenyl)but-3-en-2-one (**6**). (Yield: 63%). ^{1}H-NMR ($CDCl_3$, 500 MHz, δ ppm): 8.3 (s, 1H), 7.9 (s, 1H), 7.7 (d, J = 7 Hz, 2H), 7.6–7.5 (m, 3H),

6.9 (d, *J* = 8.9 Hz, 2H), 6.7 (d, *J* = 8.9 Hz, 2H), 3.7 (s, 3H), 2.3 (s, 3H). ^{13}C NMR ($CDCl_3$, 125 MHz, δ ppm): 194.2, 161.9, 158.0, 156.9, 155.7, 146.9, 140.2, 132.8, 132.7, 130.6, 129.5, 129.4, 128.5, 124.3, 114.4, 98.9, 55.3, 26.0. HR-MS (ESI-TOF) (*m*/*z*): calculated for $C_{22}H_{19}N_5O_2 + H^+$: 386.1612; found, 386.1573 $[M + H]^+$.

3-(4-Amino-3-phenyl-1*H*-pyrazolo[3,4-d]pyrimidin-1-yl)-4-(4-(dimethylamino)phenyl)but-3-en-2-one (**7**). (Yield: 66%). ^{1}H-NMR ($CDCl_3$, 500 MHz, δ ppm): 8.3 (s, 1H), 7.9 (s, 1H), 7.7 (d, *J* = 8 Hz, 2H), 7.6–7.5 (m, 3H), 6.8 (d, *J* = 9.1 Hz, 2H), 6.4 (d, *J* = 9.1 Hz, 2H), 2.9 (s, 6H), 2.3 (s, 3H). ^{13}C NMR ($CDCl_3$, 125 MHz, δ ppm): 194.4, 162.1, 158.2, 157.1, 155.9, 147.1, 140.4, 133.0, 132.9, 130.8, 129.7, 129.6, 128.7, 124.5, 114.6, 99.0, 41.4, 26.3. HR-MS (ESI-TOF) (*m*/*z*): calculated for $C_{23}H_{22}N_6O + H^+$: 399.1928; found, 399.1981 $[M + H]^+$.

3-(4-Amino-3-phenyl-1*H*-pyrazolo[3,4-d]pyrimidin-1-yl)-pent-3-en-2-one (**8**). (Yield: 60%). ^{1}H-NMR ($CDCl_3$, 500 MHz, δ ppm): 8.37 (s, 1H), 7.8–7.7 (m, 2H), 7.6–7.5 (m, 3H), 7.4 (q, *J* = 7.1 Hz, 1H), 2.3 (s, 3H), 1.8 (d, *J* = 7 Hz, 3H). ^{13}C NMR ($CDCl_3$, 100 MHz, δ ppm): 157.9, 156.3, 154.8, 141.7, 132.6, 129.6, 129.5, 129.5, 128.5. 128.4, 98.3, 56.2, 26.1, 14.6. HR-MS (ESI-TOF) (*m*/*z*): calcd for $C_{16}H_{15}N_5O + H^+$: 294.1349; found, 294.099 $[M + H]^+$.

3-(4-Amino-3-phenyl-1*H*-pyrazolo[3,4-d]pyrimidin-1-yl)-4-(3-nitrophenyl)but-3-en-2-one (**9**). (Yield: 44%). ^{1}H-NMR ($CDCl_3$, 500 MHz, δ ppm): 8.3 (s, 1H), 7.9 (s, 1H), 7.7 (d, *J* = 7 Hz, 2H), 7.5–7.5 (m, 3H), 6.9 (d, *J* – 8.9 Hz, 2H), 6.7 (d, *J* = 8.9 Hz, 1H), 2.3 (s, 3H). ^{13}C NMR ($CDCl_3$, 125 MHz, δ ppm): 194.2, 161.9, 158.0, 156.9, 155.7, 146.9, 140.2, 132.8, 132.7, 130.6, 129.5, 129.4, 128.5, 124.3, 114.4, 98.9, 55.3, 26.0. HR-MS (ESI-TOF) (*m*/*z*): calculated for $C_{21}H_{16}N_6O_3 + H^+$: 401.1357; found, 401.0957 $[M + H]^+$, 801.1652 $[2M + H]^+$.

3-(4-Amino-3-phenyl-1*H*-pyrazolo[3,4-d]pyrimidin-1-yl)-4-(4-chlorophenyl)but-3-en-2-one (**10**). (Yield: 57%). ^{1}H-NMR ($CDCl_3$, 500 MHz, δ ppm): 8.1 (s, 1H), 7.9 (s, 1H), 7.6 (m, 2H), 7.5–7.5 (m, 3H), 7.2 (d, *J* = 8.6 Hz, 2H), 6.9 (d, *J* = 8.6 Hz, 2H), 2.4 (s, 3H). ^{13}C NMR ($CDCl_3$, 125 MHz, δ ppm): 192.4, 153.7, 153.5, 149.5, 147.2, 140.6, 137.9, 132.5, 131.5, 131.3, 130.9, 130.4, 130.1, 129.5, 128.1, 97.6, 55.3, 25.8. HR-MS (ESI-TOF) (*m*/*z*): calculated for $C_{21}H_{16}ClN_5O + H^+$: 390.1116; found, 390.0951 $[M + 1]^+$.

3-(4-Amino-3-phenyl-1*H*-pyrazolo[3,4-d]pyrimidin-1-yl)-4-(2,4-dichlorophenyl)but-3-en-2-one (**11**). (Yield: 58%). ^{1}H-NMR ($CDCl_3$, 500 MHz, δ ppm): 8.3 (s, 1H), 7.9 (s, 1H), 7.7 (d, *J* = 7 Hz, 2H), 7.5–7.5 (m, 3H), 6.9 (s, 1H), 6.7 (d, *J* = 8.6 Hz, 2H), 2.6 (s, 3H). ^{13}C NMR ($CDCl_3$, 125 MHz, δ ppm): 192.2, 153.7, 136.9, 136.2, 130.9, 130.2, 130.1, 129.8, 129.0, 128.2, 128.1, 127.5, 127.5, 97.6, 66.4, 53.4, 25.9. HR-MS (ESI-TOF) (*m*/*z*): calculated for $C_{21}H_{15}Cl_2N_5O + H^+$: 424.0726; found, 424.1220 $[M + H]^+$.

3-(4-Amino-3-phenyl-1*H*-pyrazolo[3,4-d]pyrimidin-1-yl)-4-(2-chlorophenyl)but-3-en-2-one (**12**). (Yield: 57%). ^{1}H-NMR ($CDCl_3$, 500 MHz, δ ppm): 8.3 (s, 1H), 8.2 (s, 1H), 7.6–7.5 (m, 5H), 7.3–7.2 (m, 4H), 2.6 (s, 3H). ^{13}C-NMR ($CDCl_3$, 125 MHz, δ ppm): 153.6, 153.3, 149.1, 146.5, 138.2, 132.0, 130.8, 130.2, 130.1, 129.3, 128.9, 128.1, 126.9, 52.5, 25.9. HR-MS (ESI-TOF) (*m*/*z*): calcd for $C_{21}H_{16}ClN_5O + H^+$: 390.1116; found, 390.1427 $[M + H]^+$.

3-(4-Amino-3-phenyl-1*H*-pyrazolo[3,4-d]pyrimidin-1-yl)-4-(2-fluorophenyl)but-3-en-2-one (**13**). (Yield: 62%). ^{1}H-NMR ($CDCl_3$, 500 MHz, δ ppm): 8.3 (s, 1H), 7.9 (s, 1H), 7.7 (d, *J* = 7 Hz, 2H), 7.6–7.5 (m, 3H), 7.2–6.9 (m, 4H), 2.3 (s, 3H). ^{13}C NMR ($CDCl_3$, 125 MHz, δ ppm): 193.8, 158.1, 155.6, 147.4, 132.8, 132.7, 130.3, 131.7, 129.7, 129.5, 129.5, 129.3, 129.2, 128.4, 128.4, 128.4, 98.7, 26.2. HR-MS (ESI-TOF) (*m*/*z*): calculated for $C_{21}H_{16}FN_5O + H^+$: 374.1412; found, 374.1526 $[M + H]^+$.

3-(4-Amino-3-phenyl-1*H*-pyrazolo[3,4-d]pyrimidin-1-yl)-4-(4-fluorophenyl)but-3-en-2-one (**14**). (Yield: 64%). ^{1}H-NMR ($CDCl_3$, 500 MHz, δ ppm): 8.1 (s, 1H), 7.8 (s, 1H), 7.5–7.4 (m, 5H), 6.9 (dd, *J* = 14 Hz, *J* = 5.6 Hz, 2H), 6.8 (t, *J* = 7.6 Hz, 2H), 2.4 (s, 3H). ^{13}C NMR ($CDCl_3$, 125 MHz, δ ppm): 192.5, 153.7, 153.5, 147.2, 140.7, 132.5, 132.4, 130.9, 130.1, 130.0, 128.1, 128.1, 116.7, 116.5, 25.7. HR-MS (ESI-TOF) (*m*/*z*): calculated for $C_{21}H_{16}FN_5O + H^+$: 374.1412; found, 374.1679 $[M + H]^+$.

3-(4-Amino-3-phenyl-1*H*-pyrazolo[3,4-d]pyrimidin-1-yl)-4-phenyl but-3-en-2-one (**15**). (Yield: 59%). ^{1}H-NMR ($CDCl_3$, 500 MHz, δ ppm): 8.2 (s, 1H), 8.0 (s, 1H), 7.7–7.6 (m, 5H), 7.4–6.9 (m, 5H), 2.5 (s, 3H). ^{13}C-NMR ($CDCl_3$, 125 MHz, δ ppm): 192.5, 153.7, 153.5, 147.2, 140.7, 132.5, 132.4, 130.9, 130.1, 130.0, 128.1, 128.1, 116.7, 116.5, 25.7. HR-MS (ESI-TOF) (*m*/*z*): calculated for $C_{21}H_{17}N_5O + H^+$: 356.1506; found, 356.1703 $[M + H]^+$.

3.3. *Kinase Enzyme Assay*

3.3.1. c-Src Kinase Activity Assay

The effect of compounds on the activity of *c*-Src kinase was assessed using a Transcreener® ADP [2,8] fluorescence intensity (FI) Assay, from Bell Brook Labs, Madison, WI, USA, (catalog no. 3013-1K) according to the manufacturer's protocol. A 384-well low-volume black non-binding surface round-bottom microplate was purchased from Corning Inc. (Corning, NY, USA) (#3676). In summary, the kinase reaction was started in the 384-well low volume black microplate with the incubation of 2.5 μL of the reaction cocktail (0.7 nM of His_6-Src kinase domain in kinase buffer) with 2.5 μL of prediluted compounds (dissolved in 10% DMSO, 4× target concentration) for 10 min at room temperature using microplate shaker. The reaction cocktail was made using the kinase buffer HEPES (200 mM, pH 7.5), $MgCl_2$ (16 mM), EGTA (8 mM), DMSO (4%), Brij-35 (0.04%), and 2-mercaptoethanol (43 mM). The kinase reaction was started by adding 5 μL of ATP/substrate (40 μM/600 μM) cocktail and incubated for 30 min at room temperature on a microplate shaker. Src optimal peptide (AEEEIYGEFEAKKKK) was used as the substrate for the kinase reaction. The kinase reaction was stopped by adding 10 μL of the 1× ADP Detection Mixture to the enzyme reaction mixture and mixed using a plate shaker. The mixture was incubated at room temperature for 1 h, and the fluorescence intensity was measured. The 1× ADP Detection Mixture was prepared by adding ADP^2 Antibody-IRDyeR QC-1 (10 μg/mL) and ADP Alexa594 Tracer (8 nM) to Stop and Detect Buffer B(1×). The fluorescence Intensity measurements were performed using a fluorescence intensity optical module using the excitation of 580 nm and emission of 630 nm with bandwidths of 10 nm by Optima, BMG Labtech microplate reader (BMG Labtech, Ortenberg, Germany). The IC_{50} values of the compounds were calculated using ORIGIN 6.0 (Origin Lab, Microcal Software, Inc. Northhampton, MA, USA) software. IC_{50} is the concentration of the compound that inhibited enzyme activity by 50%. All the experiments were carried out in triplicate.

3.3.2. Evaluation of Compound **10** Against a Panel of Kinases (Abl1, Akt1, Alk, Braf, Btk, Cdk2, cSrc, Lck, and PKCa)

Compound **10** was evaluated for inhibitory activity against Abl1, Akt1, Alk, Braf, Btk, Cdk2, cSrc, Lck, and PKCa, in duplicate by Reaction Biology Corporation. Compounds were tested in a five-dose IC_{50} mode with four-fold serial dilution starting at 20 μM. Control compounds Staurosporine and GW5074 were tested in a 10-dose IC_{50} starting at 20 μM with a four-fold or three-fold serial dilution, respectively. All kinase reactions were performed at 200 μM ATP. The compounds were pre-incubated with the enzyme and substrate mixture about 20 min, and then ATP was added to start the reaction. The reaction was 2 h at room temperature. Curve fits were performed when the activities at the highest concentration of compounds were less than 65%. The detailed experimental procedure is provided here. An IC_{50} value of less than 0.04 nM or higher than 1 μM is estimated based on the best curve fitting available. The substrates for kinases are shown in Table 5.

Table 5. Substrates used for kinases.

Kinases	Kinase (Invitrogen) Cat#	Kinase Conc. in Reaction (nM)	Substrate	Substrate Conc. in Reaction
Abl1	PR4348B	0.25	ABLtide	20 μM
c-Src	P3044	0.6	pEY	0.2 mg/mL
Akt1	PR3878D	8	Crosstide	20 μM
Alk	PV3867	1.5	pEY	0.2 mg/mL
Cdk2/Cyclin A1	C29-10BG	15	Histone H1	20 μM
PKCa	PR1455C	0.5	Histone H1 + Lipid Activator	20 μM
Braf	PR6995A	30	MEK1 (K97R)	5 μM
Lck	P3043	8	pEY + Manganese	0.2 mg/mL
Btk	PV3363	8	pEY	0.2 mg/mL

Base Reaction buffer was prepared from 20 mM Hepes (pH 7.5), 10 mM $MgCl_2$, 1 mM EGTA, 0.02% Brij35, 0.02 mg/mL BSA, 0.1 mM Na_3VO_4, 2 mM DTT, and 1% DMSO. Required cofactors were added individually to each kinase reaction. Testing compounds were dissolved in 100% DMSO to a specific concentration. The serial dilution was conducted by Integra Viaflo Assist in DMSO. The substrate was prepared in a freshly prepared reaction buffer. The required cofactors for each kinase were added to the substrate solution. The kinase was added into the substrate solution, and the solution was gently mixed. The compounds in 100% DMSO were added into the kinase reaction mixture by Acoustic technology (Echo550; nanoliter range) and incubated for 20 min at room temperature. P-ATP (Specific activity 10 μCi/μl) was added into the reaction mixture to initiate the reaction. The mixture was incubated for 2 h at room temperature. The radioactivity was detected using the filter-binding method. The kinase activity data were expressed as the percentage remaining kinase activity in test samples compared to vehicle (dimethyl sulfoxide) reactions. IC_{50} values, and curve fits were obtained using GraphPad Prism software (version 7, Informer Technologies, Inc., Los Angeles, CA, USA).

3.4. Cell Culture and Cell Proliferation Assay

3.4.1. Cell Culture

Human leukemia cell line CCRF-CEM (ATCC no. CCL-119), human ovarian adenocarcinoma cell line SK-OV-3 (ATCC no. HTB-77), human breast carcinoma cell line MDA-MB-231 (ATCC no.HTB-26), and human colon adenocarcinoma cell line HT-29 (ATCC no. HTB-38) were obtained from American Type Culture Collection. Cells were grown on 75 cm^2 cell culture flasks with RPMI-16 medium (for leukemia cells) and EMEM (Eagle's minimum essential medium) (for SK-OV-3, HT-29, MDA-MB-231 cells), supplemented with 10% fetal bovine serum (FBS), and 1% penicillin-streptomycin solution (10,000 units of penicillin and 10 mg of streptomycin in 0.9% NaCl) in a humidified atmosphere of 5% CO_2, 95% air at 37 °C.

3.4.2. Cell Proliferation Assay

The cell proliferation assay was carried out using a CellTiter 96 aqueous one-solution cell proliferation assay kit (Promega, Madison, WI, USA). Briefly, upon reaching about 75–80% confluence, 5000 cells/well were plated in 96-well microplate in 100 μL of the medium. After seeding for 24 h, the cells were treated with 50 μM compound in triplicate. Doxorubicin (10 μM) was used as a positive control. At the end of the sample exposure period (72 h), 20 μL of CellTiter 96 aqueous solution was added. The plate was returned to the incubator for 1 h in a humidified atmosphere at 37 °C. The absorbance of the formazan product was measured at 490 nm using a microplate reader. The blank control was recorded by measuring the absorbance at 490 nm with wells containing medium mixed with CellTiter 96 aqueous solution but no cells. The percentage of cell survival was calculated as the OD value of cells treated with test compound − OD value of culture medium/(OD value of control cells

– OD value of culture medium) × 100%. The same strategy was used for generating a dose-response graph for compound **10**.

3.5. Molecular Modeling

3.5.1. Target Fishing

Potential targets were identified against the phenylpyrazolopyrimidine scaffold using a combination of information integration, chemometric methods, and data mining approaches. Initially, targets involved in breast, ovarian, and colorectal cancer pathways were extracted from the database of KEGG. In the next step, protein network association servers STRING, STITCH, and SEA were used to characterize the protein-ligand interactions. Similarly, the PhPP scaffold was also searched using different search engines to understand protein-ligand interactions. Based on the above-mentioned information, we selected fourteen different targets, including Btk, Itk, c-Src, EGFR [39], Braf, Fyn, Lyn, Hck, Cdk2/4, Alk, Akt1 Lck, PKC, and Abl1 kinase. To understand the binding mechanism of active compound **10** against all selected targets, molecular docking and MD simulations were performed.

3.5.2. Preparation of Complexes

Crystal structures of the Anaplastic lymphoma kinase [PDB ID: 4MKC], ABL1 kinase [PDB ID: 6HD4], Protein kinase B also known as AKT [PDB ID: 4GV1], bruton tyrosine kinase [PDB ID: 6DIS], BRAF [PDB ID: 6B8U], c-Src kinase [PDB ID: 2SRC], CDK2 [PDB ID: 4KD1], LCK [PDB ID: 2OFU], ITK [PDB ID: 4HUC], EGFR [PDB ID: 4HJO], FYN [PDB ID: 2DQ7], LYN [PDB ID: 2ZV9], HCK [PDB ID: 1QCF], and PKCa [PDB ID: 3IW4] were retrieved from RCSB Protein Databank. The missing part of the starting structures was constructed using MOE software (Molecular Operating Environment, v2016.08, 2016). Compound partial charges were derived with the MMFF94x force field. All stabilizing agents, water molecules, and ions present in the crystal structures were removed. The protonate 3D module in MOE was used for assigning the protonation state to every titratable residue at physiological conditions within the complexes. MOE docking suite was employed for docking studies. The standard default settings were used with the London dG scoring function as a fitness function in all calculations.

3.5.3. MD Simulations

After analysis of docking results, nine complexes were subjected to all-atom MD simulation using the graphics processing unit (GPU) version of the PMEMD.cuda engine provided with Amber18 [40]. The gaff [41] and ff14SB force field [42] were implemented to ligand and protein in all simulations, respectively. Each complex was neutralized by adding counter ions, and the systems were solvated by a cubic box of the TIP3P water model with a 10 Å box size from the solute. Systems were relaxed by adjusting hydrogen position, while 1000 cycles of steepest descent, and 5000 cycles of the conjugate gradient with restraints of 100 kcal·mol^{-1} were applied on heavy atoms. Finally, another minimization of 5000 steps was performed to relax the system without any restraint. It was followed by equilibration of each system by gradual heating from 0 K to 300 K in the NVT ensemble. Systems were further equilibrated under the NPT ensemble (Pressure = 1 atm). The production run of 50 ns was performed for each system using the isothermal-isobaric (NPT) ensemble at constant temperature and pressure with periodic boundary conditions. The Particle Mesh Ewald Method (PMEM) [43] was used to calculate long-range electrostatic interactions with cut off value of 8 Å for the non-bonded (electrostatics and Van der Waals) interactions. An integration time step of 2 fs was set to integrate Newton's equations of motion. The SHAKE algorithm [44] was employed to restrain the bonds involving hydrogen atoms. The trajectories were analyzed using CPPTRAJ module incorporated in AMBER suite. All visualization was performed using Chimera and VMD.

3.5.4. MM/PBSA Calculations

The binding free energy calculation for each complex was performed using the MM(GB/PB)SA method based on 1000 frames extracted from the 50 ns trajectory. The equations associated with binding free energy calculation were as follows:

$$\Delta G = G_{complex} - (G_{receptor} + G_{compound}) \quad (1)$$

$$G = H - TS \quad (2)$$

$$H = E_{vdw} + E_{ele} + E_{int} + G_{gb} + G_{surf} \quad (3)$$

The total binding free energy is ΔG, whereas the free energies for the complex, receptor, and compound are represented as $G_{complex}$, $G_{receptor}$, and $G_{compound}$, respectively. The terms H and TΔS were used for the contribution of enthalpy and entropy. The binding free energy further decomposed into electrostatic (E_{ele}), Van der Waals interaction (E_{vdw}), internal energy (E_{int}), and polar (G_{gb}) and non-polar desolvation energy (G_{surf}). The value of the dielectric constant was set to 1, and the external was set to 80 for solute protein (εin). The Generalized Born (GB) model established by Onufriev (GBOBC1) with modified Bondi radii (mbondi2) and igb = 2 implemented in AMBER18 was used to calculate the electrostatic contribution to the solvation free energy. The non-polar surface area was calculated using the LCPO model. The offset (β) and surface tension (γ) values were set to 0.92 kcal/mol and 0.00542 kcal/(mol·Å2), respectively.

4. Conclusions

A number of novel *N*1-(α,β-alkene) substituted phenylpyrazolopyrimidine (PhPP) derivatives with acetyl and functionalized phenyl groups at α- and β-positions were synthesized, and they showed modest inhibitory activity (IC_{50} = 21.7–192.1 μM) against c-Src kinases. A number of para-chlorophenyl substituted compounds, **10** and **11,** consistently inhibited the cell proliferation 72–96 h in all cell lines and were more effective against HT-29 cells. Compound **10** was also found to be modestly active against c-Src, Lck, and Btk. The target-based study of these compounds was performed by text mining, similarity search, and ligand-protein interaction pattern to identify potential targets. Further MD simulation and binding free energy calculations were carried out to discriminate the selectivity of the investigated compound with a panel of different kinases and provide more in-depth structural insight into the interaction pattern involved in the inhibition process. The structural and energetic features highlighted in this study can provide a theoretical basis for further research on selective protein kinase inhibitors.

Author Contributions: Methodology: B.S.C., N.S.J., S.A., S.M., and R.K.T.; writing—original draft preparation: B.S.C., Z.U.-H, and K.P.; supervision: Z.U.-H. and K.P.; funding acquisition: K.P.; performed the synthesis: B.S.C. and N.S.J.; conducted the antiproliferative assays: S.M. and D.M.; performed the kinase assays: R.K.T.; performed molecular modeling: S.A.; supervised, wrote, and edited the manuscript: Z.U.-H. and K.P. All authors contributed to writing the manuscript, editing, and reviewing of the manuscript. All authors read and agreed to the published version of the manuscript.

Acknowledgments: We acknowledge the financial support from the American Cancer Society Grant # RSG-07-290-01-CDD and Chapman University School of Pharmacy.

References

1. Yeatman, T.J. A renaissance for SRC. *Nat. Rev. Cancer* **2004**, *4*, 470–480. [CrossRef] [PubMed]
2. Summy JM, G.G. Src family kinases in tumor progression and metastasis. *Cancer Metastasis Rev.* **2003**, *22*, 337–358. [CrossRef] [PubMed]

3. Irby, R.B.; Yeatman, T.J. Role of Src expression and activation in human cancer. *Oncogene* **2000**, *19*, 5636–5642. [CrossRef] [PubMed]
4. Jiao, Q.; Bi, L.; Ren, Y.; Song, S.; Wang, Q.; Wang, Y.S. Advances in studies of tyrosine kinase inhibitors and their acquired resistance. *Mol. Cancer* **2018**, *17*, 36. [CrossRef] [PubMed]
5. Wagner, J.; Von Matt, P.; Sedrani, R.; Albert, R.; Cooke, N.; Ehrhardt, C.; Geiser, M.; Rummel, G.; Stark, W.; Strauss, A.; et al. Discovery of 3-(1*H*-indol-3-yl)-4-[2-(4-methylpiperazin-1-yl)quinazolin-4-yl]-pyrrole-2,5-dione (AEB071), a potent and selective inhibitor of protein kinase C isotypes. *J. Med. Chem.* **2009**, *52*, 6193–6196. [CrossRef]
6. Tsou, H.R.; Overbeek-Klumpers, E.G.; Hallett, W.A.; Reich, M.F.; Floyd, M.B.; Johnson, B.D.; Michalak, R.S.; Nilakantan, R.; Discafani, C.; Golas, J.; et al. Optimization of 6,7-disubstituted-4-(arylamino)quinoline-3-carbonitriles as orally active, irreversible inhibitors of human epidermal growth factor receptor-2 kinase activity. *J. Med. Chem.* **2005**, *48*, 1107–1131. [CrossRef] [PubMed]
7. Schenone, S.; Radi, M.; Musumeci, F.; Brullo, C.; Botta, M. Biologically driven synthesis of pyrazolo [3, 4-d] pyrimidines as protein kinase inhibitors: An old scaffold as a new tool for medicinal chemistry and chemical biology studies. *Chem. Rev.* **2014**, *114*, 7189–7238. [CrossRef]
8. Kumar, A.; Ahmad, I.; Chhikara, B.S.; Tiwari, R.; Mandal, D.; Parang, K. Synthesis of 3-phenylpyrazolopyrimidine-1,2,3-triazole conjugates and evaluation of their Src kinase inhibitory and anticancer activities. *Bioorg. Med. Chem. Lett.* **2011**, *21*, 1342–1346. [CrossRef]
9. Mukaiyama, H.; Nishimura, T.; Kobayashi, S.; Ozawa, T.; Kamada, N.; Komatsu, Y.; Kikuchi, S.; Oonota, H.; Kusama, H. Synthesis and c-Src inhibitory activity of imidazo[1,5-a]pyrazine derivatives as an agent for treatment of acute ischemic stroke. *Bioorg. Med. Chem.* **2007**, *15*, 868–885. [CrossRef]
10. Trush, V.; Cherenok, S.; Tanchuk, V.; Kalchenko, V.; Vovk, A. Evaluation of inhibition of protein tyrosine phosphatase 1B by calixarene-based α-ketophosphonic acids. *Chem. Biol. Lett.* **2015**, *2*, 1–5.
11. Rao, V.K.; Chhikara, B.S.; Tiwari, R.; Shirazi, A.N.; Parang, K.; Kumar, A. One-pot regioselective synthesis of tetrahydroindazolones and evaluation of their antiproliferative and Src kinase inhibitory activities. *Bioorg. Med. Chem. Lett.* **2012**, *22*, 410–414. [CrossRef] [PubMed]
12. Rao, M.S.; Chhikara, B.S.; Tiwari, R.; Shirazi, A.N.; Parang, K.; Kumar, A. Microwave-assisted and scandium triflate catalyzed synthesis of tetrahydrobenzo[a]xanthen-11-ones. *Monatshefte fur Chemie* **2012**, *143*, 263–268. [CrossRef]
13. Rao, V.K.; Chhikara, B.S.; Shirazi, A.N.; Tiwari, R.; Parang, K.; Kumar, A. 3-substitued indoles: One-pot synthesis and evaluation of anticancer and Src kinase inhibitory activities. *Bioorg. Med. Chem. Lett.* **2011**, *21*, 3511–3514. [CrossRef] [PubMed]
14. Nam, N.H.; Lee, S.; Ye, G.; Sun, G.; Parang, K. ATP-phosphopeptide conjugates as inhibitors of Src tyrosine kinases. *Bioorg. Med. Chem.* **2004**, *12*, 5753–5766. [CrossRef]
15. Deininger, M.; Buchdunger, E.; Druker, B.J. The development of imatinib as a therapeutic agent for chronic myeloid leukemia. *Blood* **2005**, *105*, 2640–2653. [CrossRef]
16. Shah, N.P.; Tran, C.; Lee, F.Y.; Chen, P.; Norris, D.; Sawyers, C.L. Overriding imatinib resistance with a novel ABL kinase inhibitor. *Science* **2004**, *305*, 399–401. [CrossRef]
17. Vultur, A.; Buettner, R.; Kowolik, C.; Liang, W.; Smith, D.; Boschelli, F.; Jove, R. SKI-606 (bosutinib), a novel Src kinase inhibitor, suppresses migration and invasion of human breast cancer cells. *Mol. Cancer Ther.* **2008**, *7*, 1185–1194. [CrossRef]
18. Martina Ferrari, S.; La Motta, C.; Sartini, S.; Baldini, E.; Materazzi, G.; Politti, U.; Ruffilli, I.; Ulisse, S.; Miccoli, P.; Antonelli, A. Pyrazolopyrimidine derivatives as antineoplastic agents: With a special focus on thyroid cancer. *Mini Rev. Med. Chem.* **2016**, *16*, 86–93. [CrossRef]
19. Crisci, S.; Di Francia, R.; Amitrano, F.; Saggese, M.; Mele, S.; Ronga, G.; De Filippi, R.; Berretta, M.; Rossi, P.; Pinto, A. Overview of Targeted Drugs for Mature B-Cell Non-hodgkin Lymphomas. *Front. Oncol.* **2019**, *9*, 443. [CrossRef]
20. Akinleye, A.; Chen, Y.; Mukhi, N.; Song, Y.; Liu, D. Ibrutinib and novel BTK inhibitors in clinical development. *J. Hematol. Oncol.* **2013**, *6*, 59. [CrossRef]
21. Xu, W.; Doshi, A.; Lei, M.; Eck, M.J.; Harrison, S.C. Crystal Structures of c-Src Reveal Features of Its Autoinhibitory Mechanism. *Mol. Cell* **1999**, *3*, 629–638. [CrossRef]

22. Zhu, X.; Kim, J.L.; Newcomb, J.R.; Rose, P.E.; Stover, D.R.; Toledo, L.M.; Zhao, H.; Morgenstern, K.A. Structural analysis of the lymphocyte-specific kinase Lck in complex with non-selective and Src family selective kinase inhibitors. *Structure* **1999**, *7*, 651–661. [CrossRef]

23. Bookser, B.C.; Ugarkar, B.G.; Matelich, M.C.; Lemus, R.H.; Allan, M.; Tsuchiya, M.; Nakane, M.; Nagahisa, A.; Wiesner, J.B.; Erion, M.D. Adenosine Kinase Inhibitors. 6. Synthesis, Water Solubility, and Antinociceptive Activity of 5-Phenyl-7-(5-deoxy-β-d-ribofuranosyl)pyrrolo[2,3-d]pyrimidines Substituted at C4 with Glycinamides and Related Compounds. *J. Med. Chem.* **2005**, *48*, 7808–7820. [CrossRef] [PubMed]

24. Chhikara, B.S.; Parang, K. Development of cytarabine prodrugs and delivery systems for leukemia treatment. *Expert Opin. Drug Deliv.* **2010**, *7*, 1399–1414. [CrossRef] [PubMed]

25. Chhikara, B.S.; Mandal, D.; Parang, K. Synthesis and evaluation of fatty acyl ester derivatives of cytarabine as anti-leukemia agents. *Eur. J. Med. Chem.* **2010**, *45*, 4601–4608. [CrossRef]

26. Chhikara, B.S.; Rathi, B.; Parang, K. Critical evaluation of pharmaceutical rational design of nano-delivery systems for doxorubicin in cancer therapy. *J. Mater. Nanosci.* **2019**, *6*, 47–66.

27. Nasrolahi Shirazi, A.; Tiwari, R.; Chhikara, B.S.; Mandal, D.; Parang, K. Design and biological evaluation of cell-penetrating peptide-doxorubicin conjugates as prodrugs. *Mol. Pharm.* **2013**, *10*, 488–499. [CrossRef]

28. Chhikara, B.S.; St. Jean, N.; Mandal, D.; Kumar, A.; Parang, K. Fatty acyl amide derivatives of doxorubicin: Synthesis and in vitro anticancer activities. *Eur. J. Med. Chem.* **2011**, *46*, 2037–2042. [CrossRef]

29. Chhikara, B.S.; Mandal, D.; Parang, K. Synthesis, anticancer activities, and cellular uptake studies of lipophilic derivatives of doxorubicin succinate. *J. Med. Chem.* **2012**, *55*, 1500–1510. [CrossRef]

30. Behera, D.K.; Behera, P.M.; Acharya, L.; Dixit, A. Development and validation of pharmacophore and QSAR models for influenza PB2 inhibitors. *Chem. Biol. Lett.* **2017**, *4*, 1–8.

31. Sharma, D.; Pathak, M.; Sharma, R.; Sharma, N.; Tyagi, P.; Chawla, R.; Basu, M.; Ojha, H. Homology modeling and docking studies of VP24 protein of Ebola virus with an antiviral drug and its derivatives. *Chem. Biol. Lett.* **2017**, *4*, 27–32.

32. Kanehisa, M.; Shlomi, T.; Ruppin, E.; Koonin, E.; Snoddy, J.; Gerstein, M.; Sheffer, M.; Alon, U. KEGG: Kyoto Encyclopedia of Genes and Genomes. *Nucl. Acid. Res.* **2000**, *28*, 27–30. [CrossRef] [PubMed]

33. Wang, Z.; Liang, L.; Yin, Z.; Lin, J. Improving chemical similarity ensemble approach in target prediction. *J. Cheminform.* **2016**, *8*, 20. [CrossRef] [PubMed]

34. Roth, A.; Franceschini, A.; Szklarczyk, D.; Heller, D.; Simonovic, M.; Wyder, S.; von Mering, C.; Huerta-Cepas, J.; Forslund, K.; Bork, P.; et al. STRING v10: Protein–protein interaction networks, integrated over the tree of life. *Nucl. Acid. Res.* **2014**, *43*, D447–D452.

35. Szklarczyk, D.; Santos, A.; Von Mering, C.; Jensen, L.J.; Bork, P.; Kuhn, M. STITCH 5: Augmenting protein-chemical interaction networks with tissue and affinity data. *Nucl. Acid. Res.* **2016**, *44*, D380–D384. [CrossRef] [PubMed]

36. Chandel, V.; Raj, S.; Rathi, B.; Kumar, D. In silico identification of potent FDA approved drugs against Coronavirus COVID-19 main protease: A drug repurposing approach. *Chem. Biol. Lett.* **2020**, *7*, 166–175.

37. Wencheng, X.; Zhang, L.; Yin, Y.; Yang, D.; Zhao, G. 3D-QSAR and molecular docking studies of ATP-competitive Akt inhibitors with the scaffold 4-(piperazin-1-yl)pyrimidine. *Chem. Biol. Lett.* **2014**, *1*, 44–54.

38. Kollman, P.A.; Massova, I.; Reyes, C.; Kuhn, B.; Huo, S.; Chong, L.; Lee, M.; Lee, T.; Duan, Y.; Wang, W.; et al. Calculating structures and free energies of complex molecules: Combining molecular mechanics and continuum models. *Acc. Chem. Res.* **2000**, *33*, 889–897. [CrossRef]

39. Chandel, V.; Srivastava, M.; Srivastava, A.; Asthana, S.; Kumar, D. In-silico interactions of active Phytochemicals with c-MYC EGFR and ERBB2 oncoproteins. *Chem. Biol. Lett.* **2020**, *7*, 47–54.

40. Case, D.A.; Cheatham, T.E.; Darden, T.; Gohlke, H.; Luo, R.; Merz, K.M.; Onufriev, A.; Simmerling, C.; Wang, B.; Woods, R.J. The Amber biomolecular simulation programs. *J. Comput. Chem.* **2005**, *26*, 1668–1688. [CrossRef]

41. Wang, J.; Wolf, R.M.; Caldwell, J.W.; Kollman, P.A.; Case, D.A. Development and testing of a general Amber force field. *J. Comput. Chem.* **2004**, *25*, 1157–1174. [CrossRef] [PubMed]

42. Maier, J.A.; Martinez, C.; Kasavajhala, K.; Wickstrom, L.; Hauser, K.E.; Simmerling, C. ff14SB: Improving the Accuracy of Protein Side Chain and Backbone Parameters from ff99SB. *J. Chem. Theor. Comput.* **2015**, *11*, 3696–3713. [CrossRef] [PubMed]
43. Darden, T.; York, D.; Pedersen, L. Particle mesh Ewald: An N·log(N) method for Ewald sums in large systems. *J. Chem. Phys.* **1993**, *98*, 10089–10092. [CrossRef]
44. Ryckaert, J.C.; Ciccotti, G.; Berendsen, H.J.C. Numerical Integration of the Cartesian Equations of Motion of a System with Constraints. *J. Comp. Phys.* **1977**, *23*, 327–341. [CrossRef]

6

Mechanism of the Dual Activities of Human CYP17A1 and Binding to Anti-Prostate Cancer Drug Abiraterone Revealed by a Novel V366M Mutation Causing 17,20 Lyase Deficiency

Mónica Fernández-Cancio [1,†], Núria Camats [1,2,3,†], Christa E. Flück [2,3,†], Adam Zalewski [2,3,†], Bernhard Dick [4], Brigitte M. Frey [4], Raquel Monné [5], Núria Torán [6], Laura Audí [1] and Amit V. Pandey [2,3,*]

1 Growth and Development Research Unit, Vall d'Hebron Research Institute (VHIR), Center for Biomedical Research on Rare Diseases (CIBERER), Instituto de Salud Carlos III, Autonomous University of Barcelona, Barcelona 08035, Spain; monica.fernandez.cancio@vhir.org (M.F.-C.); nuria.camats@vhir.org (N.C.); laura.audi@vhir.org (L.A.)

2 Pediatric Endocrinology Unit, Department of Paediatrics, University Children's Hospital Bern, Bern 3010, Switzerland; christa.flueck@dbmr.unibe.ch (C.E.F.); adam.zalewski@mail.com (A.Z.)

3 Department of Biomedical Research, University of Bern, Bern 3010, Switzerland

4 Department of Nephrology and Hypertension, University of Bern, Bern 3010, Switzerland; Bernhard.dick@gmx.ch (B.D.); brigitte.frey@dbmr.unibe.ch (B.M.F.)

5 Pediatric Service, Hospital Joan XXIII, Tarragona 43005, Spain; raquel.monne@urv.cat

6 Pathology Department, Hospital Universitari Vall d'Hebron, CIBERER, Barcelona 08035, Spain; toranfuentesn@gmail.com

* Correspondence: amit@pandeylab.org;

† These authors contributed equally.

Abstract: The *CYP17A1* gene regulates sex steroid biosynthesis in humans through 17α-hydroxylase/17,20 lyase activities and is a target of anti-prostate cancer drug abiraterone. In a 46, XY patient with female external genitalia, together with a loss of function mutation S441P, we identified a novel missense mutation V366M at the catalytic center of CYP17A1 which preferentially impaired 17,20 lyase activity. Kinetic experiments with bacterially expressed proteins revealed that V366M mutant enzyme can bind and metabolize pregnenolone to 17OH-pregnenolone, but 17OH-pregnenolone binding and conversion to dehydroepiandrosterone (DHEA) was impaired, explaining the patient's steroid profile. Abiraterone could not bind and inhibit the 17α-hydroxylase activity of the CYP17A1-V366M mutant. Molecular dynamics (MD) simulations showed that V366M creates a "one-way valve" and suggests a mechanism for dual activities of human CYP17A1 where, after the conversion of pregnenolone to 17OH-pregnenolone, the product exits the active site and re-enters for conversion to dehydroepiandrosterone. The V366M mutant also explained the effectiveness of the anti-prostate cancer drug abiraterone as a potent inhibitor of CYP17A1 by binding tightly at the active site in the WT enzyme. The V366M is the first human mutation to be described at the active site of CYP17A1 that causes isolated 17,20 lyase deficiency. Knowledge about the specificity of CYP17A1 activities is of importance for the development of treatments for polycystic ovary syndrome and inhibitors for prostate cancer therapy.

Keywords: P450c17; prostate cancer; abiraterone; steroidogenesis; androgens; dehydroepiandrosterone; *CYP17A1*; cytochrome P450; anti-cancer drugs; DSD

1. Introduction

The Cytochrome P450 proteins that are located in the endoplasmic reticulum are responsible for the metabolism of xenobiotics, drugs and steroid hormones (Figure 1) and are part of the microsomal mixed oxidase system [1–3]. Cytochrome P450c17 (CYP17A1) is required for the biosynthesis of steroid hormones in all vertebrates. The CYP17A1 is the qualitative regulator of the biosynthesis of sex steroid in humans (Figure 2) [4]. CYP17A1 catalyses multiple reactions in the steroid pathway [5–7]; chiefly among them, its 17α-hydroxylase activity is essential for the production of 17OH-pregnenolone (17OH-PREG) and 17OH-progesterone (17OH-PROG) which are precursors of cortisol, and its 17,20 lyase activity is required for the generation of the precursor of sex steroids, dehydroepiandrosterone (DHEA) (Figure 2). These two activities of the CYP17A1 determine the type of steroid hormone synthesized in different cells and tissues; if the CYP17A1 is absent, mineralocorticoids are produced, if only the 17α-hydroxylase activity of the CYP17A1 is present, glucocorticoids are made; and if both the 17α-hydroxylase and the 17,20 lyase activities of the CYP17A1 are present, sex steroid precursors are generated [4]. Overproduction of androgens by the specific activation of CYP17A1-17,20 lyase activity has been implicated in the pathogenesis of the polycystic ovary syndrome [4]. CYP17A1 is a target for prostate cancer therapy by inhibitor abiraterone (Zytiga by Johnson & Johnson, New Brunswick, USA) [8–12].

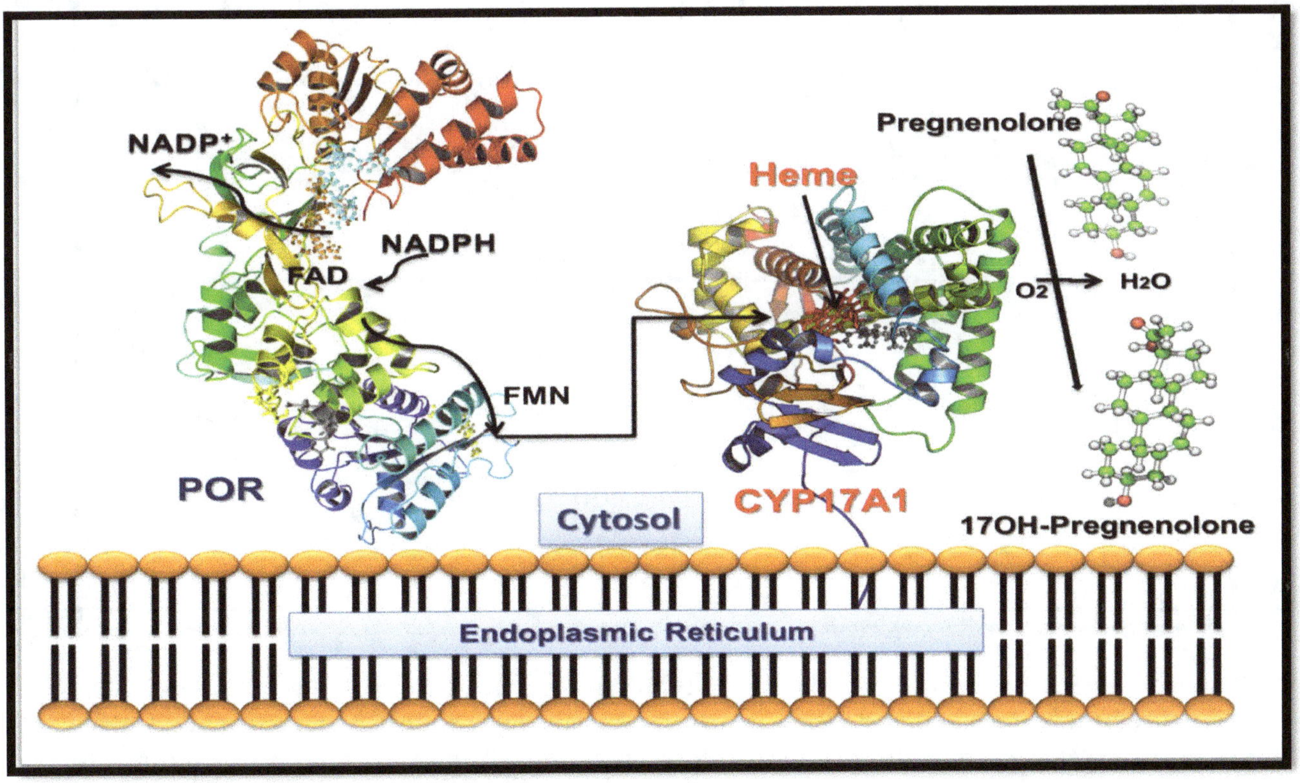

Figure 1. Schematic diagram of CYP17A1 and P450 oxidoreductase (POR) interaction in the membranes. The nicotinamide adenine dinucleotide phosphate (NADPH) molecules bind to POR, which is embedded into the membranes of endoplasmic reticulum and donate a pair of electrons, one at a time, which are received by the FAD. Transfer of electrons to FAD creates a change in conformation of POR, allowing the FAD and FMN groups to move towards each other, which facilitates the transfer of electrons from FAD to FMN. The FMN domain of POR interacts with the CYP17A1 and transfers electrons for catalytic activities.

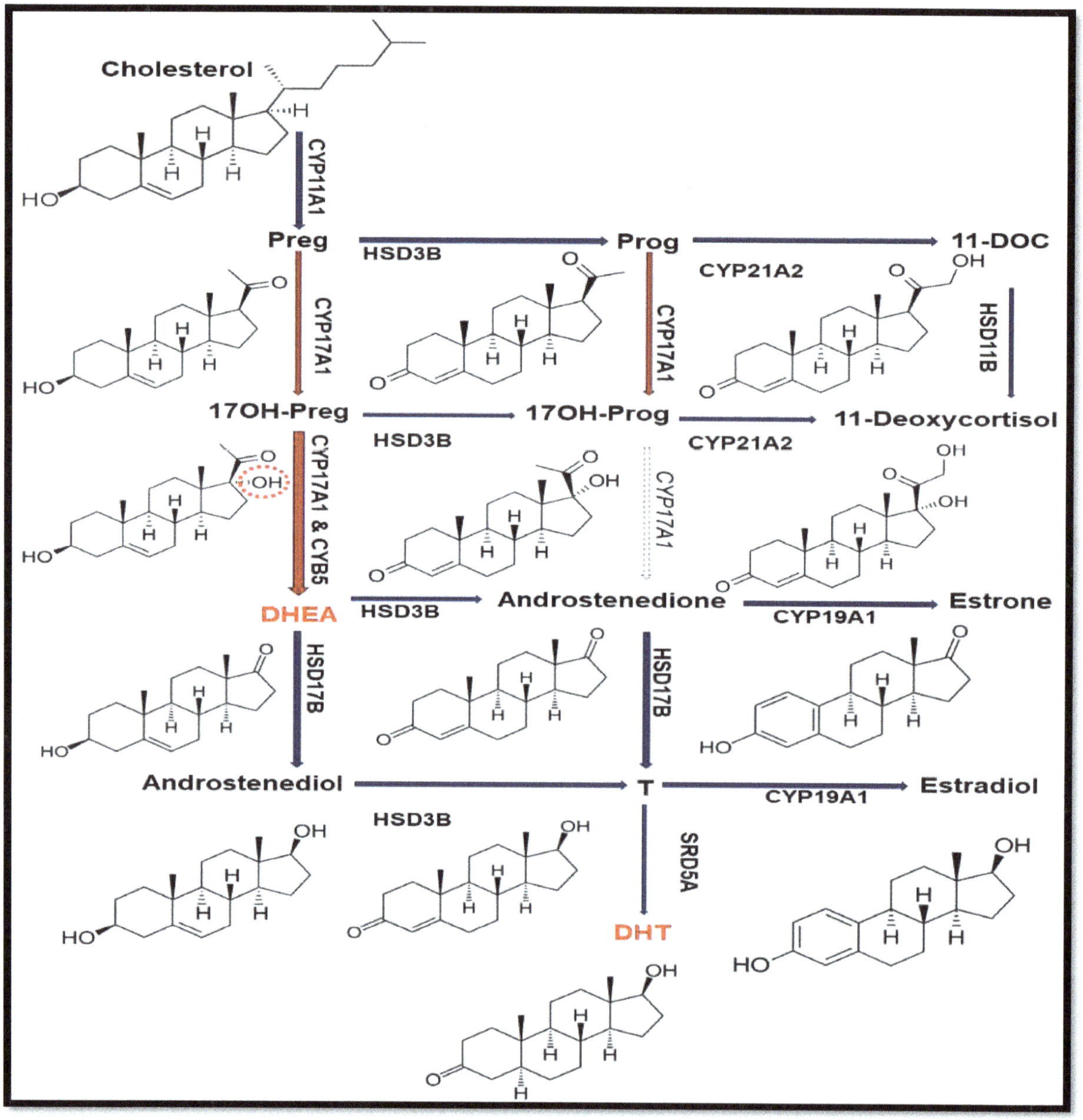

Figure 2. Steroid biosynthetic pathway. In humans, 17,20 lyase activity of *CYP17A1* converts 17α-hydroxypregnenolone (17OH-PREG) to dehydroepiandrosterone (DHEA) but does not effectively convert 17α-hydroxyprogesterone (17OH-PROG) to androstenedione. The DHEA is the precursor for androgen production and (dihydrotestosterone) DHT is the potent form of androgen with higher affinity towards androgen receptor (AR) than testosterone (T). The 17α-hydroxy position of 17OH-PREG is highlighted in red to show the difference from PREG.

Similar to other microsomal P450 proteins, CYP17A1 also requires electrons supplied from reduced nicotinamide adenine dinucleotide phosphate (NADPH) through cytochrome P450 oxidoreductase (POR) (Figure 1) [2,13–16]. The 17,20 lyase activity of CYP17A1 is influenced by the presence of cytochrome b_5 (CYB5A) in specific locations in different cells and tissues and guides the steroid hormone pathway in different directions [4] (Figure 2).

Along with CYB5A, higher molecular ratios of POR and phosphorylation of CYP17A1 also influence 17,20 lyase activity [17–21]. Recently several X-ray crystal structures of solubilized human CYP17A1 have been reported, but the structural basis of 17α-hydroxylase and 17,20, lyase activities remains unknown [22–26]. Generally, the mutations that affect the steroid-binding domain of CYP17A1 or disturb the interaction with P450 oxidoreductase (POR) for electron transfer, cause combined 17α-hydroxylase and 17,20 lyase deficiency, and are those more frequently found in humans [4,25]. Very few point mutations in CYP17A1 (R347C/H, R358Q) have been reported to cause isolated 17,20 lyase deficiency [27–30] (Table 1). These mutations are thought to interfere with CYB5A binding and/or electron transfer from POR to CYP17A1 during the 17,20 lyase reaction.

Table 1. Reported cases of *CYP17A1* mutations causing isolated 17,20 lyase deficiency [27–30]. The mutation E305G which was initially reported by Sherbet et al. [28] to cause isolated 17,20 lyase deficiency, was later reported by Tiosano et al. [30] to also result in combined 17α-hydroxylase/17,20 lyase deficiency, similar to other common mutations in *CYP17A1* [30].

17OH Steroids Basal	17OH Steroids Stimulated	Cortisol Basal	Cortisol Stimulated	Activities (% of WT)		Ref
				17OHase	17,20 lyase	
Normal	Hyperresponsive	Normal	Areactive	65	5	Geller 1997 [27]
Elevated	Hyperresponsive	Normal	Areactive	65	5	Geller 1997 [27]
Slightly elevated	Not reactive	Low normal	Areactive			van den Akker 2002 [29]
Normal	Normal	Low normal	Areactive			van den Akker 2002 [29]
Normal/Elevated	Reactive	Low normal	Hyporeactive	60	0	van den Akker 2002 [29]
Normal/Elevated	Reactive	Low normal	Hyporeactive	60	0	van den Akker 2002 [29]
Normal/Elevated	Reactive	Low	Hyporeactive	100	0	Sherbet 2003 [28]
Normal/Elevated	Normal	Low normal	Hyporeactive			Tiosano 2008 [30]
Normal/Elevated	Normal	Low normal	Hyporeactive			Tiosano 2008 [30]
Normal/Elevated	Normal	Low normal	Hyporeactive			Tiosano 2008 [30]
Normal/Elevated	Normal	Low normal	Hyporeactive			Tiosano 2008 [30]
Normal/Elevated	Normal	Low normal	Hyporeactive			Tiosano 2008 [30]
Normal/Elevated	Normal	Low normal	Hyporeactive			Tiosano 2008 [30]
Normal/low	Hyporeactive	Low normal	Areactive	43	0/0	This report

Lack of 17α-hydroxylase activity of CYP17A1 results in a compensatory overproduction of corticosterone and deoxycorticosterone with a weak glucocorticoid and significant mineralocorticoid action, which results in severe hypertension and hypokalemia. On the other hand, the 17,20 lyase deficiency results in a lack of sex steroids, leading to the 46, XY disorder of sexual development (DSD) with severe undervirilization in the "male" newborn, and deficient pubertal development and fertility in both sexes [4]. Previously, we have reported that disturbing the interaction of CYP17A1 with P450 oxidoreductase (POR) for electron transfer causes combined 17α-hydroxylase and 17,20 lyase deficiency [2,14,16,31–34]. Mutations identified on the surface of *CYP17A1* (R347C/H, R358Q) have been proposed to diminish the interaction with POR but could not explain the mechanism of their specific effect on 17,20 lyase activity [27,35].

Recently we have shown that in the earliest reported cases of apparent isolated 17,20 lyase deficiency, that were based solely on hormonal and morphological findings and without genetic analysis, the *CYP17A1* and *POR* genes were actually normal and mutations in *AKR1C2* and *AKR1C4* were found to cause a similar phenotype [36–38]. In the current report, we are describing a novel active site mutation in CYP17A1 that specifically abolishes the 17,20 lyase activity.

2. Results

2.1. Case Report and Genetic Analysis of the Patient

The patient was born at term, with normal female external genitalia, after a normal spontaneous pregnancy, whereas an older sister was the product of an insemination with donor semen to avoid retinitis pigmentosa carried by the father's family. At 2 months of age, the patient was operated for a right inguinal hernia. No female internal sex organs were found and karyotype was 46, XY. During the procedure, a gonad was detected and biopsied showing to be a testis (Figure 3). Electrolytes were normal and baseline hormone values at 3 months of age revealed moderately elevated ACTH, highly elevated PROG, normal/low 17OH-PREG, 17OH-PROG, 11-deoxycortisol and cortisol, undetectable androstenedione (Δ_4A) and normal DHEA-S and Testosterone for female sex (Table 2). At the age of 5 months a human chorionic gonadotropin (hCG) test (500 IU/d $\times$ 3) was performed which showed no increase of Δ_4A and T upon stimulation (Table 2). At 20 months of age an ACTH test (Synacthen®) revealed a moderately elevated baseline ACTH and a normal baseline plasma renin activity (PRA), Prog was highly elevated and further increased upon stimulation, whereas baseline 17OH-PREG, 17OH-PROG, cortisol, 11-deoxycortisol, and aldosterone were normal/low, and did not increase after stimulation (Table 2). Baseline DHEA-S and baseline and stimulated Δ_4A were undetectable. Because of female phenotype and obvious biochemical lack of androgens, female sex of rearing was confirmed and a gonadectomy was performed at the age of 20 months. Testes morphology showed abnormal findings similar to those found in androgen-insensitive patients (Figure 4a). Blood pressure (BP) control was recommended as a precautionary measure while hydrocortisone replacement therapy was postponed depending on follow-up. BP controls revealed normal values. Baseline BP controls revealed normal values up to 11 years of age as well a 24-h ambulatory BP monitoring performed at 8 years of age (baseline and at the end of 3 months of therapy with hydrocortisone: 6 mg/m^2 in 3 daily doses).

Initial genetic analysis of the genes for *AR* and *SRD5A2* were normal [39,40] and hormonal findings suggested partial 17α-hydroxylase and complete 17,20 lyase deficiencies (Table 2). The *CYP17A1* gene was analyzed and compound heterozygous point mutations c.1096G > A (V366M) and c.1321T > C (S441P) in exons 6 and 8 were identified (Figure 4b). The healthy fertile mother was found to carry the V366M mutation, a residue which is highly conserved across species (Figure 4c), while the father was normal. Therefore, *CYP17A1* S441P might be a de novo mutation in the patient although paternity testing was not performed. The mutations in the patient are likely to be on different alleles as even total disruption of one copy of *CYP17A1* does not result in disease. As both *CYP17A1* mutations have not been described previously, and as our patient presented with a very rare phenotype of apparent isolated 17,20 lyase deficiency, we performed further investigations to characterize these novel mutations.

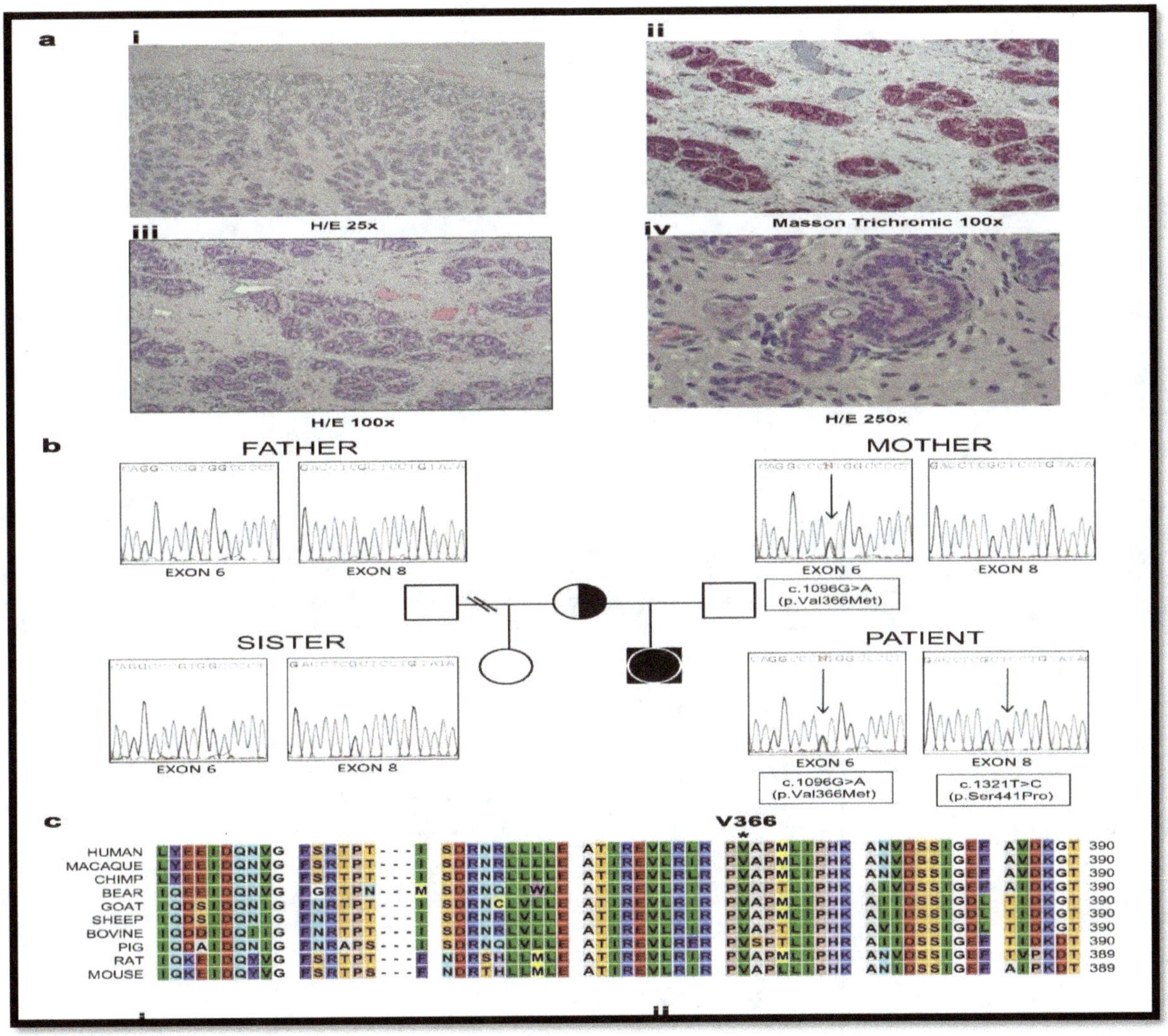

Figure 3. Genetic characterization and testis histology of the 46, XY disorder of sexual development (DSD) patient with a female phenotype. (**a**) Histopathologic studies revealed that both gonads consisted of atrophic and immature seminiferous tubules which were filled almost exclusively with pre-Sertoli cells. The fertility index was 5% with abortive and fetal type spermatogonia (i–iv); iii. in some areas, the tubules formed lobule-like structures similar to pseudo-hamartomas surrounded by collagen fibrous tissue; iv. nests of fibroblastic pre-Leydig cells were found in the interstitium. Albuginea and epidydimus were unremarkable. H/E-hematoxylin-eosin stain. (**b**) Family tree and electropherograms showing the index patient, the parents and the half-sister. Both, the patient and mother harbored the heterozygote c.1096G > A (p.Val366Met) mutation in exon 6, while the heterozygote c.1321T > C (p.Ser441Pro) mutation in exon 8 was only present in the patient. The father and the half-sister were both non-carriers of either mutation. (**c**) Alignment of human CYP17A1 amino acid sequence with a range of CYP17A1 proteins from other species found in the Universal Protein Knowledgebase (UniProt) database. The Valine 366 residue is highly conserved in all species studied.

Table 2. Laboratory findings in our patient harboring compound heterozygote *CYP17A1* mutations.

Age		3 Months		5 Months		20 Months			5 Years	6.5 Years	
Parameter	Unit	Basal	*Normal Range*	hCG Test (500 IU/d × 3)	*Normal Range*	Basal	*Normal Range*	ACTH-Stimulated	Basal	Basal	*Normal Range*
Sodium	mEq/L	140	136–145	-		141	136–145		-	144	136–145
Potassium	mEq/L	4.0	3.5–5.1	-		4.6	3.5–5.1		-	4.7	3.5–5.1
ACTH	pg/mL	81	9–50	82	9–50	66	9–50	-	62	46	9–50
Progesterone	ng/dL	222	5–80	-		251	10–50	425	522	339	10–50
17OH Preg	ng/dL	132	60–830	27	60–830	13	10–50	-	-	-	
17OHProg	ng/dL	300	40–460	40	40–460	29	19–159	35	110	80	10–470
DHEA-S	µg/dL	<5	5–62	<5	5–62	<5	5–190	-	<5	<5	5–95
11-Deoxycortisol	ng/dL	1100	1450 ± 790	200	1450 ± 790	140	186 ± 116	-	87	-	205 ± 108
Cortisol	µg/dL	3.7	4.3–22.2	8.6	4.3–22.2	8.9	4.3–22.2	7.8	7.1	4.1	4.3–22.4
Δ4A	ng/dL	<30	63 ± 39	<3	63 ± 39	<30	30–330	<30	-	<30	30–330
Testosterone	ng/dL	7	140 ± 132	<4	140 ± 132	28	15–30	16	-	-	
LH	IU/L	-		-		0.3	0.2–1.0	-	<0.07	-	0.2–1.0
FSH	IU/L	-		-		9	0.4–2.0	-	4.3	-	0.4–2.0
PRA	ng/mL/h	-		-		1.8	0.6–21.3	-	-	0.1	0.3–6.4
Aldosterone	ng/dL	-		-		12.1	14–114	11.5		6.2	9–66

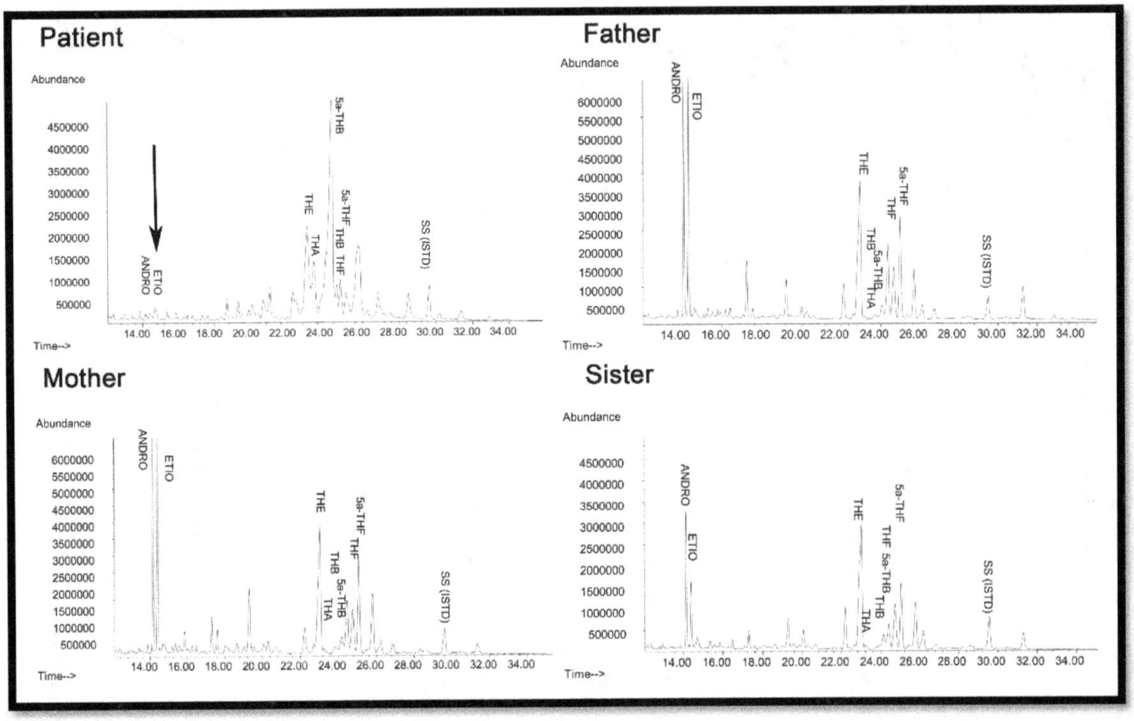

Figure 4. Urine steroid profile of the patient, heterozygote mother, father, and sister. The steroid analysis was performed on 24 h urine samples by GC/MS. Note the lack of androgens (ETIO, ANDRO) and the relative increase in corticosterone metabolites (THA, THB, 5α-THB) in the steroid profile of the patient compared to mother and father. THA—tetrahydro-11-dehydrocorticosterone; THB—tetrahydro corticosterone; 5a-THB-5α-tetrahydro corticosterone; THE—tetrahydrocortisone; THF—tetrahydrocortisol; 5a-THF-5α-tetrahydrocortisol; ETIO—etiocholanolone; ANDRO—androsterone; SS (ISTD)—internal standard.

2.2. Steroid Analysis

Urine steroid profiling of the patient revealed almost complete loss of androgen metabolites, low-normal cortisol and elevated corticosterone metabolites (Figure 5), suggesting partial 17α-hydroxylase and complete 17,20 lyase deficiency. All other family members had normal steroid profiles (Figure 4).

2.3. Loss of 17,20 Lyase Activity of CYP17A1 *by the V366M Mutation*

To investigate the molecular basis of these mutations we produced both mutant and the wild-type CYP17A1 proteins and performed enzyme kinetic assays (Table 3).

Comparison of mutant and wild-type proteins revealed that both mutations V366M and S441P affected CYP17A1 enzyme activities and therefore qualified as disease-causing mutations. The S441P mutation was found to cause a complete loss of both 17α-hydroxylase and 17,20 lyase activities of CYP17A1. Structural analysis of the S441P mutation indicated that heme binding may be affected (Figure 5), and quantification of heme in the S441P mutant revealed that it contained less than 5% of heme compared to the wild-type enzyme (Table 4).

The CYP17A1-V366M protein retained >40% of WT activity in the 17α-hydroxylase assay but had no activity in the 17,20 lyase assay using 17OH-PREG as substrate (Table 3). Therefore, S441P is a loss-of-function *CYP17A1* mutation whereas V366M qualifies as a rare mutation predominantly affecting CYP17A1-17,20 lyase activity *in vitro*. Therefore, the S441P mutation effectively created a non-functional allele and allowed us to explore the specific effects of the V366M mutation in greater detail.

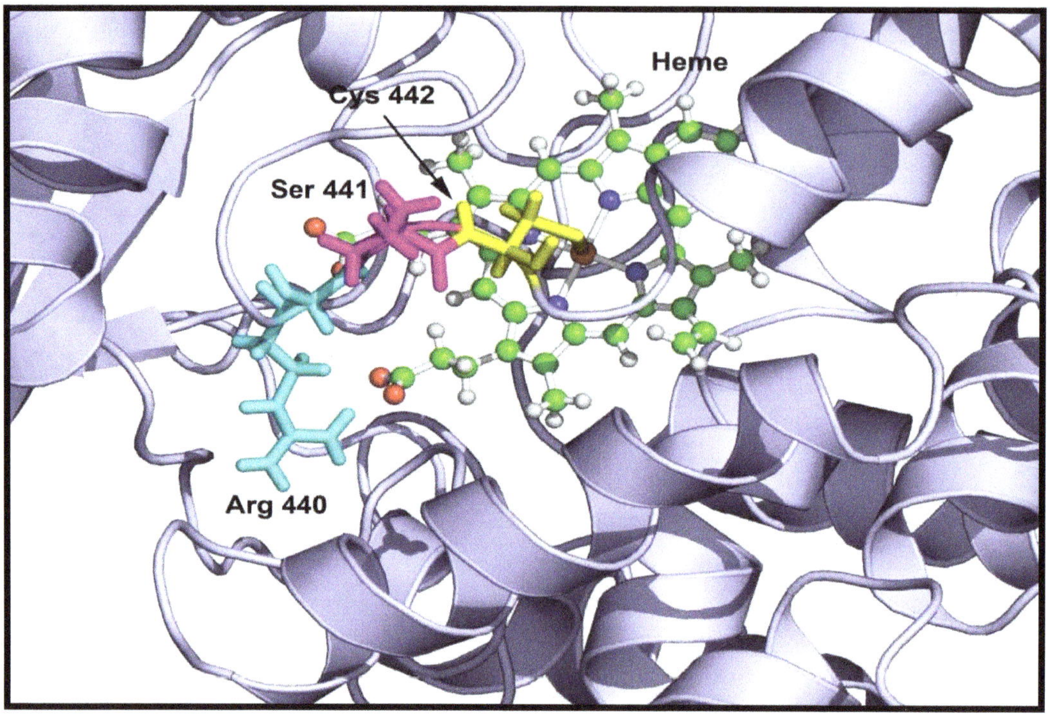

Figure 5. Location of S441P mutation in CYP17A1 structure showing the affected amino acids. The cysteine 442 is shown in yellow, serine 441 is in magenta and arginine 440 is in cyan. Both the cysteine 442 and arginine 440 are required for heme binding and the serine 441 to proline mutation creates a bend in the loop containing the cysteine 442 and arginine 440 residues, resulting in loss of heme binding that leads to an inactive enzyme.

Table 3. Kinetic parameters for the metabolism of PROG to 17OH-PROG (17hydroxylation) and 17OH-PREG to DHEA (17,20 lyase reaction) by WT and V366M mutant of CYP17A1.

CYP17A1 Variant	**17α-Hydroxylase PROG to 17OH-PROG**			**17,20 Lyase17 OH-PREG to DHEA**	
	Km (μM)	**Vmax (min^{-1})**	**Cat Eff (%)**	**Km (μM)**	**Vmax (min^{-1})**
WT	6.1 ± 0.7	0.71	100	0.92 ± 0.07	0.025 ± 0.004
V366M	8.4 ± 0.9	0.42	43	-	-
S441P	-	-	-	-	-

Table 4. Heme content of proteins used in assays.

Protein Preparation	**Heme Content (nnol/nmol of Protein)**
CYP17A1 WT	0.93
CYP17A1_V366M	0.95
CYP17A1-S441P	<0.05
CYB5A	1.0

2.4. The 17OH-PREG is Not an Effective Inhibitor of 17α-Hydroxylase Reaction by the V366M Mutant

For the human CYP17A1, PREG, 17OH-PREG, and PROG are all very good substrates and, therefore, are expected to compete for the binding to CYP17A1 when more than one substrate is present at the same time. To test if there is a difference between the WT versus the V366M mutant of CYP17A1, we used 17OH-PREG as an inhibitor for the 17α-hydroxylase reaction of CYP17A1 using radiolabeled

[^{3}H]PROG as substrate. For the WT CYP17A1, 17OH-PREG inhibited the 17α-hydroxylation of PROG with an observed IC_{50} value of 1.7 μM (Table 5).

Table 5. Binding and inhibition studies of WT and the V366M mutant of *CYP17A1*.

	CYP17A1_WT	CYP17A1_V366M
Binding studies	**Kd (nM)**	**Kd (nM)**
Binding of PROG	163 ± 29	287 ± 35
Binding of PREG	62 ± 17	92 ± 15
Binding of 17OH-PREG	142 ± 38	-
Binding of Abiraterone	85 ± 23	-
Inhibition studies	**IC_{50} (μM)**	**IC_{50} (μM)**
Inhibition of PROG 17α-hydroxylation by Abiraterone	0.04 ± 0.01	-
Inhibition of PROG 17α-hydroxylation by 17OH-PREG	1.7 ± 0.2	-
Inhibition of PROG 17α-hydroxylation by PREG	0.9 ± 0.15	1.4 ± 0.2

For the V366M mutant of *CYP17A1*, no inhibition of the 17α-hydroxylation of PROG was observed by 17OH-PREG within the range of concentration used in the assay (0–100 μM). These results indicated difficulty in the binding of 17OH-PREG to the V366M mutant of CYP17A1. By contrast, when PREG was used as an inhibitor in the 17α-hydroxylation reaction catalyzed by CYP17A1 using PROG as a substrate, both the WT as well as V366M mutant enzymes were inhibited with apparent IC_{50} values of 0.9 μM for the WT enzyme versus 1.4 μM for the V366M mutant (Table 5). This suggests that both PREG and PROG can bind and be metabolized by the V366M variant of CYP17A1 but 17OH-PREG could not be used as a substrate by the mutant enzyme.

2.5. Computational Structural Analysis by Molecular Dynamics

We used the recently solved crystal structures of the human CYP17A1 [22,23] to make in-silico mutations and analyzed the changes through molecular dynamics (MD) simulations. In the CYP17A1 crystal structure, the active site for the binding of steroids is characterized by the positioning of residues V366, N202 and E305 (Figure 6). This led us to hypothesize that the specific space requirements exist for correct positioning of 17α-hydroxysteroids. The larger side chain of methionine in the V366M mutant protruded into the active site of CYP17A1 (Figure 7). Interestingly the shape of the protruding side chain of methionine 366 indicated that it might restrict the movement of steroids only in one direction, allowing the 17-hydroxy-steroids to leave the active site by the flexibility of movement in one direction, but creating a strong steric hindrance in the path of incoming steroids.

One of the most intriguing questions about CYP17A1 activities has been whether the 17α-hydroxysteroid can stay in the catalytic site and be metabolized again to androgen precursors, or whether the product of 17α-hydroxylase reaction leaves the active site and re-enters for the second reaction (Figure 7a). The one-way valve created by V366M mutation provides some answers to this question for the human CYP17A1. The presence of 17α-hydroxylase activity in the V366M variant suggested that PREG can get into the active site and be converted to 17OH-PREG (Figure 7b). If the 17OH-PREG was not able to leave the active site, it would have created an irreversible inhibition and the enzyme would have been unable to carry out further reactions. However, the 17α-hydroxylase reaction progressed (Figure 4 and Table 3), indicating that 17OH-PREG can exit the active site. Furthermore, if the 17OH-PREG could be converted without exiting the active site, then DHEA formation should have been observed as in case of the wild-type enzyme.

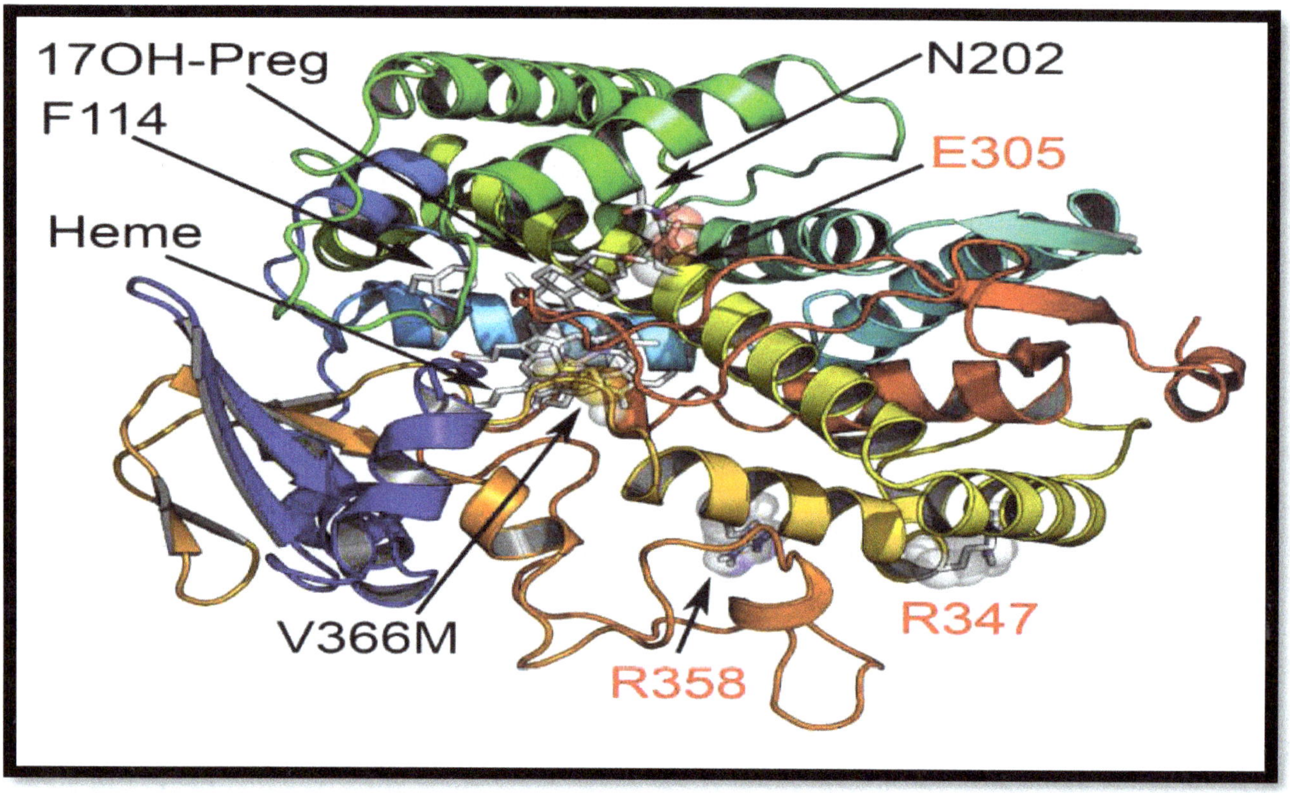

Figure 6. Comparison of novel V366M mutation with the previously reported isolated CYP17A1-17,20 lyase mutations. Only three other residues in CYP17A1 have been reported to be mutated in patients with isolated 17,20 lyase deficiency. The R347 and R358 are at the redox partner binding sites and their mutations may interfere with binding of POR and /or cytochrome b_5. The E305 residue at the active site is important for orientation of the substrate and its mutation has been shown to alter substrate specificity and lead to a preference for progesterone as the more efficient substrate. The V366 is located exactly at the active site of the CYP17A1.

However, DHEA was absent in both the *in vitro* enzyme reactions of the V366M mutant of CYP17A1 (Table 3) as well as in the urine of the patient (Figure 4), clearly indicating that 17OH-PREG must exit the active site after the 17α-hydroxylase reaction. If the problem was with the exit of DHEA, then that would also have created an irreversible inhibition by blocking the active site with one molecule of DHEA per unit of enzyme and further enzymatic activity would have come to a halt, but that was clearly not the case from the *in vitro* enzyme analysis as well as the patient's urine steroid profile (Figure 4 and Table 3). In the case of bovine CYP17A1, about 20% of pregnenolone consumed in the reaction could be converted to DHEA without exiting the active site [41]. When PROG was used as a substrate, compared to 17OH-PREG the dissociation of 17OH-PROG was 10 times faster. The release of the intermediate reaction was much faster than 17,20 lyase reaction and that prevented the direct formation of androstenedione from PROG. There are significant differences in activities of CYP17A1 between different species and the human enzyme has a very poor affinity for 17OH-PROG as substrate [25,42,43].

To further study this mechanism, we employed molecular dynamics simulations for the analysis of steroid binding in the active site of wild-type and the V366M mutant of CYP17A1. This was confirmed by the ensemble docking experiments which (for wild-type protein) yielded ligand poses in close proximity to the heme and highly resembling the co-crystallized abiraterone in the *CYP17A1* (PDB: 3RUK) structure [22]. The validity of our docking protocol was supported by a set of additional CYP17A1 crystal structures containing all the ligands of interest (PDB codes: 4NKW, 4NKX, 4NKY, and 4NKZ) in very similar poses enabling hydrogen-bonding to a distal N202 residue for PROG/PREG but not for 17OH-PREG [23]. Based on these observations, we hypothesized that the methionine side-chain could prevent a closer proximity to the heme iron necessary for the substrates undergoing lyase reaction [23,24]. To check this, we performed an additional pair of simulations with 17OH-PREG docked into the wild-type and mutant binding sites. Thus, we could indeed measure that the average distance between the ligand C17 atom and the heme iron differed in these systems (4.4 Å for wild-type and 6.3 Å for V366M mutant) (Figure 8c,d). While these results cannot be compared directly to the crystal structure of CYP17A1 with 17OH-PREG (PDB code 4NKZ; the O17-Fe distance between 3.4 and 3.9 Å depending on the chain), this hypothesis is well in line with all our experimental data and recently reported structures of human CYP17A1 in complexes with steroid substrates. In addition, the simulations, as well as the docking to the mutant protein, provided a possible explanation for the decreased reaction rates of the pregnenolone hydroxylation. Specifically, these structures (Figure 7b,d,f) hinted at an electrostatic interaction between the methionine methyl group (positively polarized by the preceding sulfur atom) and the negatively-charged carboxylate found in all ligands we studied. We propose that this added interaction slows down ligand dissociation/exit and thus slows down the reaction. Our MD simulation and docking results agree with greatly reduced Vmax but only marginally increased Km of both the wild-type and V366M mutant of CYP17A1 for the PROG (Table 3), indicating that binding of PREG and PROG is not affected but the exit of the 17α-hydroxy steroid from the active site may be slower in the V366M variant.

2.6. Substrate- and Inhibitor-Binding Analysis

Abiraterone bound to the WT CYP17A1 with a Kd value of 95 nM and showed the typical soret peak at 427 nm, indicative of nitrogen co-ordination with heme iron (Table 5). However, in case of the V366M mutant of CYP17A1, this binding pattern was not observed. To test the integrity of the protein, we used imidazole to check the binding and found that imidazole itself could bind to the V366M mutant. This confirmed our hypothesis that the introduction of the bulky methionine to replace the valine at position 366 creates steric hindrance and perturbs the binding pattern of drugs and steroids. These results also point to structural considerations for future inhibitor development which may utilize the spatial arrangement of binding-site residues to design tight-fitting inhibitors. Progesterone bound with slightly decreased affinity to the V366M mutant (Kd 287 nM compared to 162 nM for the WT enzyme). Binding of 17OH-PREG was not observed for the V366M mutation and explained the lack of 17,20 lyase activity, while for the WT CYP17A1 a Kd value 142 nM was observed. It is possible that some apparent binding of 17OH-PREG may occur at exceedingly high, non-physiological levels due to the nature of the structural hindrance from the V366M mutation which is at the very end of the binding site and close to the heme iron and water molecules that occupy the binding pocket.

Since the spectral binding of steroid substrates to CYP17A1 is observed by the replacement of water molecules at the active site, it is possible for some apparent binding to emerge from titration studies using very high enzyme and substrate concentrations, but due to unfavorable binding poses and distances, as revealed by further computational structure analysis, such apparent binding is not likely to result in an enzyme-substrate complex that can lead to product (DHEA) formation. This is further evidenced by lack of inhibition by 17OH-PREG in the 17hydroxylation reaction using PROG as substrate. In the case of inhibitor abiraterone, which needs to form an iron-nitrogen co-ordination and gets much closer to heme iron than steroid substrates (2.9 Å compared to 4.4–4.8 Å) (Figures 8 and S1), no binding was observed. Taken together these data indicate a steric hindrance for the binding of 17OH-PREG which may result in poor interaction with the enzyme and loss of 17,20 lyase activity.

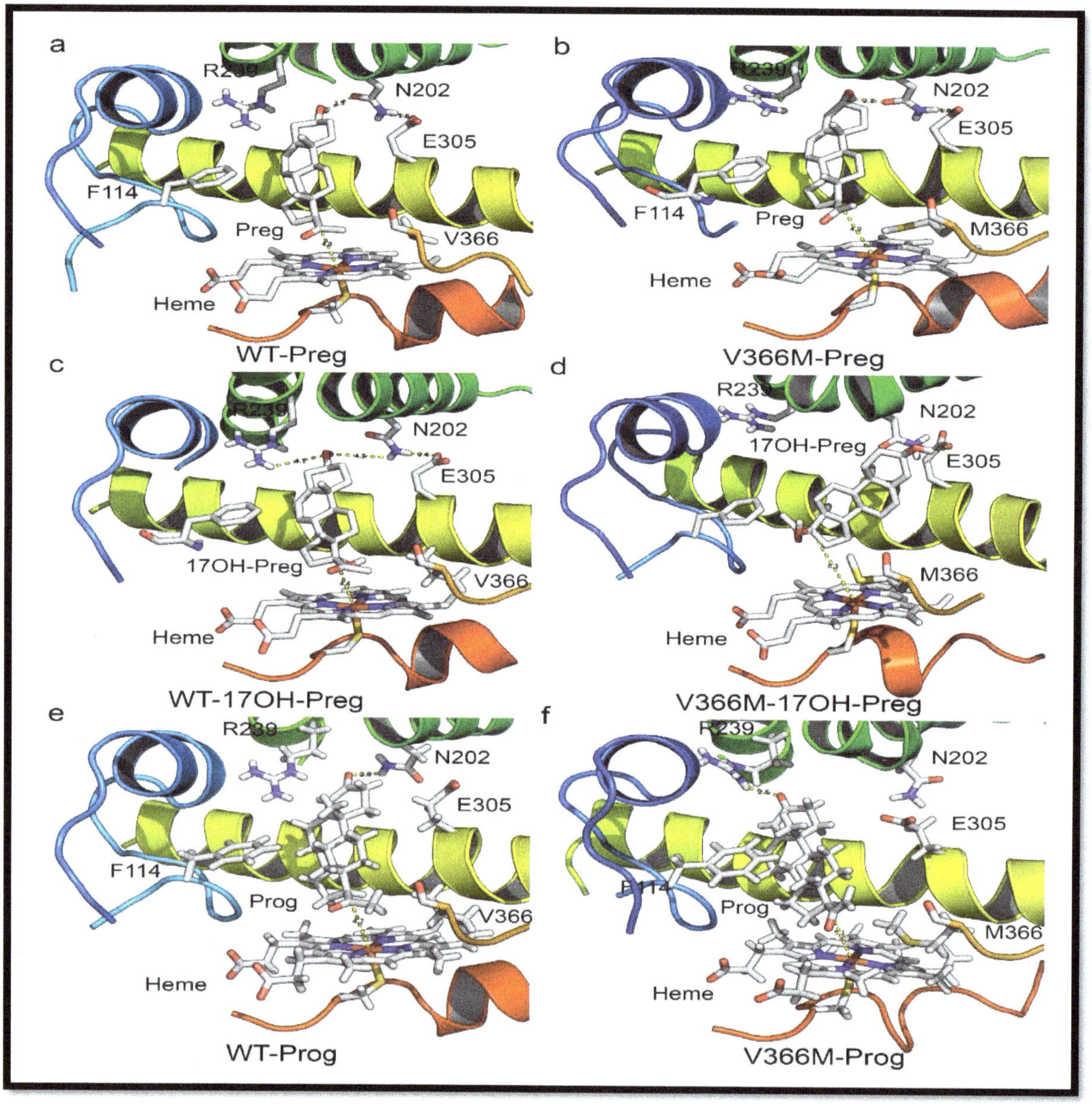

Figure 7. Structure analysis of the V366M mutation. (**a**) Binding of pregnenolone in CYP17A1 active site. Pregnenolone binds perpendicular to heme and is converted to 17OH-PREG. (**b**) Binding of pregnenolone to V366M variant of CYP17A1. Pregnenolone can still bind to V366M variant and is metabolized to 17OH-PREG. The side chain of methionine 366 in the mutant structure protrudes into the active site but still allows 17OH-PREG to exit. This is likely to slow down the reaction velocity of the 17α-hydroxylase reaction, which was confirmed by enzyme kinetic experiments (Table 1). (**c**) Binding of 17OH-PREG to WT CYP17A1. (**d**) Docking of 17OH-PREG to V366M variant of CYP17A1. The 17OH-PREG could not bind in the proximity to heme and distances between the heme iron and C17 atom increased for the mutant enzyme (6.3 Å in the mutant vs. 4.4 Å for the WT enzyme). Increased iron-C17 distances are observed together with N202-O3 interactions which are considered undesirable for optimal binding of 17hydroxy steroids for 17,20 lyase reaction. The methionine 366 side chain in the mutant protein blocks the entry of 17α-hydroxy steroid into the active site, resulting in loss of 17,20 lyase activity. (**e**,**f**) Comparison of WT and V366M variant of CYP17A1 binding to PROG.

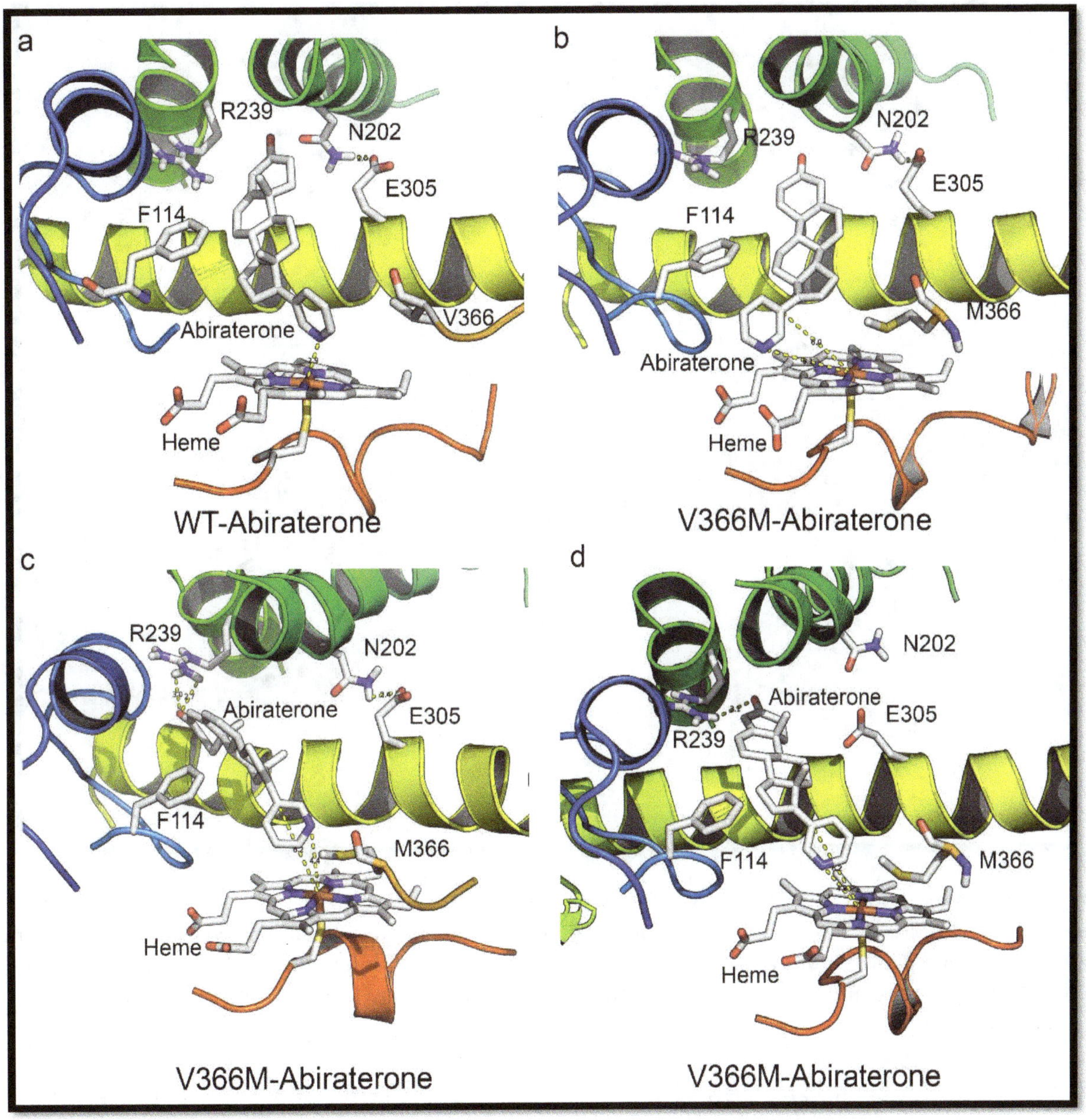

Figure 8. Comparison of abiraterone interaction with the WT and V366M variant of CYP17A1. (**a**) In the WT CYP17A1 abiraterone binds by forming a nitrogen-iron co-ordination (2.9 Å) with the central heme. (**b**–**d**) Different poses of abiraterone seen during docking into the V366M mutant of CYP17A1. In the V366M mutant, the methionine side chain prevents the binding of abiraterone and increased distances between the C17 atom and heme iron are observed together with binding poses that are different from the WT.

2.7. Mechanism of Steroid/Abiraterone Binding and Action in Relation to the V366M Mutation

Docking was performed with all ligands to WT as well as the V366M mutant of CYP17A1. Thr306 is reported to be a vital residue for the hydroxylation reaction (part of an alcohol pair donating protons). It is also very close to the heme and, like residue 366, is near the bound ligands. Asn202 is reported to interact with the distal side of the molecules. It is at the end of the cavity formed around the bound steroids/abiraterone (Figure 6) and most likely one of the residues inside the access channel. Ensemble docking of all relevant ligands implies that docking poses mimic the co-crystallized abiraterone (CH_3 groups to the left when looking from the direction of residue 366) and allow interaction with the residue 202 highlighted in recent structures of human CYP17A1 (Figures 8 and 9) [23].

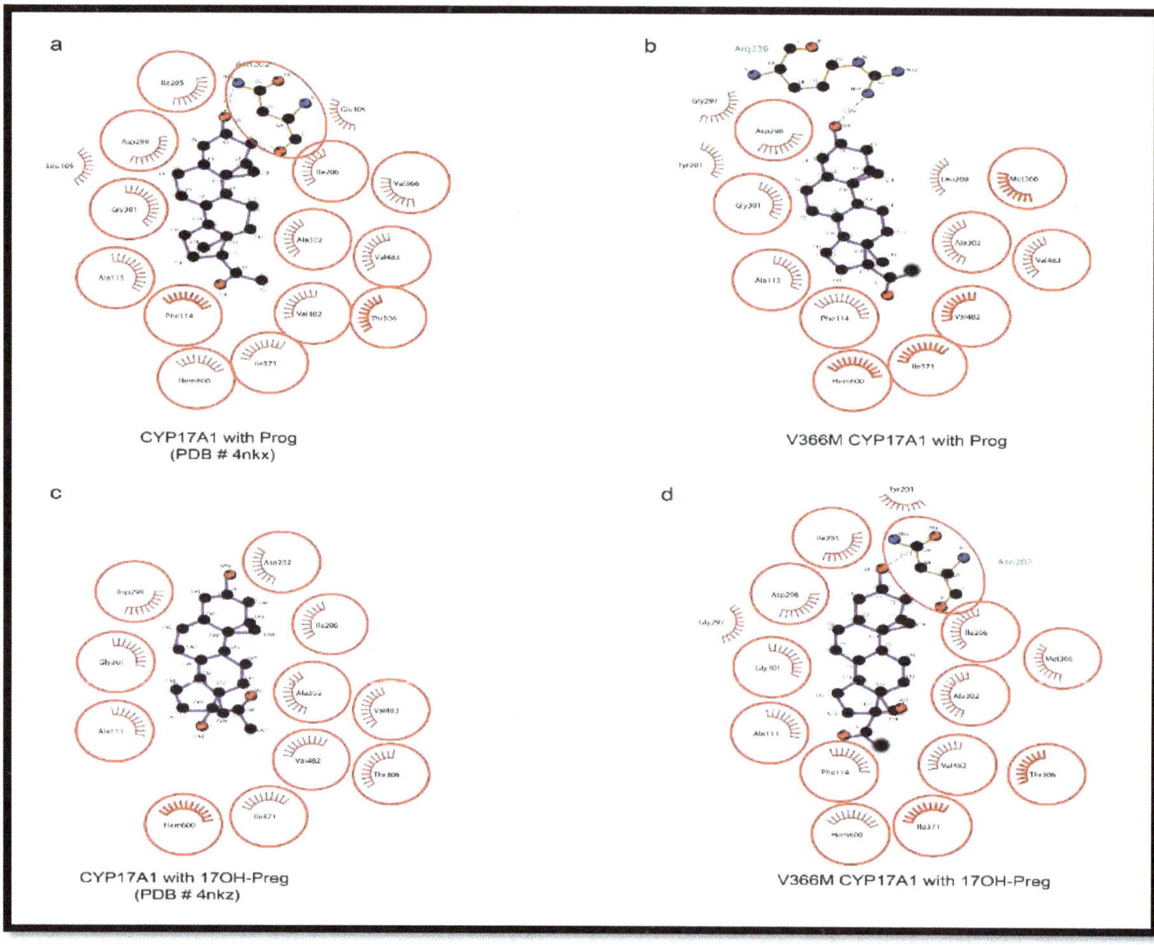

Figure 9. Comparison of PROG and 17OH-PREG bound in crystal structures of human CYP17A1 with the docked steroids into the V366M mutant. (**a**,**b**) PROG is found to bind similarly to WT as well as the mutant enzyme. (**c**,**d**) Mutation of V366 to M leads to non-optimal interactions with the N202 group in the V366M mutant compared to WT where this interaction is absent in poses which have 17OH-PREG close to the heme.

The pose from which 17α-hydroxy steroid leaves the site (after being formed) may differ from the one it assumes upon coming back. There are also possible differences between 17OH-PREG and PROG/PREG binding (Figures 7 and 9). Angular analysis of apo and relaxation V366M simulations imply that the methionine moves around a single conformation (chi2 and 3 angles roughly in 20-degree windows—a good match to the rotamers reported by http://www.dynameomics.org). It seems most likely that the CH3 group is involved in steric effects. The sulfur group in methionine may further polarize it, enhancing interaction with the carboxylate of 17α-hydroxy steroids. In some MD poses the methionine could be seen moving away from the heme, indicating it has conformational flexibility and in the presence of the metabolized PREG/PROG the 17α-hydroxylated ligand may exit without excessive hindrance. The reduced velocity of the PROG to 17OH-PROG reaction indicates that there could be an interaction between the carboxylate and the (likely-polarized) CH3 group of the methionine, which may slow down the exit of the product. Some other differences in the binding pattern were observed, like the involvement of Arg239 in the interaction of PROG with the V366M variant which may create bottlenecks during the exit of the product. Computationally calculated binding constants and binding energy calculations also supported the experimental results of reduced binding affinities for 17OH-PREG and abiraterone for the V366M mutant (Table 6). All this implies a general steric hindrance by the bigger residue (methionine vs. valine).

Table 6. Computational binding energy, computationally calculated dissociation constants, and interacting residues for steroid substrates and abiraterone with WT and the V366M mutant of *CYP17A1*. Key residues identified in different studies are shown in bold.

CYP17A1 Protein	Binding Energy (kcal/mol)	Dissociation Constant (nM)	Contacting Residues
WT with Prog	10.6	14.66	ALA113 PHE114 **ASN202** ILE205 ILE206 LEU209 **ARG239** GLY297 ASP298 GLY301 ALA302 THR306 ALA367 ILE371 VAL482 VAL483 **HEME**
M366 with Prog	9.75	43.71	ALA113 PHE114 **ASN202** ILE205 ILE206 LEU209 **ARG239** GLY297 ASP298 GLY301 ALA302 THR306 **MET366** ALA367 ILE371 VAL482 VAL483 **HEME**
WT with Preg	10.7	13.29	ALA105 ALA113 PHE114 ILE205 ILE206 LEU209 VAL236 **ARG239** GLY297 ASP298 GLY301 ALA302 **GLU305** THR306 **VAL366** ILE371 VAL482 VAL483 **HEME**
M366 with Preg	10.3	27.11	ALA105 SER106 ALA113 PHE114 ILE205 ILE206 LEU209 VAL236 **ARG239** GLY297 ASP298 GLY301 ALA302 THR306 **MET366** ILE371 VAL482 VAL483 **HEME**
WT with 17OH-Preg	11.3	5.22	ALA113 PHE114 TYR201 **ASN202** ILE205 ILE206 LEU209 LEU214 **ARG239** GLY297 ASP298 GLY301 ALA302 THR306 **VAL366** ALA367 ILE371 VAL482 VAL483 **HEME**
M366 with 17OH-Preg	7.0	60.4	ALA113 PHE114 TYR201 **ASN202** ILE205 ILE206 LEU209 **ARG239** GLY297 ASP298 GLY301 ALA302 **GLU305** THR306 **MET366** ALA367 ILE371 VAL482 VAL483
WT with Abiraterone	12.5	0.69	ALA113 PHE114 TYR201 **ASN202** ILE205 ILE206 LEU209 **ARG239** GLY297 ASP298 GLY301 ALA302 **GLU305** THR306 **VAL366** ALA367 LEU370 ILE371 VAL482 VAL483 **HEME**
V366 with Abiraterone	8.1	1112.9	ALA105 SER106 ASN107 ALA113 PHE114 TYR201 ILE205 ILE206 LEU209 **ARG239** THR294 GLY297 ASP298 GLY301 ALA302 THR306 **MET366** ILE371 VAL482 VAL483

Given the information from crystal structure of human CYP17A1 with abiraterone (nitrogen at 2.9 Å from the heme iron) (Figure 8), this implies that PREG either does not have to get this close to the heme or can accesses it from a different angle and is hence relatively unimpaired by the methionine. Recent structures of the human CYP17A1 bound with different steroid substrates confirm this hypothesis and show that 17OH-PREG binds much closer to the heme iron than PROG or PREG (Figures 7 and 9) [23,24]. For the 17OH-PREG we observed the existence of poses with the hydroxyl positioned very close to the CH3 of the methionine, indicating the bulky methionine residue could be preventing the ligand from getting close enough to the heme (Figures 7d and S2).

In addition, we also observed shorter distances suitable for hydrogen bonds with N202 and R239 groups and 17OH-PREG in the docking poses of V366M mutant (2.6 Å compared to 4.4 Å for the WT) (Figures 7d and S2, Table 6); it has been proposed that these interactions are required for PROG/PREG but are considered suboptimal for 17,20 lyase reaction and are found together with increased distances of C17 in 17α-hydroxy steroid substrate and the heme iron. Increased distances between the C17 of 17OH-PREG/Abiraterone and the heme iron, together with the extra/undesired interactions with N202/R239, were consistently observed in our simulations (Figures 7c, 8 S1 and S2).

It is more likely that the ligands cannot get into the binding site rather than have too much difficulty in leaving it since that would block the active site and prevent the 17α-hydroxylation reaction from occurring (which is not severely affected as observed by enzymatic analysis as well as the urine steroid profile of the patient). Also, DHEA is the smallest of all steroids involved, making it the most likely to leave, so it is the entry of 17OH-PREG into the active site that is likely to be impaired. Many different poses of abiraterone and 17OH-PREG were observed for the V366M mutant which illustrates the non-optimal binding pattern for the mutant enzyme (Figures 8 and S2). The inhibitor abiraterone (similar scaffold but bigger than the steroid substrates) also has trouble binding (Figures 8 and S1, Table 5) and does not act as an inhibitor for the 17α-hydroxylation reaction catalyzed by the V366M mutant of *CYP17A1* (Table 5).

3. Discussion

Among the previously reported mutations causing isolated 17,20 lyase deficiency, the R347C, R347H and R358Q are located on the redox partner binding site (Figure 6) and seem to act by altering the interaction with POR. Generally, a defect in redox partner or loss of interaction with redox partner affects all cytochrome P450 activities in the endoplasmic reticulum as well as in mitochondria [31,36,44–48]. In the case of R347H and R358Q mutations in CYP17A1, why this loss of interaction with POR affects the 17,20 lyase activity in a more severe fashion than the 17α-hydroxylase activity is not clear, since both activities of CYP17A1 require electrons supplied by NADPH through POR for their catalytic function [49]. The only other mutation in CYP17A1 that had been reported to selectively impair the 17,20 lyase activity is E305G which is part of the substrate access channel of CYP17A1 (Figures 6 and 8) [28,30]. The E305G mutation had been reported to affect the binding of 17α-hydroxy steroids while showing even higher than normal 17α-hydroxylase activities [28]; however a later analysis of the patient's steroid metabolic profile [30] showed that 17α-hydroxylase activity was also impaired, contradicting the earlier claims of isolated 17,20 lyase deficiency [30]. A more efficient coupling with POR and efficient use of NADPH have recently been proposed to favor the 17,20 lyase reaction [49]. Multiple potential mechanisms for the selectivity of the 17,20 lyase reaction have been proposed in recent works from different laboratories [23,26,49–53].

The V366M is an active site mutation in CYP17A1 that not only preferentially targets 17,20 lyase activity but also provides insights into the structural basis of the 17,20 lyase reaction, the key regulator of sex steroid biosynthesis in humans (Figures 2 and 7). The specificity of the human CYP17A1 active site allows the binding of PREG and its 17hydroxy metabolite (17OH-PREG) to bind in different conformations and exit the active site after the reactions (Figure 7a,c), and the mutation of valine 366 to methionine alters the active site and hinders the binding of 17α-hydroxy-steroids (Figure 8d). The V366M mutant also explains the effectiveness of the anti-prostate-cancer drug abiraterone as a potent inhibitor of CYP17A1. Abiraterone fills the active site of CYP17A1 (Figures 8 and S1) and becomes irreversibly bound to the enzyme (Supplementary Figure S1c), stopping any further substrate binding and activity [22]. This location of V366 at the catalytic center provides a structural basis for improving and designing novel and specific CYP17A1 inhibitors by targeting spatial selectivity of the active site with imidazole or other suitable chemical moieties added to core steroid structures.

Structural modifications based on the above information may help in designing more specific and potent inhibitors directed only towards the 17,20 lyase activity of CYP17A1 that could produce tighter binding at the active site. The 17,20 lyase-specific inhibitors will have advantages over current compounds that target both the 17α-hydroxylase and the 17,20 lyase activities of CYP17A1 and require steroid supplementation [12,54–58]. The mechanistic and structural insights revealed by these studies will help in the development of better drugs against polycystic ovary syndrome and prostate cancer. These findings will also improve our understanding of the structural basis of the dual function of CYP17A1 as both a 17α-hydroxylase and 17,20 lyase, and the role of these activities in the regulation of steroid hormone production in different tissues.

4. Materials and Methods

4.1. Human Subjects

All clinical investigations were carried out following the Declaration of Helsinki principles. Written informed consent was received from the parents for genetic work-up of 46, XY DSD in their child in the pediatric endocrinology research laboratory in Barcelona which holds ethical approval for these studies.

4.2. Genetic Analysis

DNA was extracted from the peripheral blood leucocytes of the patient. Genetic analysis of the androgen receptor gene (*AR*) and for the 5αreductase type 2 gene (*SRD5A2*) were performed as described [39,40], yielding normal results. The *CYP17A1* gene was analyzed as reported [59] and identified sequence variations were compared to National Center for Biotechnology Information (NCBI, Bethesda, USA) entry NG_007955.1 (GI:189339218). The *CYP17A1* gene was subsequently also analyzed in the parents and the older half-sister, and one mutation was found in the mother. Since the second mutation is a completely inactivating mutation, its presence on a different allele was inferred (as the presence of both mutations on one allele will give a good working copy of the *CYP17A1* gene, and that does not cause disease).

4.3. Steroid Profiling from 24-h Urine Samples

Steroid metabolites in urine were measured by the gas chromatography-mass spectrometry (GC/MS) method as described previously [60,61].

4.4. Recombinant Protein Expression

Human wild-type and mutant *CYP17A1* proteins were produced in an *E. coli* expression system and purified for enzyme kinetic assays [15,17,18,62]. The pCWH17-mod(His)4 expression plasmid (a gift from Prof. Michael Waterman, Nashville, TN) containing the cDNA for human WT or mutant CYP17A1 [15], was transformed into the *E. coli* JM109 cells and colonies were selected under ampicillin control. Bacteria were grown at 37 °C to OD_{600} 0.6 and the CYP17A1 protein expression was induced by the addition of 0.5 mM IPTG followed by further incubation at 28 °C for 48 h. Purification of CYP17A1 was performed as described [15,17,18]. In brief, the spheroplasts prepared by the lysozyme treatment of bacterial cells were ruptured by sonication and cleared by centrifugation at 4000× *g* for 10 min, then the supernatant containing the CYP17A1 protein was extracted with 1.5% Triton X-114 and centrifuged at 100,000× *g* for 30 min. A reddish-brown colored detergent-rich supernatant fraction containing the CYP17A1 was isolated, diluted to reduce the detergent concentration to 0.1%, and passed over a Ni-NTA-sepharose column. The column was washed with 5 mM histidine to remove the non-specific binding and eluted with 200 mM histidine. Further purification was carried out by gel filtration chromatography to remove histidine and other protein contaminants.

4.5. In Vitro Enzyme Kinetic Analysis of Identified CYP17A1 Mutations

To assess 17α-hydroxylase activity, 10 pmol of CYP17A1 along with 20 pmol purified human POR [17,31,32,34,62] (at a 1:2 ratio) was incubated with 0.1–15 μM [^{14}C]PROG (80,000 cpm/reaction) and 1 mM NADPH in 50 mM potassium-phosphate buffer (pH 7.4) containing 6 mM potassium acetate, 10 mM $MgCl_2$, 1 mM reduced glutathione, 20% glycerol and 20 μg phosphatidylcholine for 60 min at 37 °C. Human CYP17A1 does not use 17OH-PROG as a major substrate and, therefore, PROG is considered a better substrate to monitor only 17α-hydroxylase activity due to very little further conversion of 17OH-PROG. To assess 17,20 lyase activity, CYP17A1 and POR proteins were incubated with 0.05–5 μM [^{3}H]17OH-PREG (100,000 cpm/reaction), 1 mM NADPH and 20 pmol cytochrome b_5/reaction in 50 mM K-phosphate buffer (pH 7.4) containing 6 mM potassium acetate,

10 mM MgC_{l2}, 1 mM reduced glutathione, 20% glycerol and 20 μg phosphatidylcholine for 90 min at 37 °C. Steroids were extracted and resolved by thin layer chromatography before quantitative analysis for conversion to 17OH-PREG and DHEA respectively as described [19]. For inhibition assays, abiraterone, PREG as well as 17OH-PREG were used to compete with radioactive PROG for 17α-hydroxylase reaction. Enzyme kinetic calculations were performed using non-linear regression curve fitting with Prism (GraphPad Software Inc., San Diego, CA, USA). Data represent the mean of three independent experiments.

4.6. Heme and P450 Measurements

Heme content was measured as described previously by dissolving the protein in NaOH and measuring the heme absorbance in a triton-methanol mixture [63]. Cytochrome P450 and Cytochrome b_5 were measured as described previously [1,17]. Cytochrome b_5 content was estimated by monitoring the absorbance difference at 423–490 nm using an extinction coefficient of 181 mmol cm^{-1}.

4.7. Substrate-Binding Assay

Binding of steroid substrates to CYP17A1 was measured by recording the substrate-binding spectra in the range of 340–500 nm on a Perkin Elmer Lambda 25 spectrophotometer. A change in heme absorbance is observed when water molecules at the active site are replaced by steroid substrates [22]. In case of abiraterone, an increase in the soret peak at 427 nm is observed by co-ordination of the heme iron with pyridine nitrogen. To accurately measure the tight binding substrates and inhibitors, a cuvette with 100 mm path length was employed and protein concentration was kept at 50 nM. Binding of steroids, as well as abiraterone to CYP17A1, occurs with very high affinity and, as observed previously, Kd values measured are often close to protein concentration used in binding assays. All substrates and abiraterone were dissolved in ethanol and an equal amount of ethanol was added to the reference cuvette and the final concentration of ethanol added to the cuvettes was kept below 2%. After each addition of the compounds, cuvettes were incubated for 5 min at 22 °C before recording the spectra. The slit width was fixed at 1.0 nm and spectra were recorded at 50 nm/min with a series of increasing concentrations of different compounds (abiraterone: 0–200 nM; PREG: 0–500 nM; 17OH-PREG: 0–1000 nM; PROG: 0–1000 nM). Data were fitted with GraphPad Prism based on the tight binding pattern of substrates to a single binding site.

4.8. Protein Structure Analysis of WT and Mutant CYP17A1

The published 3D structures of human CYP17A1 [22,23] were downloaded from the protein structure repository (www.rcsb.org). We performed several rounds of multiple-sequence alignments with different CYP17A1 protein sequences from several organisms and created in-silico mutants using the programs YASARA [64] and WHATIF [65]. For all further experiments described, a 2.6 Å resolution crystal structure [22] (PDB code 3RUK) of CYP17A1 was used; with the abiraterone ligand, the membrane anchor (all residues preceding R45), and water molecules (aside from one conserved between residue 366 and the heme) removed. Missing hydrogen atoms were added to the structure with YASARA [64] which was also used for all other computations. The V366M mutant model was then constructed by replacing the original valine with the most favorable methionine conformation found with the in-built SCWALL method (rotamer library search followed by energy minimization) [66]. Afterward, both systems were subjected to 10 ns explicit solvent MD simulations at 310 K, which was preceded by 500 steps of steepest descent and simulated annealing minimization using the AMBER03 force field and the TIP3P water model [67,68]. All following MDs were performed with similar settings. The resulting simulation snapshots (100 per run) were used for the docking of steroids with the AutoDock Vina [69] ensemble-docking experiments using PREG, 17OH-PREG, PROG and 17OH-PROG (orthorhombic docking was grid-established around the central heme and the residues 105, 202, and 366 of the CYP17A1). The final selection of poses was based on their docking scores and similarities to the abiraterone ligand which was co-crystallized in the template structure (PDB: 3RUK) [22]. The docked steroid poses agreed with the binding site details highlighted by a recent set of CYP17A1 crystal structures [23]. Clustering of simulation snapshots was done using USCF Chimera [70]. Figures of the structure models were created with the program Pymol (www.pymol.org) and the chosen poses were rendered as ray-traced images with POVRAY (www.povray.org). Ligand interactions were analyzed and depicted with the program LIGPLOT+ (http://www.ebi.ac.uk/thornton-srv/software/LigPlus/).

Author Contributions: C.E.F., L.A., and A.V.P. designed the experiments. A.V.P. supervised the study. M.F.C., N.C., and R.M., N.T., and L.A. performed genetic, histochemical and biochemical analysis. A.Z. performed computational modeling and molecular dynamics simulations. A.Z. and A.V.P. performed bioinformatic analysis. C.E.F. and A.V.P. expressed and purified the proteins and performed functional assays. B.D. and B.F. performed the mass spectrometric analysis of urine samples and analysed mass spectrometry data. M.F.C., N.C., C.E.F., A.Z., B.D., B.F., R.M., N.T., L.A. and A.V.P. analysed data and critically read the manuscript. A.V.P. wrote the paper with discussion, input and editing contributions from all the authors.

Acknowledgments: We thank Walter L Miller, University of California San Francisco, CA, USA for his generous gift of anti-human CYP17A1 antibodies. We thank Michael R Waterman, Nashville, TN, USA for human CYP17A1 bacterial expression system. This study has been funded by grants from the Instituto de Salud Carlos III (FIS PI06/0903), the Centre for Biomedical Research Network on Rare Diseases (CIBERER, Madrid), and the AGAUR—University and Research Management and Evaluation Agency SGR05-00908 and 2009SGR-31, Barcelona, Spain, to M.F.-C. and L.A., and by grants from the Swiss National Science Foundation (31003A-134926) to AVP, Bern University Research Foundation (to A.V.P.), Burgergemeinde Bern (to A.V.P.) and Department of Biomedical Research intramural support (to A.V.P.). N.C. was supported by a fellowship grant of the European Society of Paediatric Endocrinology, sponsored by Novo Nordisk A/S.

References

1. Omura, T.; Sato, R. The carbon monoxide-binding pigment of liver microsomes. I. Evidence for its hemoprotein nature. *J. Biol. Chem.* **1964**, *239*, 2370–2378. [PubMed]
2. Pandey, A.V.; Flück, C.E. NADPH P450 oxidoreductase: Structure, function, and pathology of diseases. *Pharmacol. Ther.* **2013**, *138*, 229–254. [CrossRef] [PubMed]
3. Zanger, U.M.; Schwab, M. Cytochrome P450 enzymes in drug metabolism: Regulation of gene expression, enzyme activities, and impact of genetic variation. *Pharmacol. Ther.* **2013**, *138*, 103–141. [CrossRef] [PubMed]
4. Miller, W.L.; Auchus, R.J. The molecular biology, biochemistry, and physiology of human steroidogenesis and its disorders. *Endocr. Rev.* **2011**, *32*, 81–151. [CrossRef] [PubMed]
5. Zuber, M.X.; Simpson, E.R.; Waterman, M.R. Expression of bovine 17 alpha-hydroxylase cytochrome P-450 cDNA in nonsteroidogenic (COS 1) cells. *Science* **1986**, *234*, 1258–1261. [CrossRef] [PubMed]
6. Chung, B.C.; Picado-Leonard, J.; Haniu, M.; Bienkowski, M.; Hall, P.F.; Shively, J.E.; Miller, W.L. Cytochrome P450c17 (steroid 17 alpha-hydroxylase/17,20 lyase): Cloning of human adrenal and testis cDNAs indicates the same gene is expressed in both tissues. *Proc. Natl. Acad. Sci. USA* **1987**, *84*, 407–411. [CrossRef] [PubMed]
7. Nakajin, S.; Shinoda, M.; Haniu, M.; Shively, J.E.; Hall, P.F. C21 steroid side chain cleavage enzyme from porcine adrenal microsomes. Purification and characterization of the 17 alpha-hydroxylase/C17,20-lyase cytochrome P-450. *J. Biol. Chem.* **1984**, *259*, 3971–3976. [PubMed]
8. Vasaitis, T.S.; Bruno, R.D.; Njar, V.C. CYP17 inhibitors for prostate cancer therapy. *J. Steroid Biochem. Mol. Biol.* **2011**, *125*, 23–31. [CrossRef] [PubMed]
9. Attard, G.; Reid, A.H.M.; Auchus, R.; Hughes, B.A.; Cassidy, A.M.; Thompson, E.; Oommen, N.B.; Folkerd, E.; Dowsett, M.; Arlt, W.; et al. Clinical and biochemical consequences of CYP17A1 inhibition with abiraterone given with and without exogenous glucocorticoids in castrate men with advanced prostate cancer. *J. Clin. Endocrinol. Metab.* **2012**, *97*, 507–516. [CrossRef] [PubMed]
10. De Bono, J.S.; Logothetiset, C.J.; Molinaal, A.; Fizazi, K.; North, S.; Chu, L.; Chi, K.N.; Jones, R.J.; Goodman, O.B.; Saad, F.; et al. Abiraterone and Increased Survival in Metastatic Prostate Cancer. *N. Engl. J. Med.* **2011**, *364*, 1995–2005. [CrossRef] [PubMed]

11. Attard, G.; Reid, A.H.; Yap, T.A.; Raynaud, F.; Dowsett, M.; Settatree, S.; Barrett, M.; Parker, C.; Martins, V.; Folkerd, E.; et al. Phase I clinical trial of a selective inhibitor of CYP17, abiraterone acetate, confirms that castration-resistant prostate cancer commonly remains hormone driven. *J. Clin. Oncol.* **2008**, *26*, 4563–4571. [CrossRef] [PubMed]
12. Malikova, J.; Brixius-Anderko, S.; Udhane, S.S.; Parween, S.; Dick, B.; Bernhardt, R.; Pandey, A.V. CYP17A1 inhibitor abiraterone, an anti-prostate cancer drug, also inhibits the 21-hydroxylase activity of CYP21A2. *J. Steroid Biochem. Mol. Biol.* **2017**, *174*, 192–200. [CrossRef] [PubMed]
13. Lu, A.Y.; Junk, K.W.; Coon, M.J. Resolution of the cytochrome P-450-containing w-hydroxylation system of liver microsomes into three components. *J. Biol. Chem.* **1969**, *244*, 3714–3721. [PubMed]
14. Flück, C.E.; Tajima, T.; Pandey, A.V.; Arlt, W.; Okuhara, K.; Verge, C.F.; Jabs, E.W.; Mendonça, B.B.; Fujieda, K.; Miller, W.L. Mutant P450 oxidoreductase causes disordered steroidogenesis with and without Antley-Bixler syndrome. *Nat. Genet.* **2004**, *36*, 228–230. [CrossRef] [PubMed]
15. Imai, T.; Globerman, H.; Gertner, J.M.; Kagawa, N.; Waterman, M.R. Expression and purification of functional human 17 alpha-hydroxylase/17,20-lyase (P450c17) in Escherichia coli. Use of this system for study of a novel form of combined 17 alpha-hydroxylase/17,20-lyase deficiency. *J. Biol. Chem.* **1993**, *268*, 19681–19689. [PubMed]
16. Burkhard, F.Z.; Parween, S.; Udhane, S.S.; Flück, C.E.; Pandey, A.V. P450 Oxidoreductase deficiency: Analysis of mutations and polymorphisms. *J. Steroid Biochem. Mol. Biol.* **2017**, *165 Pt A*, 38–50. [CrossRef] [PubMed]
17. Pandey, A.V.; Miller, W.L. Regulation of 17,20 lyase activity by cytochrome b5 and by serine phosphorylation of P450c17. *J. Biol. Chem.* **2005**, *280*, 13265–13271. [CrossRef] [PubMed]
18. Pandey, A.V.; Mellon, S.H.; Miller, W.L. Protein phosphatase 2A and phosphoprotein SET regulate androgen production by P450c17. *J. Biol. Chem.* **2003**, *278*, 2837–2844. [CrossRef] [PubMed]
19. Auchus, R.J.; Lee, T.C.; Miller, W.L. Cytochrome b5 augments the 17,20-lyase activity of human P450c17 without direct electron transfer. *J. Biol. Chem.* **1998**, *273*, 3158–3165. [CrossRef] [PubMed]
20. Zhang, L.H.; Rodriguez, H.; Ohno, S.; Miller, W.L. Serine phosphorylation of human P450c17 increases 17,20-lyase activity: Implications for adrenarche and the polycystic ovary syndrome. *Proc. Natl. Acad. Sci. USA* **1995**, *92*, 10619–10623. [CrossRef] [PubMed]
21. Idkowiak, J.; Randell, T.; Dhir, V.; Patel, P.; Shackleton, C.H.; Taylor, N.F.; Krone, N.; Arlt, W. A missense mutation in the human cytochrome b5 gene causes 46,XY disorder of sex development due to true isolated 17,20 lyase deficiency. *J. Clin. Endocrinol. Metab.* **2012**, *97*, E465–E475. [CrossRef] [PubMed]
22. DeVore, N.M.; Scott, E.E. Structures of cytochrome P450 17A1 with prostate cancer drugs abiraterone and TOK-001. *Nature* **2012**, *482*, 116–119. [CrossRef] [PubMed]
23. Petrunak, E.M.; DeVore, N.M.; Porubsky, P.R.; Scott, E.E. Structures of human steroidogenic cytochrome P450 17A1 with substrates. *J. Biol. Chem.* **2014**, *289*, 32952–32964. [CrossRef] [PubMed]
24. Yadav, R.; Petrunak, E.M.; Estrada, D.F.; Scott, E.E. Structural insights into the function of steroidogenic cytochrome P450 17A1. *Mol. Cell Endocrinol.* **2017**, *441*, 68–75. [CrossRef] [PubMed]
25. Auchus, R.J. Steroid 17-hydroxylase and 17,20-lyase deficiencies, genetic and pharmacologic. *J. Steroid Biochem. Mol. Biol.* **2017**, *165*, 71–78. [CrossRef] [PubMed]
26. Mak, P.J.; Gregory, M.C.; Denisov, I.G.; Sligar, S.G.; Kincaid, J.R. Unveiling the crucial intermediates in androgen production. *Proc. Natl. Acad. Sci. USA* **2015**, *112*, 15856–15861. [CrossRef] [PubMed]
27. Geller, D.H.; Auchus, R.J.; Mendonça, B.B.; Miller, W.L. The genetic and functional basis of isolated 17,20-lyase deficiency. *Nat. Genet.* **1997**, *17*, 201–205. [CrossRef] [PubMed]
28. Sherbet, D.P.; Tiosano, D.; Kwist, K.M.; Hochberg, Z.; Auchus, R.J. CYP17 mutation E305G causes isolated 17,20-lyase deficiency by selectively altering substrate binding. *J. Biol. Chem.* **2003**, *278*, 48563–48569. [CrossRef] [PubMed]
29. Van Den Akker, E.L.; Koper, J.W.; Boehmer, A.L.; Themmen, A.P.; Verhoef-Post, M.; Timmerman, M.A.; Otten, B.J.; Drop, S.L.; De Jong, F.H. Differential inhibition of 17alpha-hydroxylase and 17,20-lyase activities by three novel missense CYP17 mutations identified in patients with P450c17 deficiency. *J. Clin. Endocrinol. Metab.* **2002**, *87*, 5714–5721. [CrossRef] [PubMed]
30. Tiosano, D.; Knopf, C.; Koren, I.; Wudy, S.A. Metabolic evidence for impaired 17alpha-hydroxylase activity in a kindred bearing the E305G mutation for isolate 17,20-lyase activity. *Eur. J. Endocrinol.* **2008**, *158*, 385–392. [CrossRef] [PubMed]

31. Parween, S.; Roucher-Boulez, F.; Flück, C.E.; Lienhardt-Roussie, A.; Mallet, D.; Morel, Y.; Pandey, A.V. P450 Oxidoreductase Deficiency: Loss of Activity Caused by Protein Instability From a Novel L374H Mutation. *J. Clin. Endocrinol. Metab.* **2016**, *101*, 4789–4798. [CrossRef] [PubMed]
32. Flück, C.E.; Pandey, A.V. Impact on CYP19A1 activity by mutations in NADPH cytochrome P450 oxidoreductase. *J. Steroid Biochem. Mol. Biol.* **2017**, *165 Pt A*, 64–70. [CrossRef] [PubMed]
33. Pandey, A.V.; Sproll, P. Pharmacogenomics of human P450 oxidoreductase. *Front. Pharmacol.* **2014**, *5*, 103. [CrossRef] [PubMed]
34. Udhane, S.S.; Parween, S.; Kagawa, N.; Pandey, A.V. Altered CYP19A1 and CYP3A4 Activities Due to Mutations A115V, T142A, Q153R and P284L in the Human P450 Oxidoreductase. *Front. Pharmacol.* **2017**, *8*, 580. [CrossRef] [PubMed]
35. Geller, D.H.; Auchus, R.J.; Miller, W.L. P450c17 mutations R347H and R358Q selectively disrupt 17,20-lyase activity by disrupting interactions with P450 oxidoreductase and cytochrome b5. *Mol. Endocrinol.* **1999**, *13*, 167–175. [CrossRef] [PubMed]
36. Flück, C.E.; Meyer-Böni, M.; Pandey, A.V.; Kempná, P.; Miller, W.L.; Schoenle, E.J.; Biason-Lauber, A. Why boys will be boys: Two pathways of fetal testicular androgen biosynthesis are needed for male sexual differentiation. *Am. J. Hum. Genet.* **2011**, *89*, 201–218. [CrossRef] [PubMed]
37. Flück, C.E.; Pandey, A.V. Steroidogenesis of the testis—New genes and pathways. *Ann. Endocrinol.* **2014**, *75*, 40–47. [CrossRef] [PubMed]
38. Biason-Lauber, A.; Miller, W.L.; Pandey, A.V.; Fluck, C.E. Of marsupials and men: "Backdoor" dihydrotestosterone synthesis in male sexual differentiation. *Mol. Cell Endocrinol.* **2013**, *371*, 124–132. [CrossRef] [PubMed]
39. Audi, L.; Fernández-Cancio, M.; Carrascosa, A.; Andaluz, P.; Torán, N.; Piró, C.; Vilaró, E.; Vicens-Calvet, E.; Gussinyé, M.; Albisu, M.A.; et al. Novel (60%) and recurrent (40%) androgen receptor gene mutations in a series of 59 patients with a 46,XY disorder of sex development. *J. Clin. Endocrinol. Metab.* **2010**, *95*, 1876–1888. [CrossRef] [PubMed]
40. Fernandez-Cancio, M.; Audí, L.; Andaluz, P.; Torán, N.; Piró, C.; Albisu, M.; Gussinyé, M.; Yeste, D.; Clemente, M.; Martínez-Mora, J.; et al. SRD5A2 gene mutations and polymorphisms in Spanish 46,XY patients with a disorder of sex differentiation. *Int. J. Androl.* **2011**, *34 Pt 2*, e526–e535. [CrossRef] [PubMed]
41. Yamazaki, T.; Ohno, T.; Sakaki, T.; Akiyoshi-Shibata, M.; Yabusaki, Y.; Imai, T.; Kominami, S. Kinetic analysis of successive reactions catalyzed by bovine cytochrome p450(17alpha,lyase). *Biochemistry* **1998**, *37*, 2800–2806. [CrossRef] [PubMed]
42. Soucy, P.; Van, L.-T. Conversion of pregnenolone to DHEA by human 17α-hydroxylase/17,20-lyase (P450c17). *Eur. J. Biochem.* **2000**, *267*, 3243–3247. [CrossRef] [PubMed]
43. Brock, B.J.; Waterman, M.R. Biochemical Differences between Rat and Human Cytochrome P450c17 Support the Different Steroidogenic Needs of These Two Species. *Biochemistry* **1999**, *38*, 1598–1606. [CrossRef] [PubMed]
44. Pandey, A.V.; Kempná, P.; Hofer, G.; Mullis, P.E.; Flück, C.E. Modulation of human CYP19A1 activity by mutant NADPH P450 oxidoreductase. *Mol. Endocrinol.* **2007**, *21*, 2579–2595. [CrossRef] [PubMed]
45. Flück, C.E.; Mullis, P.E.; Pandey, A.V. Reduction in hepatic drug metabolizing CYP3A4 activities caused by P450 oxidoreductase mutations identified in patients with disordered steroid metabolism. *Biochem. Biophys. Res. Commun.* **2010**, *401*, 149–153. [CrossRef] [PubMed]
46. Nicolo, C.; Flück, C.E.; Mullis, P.E.; Pandey, A.V. Restoration of mutant cytochrome P450 reductase activity by external flavin. *Mol. Cell Endocrinol.* **2010**, *321*, 245–252. [CrossRef] [PubMed]
47. Riddick, D.S.; Ding, X.; Wolf, C.R.; Porter, T.D.; Pandey, A.V.; Zhang, Q.; Gu, J.; Finn, R.D.; Ronseaux, S.; McLaughlin, L.A.; et al. NADPH-cytochrome P450 oxidoreductase: Roles in physiology, pharmacology, and toxicology. *Drug Metab. Dispos.* **2013**, *41*, 12–23. [CrossRef] [PubMed]
48. Zalewski, A.; Ma, N.S.; Legeza, B.; Renthal, N.; Flück, C.E.; Pandey, A.V. Vitamin D-Dependent Rickets Type 1 Caused by Mutations in CYP27B1 Affecting Protein Interactions With Adrenodoxin. *J. Clin. Endocrinol. Metab.* **2016**, *101*, 3409–3418. [CrossRef] [PubMed]
49. Peng, H.M.; Im, Sa.; Pearl, N.M.; Turcu, A.F.; Waskell, J.R.L.; Auchus, R.J. Cytochrome b5 Activates the 17,20-Lyase Activity of Human Cytochrome P450 17A1 by Increasing the Coupling of NADPH Consumption to Androgen Production. *Biochemistry* **2016**, *55*, 4356–4365. [CrossRef] [PubMed]

50. Yoshimoto, F.K.; Gonzalez, E.; Auchus, R.J.; Guengerich, F.P. Mechanism of 17alpha,20-Lyase and New Hydroxylation Reactions of Human Cytochrome P450 17A1: 18O Labeling And Oxygen Surrogate Evidence For A Role Of A Perferryl Oxygen. *J. Biol. Chem.* **2016**, *291*, 17143–17164. [CrossRef] [PubMed]
51. Duggal, R.; Liu, Y.; Gregory, M.C.; Denisov, I.G.; Kincaid, J.R.; Sligar, S.G. Evidence that cytochrome b5 acts as a redox donor in CYP17A1 mediated androgen synthesis. *Biochem. Biophys. Res. Commun.* **2016**, *477*, 202–208. [CrossRef] [PubMed]
52. Estrada, D.F.; Skinner, A.L.; Laurence, J.S.; Scott, E.E. Human cytochrome P450 17A1 conformational selection: Modulation by ligand and cytochrome b5. *J. Biol. Chem.* **2014**, *289*, 14310–14320. [CrossRef] [PubMed]
53. Pallan, P.S.; Nagy, L.D.; Lei, L.; Gonzalez, E.; Kramlinger, V.M.; Azumaya, C.M.; Wawrzak, Z.; Waterman, M.R.; Guengerich, F.P.; Egli, M. Structural and kinetic basis of steroid 17alpha,20-lyase activity in teleost fish cytochrome P450 17A1 and its absence in cytochrome P450 17A2. *J. Biol. Chem.* **2015**, *290*, 3248–3268. [CrossRef] [PubMed]
54. Ramudo Cela, L.; Balea-Filgueiras, J.; Vizoso-Hermida, J.R.; Martín-Herranz, I. Study of cases of abiraterone discontinuation due to toxicity in pre-chemotherapy after 1 year's experience. *J. Oncol. Pharm. Pract.* **2017**, *23*, 615–619. [CrossRef] [PubMed]
55. Li, Z.; Alyamani, M.; Li, J.; Rogacki, K.; Abazeed, M.; Upadhyay, S.K.; Balk, S.P.; Taplin, M.E.; Auchus, R.J.; Sharifi, N. Redirecting abiraterone metabolism to fine-tune prostate cancer anti-androgen therapy. *Nature* **2016**, *533*, 547–551. [CrossRef] [PubMed]
56. Bonomo, S.; Hansen, C.H.; Petrunak, E.M.; Scott, E.E.; Styrishave, B.; Jørgensen, F.S.; Olsen, L. Promising Tools in Prostate Cancer Research: Selective Non-Steroidal Cytochrome P450 17A1 Inhibitors. *Sci. Rep.* **2016**, *6*, 29468. [CrossRef] [PubMed]
57. Sharifi, N. Prostate cancer: CYP17A1 inhibitor failure-lessons for future drug development. *Nat. Rev. Urol.* **2015**, *12*, 245–246. [CrossRef] [PubMed]
58. Udhane, S.S.; Dick, B.; Hu, Q.; Hartmann, R.W.; Pandey, A.V. Specificity of anti-prostate cancer CYP17A1 inhibitors on androgen biosynthesis. *Biochem. Biophys. Res. Commun.* **2016**, *477*, 1005–1010. [CrossRef] [PubMed]
59. Monno, S.; Ogawa, H.; Date, T.; Fujioka, M.; Miller, W.L.; Kobayashi, M. Mutation of histidine 373 to leucine in cytochrome P450c17 causes 17 alpha-hydroxylase deficiency. *J. Biol. Chem.* **1993**, *268*, 25811–25817. [PubMed]
60. Quattropani, C.; Vogt, B.; Odermatt, A.; Dick, B.; Frey, B.M.; Frey, F.J. Reduced activity of 11 beta-hydroxysteroid dehydrogenase in patients with cholestasis. *J. Clin. Investig.* **2001**, *108*, 1299–1305. [CrossRef] [PubMed]
61. Shackleton, C.H. Mass spectrometry in the diagnosis of steroid-related disorders and in hypertension research. *J. Steroid Biochem. Mol. Biol.* **1993**, *45*, 127–140. [CrossRef]
62. Huang, N.; Pandey, A.V.; Agrawal, V.; Reardon, W.; Lapunzina, P.D.; Mowat, D.; Jabs, E.W.; Van Vliet, G.; Sack, J.; Flück, C.E.; et al. Diversity and function of mutations in p450 oxidoreductase in patients with Antley-Bixler syndrome and disordered steroidogenesis. *Am. J. Hum. Genet.* **2005**, *76*, 729–749. [CrossRef] [PubMed]
63. Pandey, A.V.; Joshi, S.K.; Tekwani, B.L.; Chauhan, V.S. A colorimetric assay for heme in biological samples using 96-well plates. *Anal. Biochem.* **1999**, *268*, 159–161. [CrossRef] [PubMed]
64. Krieger, E.; Darden, T.; Nabuurs, S.B.; Finkelstein, A.; Vriend, G. Making optimal use of empirical energy functions: Force-field parameterization in crystal space. *Proteins* **2004**, *57*, 678–683. [CrossRef] [PubMed]
65. Vriend, G. WHAT IF: A molecular modeling and drug design program. *J. Mol. Graph.* **1990**, *8*, 52–56. [CrossRef]
66. Canutescu, A.A.; Shelenkov, A.A.; Dunbrack, R.L. A graph-theory algorithm for rapid protein side-chain prediction. *Protein Science* **2003**, *12*, 2001–2014. [CrossRef] [PubMed]
67. Duan, Y.; Wu, C.; Chowdhury, S.; Lee, M.C.; Xiong, G.; Zhang, W.; Yang, R.; Cieplak, P.; Luo, R.; Lee, T.; et al. A point-charge force field for molecular mechanics simulations of proteins based on condensed-phase quantum mechanical calculations. *J. Comput. Chem.* **2003**, *24*, 1999–2012. [CrossRef] [PubMed]

68. Jorgensen, W.L.; Tirado-Rives, J. Potential energy functions for atomic-level simulations of water and organic and biomolecular systems. *Proc. Natl. Acad. Sci. USA* **2005**, *102*, 6665–6670. [CrossRef] [PubMed]
69. Trott, O.; Olson, A.J. AutoDock Vina: Improving the speed and accuracy of docking with a new scoring function, efficient optimization, and multithreading. *J. Comput. Chem.* **2010**, *31*, 455–461. [CrossRef] [PubMed]
70. Pettersen, E.F.; Goddard, T.D.; Huang, C.C.; Couch, G.S.; Greenblatt, D.M.; Meng, E.C.; Ferrin, T.E. UCSF Chimera—A visualization system for exploratory research and analysis. *J. Comput. Chem.* **2004**, *25*, 1605–1612. [CrossRef] [PubMed]

7

Integration of Molecular Docking and In Vitro Studies: A Powerful Approach for Drug Discovery in Breast Cancer

Claudia Cava [1,*] and Isabella Castiglioni [2]

1 Institute of Molecular Bioimaging and Physiology, National Research Council (IBFM-CNR), Via F.Cervi 93, 20090 Segrate-Milan, Italy
2 Department of Physics "Giuseppe Occhialini", University of Milan-Bicocca Piazza dell'Ateneo Nuovo, 20126 Milan, Italy; isabella.castiglioni@unimib.it
* Correspondence: claudia.cava@ibfm.cnr.it

Abstract: Molecular docking in the pharmaceutical industry is a powerful in silico approach for discovering novel therapies for unmet medical needs predicting drug–target interactions. It not only provides binding affinity between drugs and targets at the atomic level, but also elucidates the fundamental pharmacological properties of specific drugs. The purpose of this review was to illustrate newer and emergent uses of docking when combined with in vitro techniques for drug discovery in metastatic breast cancer. We grouped the selected articles into five main categories; namely, systematic repositioning of drugs, natural drugs, new synthesized molecules, combinations of drugs, and drug latentiation. We focused on new promising drugs that have a good affinity with their targets, thus inducing a favorable biological response. This review suggests that the integration of molecular docking and in vitro studies can accelerate cancer drug discovery showing a good consistency of the results between the two approaches.

Keywords: molecular docking; in vitro; metastatic breast cancer; drug discovery

1. Introduction

Breast cancer (BC) is the most common type of tumor in women, but metastases are the main cause of death. Metastasis is a complex process where cancer cells move into the blood vessels, invade other tissues, and determine a colony in secondary sites. Indeed, BC initiates as a local disease but can spread with metastases to distant sites, such as the lymph nodes and different organs [1]. This process involves the expression of a series of genes that regulate the survival and invasion of cancer cells. Therefore, drugs that modulate the genes/proteins that regulate cancer cell survival, metastasis, apoptosis, and invasion are of great importance as potential drug targets in the drug discovery process [2,3]. However, although the development of new therapies has significantly reduced mortality for metastatic BC, the resistance to anticancer agents can lead to treatment failure [4].

A drug discovery process originates because there is a clinical condition without a suitable therapy. The first step of research often begins in academia, where a hypothesis is generated; for example, the inhibition or induction of a protein or pathway as a therapeutic effect in a disease condition [5]. Indeed, a crucial point of the research process is the selection of a target, which can be a range of biological entities such as proteins, RNA, and genes that can be selected via bioinformatics analyses [6,7]. An optimal target must be accessible to the putative drug molecule and the binding drug–target complex should induce a biological response [5], which can be quantified with in vitro models. The most used in vitro BC models are cell lines, as they share many molecular and genomic features of BC. The binding affinity between the drug and the target can be calculated in silico with molecular docking. Thus, in silico and in vitro screenings may help to quickly identify the toxicity of the tested drugs/molecules, thus avoiding further steps such as in vivo and preclinical studies (in case of unfavorable results from in silico and in vitro methods) [5].

In silico approaches with docking studies require at least two elements: a protein/drug database and a molecular docking algorithm. Protein and drug databases are a collection of the structures of proteins and drugs. The rapidly increasing number of structures has created big data, which offer a wide range of biological and chemical information and are a recent opportunity to develop better knowledge of the relationships between drugs and targets (usually proteins), drugs and diseases, and targets and diseases. However, although the available data are often heterogeneous and incomplete, computational methods can exploit this knowledge to deepen these interactions [8]. Given the cost and time consumption of experimental methods, high-performing computational algorithms for drug discovery processes are needed. The computational technique known as "docking" can predict the binding of drug–target complexes, as well as the conformation of the ligand upon binding to a protein target. The binding free energy of target–drug interactions establishes the affinity of an association and the conditions for forming a complex. Ranked binding free energies are not always precise, but they can be used to select new drugs such as small molecules to be experimentally tested in a virtual screening approach [9–11]. Small molecules are promising new drugs with a low molecular weight, which allows them to penetrate cells easily [12]. In addition, molecular docking can be also used for predicting the effects of a drug; for example, the identification of an undesired interaction between a compound and off-targets. To date, 57,000 abstracts/papers have been published on molecular docking, indicating the importance of this computational method in drug development [13–15].

Despite encouraging results, the real condition of the cellular environment, such as the pH and temperature, cannot be fully replicated in a docking study. Each docking algorithm has its limitations and advantages. Therefore, it has been reported that a binding free energy that integrates the results from different docking algorithms can lead to a higher performance in a virtual screening process [16]. Moreover, molecular docking, being a structure-based method, is limited to receptors and ligands with a known stable structure. Thus, the integration of in vitro and in vivo studies as a validation step of in silico methods is an indispensable part of the drug discovery process. These techniques can study different aspects of potential drugs, such as absorption, regulation of targets, metabolic stability, and toxicity [17].

The goal of this review was to describe recent studies in metastatic BC that used molecular docking and in vitro studies for drug development.

2. Materials and Methods

Papers published on the PubMed platform on the use of in vitro and molecular docking strategies in metastatic BC were included in this review. Papers were included in the review only if: (1) they were published in the last five years (from 2015 to the end of the search on 27 August 2020); (2) they were published in full-text English language in a peer-reviewed journal (excluding short communications and abstracts); (3) they included in vitro and docking analyses in metastatic BC. Papers were excluded if: (1) only one in vitro or docking analysis was performed; (2) they did not provide in vitro studies on BC cell lines.

3. Results

We categorized the selected papers into five main groups based on the characteristics of the drugs and approaches used: systematic repositioning of drugs/molecules, natural molecules, new synthesized molecules, combinations of drugs, and drug latentiation.

3.1. Systematic Repositioning of Drugs/Molecules

Drug discovery is a time-consuming and labor-intensive work process. On average, the development of a new drug takes 10–15 years. Drug repositioning, namely, the use of old drugs for new diseases, is an efficient strategy for its low-cost and riskless characteristics [15]. Several studies have performed systematic approaches, using a combination of in silico and experimental methods, to reposition known drugs/molecules. Table 1 presents the works in the last five years that have implemented in silico and in vitro models for drug discovery using a systematic repositioning of drugs for metastatic BC.

In particular, the study of Rymbai et al. [18] focused on the similarity between the side effects of two different drugs. Indeed, the assumption of the study was that if the two drugs have common side effects, then they can also have common gene targets and clinical indications. In vitro cell line and molecular docking studies have shown that ropinirole shares many side effects with letrozole (used in the management of advanced and metastatic BC) and is efficient in the treatment of breast cancer. An in vitro study of ropinirole on MCF-7 cells by a 3-(4,5-dimethylthiazol-2-yl)-2, 5-diphenyltetrazolium bromide assay (MTT) was performed to test the ability of ropinirole to inhibit cell growth. Molecular docking showed a good interaction with a good binding affinity of −7.8 kcal/mol between ropinirole and aromatase, a well-known target of letrozole. The three-dimensional structure of aromatase (Protein Data Bank (PDB) ID: 3EQM) is available for computational docking analysis in the Protein Data Bank (PDB).

In a recent study, Liu et al. screened more than 1000 known small molecular compounds and focused on 15 compounds [19], studying their effect on breast cancer cell viability and migration with in vitro studies on MCF-7, MDA-MB-231, and BT-474 BC cell lines. Molecular docking was performed to demonstrate the ability of the binding of the 15 compounds with chemokine ligand 18 (CCL18), as previous studies suggested that CCL18 is a chemokine derived from tumor-associated macrophages (TAMs) to induce BC metastasis [20]. Therefore, CCL18 is considered a potential drug target (PDB ID: 4MHE). Narrowing the selection of ligands from more than 1000 compounds to 15 was performed by evaluating the binding energy with CCL18 obtained via molecular docking studies. In this way, 15 compounds were selected as potential drugs targeting CCL18, and the toxicity of these 15 compounds was evaluated by using cell counting kit-8 (CCK-8) assays, which indicated that most of the compounds did not influence cell viability. A total of 6 of the 15 compounds inhibited CCL18-induced cell migration; this anticancer activity was also confirmed by adherence and invasion assays [19].

In vitro, in silico, in vivo, and ex vivo analyses have been performed to evaluate the cytotoxic action of etoposide (ET), doxorubicin (DOX), pifithrin-α (PIF), and dexamethasone (DEX) in triple-negative BC (TNBC) [21]. TNBC is a molecular subtype of BC that is negative for three hormone receptors—namely, estrogen receptors (ERs), progesterone receptors (PRs), and human epidermal receptor 2 (HER2) [21]. ET, a podophyllotoxin derivative, is a chemotherapy medication used against a wide range of cancers (e.g., lung cancer, lymphoma, lung cancer, leukemia, and glioblastoma multiforme), but its efficacy against TNBC is still unknown [22]. DOX, alone or in combination with other drugs, is an effective therapy for numerous cancers, including breast cancer [23]. The antiapoptotic and non-topoisomerase inhibitors PIF and DEX were considered in a previous study as a negative control [21]. In this study, the authors identified tumor necrosis factor-related apoptosis-inducing ligand (TRAIL) and death receptor 5 (DR5) as potential drug targets (PDB ID: 4N90) [21]. Molecular docking and molecular dynamics studies have shown the ability of ET, DOX, PIF, and DEX to stabilize the TRAIL–DR5 complex. In vitro technologies have demonstrated that ET and DOX increase apoptosis, demonstrating their synergistic effect with TRAIL. These results were confirmed with the binding energy for the ternary complexes TRAIL–DR5–ET and TRAIL–DR5–DOX [21].

Thionine (TH), an organic dye, and its derivatives have been proposed as promising drugs for the photodynamic therapy of cancer [24]. Previous studies reported that TH shows possible genotoxic and cytotoxic activity in prokaryotic cells [25]. Since there is a wide range of applications of TH, it is important to evaluate the site-specific interaction of TH with human serum albumin (HSA), the main protein in plasma, which is responsible for the maintenance and regulation of the colloidal osmotic pressure of blood [24]. HSA has several binding sites to which various ligands can bind. The binding of ligands to this protein can influence drug distribution, as HSA plays a crucial role in the transport of endogenous/exogenous compounds. Therefore, HSA is widely used in clinical applications as a drug delivery system. Manivel et al. revealed that TH interacts with the hydrophobic cavity of subdomain IIA of HSA (PDB ID:1AO6) and that the complex shows a good level of cytotoxicity in cancer cells through in vitro studies [24].

Previous studies have shown the anticancer and antimetastatic effects of the microbial polyketide 2,4-diacetylphloroglucinol (DAPG) through the regulation of NF-κB activity [26]. The induction of NF-κB also mediates the expression of other antiapoptotic proteins and protein kinases in cancer cells. However, the mechanism of action of DAPG acting on metastatic proteins such as Matrix metalloproteinase 9 (MMP9), MMP2, NF-κB, and the antiapoptotic Bcl-2 family proteins are not yet known. In a recent study [27], binding energies, computed by molecular docking, revealed that MMP2, MMP9, and NF-κB achieved a higher interaction with DAPG. In vitro studies have confirmed that DAPG compounds are able to inhibit cancer cells in several cancer cell lines, including MDA-MB-231 [27].

Drug repositioning offers new clinical indications for known drugs/molecules using an efficient, low-cost and riskless strategy. However, despite encouraging results, drug repositioning is a complex process that involves different elements, such as the use of big medical data, to develop an appropriate approach for drug repositioning and a new framework for the integration of available resources.

3.2. *Natural Molecules*

Historically, natural products, which contain a wide range of compounds for drug discovery, have been considered in multiple clinical trials, especially as anticancer and antimicrobial agents [28]. The advantage of natural products with respect to synthetic compounds is that they are also metabolites. Therefore, they are biologically active and can also be substrates for transporter systems [28]. Table 2 shows the works in the last five years that have implemented in silico and in vitro models for drug discovery using natural ligands as drugs for metastatic BC.

Hypercholesterolemia has been reported to play a role in the progression of BC and resistance to hormonal therapy. High low-density lipoprotein (LDL) levels, primarily caused by familial hypercholesterolemia, are also one of the risk factors of the initiation and promotion of BC [29]. Proprotein convertase subtilisin/kexin type-9 (PCSK9) binds to LDL receptors (avoiding binding with LDL) and regulates the cholesterol metabolism, targeting the receptor for lysosomal degradation and thus leading to the degradation of LDL. Pseurotin A (PS) is a microbial secondary metabolite originally isolated from the fungal culture of *Pseudeurotium ovalis* in 1976 [30]. PS shows different biological activities, including the inhibition of the fungal chitin synthase [31], the activation of cell differentiation [32], and apomorphine antagonist activity [33]. Abdelwahed et al. showed that PS reduces PCSK9 secretion, suggesting its potential as a drug [34]. In particular, they performed predictive molecular modeling to evaluate the binding of PS to PCSK9 (PDB ID: 4NE9, 4NMX, and 3GCW). Docking analysis has revealed that PS is able to successfully bind to the PCSK9 domain, thereby disrupting PCSK9–LDL receptor interactions. Furthermore, this finding has been validated in vitro by surface plasmon resonance, confirming the capacity of PS to interfere with the PCSK9–LDL complex at their binding interface.

Table 1. Characteristics of the studies reported herein categorized as "systematic repositioning of drugs" used in metastatic breast cancer. The table reports the drug, its target with Protein Data Bank (PDB) ID, the in silico/in vitro/in vivo methods used to test the drug, clinical trials, the original use, and the reference.

Drug	Target	In Silico	In Vitro	In Vivo	Clinical Trials	Original Use	Ref.
Ropinirole	aromatase enzyme (PDB [1] ID: 3EQM)	Docking studies	MTT [2] assay	-	-	antiparkinsonism	[19]
15 small molecular compounds	CCL18 (PDB ID: 4MHE)	Docking studies	Cell viability, Boyden chamber, adherence assay	Tumor xenografts	-	CCL18 antagonist	[20]
Topoisomerase inhibitor etoposide (ET) and doxorubicin (DOX)	TRAIL-DR5 (PDB ID: 4N90)	Docking, mutational and dynamics studies	MTT assay, FACS [3]	Tumor xenografts	NCT00004 906	against a wide range of cancers	[21]
Thionine	human serum albumin (HSA) (PDB ID:1AO6)	Dockingstudies	MTT assay and Fluorescence microscopic	-	-	against bacteria, viruses and yeasts	[24]
2,4-diacetylphloroglucinol	Bcl-2 (PDB ID: 4AQ3), Bcl-xL (PDB ID: 2YQ6), Bcl-w (PDB ID: 2Y6W), MMP2 (PDB ID: 1HOV), MMP9 (PDB ID: 1GKC), NF-jB p65 (PDB ID: 1VKX)	Docking studies	MTT and invasion assay	-	-	antimicrobial, antiviral, and anticancer	[27]

[1] PDB: Protein Data Bank, [2] MTT: 3-[4, 5-dimethylthiazol-2-yl]-2, 5-diphenyltetrazolium bromide, [3] FACS: Fluorescence-activated cell sorting.

In an another study, the interactions of atranorin (ATR), a metabolite of many lichens, with the target proteins that are overexpressed in BC, such as AKT, BCL-2, BAX, BCL-W, and BCL-XL, were studied with docking and in vitro analyses [35]. Commonly, ATR is metabolite present in numerous lichens such as *Stereocaulon cacspitorim, Everniastrum vexans, Parmatrema* species, and others [35]. The complex formed by ATR and AKT shows a better binding energy, but interacting residues show minor affinities to inhibiting the overexpression of BC biomarkers. Interestingly, previous studies have reported the activation of AKT in drug resistance [36] and in vitro studies have been performed on MDA-MB-231 and MCF-7. The inhibitory activity of ATR has been tested with MTT assays, showing a downregulation of oncoproteins. Furthermore, gene expression analysis of the ATR–AKT model has shown the induction of apoptosis in BC cell lines [35].

Another natural compound, eugenol, a phenylpropanoid obtainable from honey and some essential oils with antioxidant and anticancer properties, has been tested with in silico and in vitro approaches [37]. In vivo and in vitro studies have demonstrated that eugenol promotes the inhibition of β-catenin, a biomarker associated with the progression of cancer and the development of lymph node metastasis. β-catenin accumulation in the nucleus is evident in BC because of aberrant wnt signaling. Western blot analysis has confirmed a significant modification in the expression level of total β-catenin in in vivo and in vitro models. In addition, eugenol demonstrates a downregulation of the expression of cancer stem cell biomarkers. Docking studies have revealed many binding sites of the complex and the data support a good interaction between the ligand and the β-catenin protein (PDB ID: 3BCT) [37].

Pharmacological research in recent years has also proposed the plant *Astragalus membranaceus* (AM) as a natural product for cancer treatment. A recent study using a multidisciplinary approach constituted by gene expression analysis, pharmacokinetic screening, biological network analysis, and in vitro approaches investigated the possible and novel mechanism of AM in TNBC [38]. All of the ingredients of AM were collected for a total of 87 compounds and 16 active components and *Astragalus polysaccharides* (APS) was proposed as a potential compound against BC. Indeed, docking analysis showed good results between APS and the proteins AKT, BCL2, and PIK3CG. Indeed, in vitro experiments confirmed that the compound can inhibit migration and invasion and can induce apoptosis [38].

Natural compounds can be also administrated to avoid the side effects of drugs. In a recent study, drug design methods were performed to investigate plant-derived inhibitors against sirtuin (SIRT) proteins [39]. As SIRT, which comprises seven human isoforms, is associated with the metastatic and oncogenic progression of advanced BC, its inhibition is a promising approach against tumorigenesis. A previous study considered 21 plant-derived inhibitors as ligands and the seven human isoforms of SIRT as targets [39], and molecular docking with the binding energies of the ligand–receptor complexes showed that sulforaphane, kaempferol, and apigenin can achieve the highest binding energies against SIRT1, 3, and 6, respectively. To validate these in silico results, they explored the role of these potential small molecules against BC cell lines on cellular viability using MTT assays [39].

Noscapine (NOS) is a phthalide isoquinoline alkaloid derived from the *Papaver somniferum* plant. As several studies have reported the ability of NOS to inhibit the growth of tumor cells and to activate apoptosis, there are ongoing phase I/II clinical trials for cancer management, but not for BC [40]. Maurya et al. [41] studied the interaction between NOS and carrier protein HSA using different techniques, including in vitro approaches and computational methods. The cytotoxicity findings by MTT assay indicated that NOS has good potential in cancer. Meanwhile, the in silico results showed that the main binding site for NOS was site I (subdomain II A) of HSA [41].

Shikonin (SK), a phytochemical derived from the medicinal plant *Lithospermum erythrorhizon*, has been demonstrated to induce tumor immunogenicity [42]. However, the molecular mechanisms of action and the pharmacological processes are still unknown. First, in a recent study [43] the authors performed a computation prediction analysis, applying molecular docking and a virtual screening system. They screened 27,317 human protein structures deposited in the Protein Data Bank in order to search for the molecular targets of SK. Heterogeneous nuclear ribonucleoprotein A1 (hnRNPA1) obtained the highest binding energy with SK (−15.3 kcal/mol), and this binding leads to the suppression of post-transcriptional mRNA processing in vitro [43]. In addition, the SK– hnRNPA1 complex inhibits the splicing and suppresses the nuclear export activities of specific inflammation-associated genes, resulting in a reduction in acute cytokine storms [43].

Matrix metalloproteinase 9 (MMP9) and matrix metalloproteinase 2 (MMP2) regulate the tumor microenvironment and tumor metastasis. Therefore, the inhibition of MMP9 and MMP2 could reduce invasion and tumor metastasis [44]. Currently, traditional Chinese medicines (TCMs) are proposed in the prevention and treatment of several diseases, including cancer. In a recent study, plantamajoside (PMS), a Chinese herbal medicine, was proposed as an inhibitor of MMP9 and MMP2. Indeed, molecular docking and in vitro analyses confirmed the good interaction of the molecules with the proteins and the inhibition of the proliferation, migration, and invasion of BC cell lines [44]. Specifically, in vitro studies on the MDA-MB-231 and 4T1 BC cell lines have demonstrated that PMS reduces the activity of MMP9 and MMP2. In addition, after treatment with PMS, BC cell lines show a decrease in cell proliferation.

The aryl hydrocarbon receptor (Ahr), a helix–loop–helix transcription factor, is a promising regulator of the invasiveness and metastasis of BC cells. It is regulated by a wide variety of natural molecules such as flavonoids—among which, flavipin is the least studied. Hanieh et al. [45] applied in silico and in vitro methods to investigate the relationships between flavipin and Ahr. Docking analysis revealed eight hydrogen bonds involving the Phe115, Leu116, and Ala119 residues of the Ahr molecule. The results of the in vitro analysis showed that flavipin has inhibitory effects on the migration of MDA-MB-231 and T47D cells [45].

The studies reported above show that the growing application of in silico and in vitro techniques may contribute to the recovery of interest in natural products for drug discovery.

Table 2. Characteristics of the studies reported herein categorized as "natural drugs" used in metastatic breast cancer. The table reports the drug, its target with PDB ID, the in silico/in vitro/in vivo methods used to test the drug, clinical trials, the mechanism of action, and the reference.

Drug	Target	In Silico	In Vitro	In Vivo	Clinical Trials	Mechanism of Action	Ref.
Pseurotin A	PCSK9 (PDB [1] ID: 4NE9, 4NMX, and 3GCW)	Docking studies	MTT [2] assay	Tumor xenografts	-	cholesterol metabolism	[34]
Atranorin	AKT, BCL-2, BAX, BCL-W and BCL-XL (PDB ID: NA)	Docking studies	MTT assay	-	-	apoptosis	[35]
Eugenol	β-catenin (PDB ID: 3BCT)	Docking studies	MTT assay	Tumor xenografts	-	Cancer Stem Cell	[37]
Astragalus membranaceus	AKT (PDB ID:3QKK), BCL2 (PDB ID: 4AQ3), and PIK3CG (PDB ID: CHX)	Differential expression analysis Docking, dynamics studies	CCK-8 [3], Chamber, FITC [4] assay	-	NCT03314805, NCT03634150	apoptosis	[38]
21 plant-derived inhibitors	human sirtuin (SIRTs 1-7). SIRT1 (PDB ID: 4I5I), SIRT2 (PDB ID: IJ8F), SIRT3 (PDB ID: 5D7N), SIRT5 (PDB ID: 2B4Y), SIRT6 (PDB ID: 3K35) and SIRT7 (PDB ID: 5IQZ)	Docking and dynamics studies	MTT, trypan blue, sirtuin, Anchorage-dependent clonogenic assay	-	-	sirtuin inhibitors	[39]
Noscapine	human serum albumin (HSA) (PDB ID: 1AO6)	Docking and dynamics studies	MTT assay	-	-	inhibition of cell growth	[41]
Shikonin	27,317 human protein structures	Docking studies	calorimetry analysis and electrophoretic mobility shift assay	Tumor xenografts	-	suppression of post-transcriptional mRNA processing	[42]
Plantamajoside	Matrix metalloproteinase 2 and 9 (PDB ID: NA)	Docking studies	CCK-8, chamber wound assay	Tumor allografts	-	inhibition of cell growth	[44]
Flavipin	Aryl hydrocarbon receptor (Ahr) (PDB ID: 4M4X)	Docking studies	CCK-8 and Boyden chamber	-	-	cancer cell motility	[45]

[1] PDB: Protein Data Bank, [2] MTT: 3-[4, 5-dimethylthiazol-2-yl]-2, 5-diphenyltetrazolium bromide, [3] CCK-8 cell counting kit-8, [4] FITC Annexin-V fluorescein isothiocyanate.

3.3. New Synthesized Molecules

Since there is not yet a definite solution for the treatment of cancer, there is a clear need to research new molecules with anticancer properties. The combination of in vitro techniques and molecular docking can also be used also to test new synthesized molecules. Table 3 shows the works in the last five years that have implemented in silico and in vitro models for drug discovery using new synthesized molecules as drugs for metastatic BC.

For example, Nashaat et al. [46] synthesized a new series of compounds; i.e., new benzimidazole derivatives against BC-targeting peptidylprolyl cis-trans isomerase NIMA-interacting 1 (PIN1). PIN1 proteins play a role in cell cycle regulation, and their overexpression is correlated with human cancer [46]. It has also been described that PIN1 increases DNA binding to estrogen receptors [47]. Anticancer effects have been tested in vitro with MTT assays using the MCF-7 cell line: Several synthesized compounds have shown a very strong efficacy against this BC cell line. Furthermore, the interactions of three synthesized compounds with PIN1 crystal structures (PDB: 4TYO) have been validated using molecular docking, and the formed complexes show some essential interactions for PIN1 inhibition [46]. Specifically, the interaction with Lys63 is crucial for PIN1 inhibition.

In another study, Vaz et al. [48] synthesized the new hybrid dihydroquinoline derivative (M-CNP) compound. They designed this hybrid compound composed of sulfonamide, quinoline, and chalcone. The idea behind the study was that molecules containing sulfonamide, quinoline, and chalcone could originate new hybrid architectures with novel anticancer properties. The aim is that compounds derived from more molecules can enhance the pharmacological effectiveness. Anticancer activity of the novel compound was demonstrated by regulating aldehyde dehydrogenase 1 family member A1 (ALDH1A1), which, by converting retinal (retinaldehyde) to retinoic acid (RA), plays a role in the differentiation of cells and signaling events. Interestingly, an in vivo test on a metastatic BC cell lines (i.e., MDA-MB-231) has confirmed the promising role of ALDH1A1. Indeed, cytotoxicity assays have demonstrated the specific activity of the compounds against tumor cells. Furthermore, molecular docking analyses have demonstrated that the M-CNP derivative plays a role as an anticancer drug because of its good affinity with ALDH1A1 [48].

Previous studies have shown that compounds can bind to DNA with covalent and non-covalent interactions; for example, cisplatin, a well-known anticancer drug, interacts with DNA via a covalent link. However, covalent interactions can induce serious side effects, highlighting the importance of non-covalent interactions between DNA and drugs [49]. Among metal complexes, nickel aroylhydrazone Schiff base complexes show non-covalent interactions. Following this assumption, Li et al. [49] synthesized two nickel-derived complexes, and molecular docking revealed that both compounds could bind to DNA through the interaction of the phenyl rings with the double helix. In addition, the association between DNA and bovine serum albumin (BSA) is able to modify the secondary structure of BSA. The anticancer activity of individual complexes was also evaluated with in vitro cytotoxicity assays on the A549, MCF-7, and L-02 cell lines [49]. Both complexes obtained a lower cytotoxic effect than cisplatin against normal cell lines. Thus, in vitro analysis suggests more selective effects of the compounds against cancer cell lines.

Ruarene complexes have been observed to be possible agents against cisplatin resistance with fewer side effects, demonstrating a different mechanism of action. Acharya et al. synthesized four ruarene complexes and characterized them using X-ray crystallography [50], and molecular docking was performed to demonstrate their ability to bind tubulin proteins (PDB: 1SA0). The cytotoxicity of the molecules was tested in vitro by MTT assays in three different cancer cell lines, including MDA-MB-231. The complexes that demonstrated a lower toxicity were selected to test their effect on the inhibition of the microtubule network in the MDA-MB-231 cell line. In silico and in vitro studies demonstrated good binding between the compounds and the tubulin, as well as antiproliferative action against advanced subtypes of cancer, such as triple-negative metastatic BC [50].

Glycyrrhiza glabra, an Indian therapeutic herb, contains a diglucopyranosiduronic acid of glycyrrhetinic acid (GA). GA plays a role in immune responses, cell cycle, apoptosis, and autophagy [51]. Shukla et al. [52] designed five glycyrrhetinic acid (GA) derivatives and analyzed their in vitro action in a metastatic breast cancer cell line (i.e., MDA-MB-231). Molecular docking studies have been carried out to investigate the action of compounds on BC targets such as glyoxalase-I (GLO-I). BC receives energy from glycolysis based on the Warburg effect, and GLO-1 is able to inhibit and inactivate methyl glyoxalases, a compound formed during glycolysis, making GLO-I inhibitors potential anticancer agents. It has been shown that GA-1 increases cytotoxic action, and a study using molecular docking confirmed the binding of GA derivatives with GLO-I [52].

As previous studies have described that epidermal growth factor receptor tyrosine kinase (EGFR-TK) is upregulated in BC, it has been suggested as a potential drug target for novel therapy agents. The EGFR-TK inhibitory activity of known 1,3,5-triazines derivatives against BC has been examined [53]. In addition, the effects of the compounds on several BC cell lines have been estimated, including MDA-MB-231, a metastatic BC cell line. The consequence of the compounds on β-catenin expression has also been evaluated: all designed compounds achieved a good binding energy against the target protein. Furthermore, in vitro experiments have confirmed the docking analysis since the synthesized derivatives demonstrated an inhibitory effect on EGFR-TK [53].

Rac family small GTPase 1 (RAC1) is involved in the migration and invasion of BC cells. Therefore, therapeutic strategies that silence RAC1 could be a new challenge [54]. A new series of carbazole derivatives have been designed for their antitumor properties. Vlaar et al. evaluated the role of the compounds via interactions with RAC1 through molecular docking: the molecular docking results indicated a favorable conformation of the receptor–ligand complex. The compounds also demonstrated moderate antiproliferative activity using in vitro techniques [54].

The main site of BC metastasis is bone, and bone metastases often lead to complications, including fractures, bone pain, and hypercalcemia. However, to date, no biomarkers have been identified that are able to predict bone metastases. A first circulating fragment of parathyroid hormone-related protein (PTHrP), PTHrP(12-48), has been proposed as a biomarker associated with the presence of bone metastases. Kamalakar et al. [55] investigated the biological processes and mechanisms of action of PTHrP(12-48). First of all, they predicted the tertiary structure of PTHrP(12-48) through bioinformatics analyses, and the molecular modeling found that PTHrP(12-48) interacts via a weak binding with the PTH1 receptor (PTHR1). In vitro analysis supported this model: PTHrP(12-48) treatment does not promote an increase in cAMP in PTHR1-expressing SaOS2 cells. In conclusion, these data indicate that PTHrP(12-48) acts in the regulation of the differentiation of hematopoietic cells and regulates the osteoclasts within the tumor–bone marrow microenvironment, possibly to induce bone metastasis [55].

Angiogenesis, a physiological process that produces new blood vessels from pre-existing blood cells, consists of a series of steps such as the production of protease, endothelial cell migration and proliferation, vascular tube formation, and the maturation of cells [56]. Accelerated angiogenesis is correlated with several diseases, including cancer. The inhibitors of angiogenesis that target several proteins, such as vascular endothelial growth factor (VEGF), epidermal growth factor (EGF), platelet-derived growth factor (PDGF), and basic fibroblast growth factor (bFGF), that are involved in the regulation of the process can be used as a therapeutic strategy. The main factor in the angiogenesis process is VEGF [56]. Aboul-Enein et al. [57] designed 7-chloro-4-(piperazin-1-yl)quinoline derivatives as VEGFR-II inhibitors, and the anticancer abilities of these compounds were tested in vitro using breast cancer and prostate cancer cell lines. These analyses demonstrated that compound **4q** is the most active on both cell lines, and molecular modeling revealed that **4q** has similar sites of binding as sorafenib and lenavatinib at the ATP binding site of VEGFR-II. Furthermore, the binding energy of **4q** is slightly better than that of lenavatinib but lower than that of sorafenib [57].

Apoptosis is one of the key hallmarks of cancer. The BCL-2 family is a group of proteins that have a fundamental role in the regulation of apoptosis. For this reason, BCL-2 has become one of the most studied drug targets over recent years. Ziedan et al. [58] designed a 3D pharmacophore model to act as an inhibitor of the antiapoptotic BCL-2 protein. The 15 oxadiazole derivative compounds were tested to demonstrate their inhibitory activity in two cancer cell lines (i.e., cervical HeLa and breast MDA-MB-231). Molecular docking was carried out to evaluate the interaction scores between the compounds and the BCL-2 protein. Some of the proposed compounds obtained good antiproliferative activity and good binding energy with the BCL-2 protein (compounds **1** and **16j**) [58]. The simplicity of the synthesis of these compounds and their low molecular weight is promising; therefore, additional studies should be employed based on this novel class of BCL-2 inhibitors.

Oncogenic proteins such as tyrosine kinases, cell cycle regulators, and transcriptional factors are implicated in metastatic pathways in cancer. Many of them interact with heat shock protein 90 (Hsp90). Therefore, Hsp90 inhibitors have been proposed as novel cancer treatment methods, although they can lead to adverse effects in clinical trials. To overcome these disadvantages, Koca et al. [59] designed novel molecular Hsp90 inhibitors. Specifically, they designed novel pyrimidinyl acyl thiourea derivatives as Hsp90 inhibitors, and in vitro analyses revealed that these compounds can inhibit cell proliferation and demonstrate cytotoxic effects in BC and human bone osteosarcoma cell lines. Molecular docking confirmed the interaction of these compounds with the Hsp90 domain [59].

Previous studies have suggested KDM5A and KDM5B as oncogenic regulators [60]. The catalytic domain of KDM5 proteins has an unusual inclusion of an ARID and PHD1 domain that divides the catalytic domain into two subdomains—namely, JmjN and JmjC. Horton et al. demonstrated that a deletion of the ARID and PHD1 domains has a negative impact on the in vitro enzymatic kinetics of the KDM5 family. Thus, the challenge is finding inhibitors that act on the catalytic domain of the KDM5 family; to this end, the authors proposed GSK-J1 as an inhibitor of the KDM family through in silico studies [61].

EPH receptor A2 (EphA2) is a receptor tyrosine kinase that is involved in drug resistance and metastatic processes [62]. Gambini et al. designed agonistic peptides that target the ligand-binding domain of the EphA2 receptor, called 135H11 and 135H12 [63]. In vitro approaches and computational methods have suggested that both are effective agonistic EphA2 agents and are effective in inhibiting cell migration and invasion [63]. In addition, both dimeric agents are able to induce EphA2 receptor degradation.

The use of drugs to treat or manage the progression of BC is the best strategy. However, the efficacy of traditional drugs has been seriously compromised due to the phenomenon of resistance. Therefore, it is essential to discover new synthesized drugs that target novel sites and regulate biological processes involved in the progression of cancer.

Table 3. Characteristics of studies reported in the review categorized as "new synthesized molecules" used in metastatic breast cancer. The table reports the drug, its target with PDB ID, in silico/in vitro/in vivo methods used to test the drug, clinical trials, mechanism of action and reference.

Drug	Target	In Silico	In Vitro	In Vivo	Clinical Trials	Mechanism of Action	Ref.
new benzimidazole derivatives	PIN1 (PDB [1]: 4TYO)	Docking studies	MTT [2] and apoptosis assay	-	-	apoptosis	[46]
Dihydroquinoline derivate, M-CNP	ALDH1A1 (PDB ID: NA)	Docking studies	MTT assay	-	-	cell viability	[48]
Two new nickel (II) triphenylphosphine complexes	DNA (PDB ID:1Z3F), BSA (PDB ID: 4F5S)	Docking studies	CCK-8 [3] assay	-	-	antioxidant activity	[49]
Ruarene complexes	Tubulin (PDB ID: 1SA0)	Docking studies	MTT, Annexin-V/PE assays	-	-	proliferation	[50]
5 glycyrrhetinic acid (GA) derivates	GLO-I (PDB: 4PV5)	Docking studies	cytotoxicity assay	-	-	metabolism	[52]
1,3,5-triazine derivatives	epidermal growth factorreceptor-tyrosine kinase (EGFR-TK) (PDB ID: 1M17)	Docking studies	MTT and apoptosis assay	-	-	apoptosis	[53]
carbazole derivatives	RAC1 (PDB ID: NA)	Docking studies	Wound healing	-	-	migration	[54]
PTHrP(12-48)	PTH1 receptor (PDB ID: NA)	Docking studies	Immunofluorescence assays	-	NCT00051779	activity of osteoclasts	[55]
Certain 7-Chloro-4-(piperazin-1-yl)quinoline Derivatives	VEGFR-II (PDB ID: NA)	Docking studies	SRB [4] assay	-	-	proliferation	[57]
Oxadiazole derivates	BCL-2 protein (PDB ID: 1YSW)	Docking studies	MTT assay	-	-	apoptosis	[58]
novel pyrimidinyl acyl thiourea derivatives	Heat Shock Protein 90(Hsp90) (PDB ID: 1UYM)	Docking studies	XTT [5] assay	-	-	ATPase function	[59]
crystalstructure of the linked JmjN-JmjC domain	KDM5A and KDM5B (PDB ID: NA)	Docking studies	SRB assay	-	-	cell growth	[61]
135H11 and 135H12	EphA2 (PDB ID: 6B9L)	Docking studies	Wound healing	-	-	migration	[63]

[1] PDB: Protein Data Bank, [2] MTT: 3-[4, 5-dimethylthiazol-2-yl]-2, 5-diphenyltetrazolium bromide, [3] CCK-8 cell counting kit-8, [4] SRB: SulfoRhodamine-B stain, [5] XTT: 2,3-bis[2-methoxy-4-nitro-5-sulfophenyl]-2H-tetrazolium-5-carboxanilide.

3.4. Combination of Drugs

Current chemotherapeutic agents can lead to many adverse effects and can be toxic to healthy cells. For this reason, the identification of new agents that can effectively eradicate tumorigenic cells without damaging normal cells is necessary. A possible solution could be the use of combinations of drugs. Indeed, the efficacy of treatment could be improved, as individual drugs can target different biological pathways. Moreover, combinations of drugs could also potentially reduce drug resistance [64]. In silico and in vitro approaches have been used to test combinations of small molecules against cancer. Table 4 shows the studies in the last five years that have implemented in silico and in vitro models for drug discovery using combinations of drugs/molecules for metastatic BC.

For example, Nayak et al. [65] showed the ability of quinacrine and curcumin to regulate the apoptosis of cancer stem cells with an in vitro model. Curcumin is a diarylheptanoid, which is a natural phenol isolated from the *Curcuma longa* plant, and has multiple pleiotropic effects, such as the suppression of multiple signaling pathways, the inhibition of cell proliferation, and antimetastatic properties [66]. Quinacrine, a 9-aminoacridine (9-AA) derivative, shows anticancer properties against several cancers, such as breast, pancreatic, and lung cancers. Its antiapoptotic activity is shown by its ability to arrest the cell cycle in the S-phase via the inactivation of topoisomerase activity, the activation of p53 and p21, and the inhibition of NF-kβ [67]. The study of Nayak et al. [65] analyzed the anticancer effects of curcumin and quinacrine, as well as their combination, using in vitro and molecular modeling. Multiple BC cells were used to characterize a metastatic model that demonstrated the effects of the combination of molecules on decreasing the migration and invasion and inducing apoptosis. The cytotoxic and antiproliferative activity results showed the synergistic action of the drugs, and molecular docking showed a good affinity of the molecules with ABCG2, a biomarker of BC. Specifically, the binding site is in the transmembrane domain of ABCG2 [65].

Table 4. Characteristics of studies reported in the review categorized as "combination of drugs" used in metastatic breast cancer. The table reports the drug, its target with PDB ID, in silico/in vitro/in vivo methods used to test the drug, clinical trials, mechanism of action and reference.

Drug	Target	In Silico	In Vitro	In Vivo	Clinical Trials	Mechanism of Action	Ref.
Quinacrine and curcumin	ABCG2 (PDB [1] ID: NA)	Docking studies	MTT [2] assay	-	-	DNA damage and repair	[65]
ITH-47 and ESE-15-ol	bromodomain-containing protein 4 32(BRD4) (PDB ID: NA)	Docking and dynamics Studies	Annexin V-FITC [3] and caspase activation assays	-	-	apoptosis	[68]
Vitamin E and Paclitaxel	Bovine serum albumin: (PDB ID: 4OR0)	Docking studies	MTT assay	Tumor xenografts	-	proliferation	[69]

[1] PDB: Protein Data Bank, [2] MTT: 3-[4, 5-dimethylthiazol-2-yl]-2, 5-diphenyltetrazolium bromide [3] FITC Annexin-V fluorescein isothiocyanate.

In another study [68], the authors investigated the combination of two novel compounds, namely, ITH-47 (a BRD4 inhibitor) and ESE-15-ol (an antimitotic agent). The in vitro study revealed that the combination of these two compounds inhibits the growth of MDA-MB-231. To compare the binding energy of the two molecules, they performed molecular docking with a known drug—i.e., JQ1—which revealed that, compared to JQ1, the molecules can achieve similar binding energies and sites as bromodomain-containing protein 4 (BRD4). BRD4 plays a role in regulating c-Myc, a key regulator of cell growth and apoptosis [68].

Paclitaxel (PTX), also known as Taxol, is used as a drug in clinical treatment against different cancers. However, as it causes different side effects, Tang et al. [69] suggested vitamin E (VE)–albumin core–shell nanoparticles (NPs) to improve the efficacy of PTX in BC models. They also investigated the cytotoxicity with in vitro approaches on MCF-7 BC cell lines. Docking studies were performed to analyze the interaction between PTX or VE and BSA, and the results demonstrated a strong receptor–ligand interaction and PTX–VE NPs exhibited better cytotoxic effects than PTX NPs [69].

The antitumor effect was also studied using the xenograft model, showing that treatment with PTX–VE NPs is more effective and lowers the toxicity of the molecules.

3.5. Drug Latentiation

Drug latentiation is a procedure where a compound is chemically modified to improve its binding affinity with a target in order to increase its therapeutic activity.

Gefitinib is one of the more effective and specific epidermal growth factor receptor (EGFR) inhibitors, which interacts with the adenosine triphosphate (ATP)-binding site of the EGFR tyrosine kinase enzyme. Sharma et al. designed three gefitinib-based derivatives to improve the ligand–receptor interaction [70]. Molecular docking studies were also presented for the study of the interactions of the gefitinib derivatives with EGFR, DNA, and BSA. Synthesized compounds were further screened in different cancer cell lines, including MDA-MB-231, to evaluate the cytotoxicity of the new compounds. The results demonstrated a similar effect between experimental and molecular docking analyses, suggesting the important role of gefitinib-based derivatives [70]. Indeed, the in vitro cytotoxicity and antiproliferative activity demonstrated that the derivatives are more potent than gefitinib.

4. Conclusions

In this review, we reported recent studies that have used molecular docking and in vitro studies in metastatic BC for drug discovery. We divided the studies into five main categories: "Systematic repositioning of drugs/molecules", "natural drugs", "new synthesized molecules", "combinations of drugs", and "drug latentiation".

The studies in the systematic repositioning of drugs/molecules category generated new clinical indications for old known drugs or molecules, such as ropinirole, small molecular compound SYSU-21598, etoposide, thionine, and 2,4-diacetylphloroglucinol, reporting a new possible application in metastatic BC. In addition, natural products such as pseurotin A, atranorin, eugenol, astragalus membranaceus, 21 plant-derived inhibitors, noscapine, shikonin, plantamajoside, flavipin, and 13 new synthesized molecules were analyzed and proposed as effective drugs.

Another possible application of molecular docking is studying combinations of drugs and drug latentiation in metastatic BC. We proposed, as promising combinations of drugs, quinacrine and curcumin, ITH-47 and ESE-15-ol, and vitamin E and paclitaxel. The drug latentiation procedures demonstrated that the three gefitinib-based derivatives are more potent than gefitinib.

Overall, the computational and experimental results included herein reported a good consistency and demonstrated that molecular docking and in vitro studies should be used as complementary methods, which, together, can increase the knowledge for drug discovery and development. Indeed, molecular docking generates a binding score that shows the affinity between drugs and targets and in vitro studies investigate the biological responses. However, the binding affinity energy obtained by a single docking algorithm could be inaccurate due to incorrect ligand poses. A better strategy could be the use of combined scores obtained by two or more docking algorithms and/or the use of molecular dynamics. Molecular dynamics is a computational method that describes the dynamic behavior of a biological complex as a function of time. These methods could be more powerful approaches to investigate the novel biological aspects of disease mechanisms, providing a combined procedure to increase innovation in the pharmaceutical industry and to discovery novel therapies for unmet medical needs.

Author Contributions: Conceptualization, C.C.; methodology, C.C.; writing—original draft preparation, C.C.; supervision, I.C.; project administration, I.C.; funding acquisition, I.C. All authors have read and agreed to the published version of the manuscript.

References

1. Weigelt, B.; Peterse, J.L.; Veer, L.J.V. Breast cancer metastasis: Markers and models. *Nat. Rev. Cancer* **2005**, *5*, 591–602. [CrossRef]
2. Cava, C.; Pini, S.; Taramelli, D.; Castiglioni, I. Perturbations of pathway co-expression network identify a core network in metastatic breast cancer. *Comput. Biol. Chem.* **2020**, *87*, 107313. [CrossRef] [PubMed]
3. Bravatà, V.; Cava, C.; Minafra, L.; Cammarata, F.P.; Russo, G.; Gilardi, M.C.; Castiglioni, I.; Forte, G.I. Radiation-Induced Gene Expression Changes in High and Low Grade Breast Cancer Cell Types. *Int. J. Mol. Sci.* **2018**, *19*, 1084. [CrossRef] [PubMed]
4. Ponnusankar, S.; Mohan, A. Newer therapies for the treatment of metastatic breast cancer: A clinical update. *Indian J. Pharm. Sci.* **2013**, *75*, 251–261. [CrossRef] [PubMed]
5. Hughes, J.; Rees, S.; Kalindjian, S.; Philpott, K. Principles of early drug discovery. *Br. J. Pharmacol.* **2011**, *162*, 1239–1249. [CrossRef]
6. Cava, C.; Colaprico, A.; Bertoli, G.; Bontempi, G.; Mauri, G.; Castiglioni, I. How interacting pathways are regulated by miRNAs in breast cancer subtypes. *BMC Bioinform.* **2016**, *17*, 111–133. [CrossRef]
7. Cava, C.; Novello, C.; Martelli, C.; Lodico, A.; Ottobrini, L.; Piccotti, F.; Truffi, M.; Corsi, F.; Bertoli, G.; Castiglioni, I. Theranostic application of miR-429 in HER2+ breast cancer. *Theranostics* **2020**, *10*, 50–61. [CrossRef]
8. Yang, Y.; Adelstein, S.J.; Kassis, I.A. Target discovery from data mining approaches. *Drug Discov. Today* **2009**, *14*, 147–154. [CrossRef]
9. Meng, X.-Y.; Zhang, H.-X.; Mezei, M.; Cui, M. Molecular docking: A powerful approach for structure-based drug discovery. *Curr. Comput. Drug Des.* **2011**, *7*, 146–157. [CrossRef]
10. McConkey, B.J.; Sobolev, V.; Edelman, M. The performance of current methods in ligand-protein docking. *Curr. Sci.* **2002**, *83*, 845–855.
11. Csermely, P.; Korcsmáros, T.; Kiss, H.J.; London, G.; Nussinov, R. Structure and dynamics of molecular networks: A novel paradigm of drug discovery: A comprehensive review. *Pharmacol. Ther.* **2013**, *138*, 333–408. [CrossRef] [PubMed]
12. Ngo, H.X.; Garneau-Tsodikova, S. What are the drugs of the future? *MedChemComm* **2018**, *9*, 757–758. [CrossRef] [PubMed]
13. Lin, X.; Li, X.; Lin, X. A Review on Applications of Computational Methods in Drug Screening and Design. *Molecules* **2020**, *25*, 1375. [CrossRef] [PubMed]
14. Bafna, D.; Ban, F.; Rennie, P.S.; Singh, K.; Cherkasov, A. Computer-Aided Ligand Discovery for Estrogen Receptor Alpha. *Int. J. Mol. Sci.* **2020**, *21*, 4193. [CrossRef]
15. Xue, H.; Xie, H.; Xie, H.; Wang, Y. Review of Drug Repositioning Approaches and Resources. *Int. J. Biol. Sci.* **2018**, *14*, 1232–1244. [CrossRef]
16. Palacio-Rodríguez, K.; Lans, I.; Cavasotto, C.N.; Cossio, P. Exponential consensus ranking improves the outcome in docking and receptor ensemble docking. *Sci. Rep.* **2019**, *9*, 5142. [CrossRef]
17. Bajpai, M.; Esmay, J.D. In Vitro Studies in Drug Discovery and Development: An Analysis of Study Objectives and Application of Good Laboratory Practices (GLP). *Drug Metab. Rev.* **2002**, *34*, 679–689. [CrossRef]
18. Rymbai, E.; Sugumar, D.; Saravanan, J.; Divakar, S. Ropinirole, a potential drug for systematic repositioning based on side effect profile for management and treatment of Breast Cancer. *Med. Hypotheses* **2020**, *144*, 110156. [CrossRef]
19. Liu, Y.; Zheng, H.; Li, Q.; Li, S.; Lai, H.; Song, E.; Li, D.; Chen, J. Discovery of CCL18 antagonist blocking breast cancer metastasis. *Clin. Exp. Metastasis* **2019**, *36*, 243–255. [CrossRef]
20. Chen, J.; Yao, Y.; Gong, C.; Yu, F.; Su, S.; Chen, J.; Liu, B.; Deng, H.; Wang, F.; Lin, L.; et al. CCL18 from Tumor-Associated Macrophages Promotes Breast Cancer Metastasis via PITPNM3. *Cancer Cell* **2011**, *19*, 541–555. [CrossRef]
21. Das, S.; Tripathi, N.; Siddharth, S.; Nayak, A.; Nayak, D.; Sethy, C.; Bharatam, P.V.; Kundu, C.N. Etoposide and doxorubicin enhance the sensitivity of triple negative breast cancers through modulation of TRAIL-DR5 axis. *Apoptosis* **2017**, *22*, 1205–1224. [CrossRef] [PubMed]
22. Baldwin, E.L.; Osheroff, N. Etoposide, Topoisomerase II and Cancer. *Curr. Med. Chem. Anti Cancer Agents* **2005**, *5*, 363–372. [CrossRef] [PubMed]

23. Zhao, N.; Woodle, M.C.; Mixson, A.J. Advances in Delivery Systems for Doxorubicin. *J. Nanomed. Nanotechnol.* **2018**, *9*, 1–9. [CrossRef] [PubMed]
24. Manivel, P.; Paulpandi, M.; Murugan, K.; Benelli, G.; Ilanchelian, M. Probing the interaction of thionine with human serum albumin by multispectroscopic studies and its in vitro cytotoxic activity toward MCF-7 breast cancer cells. *J. Biomol. Struct. Dyn.* **2016**, *35*, 3012–3031. [CrossRef]
25. Dohno, C.; Stemp, E.D.A.; Barton, J.K. Fast Back Electron Transfer Prevents Guanine Damage by Photoexcited Thionine Bound to DNA. *J. Am. Chem. Soc.* **2003**, *125*, 9586–9587. [CrossRef]
26. Veena, V.K.; Popavath, R.N.; Kennedy, K.; Sakthivel, N. In vitro antiproliferative, pro-apoptotic, antimetastatic and anti-inflammatory potential of 2,4-diacteylphloroglucinol (DAPG) by Pseudomonas aeruginosa strain FP10. *Apoptosis* **2015**, *20*, 1281–1295. [CrossRef]
27. Veena, V.K.; Kennedy, K.; Lakshmi, P.; Krishna, R.; Sakthivel, N. Anti-leukemic, anti-lung, and anti-breast cancer potential of the microbial polyketide 2, 4-diacetylphloroglucinol (DAPG) and its interaction with the metastatic proteins than the antiapoptotic Bcl-2 proteins. *Mol. Cell. Biochem.* **2016**, *414*, 47–56. [CrossRef]
28. Harvey, A.L.; Edrada-Ebel, R.; Quinn, R.J. The re-emergence of natural products for drug discovery in the genomics era. *Nat. Rev. Drug Discov.* **2015**, *14*, 111–129. [CrossRef]
29. Nelson, E.R.; Chang, C.-Y.; McDonnell, D.P. Cholesterol and breast cancer pathophysiology. *Trends Endocrinol. Metab.* **2014**, *25*, 649–655. [CrossRef]
30. Bloch, P.; Tamm, C.; Bollinger, P.; Petcher, T.J.; Weber, H.P. Pseurotin, a new metabolite of Pseudeurotium ovalis Stolk having an unusual hetero-spirocyclic system. *Helv. Chim. Acta* **1976**, *7*, 133–137. [CrossRef]
31. Wenke, J.; Anke, H.; Sterner, O. Pseurotin A and 8-Odemethylpseurotin A from Aspergillus fumigatus and their inhibitory activities on chitin synthase. *Biosci. Biotech. Biochem.* **1993**, *57*, 961–964. [CrossRef]
32. Komagata, D.; Fujita, S.; Yamashita, N.; Saito, S.; Morino, T. Novel Neuritogenic Activities of Pseurotin A and Penicillic Acid. *J. Antibiot.* **1996**, *49*, 958–959. [CrossRef] [PubMed]
33. Wink, J.; Grabley, S.; Gareis, M.; Zeeck, A.; Phillips, S. Biologically active pseurotin A and D, new metabolites from Aspergillus fumigatus, process for their preparation and their use as apomorphine antagonists. *Eur. Pat. Appl.* **1993**, ep546475.
34. Abdelwahed, K.S.; Siddique, A.B.; Mohyeldin, M.M.; Qusa, M.H.; Goda, A.A.; Singh, S.S.; Ayoub, N.M.; King, J.A.; Jois, S.D.; El Sayed, K.A. Pseurotin A as a novel suppressor of hormone dependent breast cancer progression and recurrence by inhibiting PCSK9 secretion and interaction with LDL receptor. *Pharmacol. Res.* **2020**, *158*, 104847. [CrossRef] [PubMed]
35. Harikrishnan, A.; Veena, V.; Lakshmi, B.; Shanmugavalli, R.; Theres, S.; Prashantha, C.N.; Shah, T.; Oshin, K.; Togam, R.; Nandi, S.; et al. Atranorin, an antimicrobial metabolite from lichen Parmotrema rampoddense exhibited in vitro anti-breast cancer activity through interaction with Akt activity. *J. Biomol. Struct. Dyn.* **2020**, *9*, 1–11. [CrossRef]
36. Kaboli, P.J.; Salimian, F.; Aghapour, S.; Xiang, S.; Zhao, Q.; Li, M.; Wu, X.; Du, F.; Zhao, Y.; Shen, J.; et al. Akt-targeted therapy as a promising strategy to overcome drug resistance in breast cancer—A comprehensive review from chemotherapy to immunotherapy. *Pharmacol. Res.* **2020**, *156*, 104806. [CrossRef]
37. Choudhury, P.; Barua, A.; Roy, A.; Pattanayak, R.; Bhattacharyya, M.; Saha, P. Eugenol restricts Cancer Stem Cell population by degradation of β-catenin via N-terminal Ser37 phosphorylation-an in vivo and in vitro experimental evaluation. *Chem. Biol. Interact.* **2020**, *316*, 108938. [CrossRef]
38. Liu, C.; Wang, K.; Zhuang, J.; Gao, C.; Li, H.; Liu, L.; Feng, F.; Zhou, C.; Yao, K.; Deng, L.; et al. The Modulatory Properties of Astragalus membranaceus Treatment on Triple-Negative Breast Cancer: An Integrated Pharmacological Method. *Front. Pharmacol.* **2019**, *10*. [CrossRef]
39. Sinha, S.; Patel, S.; Athar, M.; Vora, J.; Chhabria, M.T.; Jha, P.C.; Shrivastava, N. Structure-based identification of novel sirtuin inhibitors against triple negative breast cancer: An in silico and in vitro study. *Int. J. Biol. Macromol.* **2019**, *140*, 454–468. [CrossRef]
40. Stanton, R.A.; Gernert, K.M.; Nettles, J.H.; Aneja, R. Drugs that target dynamic microtubules: A new molecular perspective. *Med. Res. Rev.* **2011**, *31*, 443–481. [CrossRef]
41. Maurya, N.; Maurya, J.K.; Singh, U.K.; Dohare, R.; Yab, Z.; Alam Rizvi, M.M.; Kumari, M.; Patel, R. In Vitro Cytotoxicity and Interaction of Noscapine with Human Serum Albumin: Effect on Structure and Esterase Activity of HSA. *Mol. Pharm.* **2019**, *16*, 952–966. [CrossRef] [PubMed]

42. Chen, H.M.; Wang, P.H.; Chen, S.S.; Wen, C.C.; Chen, Y.H.; Yang, W.C.; Yang, N.S. Shikonin induces immunogenic cell death in tumor cells and enhances dendritic cell-based cancer vaccine. *Cancer Immunol. Immunother.* **2012**, *61*, 1989–2002. [CrossRef] [PubMed]
43. Yin, S.-Y.; Efferth, T.; Jian, F.-Y.; Chen, Y.-H.; Liu, C.-I.; Wang, A.H.; Chen, Y.-R.; Hsiao, P.-W.; Yang, N.S. Immunogenicity of mammary tumor cells can be induced by shikonin via direct binding-interference with hnRNPA1. *Oncotarget* **2016**, *7*, 43629–43653. [CrossRef] [PubMed]
44. Pei, S.; Yang, X.; Wang, H.; Zhang, H.; Zhou, B.; Zhang, D.; Lin, D. Plantamajoside, a potential anti-tumor herbal medicine inhibits breast cancer growth and pulmonary metastasis by decreasing the activity of matrix metalloproteinase-9 and-2. *BMC Cancer* **2015**, *15*, 965. [CrossRef]
45. Hanieh, H.; Mohafez, O.; Hairul-Islam, V.I.; Alzahrani, A.; Ismail, M.B.; Thirugnanasambantham, K. Novel Aryl Hydrocarbon Receptor Agonist Suppresses Migration and Invasion of Breast Cancer Cells. *PLoS ONE* **2016**, *11*, e0167650. [CrossRef]
46. Nashaat, S.; Henen, M.A.; El-Messery, S.M.; Eisa, H. Synthesis, state-of-the-art NMR-binding and molecular modeling study of new benzimidazole core derivatives as Pin1 inhibitors: Targeting breast cancer. *Bioorganic Med. Chem.* **2020**, *28*, 115495. [CrossRef]
47. Bacharaju, K.; Jambula, S.R.; Sivan, S.; JyostnaTangeda, S.; Manga, V. Design, synthesis, molecular docking and biological evaluation of new dithiocarbamates substituted benzimidazole and chalcones as possible chemotherapeutic agents. *Bioorganic Med. Chem. Lett.* **2012**, *22*, 3274–3277. [CrossRef]
48. Vaz, W.F.; Custodio, J.M.F.; D'Oliveira, G.D.C.; Neves, B.J.; Junior, P.S.C.; Filho, J.T.M.; Andrade, C.H.; Perez, C.N.; Silveira-Lacerda, E.P.; Napolitano, H.B. Dihydroquinoline derivative as a potential anticancer agent: Synthesis, crystal structure, and molecular modeling studies. *Mol. Divers.* **2020**, 1–12. [CrossRef]
49. Li, Y.; Li, Y.; Wang, N.; Lin, D.; Liu, X.; Yang, Y.; Gao, Q. Synthesis, DNA/BSA binding studies and in vitro biological assay of nickel(II) complexes incorporating tridentate aroylhydrazone and triphenylphosphine ligands. *J. Biomol. Struct. Dyn.* **2019**, 1–20. [CrossRef]
50. Acharya, S.; Maji, M.; Ruturaj; Purkait, K.; Gupta, A.; Mukherjee, A. Synthesis, Structure, Stability, and Inhibition of Tubulin Polymerization by RuII–p-Cymene Complexes of Trimethoxyaniline-Based Schiff Bases. *Inorg. Chem.* **2019**, *58*, 9213–9224. [CrossRef]
51. Cai, Y.; Zhao, B.; Liang, Q.-Y.; Zhang, Y.; Cai, J.; Li, G. The selective effect of glycyrrhizin and glycyrrhetinic acid on topoisomerase IIα and apoptosis in combination with etoposide on triple negative breast cancer MDA-MB-231 cells. *Eur. J. Pharmacol.* **2017**, *809*, 87–97. [CrossRef] [PubMed]
52. Shukla, A.; Tyagi, R.; Meena, S.; Datta, D.; Srivastava, S.K.; Khan, F. 2D- and 3D-QSAR modelling, molecular docking and in vitro evaluation studies on 18β-glycyrrhetinic acid derivatives against triple-negative breast cancer cell line. *J. Biomol. Struct. Dyn.* **2019**, *38*, 168–185. [CrossRef] [PubMed]
53. Yan, W.; Zhao, Y.; He, J. Anti-breast cancer activity of selected 1,3,5-triazines via modulation of EGFR-TK. *Mol. Med. Rep.* **2018**, *18*, 4175–4184. [CrossRef] [PubMed]
54. Vlaar, C.P.; Castillo-Pichardo, L.; Medina, J.I.; Marrero-Serra, C.M.; Velez, E.; Ramos, Z.; Hernández, E. Design, synthesis and biological evaluation of new carbazole derivatives as anti-cancer and anti-migratory agents. *Bioorganic Med. Chem.* **2018**, *26*, 884–890. [CrossRef] [PubMed]
55. Kamalakar, A.; Washam, C.L.; Akel, N.S.; Allen, B.J.; Williams, D.K.; Swain, F.L.; Leitzel, K.; Lipton, A.; Gaddy, D.; Suva, L. PTHrP(12-48) Modulates the Bone Marrow Microenvironment and Suppresses Human Osteoclast Differentiation and Lifespan. *J. Bone Miner. Res.* **2017**, *32*, 1421–1431. [CrossRef]
56. Rajabi, M.; Mousa, S.A. The Role of Angiogenesis in Cancer Treatment. *Biomedicines* **2017**, *5*, 34. [CrossRef]
57. Aboul-Enein, M.N.; El Azzouny, A.; Ragab, F.A.-F.; Hamissa, M.F. Design, Synthesis, and Cytotoxic Evaluation of Certain 7-Chloro-4-(piperazin-1-yl)quinoline Derivatives as VEGFR-II Inhibitors. *Arch. Pharm.* **2017**, *350*, 1600377. [CrossRef]
58. Ziedan, N.I.; Hamdy, R.; Cavaliere, A.; Kourti, M.; Prencipe, F.; Brancale, A.; Jones, A.T.; Westwell, A.D. Virtual screening, SAR, and discovery of 5-(indole-3-yl)-2-[(2-nitrophenyl)amino] [1,3,4]-oxadiazole as a novel Bcl-2 inhibitor. *Chem. Biol. Drug Des.* **2017**, *90*, 147–155. [CrossRef]
59. Koca, I.; Özgür, A.; Er, M.; Gümüş, M.; Coşkun, K.A.; Tutar, Y. Design and synthesis of pyrimidinyl acyl thioureas as novel Hsp90 inhibitors in invasive ductal breast cancer and its bone metastasis. *Eur. J. Med. Chem.* **2016**, *122*, 280–290. [CrossRef]

60. Nie, Z.; Shi, L.; Lai, C.; O'Connell, S.M.; Xu, J.; Stansfield, R.K.; Hosfield, D.J.; Veal, J.M.; Stafford, J.A. Structure-based design and discovery of potent and selective KDM5 inhibitors. *Bioorganic Med. Chem. Lett.* **2018**, *28*, 1490–1494. [CrossRef]
61. Horton, J.R.; Engstrom, A.; Zoeller, E.L.; Liu, X.; Shanks, J.R.; Zhang, X.; Johns, M.A.; Vertino, P.M.; Fu, H.; Cheng, X. Characterization of a Linked Jumonji Domain of the KDM5/JARID1 Family of Histone H3 Lysine 4 Demethylases. *J. Biol. Chem.* **2015**, *291*, 2631–2646. [CrossRef] [PubMed]
62. Salem, A.F.; Wang, S.; Billet, S.; Chen, J.-F.; Udompholkul, P.; Gambini, L.; Baggio, C.; Tseng, H.-R.; Posadas, E.M.; Bhowmick, N.A.; et al. Reduction of Circulating Cancer Cells and Metastases in Breast-Cancer Models by a Potent EphA2-Agonistic Peptide–Drug Conjugate. *J. Med. Chem.* **2018**, *61*, 2052–2061. [CrossRef] [PubMed]
63. Gambini, L.; Salem, A.F.; Udompholkul, P.; Tan, X.-F.; Baggio, C.; Shah, N.; Aronson, A.; Song, J.; Pellecchia, M. Structure-Based Design of Novel EphA2 Agonistic Agents with Nanomolar Affinity in Vitro and in Cell. *ACS Chem. Biol.* **2018**, *13*, 2633–2644. [CrossRef]
64. Cava, C.; Bertoli, G.; Castiglioni, I. In silico identification of drug target pathways in breast cancer subtypes using pathway cross-talk inhibition. *J. Transl. Med.* **2018**, *16*, 154. [CrossRef]
65. Nayak, D.; Tripathi, N.; Kathuria, D.; Siddharth, S.; Nayak, A.; Bharatam, P.V.; Kundu, C.N. Quinacrine and curcumin synergistically increased the breast cancer stem cells death by inhibiting ABCG2 and modulating DNA damage repair pathway. *Int. J. Biochem. Cell Biol.* **2020**, *119*, 105682. [CrossRef]
66. Minafra, L.; Porcino, N.; Bravatà, V.; Gaglio, D.; Bonanomi, M.; Amore, E.; Cammarata, F.P.; Russo, G.; Militello, C.; Savoca, G.; et al. Radiosensitizing effect of curcumin-loaded lipid nanoparticles in breast cancer cells. *Sci. Rep.* **2019**, *9*, 11134. [CrossRef] [PubMed]
67. Gurova, K.V.; Hill, J.E.; Guo, C.; Prokvolit, A.; Burdelya, L.G.; Samoylova, E.; Khodyakova, A.V.; Ganapathi, R.; Tararova, N.D.; Bosykh, D.; et al. Small molecules that reactivate p53 in renal cell carcinoma reveal a NF-B-dependent mechanism of p53 suppression in tumors. *Proc. Natl. Acad. Sci. USA* **2005**, *102*, 17448–17453. [CrossRef] [PubMed]
68. Mqoco, T.; Stander, A.; Engelbrecht, A.-M.; Joubert, A.M. A Combination of an Antimitotic and a Bromodomain 4 Inhibitor Synergistically Inhibits the Metastatic MDA-MB-231 Breast Cancer Cell Line. *BioMed Res. Int.* **2019**, *2019*, 1850462. [CrossRef]
69. Tang, B.; Qian, Y.; Gou, Y.; Cheng, G.; Fang, G. VE-Albumin Core-Shell Nanoparticles for Paclitaxel Delivery to Treat MDR Breast Cancer. *Molecules* **2018**, *23*, 2760. [CrossRef]
70. Sharma, M.J.; Kumar, M.S.; Murahari, M.; Mayur, Y.C. Synthesis of novel gefitinib-based derivatives and their anticancer activity. *Arch. Pharm.* **2019**, *352*, e1800381. [CrossRef]

8

From a Medicinal Mushroom Blend a Direct Anticancer Effect on Triple-Negative Breast Cancer: A Preclinical Study on Lung Metastases

Elisa Roda [1,2,*,†], Fabrizio De Luca [1,†], Carlo Alessandro Locatelli [2], Daniela Ratto [1], Carmine Di Iorio [1], Elena Savino [3], Maria Grazia Bottone [1] and Paola Rossi [1,*]

1 Department of Biology and Biotechnology "L. Spallanzani", University of Pavia, 27100 Pavia, Italy; fabrizio.deluca01@universitadipavia.it (F.D.L.); daniela.ratto01@universitadipavia.it (D.R.); carmine.diiorio01@universitadipavia.it (C.D.I.); mariagrazia.bottone@unipv.it (M.G.B.)
2 Laboratory of Clinical & Experimental Toxicology, Pavia Poison Centre, National Toxicology Information Centre, Toxicology Unit, Istituti Clinici Scientifici Maugeri IRCCS, 27100 Pavia, Italy; carlo.locatelli@icsmaugeri.it
3 Department of Earth and Environmental Science, University of Pavia, 27100 Pavia, Italy; elena.savino@unipv.it
* Correspondence: elisa.roda@unipv.it (E.R.); paola.rossi@unipv.it (P.R.);

† These authors contributed equally to this work.

Academic Editors: José Antonio Lupiáñez, Amalia Pérez-Jiménez and Eva E. Rufino-Palomares

Abstract: Bioactive metabolites isolated from medicinal mushrooms (MM) used as supportive treatment in conventional oncology have recently gained interest. Acting as anticancer agents, they interfere with tumor cells and microenvironment (TME), disturbing cancer development/progression. Nonetheless, their action mechanisms still need to be elucidated. Recently, using a 4T1 triple-negative mouse BC model, we demonstrated that supplementation with Micotherapy U-Care, a MM blend, produced a striking reduction of lung metastases density/number, paralleled by decreased inflammation and oxidative stress both in TME and metastases, together with QoL amelioration. We hypothesized that these effects could be due to either a direct anticancer effect and/or to a secondary/indirect impact of Micotherapy U-Care on systemic inflammation/immunomodulation. To address this question, we presently focused on apoptosis/proliferation, investigating specific molecules, i.e., PARP1, p53, BAX, Bcl2, and PCNA, whose critical role in BC is well recognized. We revealed that Micotherapy U-Care is effective to influence balance between cell death and proliferation, which appeared strictly interconnected and inversely related (p53/Bax vs. Bcl2/PARP1/PCNA expression trends). MM blend displayed a direct effect, with different efficacy extent on cancer cells and TME, forcing tumor cells to apoptosis. Yet again, this study supports the potential of MM extracts, as adjuvant supplement in the TNBC management.

Keywords: breast cancer; lung metastases; in vivo; apoptosis; complementary medicine; medicinal mushrooms

1. Introduction

Breast cancer (BC) is the most frequently diagnosed malignant neoplasm in women [1]. Due to the progress achieved both in early diagnosis and in novel therapeutic treatments, the death rate of BC is progressively decreasing, but BC still remains one of the leading causes of morbidity and mortality in females worldwide [2]. In particular, in Western countries BC metastases are the second cause of mortality among tumor patients [3,4].

Triple-negative breast cancer (TNBC) is characterized by the lack of expression of specific receptors, i.e., estrogens, progesterone, and epidermal growth factor 2, and represents about 15–20% of all BC diagnoses. Indeed, TNBC differs from other subgroups of BC for its increased growth and fast spreading, with reduced treatment possibilities (due to the absence of the three above reported receptors) and a worse outcome [5,6]. Actually, TNBC patients are extremely prone to metastasis and relapse [7] which mainly affect brain, liver, and, in particular, lungs [8]. Tumor progression to metastasis is a complex and many-sided process, affected by both intrinsic cellular mutational burden and several interactions between malignant and non-malignant cell types, and also constantly regulated by the various extrinsic microenvironmental niches [9].

The tumor microenvironment (TME), consisting of immune cells, fibroblasts, satellite cells, as well as blood and lymphatic vessels, plays a fundamental role in the tumor biology, i.e., the behavior of a bulk tumor, co-evolving in a delicate ecosystem with the tumor niche. This never-ending evolving process is governed by local and distant microenvironments, being also regulated by systemic inflammation. In fact, under cytokines, growth factors, and chemotactic stimuli induction, cancer cells recruit and transform stromal fibroblasts into malignant cells, which alter the extracellular matrix by secreting tumor-stimulating factors to facilitate tumor invasion and metastasis. Thus, based on the strict interaction between tumor cells and multicellular proinflammatory TME, cancer typical features also include the evasion of immune destruction, tumor promoting inflammation, and angiogenesis induction. Indeed, nowadays it is well-known that TME plays a crucial role in cancer progression, therapeutic response, and patient outcome [9–11]. Immunotherapy is a recent approach in cancer therapy, specifically addressed on TME [12]. Currently, the elite therapy for treating TNBC is the cytotoxic chemotherapy, characterized by several side effects [13,14]. A bulk of literature demonstrated that chemotherapy induces apoptosis and cancer is a pathology characterized by a dysregulation in cell cycle/death, in which the disruption of the apoptotic pathway leads to uncontrolled cell proliferation [15]. Anomalies in the apoptotic pathway are crucial for cancer genesis, evolution, and regression after treatment [16]. Indeed, the apoptosis rate is crucial in determining the fate between cancer progression and regression as well as in response to current available treatments, i.e., chemotherapy, radiotherapy, surgery, and hormonal therapies.

As a matter of fact, cells undergo apoptosis by changing the balance of proapoptotic and antiapoptotic genes [17]. The main actors involved in apoptosis pathway can be reduced to a few crucial proteins largely preserved through species [18]. In humans and mice, these key proteins belong to the Bcl-2 family [18], Poly (ADP-ribose) polymerase (PARP) [19], and p53 [20]. Bcl-2 family contains both inhibitors and promoters of apoptosis [18]. Acting as proapoptotic protein, Bax is an important tumor suppressor factor, and its reduced levels provide tumor cells with a selective survival advantage, contributing to their expansion [21]. Contrarily, acting as antiapoptotic protein, Bcl-2 plays an essential role as a cell survivor enhancer, and its increased expression level gives cancer cells with a selective survival gain [22]. Concerning PARPs, PARP1 is a nuclear protein which contributes in DNA single-strand break repair, and its dysregulation is involved in tumorigenesis phenomena to such a degree that PARP1 inhibitors have been authorized for the treatment of some types of BC, stimulating both apoptosis induction and synthetic lethality mechanism/DNA repair [23–27]. p53 protein is a nuclear protein known as tumor suppression factor, which plays a critical role deciding whether DNA would be repaired or the damaged cell will self-destruct, inducing programmed cell death [20,28]. Dysregulation of these mentioned proteins is a frequent feature of human malignant diseases and causal for therapy resistance. Tumor cells usually escape from apoptosis by downregulation of proapoptotic genes and/or hyperactivation of antiapoptotic genes. Therefore, apoptosis induction in cancer cells is considered an excellent approach for treating tumors [29].

It has also to be mentioned the PCNA pivotal role in cancer, owing to its function in cell proliferation. Since cancer is caused by and manifest through multiple mechanisms, many of which converging to deregulated proliferation at primary and metastatic sites, and PCNA is an indispensable factor for cell cycle control, DNA replication, DNA nucleotide excision repair, and chromatin assembly, PCNA inhibition is considered to be another viable anticancer strategy [30,31].

In the last decades, considerable attention has been focused on developing/identifying new compounds for TNBC treatment with absent/minimal side adverse effects. Interestingly, in recent years the importance of naturally derived compounds has been highlighted as a source of anticancer and proapoptotic drugs [32]. One of the most promising sources for drug discovery in integrative oncology are medicinal mushrooms (MM), which have an established story of use in traditional oriental medicine and as nutritionally functional foods. MM display antitumor, proapoptotic, onco-immunological, and immunomodulatory effects in vitro and improve the quality of life in cancer patients during conventional anticancer treatments [33,34]. Indeed, in the last years, the use of several MM has been approved as adjuvant supplements in antitumor therapy in different countries.

Different MM produce hundreds of bioactive compounds which are able to influence, often in a synergistic way, numerous cancer-related pathways, also modulating cellular targets typically involved in cell proliferation, survival, and angiogenesis [33,35].

Several studies showed that the use of MM extracts or their compounds, alone or combined with conventional anticancer treatments, is safe and beneficial [33,35].

The present investigation is strictly linked to a previous study employing a 4T1 triple-negative mouse BC model to explore the effects of an oral supplementation with "Micotherapy U-care" (M. U-care), a medicinal mushroom blend, consisting of a mixture of 20% extracts of mycelia and sporophores of five MM, i.e., *Agaricus blazei*, *Ophiocordyceps sinensis*, *Ganoderma lucidum*, *Grifola frondosa*, and *Lentinula edodes* [36]. Each of these MM have been shown displays anticancer and immunomodulatory effects, both in vitro and in vivo, and in preclinical and clinical studies [34,37].

Using a syngeneic tumor-bearing mouse model of TNBC, we demonstrated that M. U-Care supplementation, starting before 4T1 cells injection and lasting throughout the whole experimental time (about 3 months), elicited (i) an increase in the quality of life, (ii) a dramatic decrease of lung metastases density and nodules number, and (iii) a substantial decrease of inflammatory and oxidative stress pathways, characterized by a similar protein expression trend in both lung TME and metastases [36]. Based on these results, we hypothesized that the supplement effects could have been ascribable either to a direct M. U-care anticancer effect on lung cells and/or to secondary/indirect impacts of the MM blend on systemic inflammation and immunomodulation. To punctually address this question, in the present study, we focused on the programmed cell death pathway, namely, apoptosis, by investigating specific molecules whose critical role in human BC is well known. With this aim, using immunohistochemistry, we evaluated the expression, localization and changes of the following proteins, i.e., PARP1, p53, Bax, and Bcl2, performing a comparative assessment on lung metastases and pulmonary parenchyma, namely, TME. For the sake of clarity, we focused on the pathological outcomes in the murine pulmonary tissue, as the lung is the one of the distant organs recurrently implicated in typical metastatic pattern of primary TNBC [7]. The apoptotic cell death was also examined by in situ detection of DNA fragmentation using the terminal deoxynucleotidyl-transferase (TUNEL) assay. In addition, based on the notion that proliferative activity of cancer cells is also a crucial prognostic marker in the tumor diagnosis, we investigated the role of Proliferating Cell Nuclear Antigen (PCNA), being a pivotal protein directly related to the degrees of tumor malignancy and diagnosis [38,39].

2. Results

Figure 1 emphasizes the key outcomes of the present investigation and also summarizes some major results of our previous study (for details see the work in [36]).

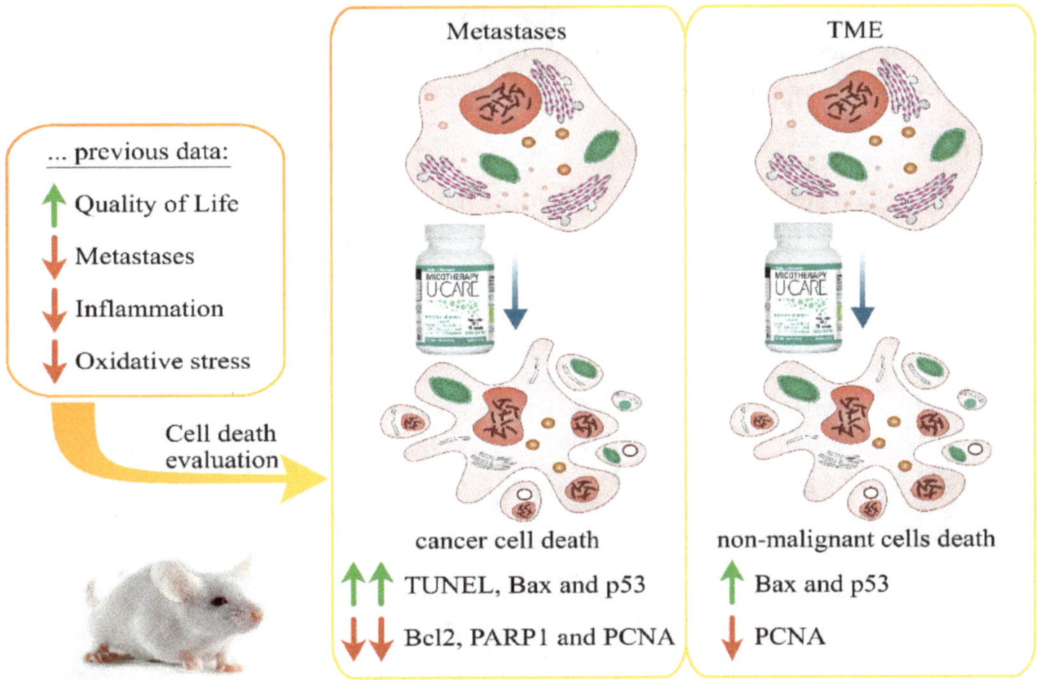

Figure 1. Graphic illustration underlining the main results.

2.1. *Raw Materials, Extract Procedure, and Main Active Metabolites of Micotherapy U-Care Blend*

The MM blend Micotherapy U-care was produced and supplied by A.V.D. Reform s.r.l. (Noceto, Parma, Italy) and it consists of a mixture of five fungal species, as reported in Table 1.

Table 1. Details on Micotherapy U-care supplement composition.

Medicinal Mushroom	Fungal Part Used in Micotherapy U-Care	% Contained in Micotherapy U-Care	ID Code
Agaricus blazei	Fruiting body	20%	7700
Ophiocordyceps sinensin	Fruiting body and mycelium	20%	Cm2
Ganoderma lucidum	Fruiting body	20%	Gač
Grifola frondosa	Fruiting body	20%	Gf3
Lentinula edodes	Fruiting body	20%	Le.ed.1

The specific MM species strains were established by genetic analyses, sequencing ITS regions and confirming the ID code. Each MM was ground, and total genomic DNA was extracted through the DNeasy mini plant kit (Qiagen NV, Venlo, Netherlands). The Internal Transcribed Spacer (ITS) regions of nuclear DNA were amplified by using PCR, applying two set of primers: ITS F 5′-AGAAAGTCGTAACAAGGTTTCCGTAG-3′, ITS R 5′-TTTTCCTCCGCTCATTGATATGCTT-3′, ITS-g F 5′-TCCGTAGGTGAACCTGCGG-3′, and ITS-g R 5′-TCCTCCGCTTATTGATATGC-3′. Next, the PCR products were purified, sequenced by Eurofins Genomics (Konstanz, Germany), and identified by using NCBI Nucleotide Blast software, version 2.9.0 (Table 1, ID code).

Next, the sporophores and/or mycelia were cultivated, harvested, and the fresh material was extracted for 3 h at 95 °C in distilled water with ethanol 10% (for 1 kg of raw material, 15 L of water-ethanol solution was used). After water-ethanol extraction, solid and liquid components were divided, and the fluid part was dehydrated until the humidity amount was smaller than 7%. Dry extracts were ground and blended to have the 20% of each selected mushroom in the MM blend Micotheraphy U-care (Table 1).

Finally, the polysaccharide content of Micotherapy U-care was determined by using a β-Glucan Assay Kit, and the polysaccharide content was more than 30%. Of this 30%, more than 15% of the polysaccharides were 1,3-1,6 β-glucans, the main active metabolites in Micotherapy U-care.

2.2. TUNEL Assay

TUNEL staining, as a typical marker of apoptotic events [40], revealed an extensive spreading in alveolar pneumocytes (both type I and II) and bronchiolar epithelial cells as well as in metastatic nodules (Figure 2).

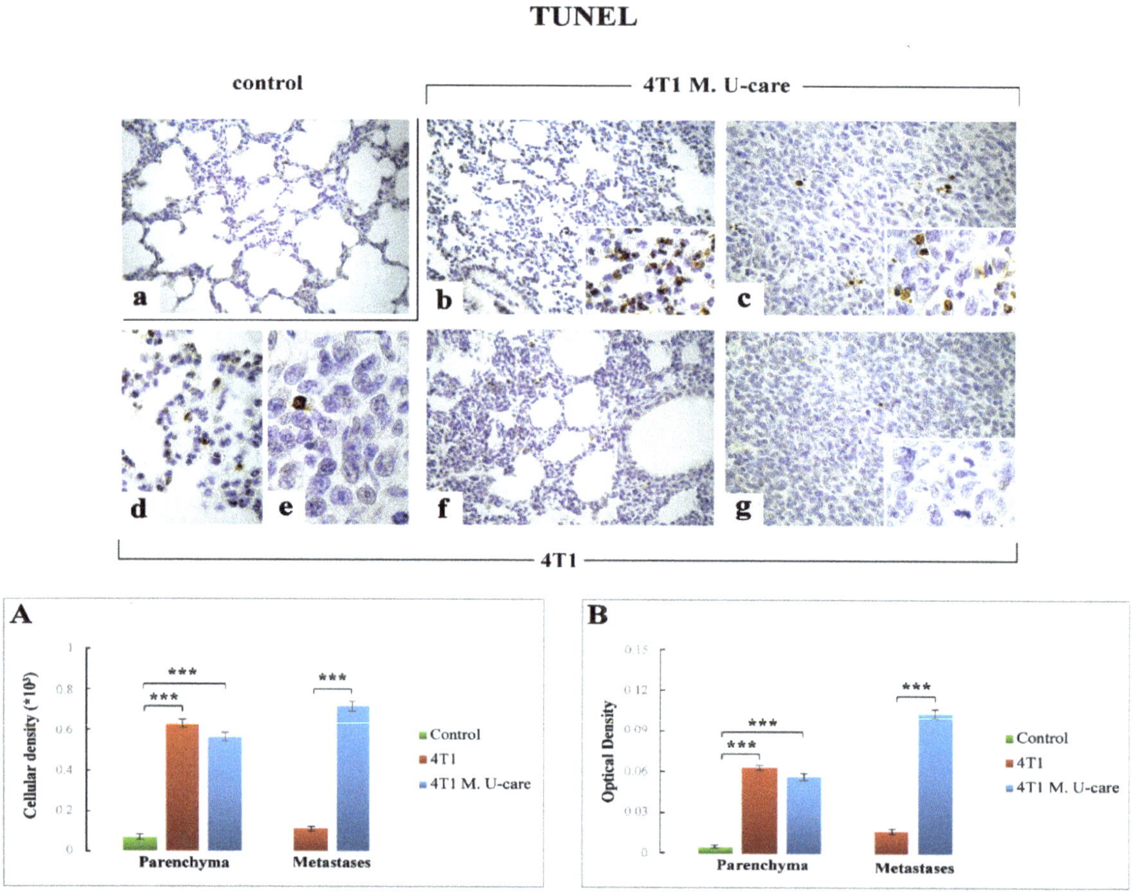

Figure 2. Terminal deoxynucleotidyl-transferase (TUNEL) immunostaining in healthy control (**a**), 4T1 M. U-care (**b**,**c**) and 4T1 (**d**–**g**) mice. Light microscopy magnification: 40× (**a**–**c**,**f**,**g**); 100× (**d**,**e**, insert in panels (**b**,**c**,**g**)). Panel (**A**) and (**B**): Histograms presenting immunopositive cell density and OD, respectively. p values calculated by unpaired Student's t-test: (***) < 0.001.

In particular, concerning the TME, TUNEL-immunoreactivity significantly increased in both 4T1 and 4T1 M. U-care mice (Figure 2b,d,f, respectively) compared to controls (Figure 2a).

The quantitative analysis showed an extremely significant increase of TUNEL-immunopositive cell density and OD comparing 4T1 animals to controls (0.63 ± 0.02 vs. 0.07 ± 0.01 and 0.06 ± 0.00 vs. 0.01 ± 0.00, for cell density and OD, respectively) (Figure 2, Panels (A,B)). In a similar manner, an extremely significant immunoreactivity enhancement was detected when comparing 4T1 M. U-care mice to controls (0.56 ± 0.02 vs. 0.07 ± 0.01 and 0.06 ± 0.00 vs. 0.01 ± 0.00, for cell density and OD, respectively). Diversely, a slight decrease of TUNEL-immunopositive cell density and OD was revealed in 4T1 M. U-care animals compared to 4T1 mice (0.56 ± 0.02 vs. 0.63 ± 0.02 and 0.06 ± 0.00 vs. 0.06 ± 0.00, for cell density and OD, respectively) (Figure 2, Panels (A,B)).

Regarding metastases, an extremely significant increase of TUNEL-immunopositive cell density and OD was detected in 4T1 M. U-care mice compared to 4T1 animals (Figure 2c,e,g, respectively):

0.72 ± 0.02 vs. 0.11 ± 0.01 and 0.10 ± 0.00 vs. 0.02 ± 0.00, for density and OD, respectively (Figure 2, Panels (A,B)). Notably, in 4T1 mice several mitoses were also observable (Figure 2, insert in Figure 2g).

2.3. *PARP1, p53, Bax, Bcl2, and PCNA Immunohistochemical Assessment*

The cellular expression, localization, and distribution of PARP1, p53, Bax, Bcl2, and PCNA, all involved in cell death and proliferation pathways, were explored.

The immunohistochemical evaluation of all these molecules revealed a widespread labeling in the metastatic nodules and/or in TME, at bronchiolar and alveolar level, evidencing a different efficacy of the MM blend, with the more marked effect on tumor cells.

2.3.1. PARP1

A very significant increase of PARP1-immunoreactive cell density was measured in the TME of 4T1 animals (Figure 3d,f) compared to controls (Figure 2a): 7.46 ± 0.83 vs. 1.85 ± 0.14, respectively (Figure 3, Panel (A)); similarly, a significant increase was detected when comparing 4T1 M. U-care mice (Figure 3b) to controls (6.14 ± 0.87 vs. 1.85 ± 0.14, respectively). Notably, any difference was determined evaluating PARP1-immunopositive cell density in 4T1 animals and 4T1 M. U-care mice (7.46 ± 0.83 vs. 6.14 ± 0.87, respectively) (Figure 3, Panel (A)).

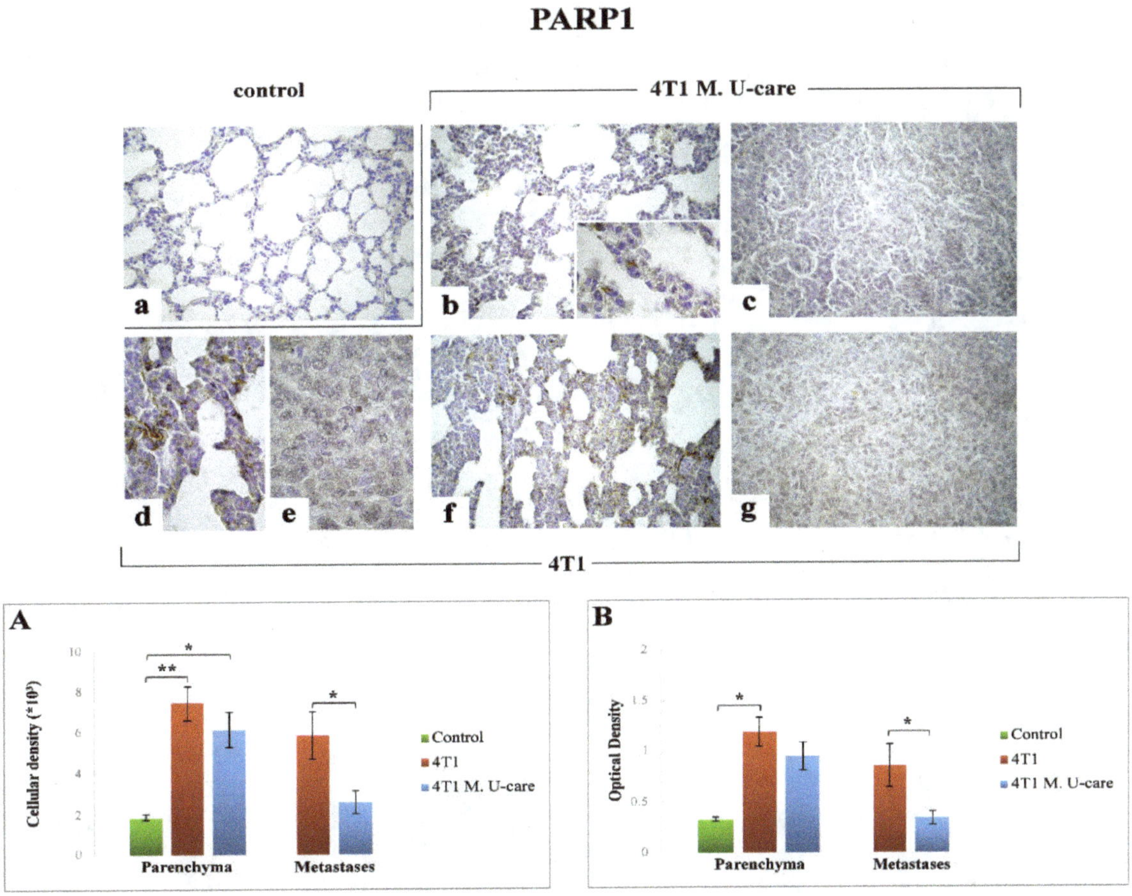

Figure 3. Immunostaining reaction for PARP1 in healthy control (**a**), 4T1 M. U-care (**b**,**c**) and 4T1 (**d**–**g**) mice. Light microscopy magnification: 40× (**a**–**c**,**f**,**g**); 100× (**d**,**e**, insert in panel (**b**)). Panels (**A**) and (**B**): Histograms displaying immunopositive cell density and OD, respectively. *p* values calculated by Unpaired Student's *t*-test: (*) < 0.05 and (**) < 0.01.

Likewise, a significant increase of PARP1-immunoreactive OD was measured in 4T1 animals compared to controls (1.19 ± 0.14 vs. 0.32 ± 0.02, respectively) (Figure 3, Panel (B)), while, differently, any difference was revealed evaluating PARP1-immunopositive OD in 4T1 animals compared to 4T1

M. U-care mice (1.19 ± 0.14 vs. 0.95 ± 0.14, respectively), or even between 4T1 M. U-care and controls (0.95 ± 0.14 vs. 0.32 ± 0.02, respectively) (Figure 3, Panel (B)).

Concerning the metastatic tissue, a significant increase of PARP1-immunopositive cell density and OD was determined in 4T1 mice compared to 4T1 M. U-care animals (5.85 ± 1.16 vs. 2.57 ± 0.57 and 0.85 ± 0.21 vs. 0.34 ± 0.07, for cell density and OD, respectively) (Figure 3, Panels (A,B)).

2.3.2. p53

Comparably to the above reported TUNEL immunostaining trend, p53 immunoreactivity was significantly increased in 4T1 M. U-care mice (Figure 4b,c) compared to both 4T1 animals (Figure 4d–g) and controls (Figure 4a). Specifically, a very significant increase of p53-immunopositive cell density and OD was determined in 4T1 M. U-care animals compared to 4T1 mice (6.42 ± 0.78 vs. 3.09 ± 0.65 and 1.11 ± 0.14 vs. 0.53 ± 0.12, for cell density and OD, respectively). A significant increase of p53-immunopositive cell density and OD was also observed when comparing 4T1 M. U-care animals to control (6.42 ± 0.78 vs. 2.93 ± 0.59 and 1.11 ± 0.14 vs. 0.49 ± 0.11, for cell density and OD, respectively). Differently, any significant difference was calculated when comparing 4T1 mice to controls (3.09 ± 0.65 vs. 2.93 ± 0.59 and 0.53 ± 0.12 vs. 0.49 ± 0.11, for cell density and OD, respectively) (Figure 4, Panel (A,B)).

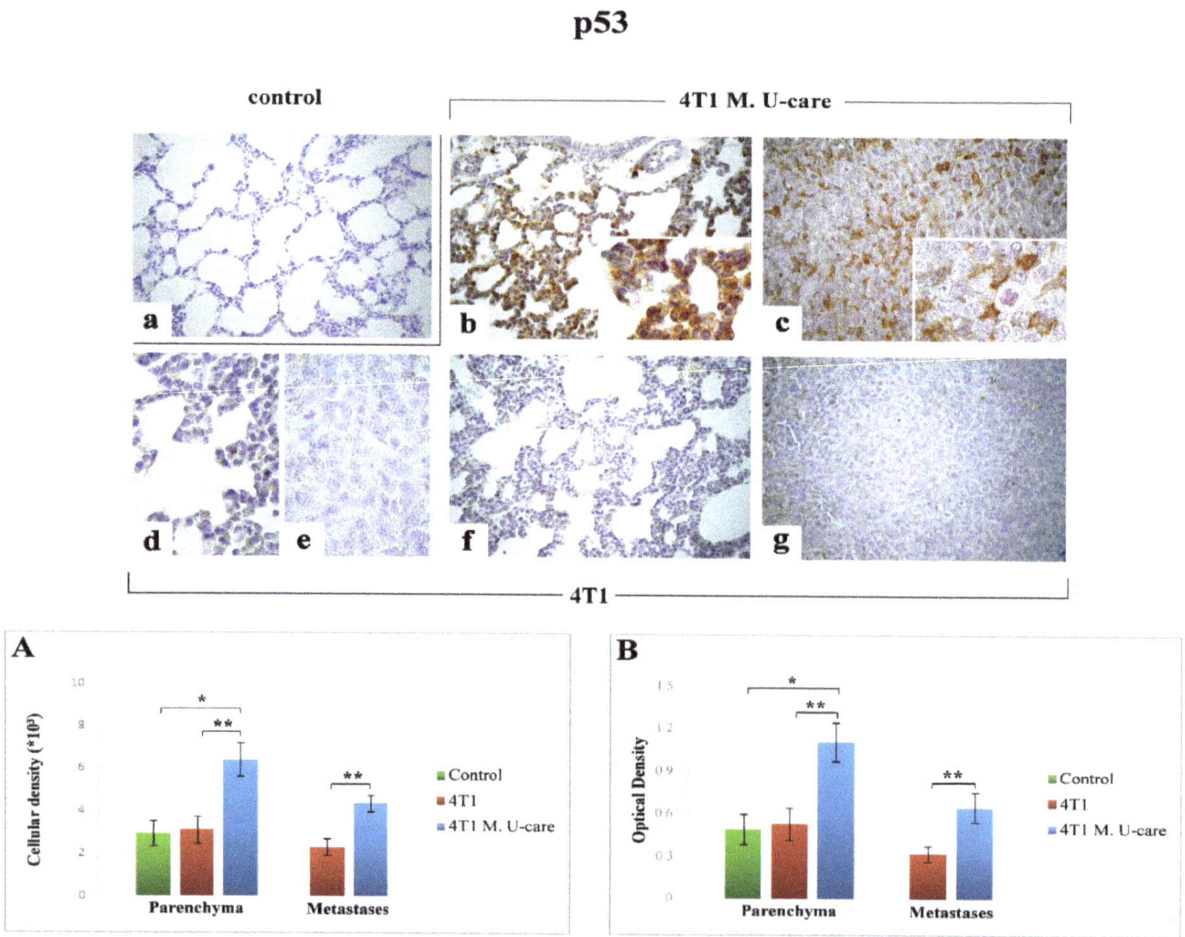

Figure 4. p53-immunostaining reaction in healthy control (**a**), 4T1 M. U-care (**b**,**c**) and 4T1 (**d**–**g**) mice. Light microscopy magnification: 40× (**a**–**c**,**f**,**g**); 100× (**d**,**e**, insert in panels (**b**,**c**)). Panels (**A**) and (**B**): Histograms showing immunopositive cell density and OD, respectively. p values calculated by Unpaired Student's t-test: (*) < 0.05 and (**) < 0.01.

With regard to metastatic tissue, a very significant increase of both p53-immunoreactive cell density and OD was determined in 4T1 M. U-care mice compared to 4T1 animals (4.38 ± 0.63 vs. 2.29 ± 0.39 and 0.64 ± 0.10 vs. 0.32 ± 0.06, for density and OD, respectively) (Figure 4, Panels (A,B)).

2.3.3. Bax

Similarly to p53, a significant increase in Bax immunopositivity was observed in the TME of 4T1 M. U-care mice at alveolar and stromal level, with several immunopositive endothelial cells in bronchiolar areas (Figure 5b), compared to both 4T1 mice (Figure 5d,f) and controls (Figure 5a). In the same manner, Bax resulted overexpressed in metastatic nodules 4T1 M. U-care mice (Figure 5c), compared to 4T1 animals (Figure 5e,g). Notably, a significant increase of Bax-immunoreactive cell density was measured in 4T1 M. U-care animals compared to 4T1 mice (4.75 ± 0.48 vs. 3.13 ± 0.40, respectively). Likewise, a significant increase was observed in 4T1 M. U-care mice compared to control (4.75 ± 0.48 vs. 2.47 ± 0.28, respectively), while any difference was determined when comparing 4T1 animals and controls (3.13 ± 0.4 and 2.47 ± 0.28, respectively) (Figure 5, Panel (A)). Moreover, a significant increase of Bax-immunostaining OD was evidenced in 4T1 M. U-care mice, compared to both 4T1 and controls (0.76 ± 0.09 vs. 0.48 ± 0.07 and 0.76 ± 0.09 vs. 0.37 ± 0.04, respectively). Any significant difference was measured when comparing 4T1 mice to controls (0.48 ± 0.07 vs. 0.37 ± 0.04, respectively) (Figure 5, Panel (B)).

Concerning the metastases, an extremely significant increase of both Bax-immunopositive cell density and OD was determined in 4T1 M. U-care mice compared to 4T1 animals (4.47 ± 0.40 vs. 1.59 ± 0.31, and 0.58 ± 0.07 vs. 0.24 ± 0.06, respectively) (Figure 5, Panels (A,B)).

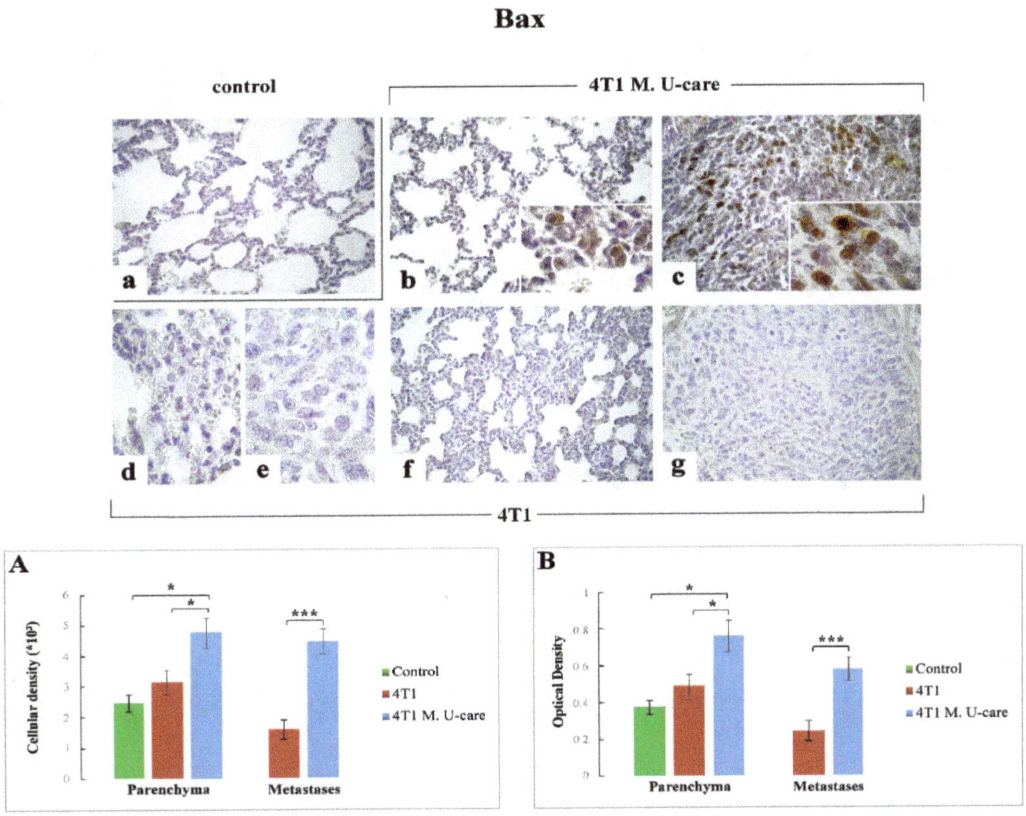

Figure 5. Immunohistochemical staining for Bax in healthy control (**a**), 4T1 M. U-care (**b**,**c**) and 4T1 (**d**–**g**) mice. Light microscopy magnification: 40× (**a**–**c**,**f**,**g**); 100× (**d**,**e**, insert in panels (**b**,**c**)). Panels (**A**) and (**B**): Histograms showing immunopositive cell density and OD, respectively. p values calculated by Unpaired Student's t-test: (*) < 0.05 and (***) < 0.001.

2.3.4. Bcl2

Concerning the TME, Bcl2-immunoreactivity appeared slightly enhanced in both 4T1 and 4T1 M. U-care mice (Figure 6b,d,f, respectively) compared to controls (Figure 6a). Notably, a slight non-significant increase of Bcl2-immunoreactive cell density and OD was measured both in 4T1 and 4T1 M. U-care animals compared to controls (4.88 ± 0.69 vs. 4.89 ± 0.68 vs. 1.74 ± 0.15 and 0.86 ± 0.12 vs. 0.89 ± 0.13 vs. 0.32 ± 0.03, for density and OD, respectively). Any difference was evidenced evaluating Bcl2-immunopositive cell density and OD in 4T1 animals and 4T1 M. U-care mice (4.88 ± 0.69 vs. 4.89 ± 0.68 and 0.86 ± 0.12 vs. 0.89 ± 0.13, for density and OD, respectively) (Figure 6, Panels (A,B)).

Regarding the metastatic nodules (Figure 6c,e,g), contrarily to Bax, a very significant decrease of Bcl2-immunopositive cell density and OD was detected in 4T1 M. U-care mice compared to 4T1 (1.77 ± 0.32 vs. 3.29 ± 0.34 and 0.24 ± 0.04 vs. 0.52 ± 0.06, for density and OD, respectively) (Figure 6, Panels (A,B)).

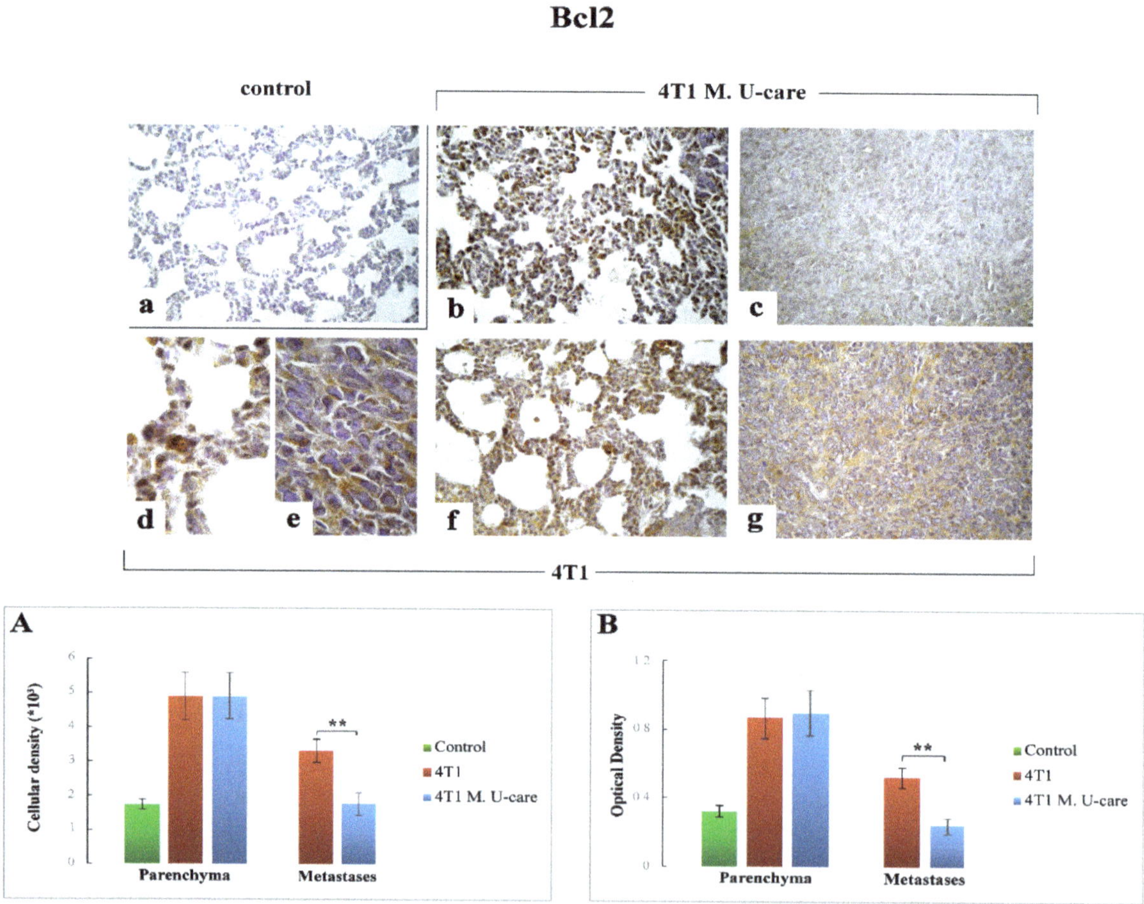

Figure 6. Bcl2-immunostaining reaction in healthy control (**a**), 4T1 M. U-care (**b**,**c**) and 4T1 (**d**–**g**) mice. Light microscopy magnification: 40× (**a**–**c**,**f**,**g**); 100× (**d**,**e**). Panels (**A**) and (**B**): Histograms showing immunopositive cell density and OD, respectively. p values calculated by Unpaired Student's t-test: (**) < 0.01.

2.3.5. PCNA

PCNA-immunopositivity was extremely enhanced in TME of 4T1 mice (Figure 7d,f) compared to both 4T1 M. U-care (Figure 7b) and controls (Figure 7a). In particular, the quantitative analysis highlighted an extremely significant increase in PCNA-immunoreactive cell density and OD when comparing 4T1 animals to controls (0.40 ± 0.03 vs. 0.06 ± 0.01 and 0.93 ± 0.01 vs. 0.01 ± 0.00, for cell density and OD, respectively). In a similar manner, an extremely significant enhancement was detected when comparing 4T1 mice to 4T1 M. U-care animals (0.40 ± 0.03 vs. 0.17 ± 0.02 and 0.93 ± 0.01 vs.

0.02 ± 0.00, for cell density and OD, respectively). No significant differences were revealed in 4T1 M. U-care animals compared to control (0.17 ± 0.02 vs. 0.06 ± 0.01 and 0.02 ± 0.00 vs. 0.01 ± 0.00, for cell density and OD, respectively) (Figure 7, Panels (A,B)).

Concerning the metastatic tissue, an extremely significant decrease of PCNA-immunopositive cell density and OD was detected in 4T1 M. U-care mice (Figure 7c) compared to 4T1 animals (Figure 7e,g): 4.74 ± 0.28 vs. 9.57 ± 0.44 and 0.64 ± 0.04 vs. 1.77 ± 0.08, for density and OD, respectively (Figure 7, Panels (A,B)).

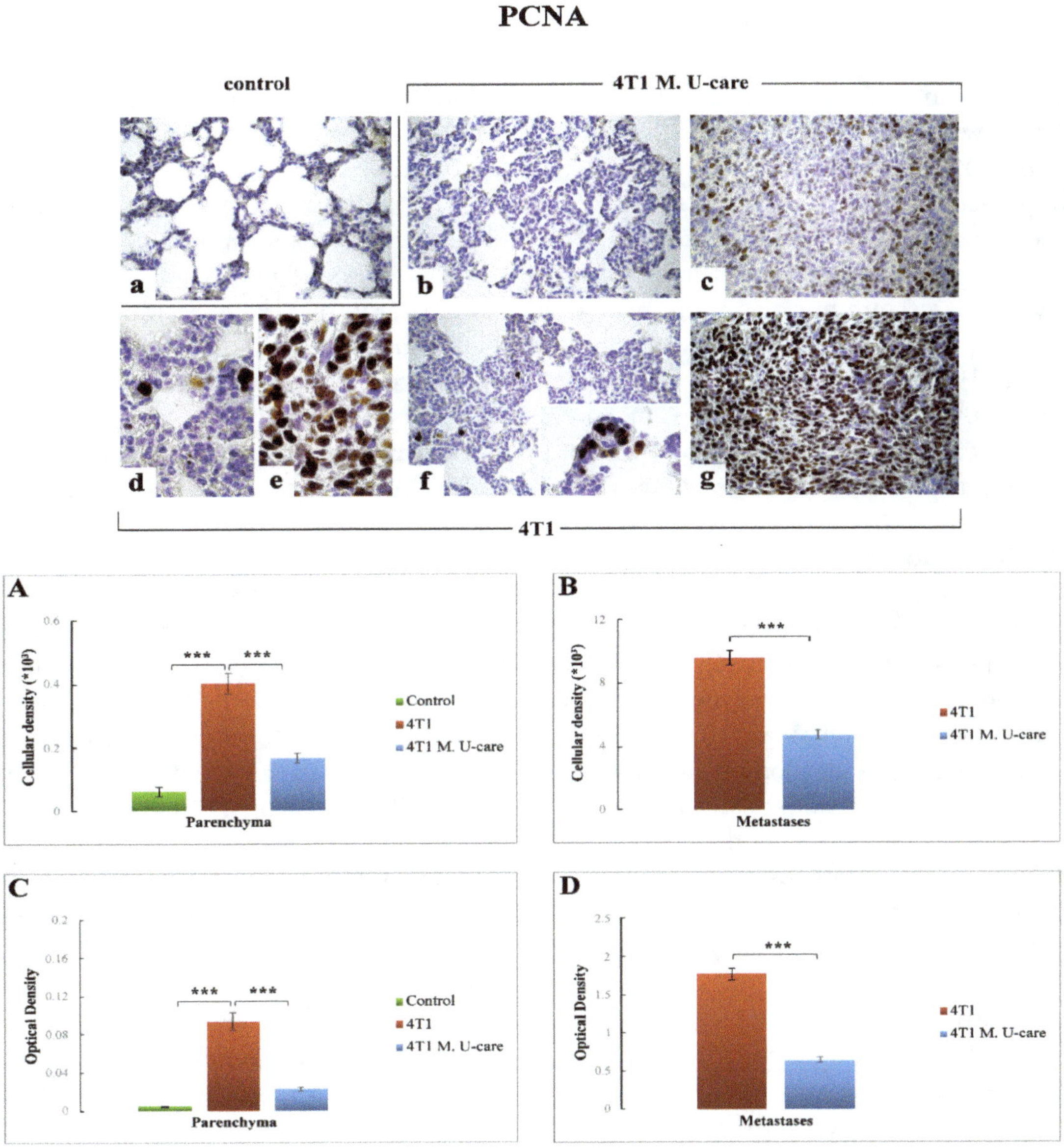

Figure 7. DAB-immunostaining reaction for PCNA in healthy control (**a**) 4T1 M. U-care (**b**,**c**), and 4T1 (**d**–**g**) mice. Light microscopy magnification: 40× (**a**–**c**,**f**,**g**); 100× (**d**,**e**, insert in panel (**f**)). Panels (**A**) and (**B**): Histograms showing immunopositive cell density. Panels (**C**) and (**D**): histograms exhibiting immunoreactive OD. p values calculated by Unpaired Student's t-test: (***) < 0.001.

3. Discussion

Tumor development and progression are influenced by rearrangement of TME components, e.g., immune cells, fibroblasts, satellite cells, blood, and lymphatic vessels. Tumor cells are known to manipulate the function of cellular and non-cellular components through a complex signaling network to gain tumorigenesis, tumor maintenance, and drug resistance (MDR), taking advantage of the non-malignant cells. Experimental and clinical data evidence that an in-depth analysis of the bidirectional communications and interactions between tumor cells and their surrounding dynamic TME is essential to identify the existing mechanisms of tumor expansion and invasion [41]. This complex network moreover involved apoptosis, also engaged to efficiently eliminate dysfunctional cells, plays an important role in both carcinogenesis and cancer treatment [42]. In particular, to guarantee its nourished growth, cancer is able to provide both endurance signals as well as mechanisms saving malignant cells from apoptosis. It is well known that an imbalance between cell proliferation and cell death typically characterizes cancer condition, in which several genetic aberrations may drive malignant cells to an uncontrolled progression and survival [43,44].

In our previous paper using the same preclinical model, i.e., 4T1 triple-negative mouse BC, we demonstrated that M. U-Care supplementation, starting 2 months before 4T1 injection and lasting throughout the whole experimental time (including tumor development and metastatization), produced a dramatic reduction of both lung metastases density and number. These effects were accompanied by a substantial decrease of inflammation and oxidative stress both in lung TME and metastases, together with a bettering of the QoL [36]. Therefore, we hypothesized that the supplement effects could have been ascribable either to a direct anticancer effect and/or to the secondary/indirect impacts of the MM blend on systemic inflammation and immunomodulation. Therefore, aiming at addressing this crucial question, in the present investigation, we focused on the programmed cell death, investigating specific molecules, i.e., PARP1, p53, BAX, and Bcl2, pivotally involved in apoptotic pathway, whose critical role in human BC is well known. Further, in parallel we investigated PCNA expression pathway, based on the great interest on the pivotal role of PCNA in cancer cells proliferation, also taking into consideration that PCNA modifications may determine both tumor progression as well as the outcome of anticancer treatment.

Firstly, it has to be highlighted that performing a comparative assessment on cancer tissue, i.e., lung metastases, and surrounding TME by TUNEL assay, we revealed the existence of a different expression trend in 4T1 animals compared to 4T1 M. U-care mice. In detail, in these latter animals, an extremely intense immunopositivity was observed in the metastases, indicating an evident activation of the apoptotic pathway in cancer cells after the oral supplementation with the MM blend. Interestingly, this effect was definitely weaker in 4T1 animals, in which several mitoses were clearly observed in the tumor nodules, thus demonstrating the occurrence of an already active proliferation process. Concerning the TME, any statistical difference was measured comparing 4T1 M. U-care animals and 4T1 mice. These data corroborate the action of the MM blend, who display a powerful action able to drive metastatic cells to apoptosis, whereas was less effective with regards to the surrounding TME.

Concerning all evaluated apoptotic and proliferation markers, the comparative assessment of TME and metastases revealed diverse trends of protein expression, with the metastatic nodules being the most affected.

With regards to PARP1 levels, crucially implicated in tumorigenesis phenomena [24,26,27], the significant reduction observed in metastatic nodules of 4T1 M. U-care mice compared to 4T1 animals seemed to demonstrate a valuable action of the adjuvant micotherapic supplementation, suggesting a direct influence of the blend on tumor cells.

Our putative idea of a direct MM blend action able to determine an imbalance between proliferation and apoptosis, driving to a significant increase in apoptotic events, was further supported by p53 and Bax high expression levels measured in 4T1 M. U-care mice, showing the most striking effect in the metastatic nodules. By contrast, concerning both Bax and p53, an almost complete lack of effect was determined in 4T1 animals, in which the protein expression levels were similar to that observed in controls. Acting as proapoptotic protein, Bax should essentially play as a tumor suppressor factor. Consequently, reductions in its expression levels would provide tumor cells with a selective survival advantage, contributing to their expansion and invasion [21]. In particular, the reduced Bax expression levels can be traced back to an alteration of the p53 function which, by itself, is able to alter the levels of this proapoptotic protein [21]. Certainly, TP53 mutations are the most common genetic alterations in breast cancer [28]. Notably, the increased immunopositivity for the wild type p53 isoform detected in 4T1 M. U-care mice could indicate a possible attempt to cell cycle arrest, in order to allow cellular repair processes and inhibit the proliferation of damaged cells.

Based on the notion that (i) several apoptotic stimuli induce cell death through a Bcl-2-regulated pathway and (ii) proteins belonging to Bcl2 family can play a dichotomous role, acting both as promoters as well as inhibitors of apoptotic events [21,45,46], we may suppose that the lower expression of Bcl-2 determined in metastatic tissue of 4T1 M. U-care mice could be related to a decrease in cancer cell proliferation, evidencing an alteration of the proliferation/apoptosis balance. This effect could also counteract the capacity of Bcl2 to trigger drug resistance at high expression [21,47]. Moreover, the overexpression of p53 in 4T1 M. U-Care mice may support a possible role of p53 in downregulating Bcl-2, feasibly explaining the apoptosis induction by wild type p53. Notably, it has to be underlined that, differently to all other evaluated markers, but similarly to TUNEL staining, we determined any difference in the Bcl-2 expression trend comparing metastases and TME in 4T1 M. U-care mice and 4T1 animals. Specifically, TME appeared to be unaffected by the mycotherapic oral supplementation, whereas the MM blend display a specific and selective effect restricted to the metastatic area.

In addition, concerning the proliferation marker PCNA, we evidenced a reduced expression in metastatic nodules in 4T1 M. U-care mice, thus highlighting an evident inhibitory effect of the MM blend on proliferation activity in tumor cells. Notably, a strong positive correlation between the expression of PCNA and COX2 in breast cancer has been recently highlighted [48], also in accordance with our previous findings [36].

Taken together the present data supported that the oral supplementation is effective to induce a peculiar swinging balance of cell death and proliferation, in which these two essential mechanisms appeared strictly interconnected and inversely related (see p53 and Bax vs. Bcl2 and PCNA expression trends). Notably, the MM blend bettered the cancer state with a direct effect, able to force tumor metastatic cells to an apoptotic fate.

In summary, all the present findings confirmed the protective role played by Micotherapy U-care blend in the lung metastases and surrounding TME. Our data further suggest that both an immunomodulatory anti-inflammatory systemic effect and a direct, selective anticancer effect act in a positive pleiotropic way. This double action mechanism, which (i) disturbs the TME signaling and (ii) targets the complex apoptotic pathway, could represent a promising approach for patient's treatment. In fact, in the search for novel therapeutic agents targeting tumor development and progression, MM-derived natural bioactive compounds, displaying multi-targeting potential, can overcome the disadvantages of monotherapy such as side effects and drug resistance. In particular, TNBC is the most aggressive malignant BC, difficult to treat due to its unresponsiveness to current clinical targeted treatments (e.g., hormonal therapy protocols or chemotherapeutics targeting HER2 protein receptors) and high rate of recurrence. In this scenario, the biological effects of combining M. U-care supplement with conventional therapies to target crucial cancer signaling pathways, i.e., proliferation and apoptosis, may interfere with cellular and molecular processes fueling TNBC growth, trying to create a new joint medical protocol able to hinder the typical TNBC metastatic pattern, i.e., frequent occurrence of distant metastases, mainly localized in lung, central nervous system, and bones, often associated with poor prognosis.

4. Materials and Methods

4.1. Cell Culture

The mice breast cancer cell line, 4T1, was acquired from American Type Culture Collection (ATCC) and maintained at 37 °C in a humidified atmosphere (95% air/5% CO_2) [36].

4.2. Animals and Experimental Plan

The detailed experimental design was previously describe in Roda et al. [36]. Briefly, 34 two-month-old wild type female BALB/c mice were obtained from Charles River Italia (Calco, Italy) and acclimatized for at least 3 weeks before the experiments.

All experiments were achieved in agreement with the European Council Directive 2010/63/EU and the Ethics Committee of Pavia University guidelines (Ministry of Health, License number 364/2018-PR). Therefore, all mice have been treated humanely, with due consideration for the reduction of pain and distress.

For execution of experiments and subsequent analyses, researchers were blinded to the designed group.

Sixteen (4T1 M. U-care mice) out of thirty-four mice were supplemented until sacrifice with a medicinal mushroom blend, namely, Micotherapy U-care (provided by A.V.D. Reform s.r.l., Noceto, Parma, Italy) consisting of a mixture of 20% extracts of sporophores and mycelia of five fungal species: *Agaricus blazei*, *Cordyceps sinensis*, *Ganoderma lucidum*, *Grifola frondosa*, and *Lentinula edodes* (see Table 1 and Results section). The mycotherapic blend was solubilized in water, selecting a dose of 4 mg supplement/mice per day to mimic the oral supplementation in humans (about 1.5 g/day). Otherwise, control ($n = 4$) and non-treated (4T1, $n = 14$) mice did not received any diet supplementation.

For the syngeneic tumor-bearing mice (4T1 and 4T1 M. U-care) generation see the work in [36].

The syngeneic tumor-bearing mice (4T1 and 4T1 M. U-care) were generated by injecting 1×10^6 of the 4T1 cells into the nape of the neck of the female Balb/C mice. Control animals were injected with phosphate-buffer saline (PBS). A survival rate of 100% was kept in all experimental groups, throughout the whole experimental time course.

Lung preparation was done by vascular perfusion of fixative [49]. Then, lungs were accurately removed, sectioned and then processed for immunohistochemistry.

4.3. Tissue Sampling and Immunohistochemistry

4.3.1. Lung Specimens Preparation

The lung specimens preparation was previously described in detail [36]. Briefly, the top and the bottom regions of the right lungs of mice from each experimental group were dissected. Tissue samples were obtained according to a stratified random sampling scheme, fixed and processed as previously described [36]. Eight micrometer thick sections were cut in transversal plane and placed on silane-coated slides.

4.3.2. TUNEL Staining

The reaction was performed using the terminal deoxynucleotidyl-transferase (TUNEL) assay (Oncogene Res. Prod., Boston, MA, USA). The lung sections were incubated for 5 min with 20 μg mL^{-1} proteinase-K solution at room temperature, followed by treatment with 3% H_2O_2 to quench endogenous peroxidase activity. After incubation with the TUNEL solution (90 min with TdT/biotinylated dNTP and 30 min with HRP-conjugate streptavidin) in a humidified chamber at 37 °C, the reaction was developed using a 0.1% DAB solution. After nuclear counterstaining employing Carazzi's Hematoxylin, the sections were dehydrated in ethanol, cleared in xylene, and finally mounted in Eukitt (Kindler, Freiburg, Germany).

As a negative control, the TdT incubation was omitted; no staining was observed in these conditions.

4.3.3. Immunohistochemistry: Apoptotic Pathway Assessment

Commercial antibodies were employed on murine lung specimens to investigate the expression of different specific apoptotic markers: (i) Poly (AD-ribose) polymerase 1(PARP1), (ii) p53, (iii) Bcl2 associated X-protein (Bax), (iv) B-cell lymphoma/leukemia protein (Bcl2), and (v) the proliferating cell nuclear antigen (PCNA). Table 2 shows both primary and secondary antibodies as well as respective dilutions used for immunohistochemical experiments.

Immunohistochemical procedures have been conducted exactly as previously described [36].

Table 2. Primary/secondary antibodies and respective dilution used for immunohistochemical experimental procedures.

	Antigen	Immunogen	Manufacturer, Species, Mono-Polyclonal, Cat./Lot. No., RRID	Dilution
Primary Antibodies	Anti-poly (ADP-ribose) polymerase (46D11)	Purified antibody raised against the residues surrounding Gly623 of human PARP-1	Cell Signaling Technology (Danvers, MA, USA), Rabbit monoclonal IgG, Cat# 9532, RRID:AB_659884	1:100
	Anti-p53 (Ab-5)	Purified antibody raised against the ~53 kDa wild type p53 protein of mouse origin	Sigma-Aldrich (St. Louis, MO, USA), Mouse monoclonal IgG2a, Cat# OP33-100UG, RRID:AB_564977	1:100
	Anti-Bcl-2-associated X protein (P-19)	Purified antibody Raised against a peptide mapping at the amino terminus of Bax of mouse origin	Santa Cruz Biotechnology (Santa Cruz, CA, USA), Rabbit polyclonal IgG, Cat# sc-526, RRID:AB_2064668	1:100
	Anti-B-Cell Leukemia/Lymphoma 2 protein (N-19)	Purified antibody raised against a peptide mapping at the N-terminus of Bcl-2 of human origin	Santa Cruz Biotechnology (Santa Cruz, CA, USA), Rabbit polyclonal IgG, Cat# sc-492, RRID:AB_2064290	1:100
	Anti-Proliferating Cell Nuclear Antigen (Ab-1)	Purified antibody raised against the ~37 kDa PCNA protein of mouse origin	Sigma-Aldrich (St. Louis, MO, USA), Mouse monoclonal IgG2a, Cat# NA03-200UG, RRID:AB_213111	2:1000
Secondary Antibodies	Biotinylated horse anti-mouse IgG	Gamma immunoglobulin	Vector Laboratories (Burlingame, CA, USA), Horse, Cat# PK-6102, RRID:AB_2336821	1:200
	Biotinylated goat anti-rabbit IgG	Gamma immunoglobulin	Vector Laboratories (Burlingame, CA, USA), Goat, lot# PK-6101, RRID: AB_2336820	1:200

4.3.4. Immunohistochemical Evaluations

To prevent differences due to small procedural changes, immunohistochemical reactions were performed simultaneously on samples from different experimental groups. The expression of each selected marker was examined in six slides (about 30 sections) per mouse. The shown micrographs display the most representative pulmonary conditions and modifications for each immunohistochemical reaction.

Immunohistochemical labeling extent evaluation was previously described in detail [36].

The optical density (OD), intended as immunohistochemical intensity, was assessed in 30 cells/section per six slides/mouse. OD was related to the immunopositive cell density. In addition, immunopositive cells density count was evaluated, intended as number of immunopositive cells/area in mm^2.

4.4. Statistics

Data were expressed as mean ± standard error of the mean (SEM). Regarding the TME, the statistical differences among the three experimental groups were calculated by using one-way ANOVA followed by Bonferroni's post hoc test. Otherwise, for metastases, the statistical differences between 4T1 and 4T1 M. U-care mice were evaluated by using unpaired Student's *t*-test.

The differences were considered statistically significant for $p < 0.05$ (*), $p < 0.01$ (**), and $p < 0.001$ (***). Statistical analyses were performed by using GraphPad Prism 7.0 (GraphPad Software Inc., La Jolla, CA, USA).

5. Conclusions

Overall, these results support the use of oral supplementation with Micotherapy U-care blend as a new effective strategy to be used in the field of integrative oncology to decrease adverse side effects caused by conventional cancer therapies. All obtained results corroborated the Micotherapy U-care protective role in metastases and TME, in which an immunomodulatory anti-inflammatory systemic action together with a direct, selective anticancer mechanism exerted a positive pleiotropic effect. The Micotherapy U-care preventive and protective effect could affect the TME signaling and, at the same time, target the multifaceted apoptotic pathway. Once again, the present investigation highlights the importance of translational research in the development of clinically relevant therapeutic strategies. In particular, the growing use of translational research "from bench to bedside" in cancer medicine, could allow to overcome challenges which everlastingly hinder medicinal advancements, yielding significant advances in cancer therapeutics and also improvements in the ability to predict clinical course of patient's disease based on individual tumor characteristics. In this view, medicinal mushrooms extracts, being natural sources of novel drugs, could be used as effective adjuvant therapy in the critical management of TNBC.

Author Contributions: Conceptualization, E.R., E.S. and P.R.; methodology, F.D.L., D.R. and C.D.I.; software, F.D.L. and D.R.; formal analysis, E.R., F.D.L. and P.R.; investigation, E.R., F.D.L. and C.D.I.; writing—original draft preparation, E.R. and P.R.; writing—review and editing, F.D.L. and D.R.; supervision, E.R., C.A.L., M.G.B. and P.R. All authors have read and agreed to the published version of the manuscript.

Acknowledgments: We thank Andrei Gregori (Biotechnical Faculty, University of Ljubljana, Slovenia) for raw materials, extract procedure, and main active metabolites of MM blend Micotherapy U-care. We thank A.V.D. Reform s.r.l. (Noceto, Parma) for providing us the supplement "Micotherapy U-Care". We thank Rita Vaccarone, Department of Biology and Biotechnology, University of Pavia, for her excellent technical assistance.

References

1. Jemal, A.; Bray, F.; Center, M.M.; Ferlay, J.; Ward, E.; Forman, D. Global cancer statistics. *CA Cancer J. Clin.* **2011**, *61*, 69–90. [CrossRef] [PubMed]
2. Cardoso, F.; Harbeck, N.; Fallowfield, L.; Kyriakides, S.; Senkus, E.; ESMO Guidelines Working Group. Locally recurrent or metastatic breast cancer: ESMO Clinical Practice Guidelines for diagnosis, treatment and follow-up. *Ann. Oncol.* **2012**, *23*, vii11–vii19. [CrossRef] [PubMed]
3. Zeeshan, R.; Mutahir, Z. Cancer metastasis: Tricks of the trade. *Bosn. J. Basic Med. Sci.* **2017**, *17*, 172–182. [CrossRef] [PubMed]
4. Schito, L.; Rey, S. Hypoxic pathobiology of breast cancer metastasis. *Biochim. Biophys. Acta Rev. Cancer* **2017**, *1868*, 239–245. [CrossRef]
5. Yadav, B.S.; Chanana, P.; Jhamb, S. Biomarkers in triple negative breast cancer: A review. *World J. Clin. Oncol.* **2015**, *6*, 252. [CrossRef]
6. Yeo, S.K.; Guan, J.L. Breast Cancer: Multiple Subtypes within a Tumor? *Trends Cancer* **2017**, *3*, 753–760. [CrossRef]

7. Yao, Y.; Chu, Y.; Xu, B.; Hu, Q.; Song, Q. Risk factors for distant metastasis of patients with primary triple-negative breast cancer. *Biosci. Rep.* **2019**, *39*. [CrossRef]
8. Iriondo, O.; Liu, Y.; Lee, G.; Elhodaky, M.; Jimenez, C.; Li, L.; Lang, J.; Wang, P.; Yu, M. TAK1 mediates microenvironment-triggered autocrine signals and promotes triple-negative breast cancer lung metastasis. *Nat. Commun.* **2018**, *9*, 1994. [CrossRef]
9. Chitty, J.L.; Filipe, E.C.; Lucas, M.C.; Herrmann, D.; Cox, T.R.; Timpson, P. Recent advances in understanding the complexities of metastasis. *F1000Research* **2018**, *7*, 1169. [CrossRef]
10. Katsuta, E.; Rashid, O.M.; Takabe, K. Clinical relevance of tumor microenvironment: Immune cells, vessels, and mouse models. *Hum. Cell* **2020**, *33*, 930–937. [CrossRef]
11. Buhrmann, C.; Shayan, P.; Banik, K.; Kunnumakkara, A.B.; Kubatka, P.; Koklesova, L.; Shakibaei, M. Targeting NF-κB Signaling by Calebin A, a Compound of Turmeric, in Multicellular Tumor Microenvironment: Potential Role of Apoptosis Induction in CRC Cells. *Biomedicines* **2020**, *8*, 236. [CrossRef] [PubMed]
12. Cacho-Diaz, B.; García-Botello, D.R.; Wegman-Ostrosky, T.; Reyes-Soto, G.; Ortiz-Sánchez, E.; Herrera-Montalvo, L.A. Tumor microenvironment differences between primary tumor and brain metastases. *J. Transl. Med.* **2020**, *18*, 1. [CrossRef] [PubMed]
13. Nounou, M.I.; Elamrawy, F.; Ahmed, N.; Abdelraouf, K.; Goda, S.; Syed-Sha-Qhattal, H. Breast Cancer: Conventional Diagnosis and Treatment Modalities and Recent Patents and Technologies. *Breast Cancer* **2015**, *9*, 17–34. [CrossRef] [PubMed]
14. Zhao, Y.; Jing, Z.; Li, Y.; Mao, W. Berberine in combination with cisplatin suppresses breast cancer cell growth through induction of DNA breaks and caspase-3-dependent apoptosis. *Oncol. Rep.* **2016**, *36*, 567–572. [CrossRef] [PubMed]
15. Czabotar, P.E.; Lessene, G.; Strasser, A.; Adams, J.M. Control of apoptosis by the BCL-2 protein family: Implications for physiology and therapy. *Nat. Rev. Mol. Cell Biol.* **2014**, *15*, 49–63. [CrossRef]
16. Kadam, C.Y.; Abhang, S.A. Apoptosis Markers in Breast Cancer Therapy. *Adv. Clin. Chem.* **2016**, *74*, 143–193. [CrossRef]
17. Elmore, S. Apoptosis: A Review of Programmed Cell Death. *Toxicol. Pathol.* **2007**, *35*, 495–516. [CrossRef]
18. Parton, M.; Dowsett, M.; Smith, I. Studies of apoptosis in breast cancer. *BMJ* **2001**, *322*, 1528–1532. [CrossRef]
19. Hong, S.J.; Dawson, T.M.; Dawson, V.L. PARP and the Release of Apoptosis-Inducing Factor from Mitochondria; Madame Curie Bioscience Database. 2013. Available online: https://www.ncbi.nlm.nih.gov/books/NBK6179/ (accessed on 8 October 2020).
20. Aubrey, B.J.; Kelly, G.L.; Janic, A.; Herold, M.J.; Strasser, A. How does p53 induce apoptosis and how does this relate to p53-mediated tumour suppression? *Cell Death Differ.* **2018**, *25*, 104–113. [CrossRef]
21. Krajewski, S.; Thor, A.D.; Edgerton, S.M.; Moore, D.H.; Krajewska, M.; Reed, J.C. Analysis of Bax and Bcl-2 expression in p53-immunopositive breast cancers. *Clin. Cancer Res.* **1997**, *3*, 199–208.
22. Frenzel, A.; Grespi, F.; Chmelewskij, W.; Villunger, A. Bcl2 family proteins in carcinogenesis and the treatment of cancer. *Apoptosis* **2009**, *14*, 584–596. [CrossRef] [PubMed]
23. Slade, D. PARP and PARG inhibitors in cancer treatment. *Genes Dev.* **2020**, *34*, 360–394. [CrossRef] [PubMed]
24. Ossovskaya, V.; Koo, I.C.; Kaldjian, E.P.; Alvares, C.; Sherman, B.M. Upregulation of poly (ADP-Ribose) polymerase-1 (PARP1) in triple-negative breast cancer and other primary human tumor types. *Genes Cancer* **2010**, *1*, 812–821. [CrossRef] [PubMed]
25. Yu, S.W.; Andrabi, S.A.; Wang, H.; No, S.K.; Poirier, G.G.; Dawson, T.M.; Dawson, V.L. Apoptosis-inducing factor mediates poly(ADP-ribose) (PAR) polymer-induced cell death. *Proc. Nat. Acad. Sci. USA* **2006**, *103*, 18314–18319. [CrossRef]
26. Domagala, P.; Huzarski, T.; Lubinski, J.; Gugala, K.; Domagala, W. PARP-1 expression in breast cancer including BRCA1-associated, triple negative and basal-like tumors: Possible implications for PARP-1 inhibitor therapy. *Breast Cancer Res. Treat.* **2011**, *127*, 861–869. [CrossRef]
27. Schreiber, V.; Dantzer, F.; Amé, J.C.; De Murcia, G. Poly(ADP-ribose): Novel functions for an old molecule. *Nat. Rev. Mol. Cell Biol.* **2006**, *7*, 517–528. [CrossRef]
28. Bertheau, P.; Lehmann-Che, J.; Varna, M.; Dumay, A.; Poirot, B.; Porcher, R.; Turpin, E.; Plassa, L.F.; De Roquancourt, A.; Bourstyn, E.; et al. P53 in breast cancer subtypes and new insights into response to chemotherapy. *Breast* **2013**, *22*, S27–S29. [CrossRef]
29. Hanahan, D.; Weinberg, R.A. The hallmarks of cancer. *Cell* **2000**, *100*, 57–70. [CrossRef]

30. Wang, S.-C. PCNA: A silent housekeeper or a potential therapeutic target? *Trends Pharmacol. Sci.* **2014**, *35*, 178–186. [CrossRef]
31. Juríková, M.; Danihel, L'.; Polák, Š.; Varga, I. Ki67, PCNA, and MCM proteins: Markers of proliferation in the diagnosis of breast cancer. *Acta Histochem.* **2016**, *118*, 544–552. [CrossRef]
32. Varghese, E.; Samuel, S.M.; Sadiq, Z.; Kubatka, P.; Liskova, A.; Benacka, J.; Pazinka, P.; Kruzliak, P.; Büsselberg, D. Anti-Cancer Agents in Proliferation and Cell Death: The Calcium Connection. *Int. J. Mol. Sci.* **2019**, *20*, 3017. [CrossRef] [PubMed]
33. Rossi, P.; Difrancia, R.; Quagliariello, V.; Savino, E.; Tralongo, P.; Randazzo, C.L.; Berretta, M. B-glucans from Grifola frondosa and Ganoderma lucidum in breast cancer: An example of complementary and integrative medicine. *Oncotarget* **2018**, *9*, 24837–24856. [CrossRef] [PubMed]
34. Wasser, S.P. Medicinal mushrooms in human clinical studies. Part I. anticancer, oncoimmunological, and immunomodulatory activities: A review. *Int. J. Med. Mush.* **2017**, *19*, 279–317. [CrossRef]
35. Blagodatski, A.; Yatsunskaya, M.; Mikhailova, V.; Tiasto, V.; Kagansky, A.; Katanaev, V.L. Medicinal mushrooms as an attractive new source of natural compounds for future cancer therapy. *Oncotarget* **2018**, *9*, 29259–29274. [CrossRef] [PubMed]
36. Roda, E.; De Luca, F.; Di Iorio, C.; Ratto, D.; Siciliani, S.; Ferrari, B.; Cobelli, F.; Borsci, G.; Priori, E.C.; Chinosi, S.; et al. Novel medicinal mushroom blend as a promising supplement in integrative oncology: A multi-tiered study using 4t1 triple-negative mouse breast cancer model. *Int. J. Mol. Sci.* **2020**, *21*, 3479. [CrossRef]
37. Zmitrovich, I.V.; Belova, N.V.; Balandaykin, M.E.; Bondartseva, M.A.; Wasser, S.P. Cancer without Pharmacological Illusions and a Niche for Mycotherapy (Review). *Int. J. Med. Mush.* **2019**, *21*, 105–119. [CrossRef]
38. Bechtel, P.E.; Hickey, R.J.; Schnaper, L.; Sekowski, J.W.; Long, B.J.; Freund, R.; Liu, N.; Rodriguez-Valenzuela, C.; Malkas, L.H. A Unique Form of Proliferating Cell Nuclear Antigen Is Present in Malignant Breast Cells. *Cancer Res.* **1998**, *58*, 3264–3269.
39. Malkas, L.H.; Herbert, B.S.; Abdel-Aziz, W.; Dobrolecki, L.E.; Liu, Y.; Agarwal, B.; Hoelz, D.; Badve, S.; Schnaper, L.; Arnold, R.J.; et al. A cancer-associated PCNA expressed in breast cancer has implications as a potential biomarker. *Proc. Natl. Acad. Sci. USA* **2006**, *103*, 19472–19477. [CrossRef]
40. Coccini, T.; Manzo, L.; Roda, E. Safety Evaluation of Engineered Nanomaterials for Health Risk Assessment: An Experimental Tiered Testing Approach Using Pristine and Functionalized Carbon Nanotubes. *ISRN Toxicol.* **2013**, *2013*, 825427. [CrossRef]
41. Baghban, R.; Roshangar, L.; Jahanban-Esfahlan, R.; Seidi, K.; Ebrahimi-Kalan, A.; Jaymand, M.; Kolahian, S.; Javaheri, T.; Zare, P. Tumor microenvironment complexity and therapeutic implications at a glance. *Cell Commun. Signal.* **2020**, *18*, 59. [CrossRef]
42. Liu, Z.; Ding, Y.; Ye, N.; Wild, C.; Chen, H.; Zhou, J. Direct Activation of Bax Protein for Cancer Therapy. *Med. Res. Rev.* **2016**, *36*, 313–341. [CrossRef] [PubMed]
43. Wong, R.S. Apoptosis in cancer: From pathogenesis to treatment. *J. Exp. Clin. Cancer Res.* **2011**, *30*, 87. [CrossRef] [PubMed]
44. Yaacoub, K.; Pedeux, R.; Tarte, K.; Guillaudeux, T. Role of the tumor microenvironment in regulating apoptosis and cancer progression. *Cancer Lett.* **2016**, *378*, 150–159. [CrossRef] [PubMed]
45. Oltval, Z.N.; Milliman, C.L.; Korsmeyer, S.J. Bcl-2 heterodimerizes in vivo with a conserved homolog, Bax, that accelerates programed cell death. *Cell* **1993**, *74*, 609–619. [CrossRef]
46. Bodrug, S.E.; Aimé-Sempé, C.; Sato, T.; Krajewski, S.; Hanada, M.; Reed, J.C. Biochemical and functional comparisons of Mcl-1 and Bcl-2 proteins: Evidence for a novel mechanism of regulating Bcl-2 family protein function. *Cell Death Diff.* **1995**, *2*, 173–182.
47. Teixeira, C.; Reed, J.C.; Pratt, M.A. Estrogen promotes chemotherapeutic drug resistance by a mechanism involving Bcl-2 proto-oncogene expression in human breast cancer cells. *Cancer Res.* **1995**, *55*, 3902–3907.
48. Qiu, X.; Mei, J.; Yin, J.; Wang, H.; Wang, J.; Xie, M. Correlation analysis between expression of PCNA, Ki-67 and COX-2 and X-ray features in mammography in breast cancer. *Oncol. Lett.* **2017**, *14*, 2912–2918. [CrossRef]
49. Roda, E.; Bottone, M.; Biggiogera, M.; Milanesi, G.; Coccini, T. Pulmonary and hepatic effects after low dose exposure to nanosilver: Early and long-lasting histological and ultrastructural alterations in rat. *Toxicol. Rep.* **2019**, *6*, 1047–1060. [CrossRef]

9

Protective Effect of Cashew Gum (*Anacardium occidentale* L.) on 5-Fluorouracil-Induced Intestinal Mucositis

João Antônio Leal de Miranda [1,2,*], João Erivan Façanha Barreto [1], Dainesy Santos Martins [1], Paulo Vitor de Souza Pimentel [1], Deiziane Viana da Silva Costa [1], Reyca Rodrigues e Silva [2], Luan Kelves Miranda de Souza [2], Camila Nayane de Carvalho Lima [3], Jefferson Almeida Rocha [4], Ana Paula Fragoso de Freitas [1], Durcilene Alves da Silva [2], Ariel Gustavo Scafuri [1], Renata Ferreira de Carvalho Leitão [1], Gerly Anne de Castro Brito [1], Jand Venes Rolim Medeiros [2] and Gilberto Santos Cerqueira [1,2]

1 Department of Morphology, Faculty of Medicine, Federal University of Ceará, s/n Delmiro de Farias Street, Porangabuçu Campus, Fortaleza 60416-030, Brazil; erivanfacanha@yahoo.com.br (J.E.F.B.); dainy.santos@gmail.com (D.S.M.); paulo_vitordesouza@hotmail.com (P.V.d.S.P.); deiziane2009@gmail.com (D.V.d.S.C.); paulinhaff2@hotmail.com (A.P.F.d.F.); urologia@gmail.com (A.G.S.); leitao_renata@yahoo.com.br (R.F.d.C.L.); gerlybrito@hotmail.com (G.A.d.C.B.); giufarmacia@hotmail.com (G.S.C.)

2 Biotechnology and Biodiversity Center Research, BIOTEC, Federal University of Piauí, Parnaíba, Piauí 64202-020, Brazil; reyca_14@hotmail.com (R.R.e.S.); luankelves11@gmail.com (L.K.M.d.S.); durcileneas@yahoo.com.br (D.A.d.S.); jandvenes@ufpi.edu.br (J.V.R.M.)

3 Nucleus of Research and Development of Medications (NPDM), Federal University of Ceará, Coronel Nunes de Melo Street, 100, Fortaleza 60430-275, Brazil; camilacarvalhoenf@yahoo.com.br

4 Research Group in Natural Sciences and Biotechnology, Federal University of Maranhão, s/n Avenue Aurila Maria Santos Barros de Sousa, Frei Alberto Beretta, Grajaú-MA 65940-000, Brazil; jeffersonkalel@hotmail.com

* Correspondence: joaoantonio@ufpi.edu.br;

Abstract: Intestinal mucositis is a common complication associated with 5-fluorouracil (5-FU), a chemotherapeutic agent used for cancer treatment. Cashew gum (CG) has been reported as a potent anti-inflammatory agent. In the present study, we aimed to evaluate the effect of CG extracted from the exudate of *Anacardium occidentale* L. on experimental intestinal mucositis induced by 5-FU. Swiss mice were randomly divided into seven groups: Saline, 5-FU, CG 30, CG 60, CG 90, Celecoxib (CLX), and CLX + CG 90 groups. The weight of mice was measured daily. After treatment, the animals were euthanized and segments of the small intestine were collected to evaluate histopathological alterations (morphometric analysis), levels of malondialdehyde (MDA), myeloperoxidase (MPO), and glutathione (GSH), and immunohistochemical analysis of interleukin 1 beta (IL-1β) and cyclooxygenase-2 (COX-2). 5-FU induced intense weight loss and reduction in villus height compared to the saline group. CG 90 prevented 5-FU-induced histopathological changes and decreased oxidative stress through decrease of MDA levels and increase of GSH concentration. CG attenuated inflammatory process by decreasing MPO activity, intestinal mastocytosis, and COX-2 expression. Our findings suggest that CG at a concentration of 90 mg/kg reverses the effects of 5-FU-induced intestinal mucositis.

Keywords: intestinal mucositis; heteropolysaccharide; 5-fluorouracil; inflammation

1. Introduction

Cancer, a complex disease characterized by uncontrolled cell growth, is one of the main causes of morbidity and mortality in both developed and developing countries [1–3]. Chemotherapeutic agents can controlled the dissemination of several tumors and improve the quality of life in most patients with cancer. Currently, 5-fluorouracil (5-FU) is one of the major chemotherapeutic agents used for the treatment of cancer. 5-FU is a fluorinated pyrimidine with antimetabolite activity. However, it can cause side effects such as nausea, vomiting, diarrhea, myelosuppression, and intestinal mucositis [4–9].

Mucositis is initiated by basal cell lesions in the gastrointestinal tract, resulting in mucosal damage, intense inflammatory reaction, and consequent ulceration. It affects around 40% of patients treated with chemotherapeutic agents [10,11]. Intestinal mucositis can increase the risk of bacterial translocation and sepsis, thus impairing the continuity of anticancer treatment.

Owing to the lack of efficacious therapeutic tools for the treatment of intestinal mucositis, new alternative therapeutics that can reduce the side effects of 5-FU, without impairing cancer treatment, have been investigated.

Cashew gum (CG), a high-molecular weight complex heteropolysaccharide, is obtained from the exudate of cashew tree (*Anacardium occidentale* L.) through condensation of a large number of aldose and ketose molecules [12,13]. Its anti-inflammatory, antiulcerogenic, and antidiarrheal activity have been reported in previous studies [14–17]. In this study, we investigated the effect of CG on 5-FU-induced experimental intestinal mucositis. In addition, we evaluated its effect on inflammatory process and oxidative stress, as well as the involvement of cyclooxygenase 2 (COX-2).

2. Results

2.1. Weight Analysis

As expected, from the second day, all mice subjected to 5-FU-induced intestinal mucositis presented progressive weight loss, which was significant compared to the saline group ($p < 0.05$). Notably, only CG 60 pretreatment prevented weight loss induced by 5-FU ($p < 0.05$). CG 30 and CG 90 were unable to reverse 5-FU-induced weight loss (Figure 1).

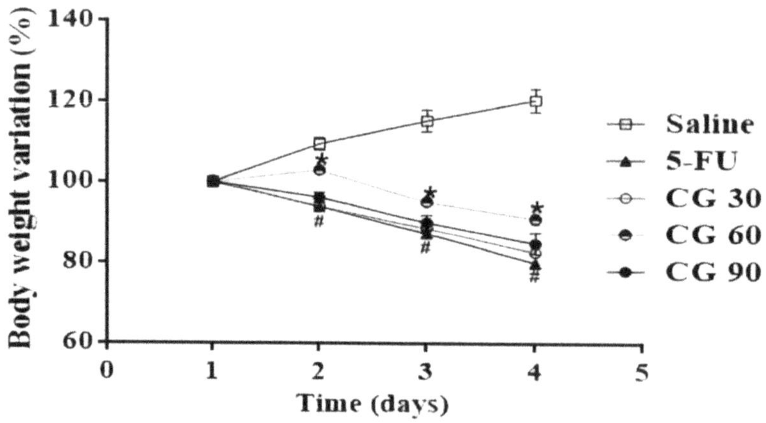

Figure 1. Body weight variation in mice subjected to intestinal mucositis (5-FU, 450 mg/kg, ip, single dose) and treated with CG (30, 60 and 90 mg/kg for 4 days). The results are expressed as the mean ± SEM of the weight evaluation percentage of the initial weight, of a minimum of 6 animals per group. Two-way ANOVA followed by the Tukey's test were used for the statistical analysis, where # $p < 0.05$ vs. saline and * $p < 0.05$ vs. 5-FU.

2.2. Histopathological and Morphometric Analysis

The 5-FU group showed intense inflammatory cell infiltration, disruption of intestinal mucosal architecture, and a significant reduction in villus height, crypt depth, and villus/crypt ratio compared to saline group ($p < 0.05$) (Figure 2B). Notably, all doses of CG attenuated the effects induced by 5-FU ($p < 0.05$) (Figure 2C–H). Moreover, a significant increase in histopathological scores was found in 5-FU group ($p < 0.05$) compared to the saline group (Table 1). CG 90 pretreatment decreased the histopathological scores compared to the 5-FU group ($p < 0.05$). However, CG 30 and CG 60 pretreatment did not reduce histopathological scores.

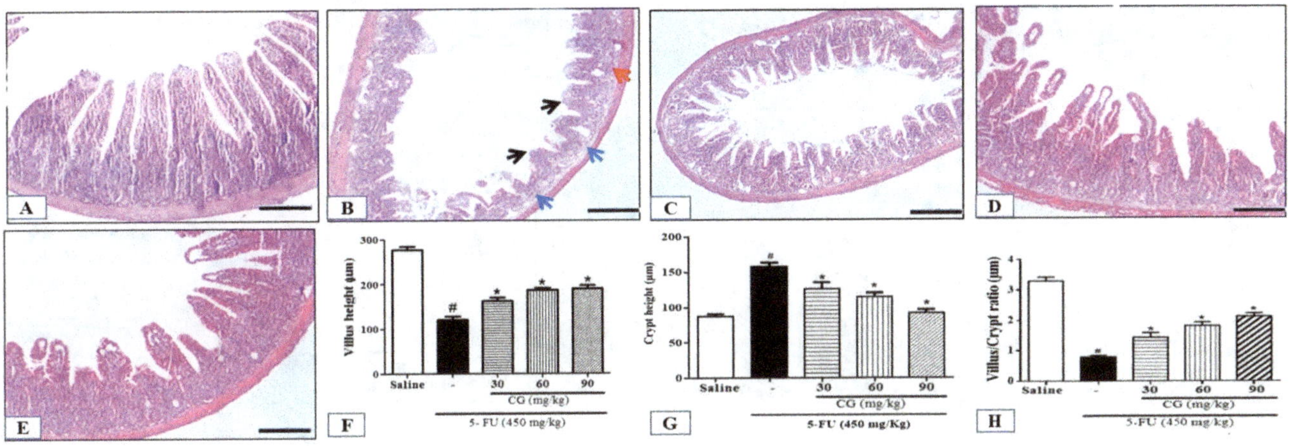

Figure 2. Histopathological analysis. (**A**) Saline; (**B**) 5-FU; (**C**) CG 30; (**D**) CG 60; (**E**) CG 90. 5 FU induced inflammatory cell infiltrate (red arrow), decreased intestinal villi (black arrow), loss of intestinal crypt architecture (blue arrow). Pretreatment with CG (30, 60 and 90 mg/kg) decreased the inflammatory infiltrate and prevented the shortening of the villi (**F**), increased crypt depth (**G**) and decreased villus/crypt ratio (**H**), with greater reversion of the 5-FU effect in the CG 90 + 5-FU group. All panels were obtained on the 100 µm scale (×200). Values were expressed as mean ± SEM. One-way ANOVA followed by the Tukey's test were used for the statistical analysis was used, where # $p < 0.05$ vs. saline group and * $p < 0.05$ vs. group 5-FU.

Table 1. Histopathological scores of mice subjected to 5-FU-induced intestinal mucositis and pretreated with CG.

Groups	Scores
Saline	0 (0-0)
5-FU	2 (1-3) #
CG 30	3 (3-3)
CG 60	1 (1-2)
CG 90	1 (0-1) *

Values were expressed as median, where # $p < 0.05$ vs. saline and * $p < 0.05$ vs. 5-FU ($n = 6$/group). The data was analyzed by the Kruskal-Wallis test followed by the Dunns multiple comparisons test.

2.3. Leukocyte Count

Analysis of leukocyte count in blood showed a significant decrease ($p < 0.05$) in the number of total leukocytes in 5-FU group compared to that in the saline group. In contrast, CG pretreatment reduced 5-FU-induced leukopenia ($p < 0.05$) (Figure 3A).

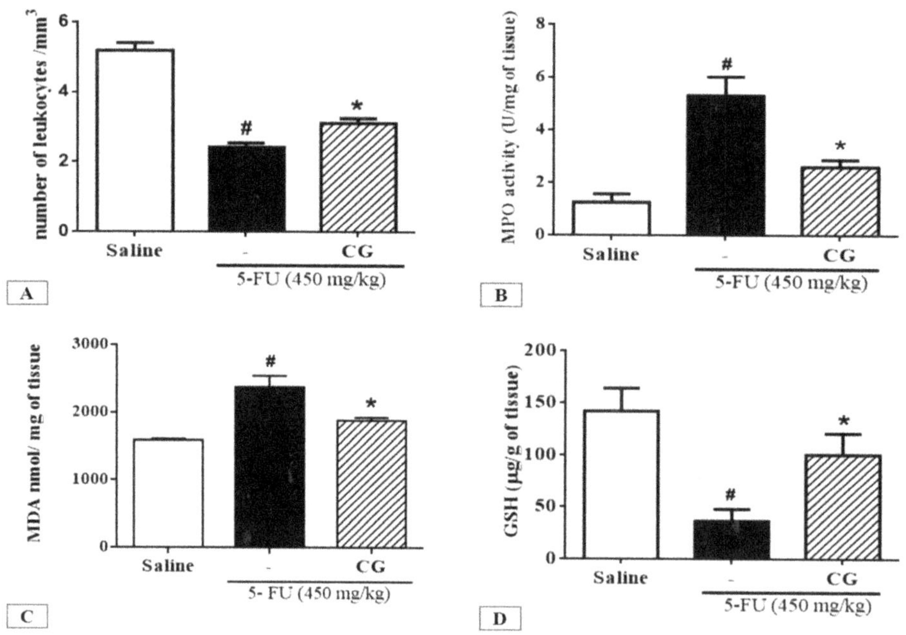

Figure 3. (**A**) Total leukocyte count; (**B**) Activity of myeloperoxidase (MPO); (**C**) Level of malondialdehyde (MDA); (**D**) concentration of glutathione (GSH). Values were presented as mean ± SEM. For the statistical analysis, one-way ANOVA followed by Tukey's test was used, where # $p < 0.05$ vs. saline group and * $p < 0.05$ vs. group 5-FU.

2.4. Myeloperoxidase Assay (MPO)

To investigate the effects of CG pretreatment on neutrophil recruitment in 5-FU-induced intestinal mucositis, we determined the activity of myeloperoxidase (MPO), a neutrophil marker. The 5-FU group presented a significant increase in MPO levels in the duodenum compared to the saline group ($p < 0.05$). CG (90 mg/kg) pretreatment decreased MPO levels in the duodenum of mice subjected to 5-FU-induced intestinal mucositis ($p < 0.05$), which in turn decreased polymorphonuclear leukocyte infiltration (Figure 3B).

2.5. Malondialdehyde (MDA) and Glutathione (GSH) Levels

To investigate the effect of CG pretreatment on 5-FU-induced oxidative stress in the duodenum, MDA and GSH levels (end products of oxidative stress) were evaluated. We found that 5-FU elevated MDA levels in the duodenum compared to the saline group (Figure 3C). CG (90 mg/kg) pretreatment reduced MDA levels compared to the 5-FU group ($p < 0.05$), thereby reducing 5-FU-induced oxidative stress (Figure 3C). Animals treated with 5-FU showed a significant ($p < 0.05$) decrease in GSH levels compared to the saline group. In contrast, CG (90 mg/kg) increased GSH levels compared to the 5- FU group ($p < 0.05$) (Figure 3D).

2.6. Mast Cell Concentration Analysis

To evaluate the effect of CG pretreatment on 5-FU-induced mastocytosis, the number of mast cells in the duodenum was measured. 5-FU (Figure 4B) increased the number of mast cells per field in the duodenum compared to the saline group (Figure 4A) ($p < 0.05$). CG (90 mg/kg) pretreatment (Figure 4C) decreased the number of mast cells compared to the 5-FU group ($p < 0.05$) (Figure 4D).

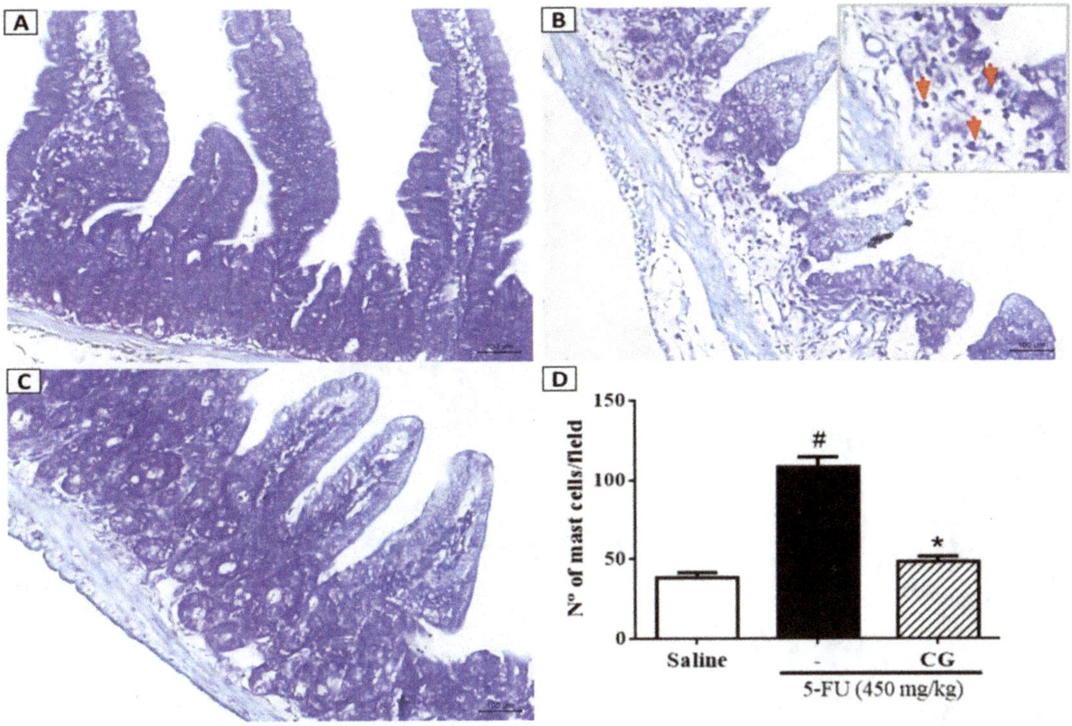

Figure 4. Mast cell counts in the duodenum samples. In (**B**) demonstrates that 5-FU promoted increased mast cell counts (red arrows) when compared to saline group (**A**). CG 90 (**C**) reversed the 5-FU-induced mastocytosis. All the panels were obtained at ×400 magnification. (**D**) Values were presented as mean ± SEM of the number of mast cells per field. For the statistical analysis, tone-way ANOVA followed by Tukey's test was used, where # p <0.05 vs. saline group and * $p < 0.05$ vs. group 5-FU.

2.7. *Effect of CG on Cyclooxygenase-2 Pathway in Histopathological and Morphometric Analyses*

To investigate whether the effects of CG on reduction of 5-FU-induced intestinal injury, oxidative stress, and inflammation are mediated by cyclooxygenase-2 (COX-2) pathway, we blocked COX-2 by injecting celecoxib (CLX) in the presence or absence of CG in mice subjected to 5-FU-induced intestinal mucositis. Pretreatment with COX-2 blocker (CLX) (Figure 5D), as well as pretreatment with the combination of CLX and CG (90 mg/kg) (Figure 5E) prevented 5-FU-induced shortening of villus, cellular vacuolization, infiltration of inflammatory cells, edema, and loss of cellular architecture (Figure 5B).

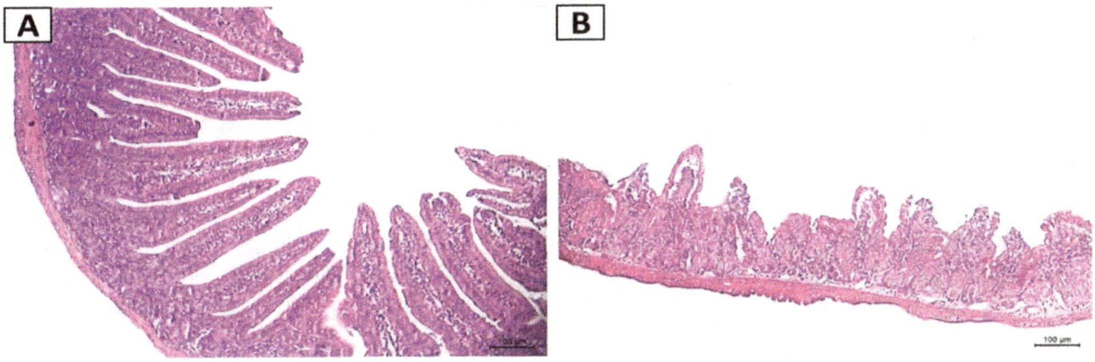

Figure 5. *Cont.*

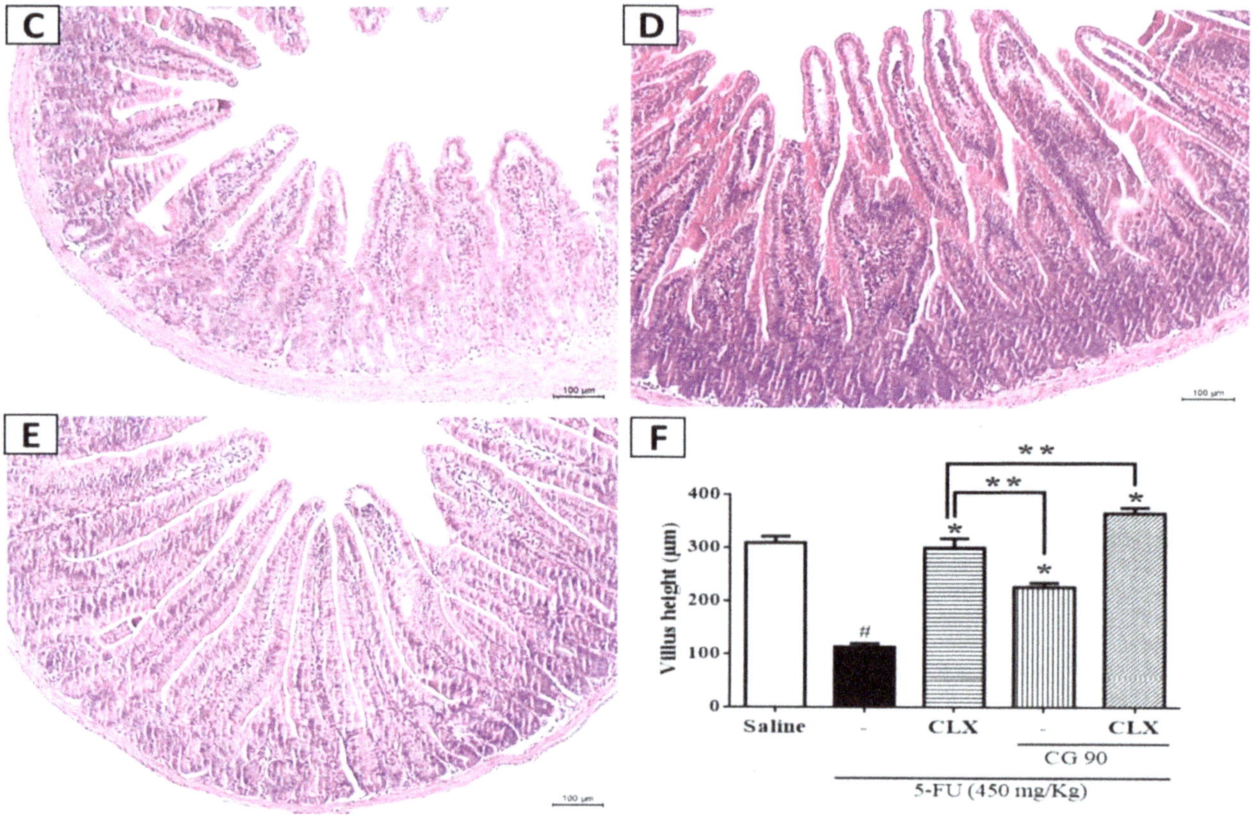

Figure 5. Effect of GC on the cyclooxygenase-2 pathway (COX-2) in histopathological and morphometric. The histopathological analysis represented by the groups (**A**) Saline; (**B**) 5-FU; (**C**) CG 90; (**D**) Celecoxib (CLX); (**E**) CLX and CG 90, as well as morphometric analysis of villus height (**F**) showed that 5-FU caused a decrease in villi and loss of cellular architecture when compared to the saline group. C, D, and E reversed the effect of 5-FU. All panels were obtained at ×200 magnification. Values were expressed as mean ± SEM for villi height in µm. For statistical analysis, one-way ANOVA followed by Tukey's test was used, where # $p < 0.05$ vs. saline group, * $p < 0.05$ vs. group 5-FU, ** $p < 0.05$ vs. group CLX.

CLX pretreatment decreased 5-FU-induced villus shortening ($p < 0.05$). In addition, pretreatment with the combination of CLX and CG (90 mg/kg) reverted villus shortening induced by 5-FU ($p < 0.05$). Moreover, the combination of CLX and CG (90 mg/kg) (Figure 5F) showed a greater effect on the recovery of duodenal villus in mice subjected to 5-FU-induced intestinal mucositis than pretreatment with CG 90 (Figure 5C) or CLX alone (Figure 5C) ($p < 0.05$).

2.8. *Immunohistochemistry for the Detection of COX-2 and IL-1β*

We investigated the effects of CG (90 mg/kg) in the presence or absence of CLX on COX-2 and IL-1β expression during 5-FU-induced intestinal mucositis through immunohistochemical analysis. 5-FU promoted intense immunostaining of COX-2 (Figure 6C) and IL-1β (Figure 6D) in the duodenal mucosa compared to the saline group (Figure 6A,B,K,L, $p < 0.05$). As shown in Figure 6E,F CG (90 mg/kg) pretreatment decreased immunostaining for COX-2 and IL-1β, respectively, compared to 5-FU group (Figure 6K,L, $p < 0.05$). Similarly, CLX alone (Figure 6G,H) or the combination of CLX and CG (90 mg/kg) (Figure 6I,J) decreased cell immunostaining forproinflammatory molecules in mice subjected to 5-FU-induced intestinal mucositis compared to the 5-FU group (Figure 6K,L, $p < 0.05$). Intense immunostaining was evidenced for the 5-FU lesion group, on the lamina followed by mild mucosal immunostaining, also was observed an absence of labeling in the epithelial cells.

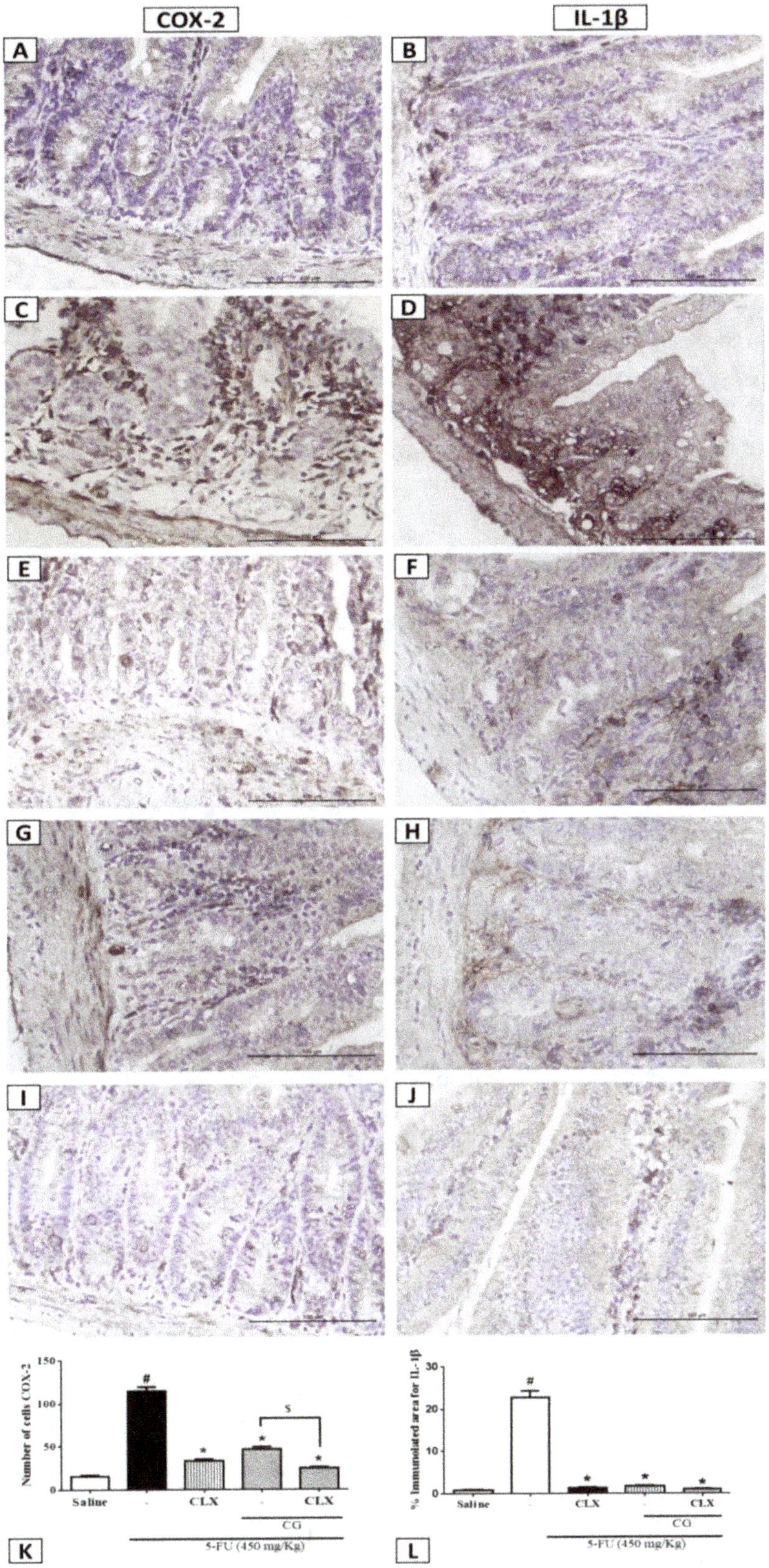

Figure 6. Immunohistochemistry analysis for COX-2 and IL-1β. (**A**,**B**) Saline; (**C**,**D**) 5-FU; (**E**,**F**) CLX; (**G**,**H**) CG 90; (**I**,**J**) CLX + CG 90. (**K**) a number of cells immunolabelled for cox-2. (**L**) % immunolabelled for IL-1β. Values were expressed as mean ± SEM. For statistical analysis, one-way ANOVA followed by Tukey´s test was used, where # $p < 0.05$ vs. saline group, * $p < 0.05$ vs. group 5-FU, $ $p < 0.05$ vs. group CLX.

3. Discussion

In the present study, we evaluated the effects of CG on intestinal mucositis induced by 5-FU and found that CG reversed the effects of 5-FU-induced intestinal mucositis at a concentration of 90 mg/kg. With the continuous expanded use of medicinal plants for the prevention and treatment of different pathologies worldwide, there has been increasing interest in the discovery of natural products with pharmacological effects. In Brazil, many herbal extracts are used in folk medicine to treat various digestive disorders, and several studies have documented the benefits of Brazilian plants in the prevention of gastrointestinal lesions [18,19].

A previous study reported that the extract of *Spondias pinnata,* belonging to the family Anacardiaceae, decreased histological severity scores and intestinal inflammation, and altered the mucosal architecture after chemotherapy. This indicated that *S. pinnata* extract could be an important pharmacological agent in promoting healing of damaged intestine after chemotherapy [20]. *A. occidentale* L. has been reported to possess diverse pharmacological properties. Its bark, leaves, and bark oil are used in anti-inflammatory and astringent preparations for the treatment of diarrhea [21]. Previous studies using the extracts of cashew tree bark have reported hypoglycemic [22,23], antioxidant and anti-inflammatory [24], antimicrobial [25], antihypertensive [26], and anticancer effects. It also showed beneficial effects in the treatment of gastritis, diarrhea, and wounds [22,27]. The anti-inflammatory activities and wound healing potential of cashew nuts have also been reported [28].

Weight loss is considered one of the common side effects of 5-FU chemotherapy. Therefore, body mass measure is one of the daily evaluated parameters to confirm the model of intestinal mucositis induced by 5-FU. Similar to our results, previous studies showed a decrease in body weight of animals after 5-FU-induced intestinal mucositis [29–31]. In this study, we showed that CG 60mg/kg decreased 5-FU-induced weight loss in mice, instead of the other CG doses which the loss weight was irreversible. Studies with probiotics and olmesartan showed that doses of these drugs were considered effective in reversing the harmful effects promoted by chemotherapy in mucositis model, after evaluation of histopathological parameters and inflammatory markers, however they were not effective in reverse weight loss as presented in ours studies [32,33].

Previous studies reported that 5-FU promoted decrease and vacuolization of intestinal villi, cryptic necrosis, infiltration of inflammatory cells, loss of cell architecture, and a decrease in villus/crypt ratio [34–37]. These findings are consistent with those of the present study. In addition, we found that CG at a concentration of 90 mg/kg was able to reduce the harmful effects of 5-FU on the duodenal mucosa. The anti-inflammatory effect of CG has been reported in skin lesions [15]. Araújo et al. [17] reported that 90 and 60 mg/kg of CG were effective in the treatment of acute inflammatory diarrhea. Similarly, 90 mg/kg was the best treatment concentration to prevent histopathological changes in 5-FU-induced intestinal mucositis.

Mucositis and myelosuppression are the main adverse effects related to 5-FU treatment [7,9,38]. In the present study, we showed that CG (90 mg/kg) attenuated leukopenia, the decrease in a number of total leukocytes, induced by 5-FU. Soares et al. [39] and Quaresma [40] demonstrated leukopenia in mice following a single administration of 5-FU (450 mg/kg).

The ulcerative phase of mucositis is characterized by loss of epithelial integrity of the mucosa, which facilitates a propitious environment for the invasion of bacteria. In addition, leucopenia may potentialize this process, resulting in bacteremia or sepsis [11,41,42]. We suggested that CG can be fundamental in preventing potential generalized bacterial infections during 5-FU treatment because it attenuated 5-FU-induced leukopenia. However, further investigations are needed to confirm this.

CG 90 prevented a 5-FU-induced increase in MPO levels in the duodenum. Similar to the present study, Bastos et al. [43], Justino et al. [44], Ávila et al. [45], Al-Asmari et al. [46], and Carvalho et al. [30]

showed an increase in MPO activity after induction of intestinal mucositis by 5-FU. MPO has been used as a quantitative marker of neutrophil infiltration into various organs, including the gastrointestinal tract.

We showed that CG exerted antioxidant effects against intestinal mucositis by increasing GSH levels and decreasing MDA levels in the duodenum of mice subjected to 5-FU-induced intestinal mucositis. This finding is in agreement with the result of a previous study demonstrating that CG formulations exerted an antioxidant effect by decreasing MDA levels [47].

Our findings showed that CG reversed 5-FU-induced mastocytosis (increase in a number of mast cells) in the duodenum, indicating potent anti-inflammatory effects of CG in mice with 5-FU-induced intestinal mucositis. Previous studies have shown intense mastocytosis during intestinal mucositis induced by chemotherapeutics in mice [46,48]. The role of mast cells in the gastrointestinal tract is paradoxical, as their function depends on the mediators released and receptors activated. Mast cells contribute to intestinal homeostasis through immune protection, regulation of architecture and permeability of the epithelial barrier, and mucosal tissue remodeling through stimulation of fibroblast growth [49]. However, they are considered critical in the pathogenesis of inflammatory processes such as mucositis, because their overexpression consequently leads to amplification of inflammatory response caused by the selective release of mediators [50,51]. Besides exacerbation of inflammation, mastocytosis in the gastrointestinal tract has been reported to culminate in alteration of architecture and impairment of the gastrointestinal barrier, such as villus enlargement and changes in crypt size in the small intestine [52,53].

In the present study, we evaluated the effect of CG on COX-2 pathway by pretreating mice subjected to intestinal mucositis with a combination of CLX (a COX-2 blocker) and CG (90 mg/kg). In addition, we investigated whether the protective effect of CG on morphometric and histopathological changes induced by 5-FU was related to COX-2 inhibition. We found that the combination of CLX and CG (90 mg/kg) completely reverted 5-FU-induced decrease in villi, cryptic necrosis, inflammatory cell infiltration, and loss of cellular architecture in the duodenum. Our findings demonstrated that pretreatment with the combination of CG and CLX during 5-FU-induced intestinal mucositis was more effective in reversing histopathological effects than treatment with CLX alone, a commercially available nonsteroidal anti-inflammatory drug that acts as a selective inhibitor of COX-2. Short et al. [54] suggested that low doses of CLX can be used therapeutically for the protection of the intestinal barrier in patients with inflammatory bowel disorders, because of its ability to reduce COX-2 expression. Javle et al. [55] found that the combination of irinotecan (CPT-11) and CLX resulted in antitumor effects, with improvement in irinotecan-induced diarrhea and lethality. Furthermore, CG (90 mg/kg) alone or in combination with CLX was able to decrease 5-FU-induced COX-2 and IL-1β immunostaining in the duodenum. It is known that IL-1β is produced by macrophages, monocytes, and glial cells. This proinflammatory cytokine induces the expression of inflammatory mediators, such as COX-2 with subsequent release of prostaglandins, and the onset of primary tissue damage and progression [56–58]. The gene expression and tissue levels of IL-1β are correlated with intestinal mucosal injury induced by chemotherapy [59].

The study and use of natural polysaccharides in inflammatory bowel diseases, especially mucositis, is a current reality and future promise for the development of effective drugs in the treatment of 5-FU-induced intestinal mucositis. The present study has however a limitation. As intestinal inflammation is a complex process involving multiple mechanisms of activation and maintenance of the inflammatory process, the hypothetical model of action of CG on 5-FU-induced intestinal mucositis in mice proposed using the results of the present study (Figure 7) may be inadequate. Further studies are needed to elucidate the other possible mechanisms of CG action in intestinal mucositis.

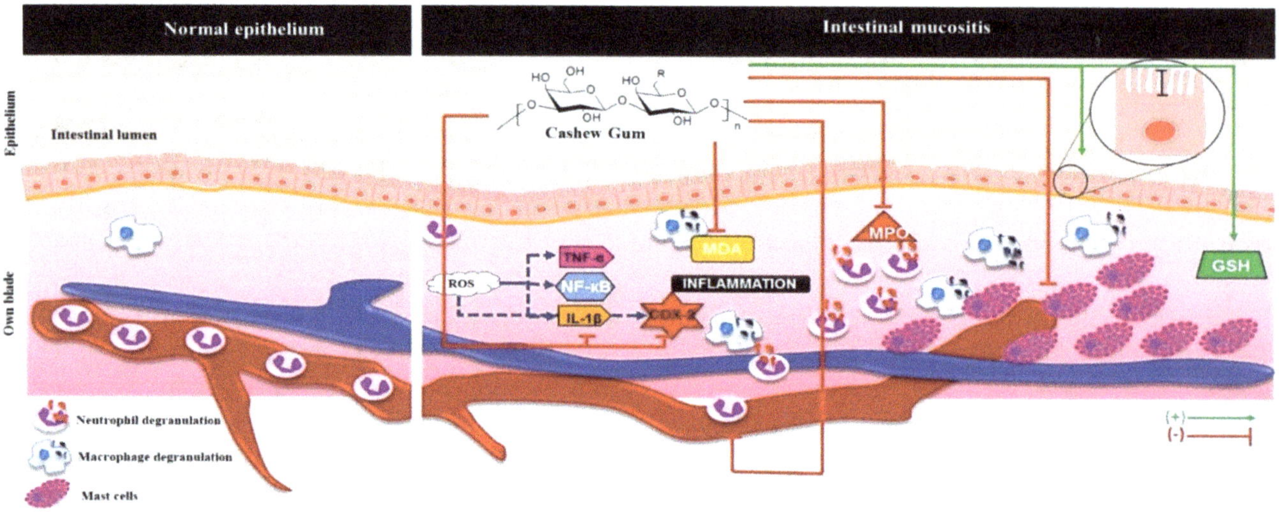

Figure 7. Hypothetical model of action of CG in intestinal mucositis induced by 5-FU. CG prevented the 5-FU-induced injury intestinal through inhibition of MDA formation, neutrophil recruitment (decreasing MPO levels), mast cells activation and IL-1β and COX-2 immunostaining marker and inhibited leucopenia. CG also stimulate villus enlargement and increase levels of GSH, an antioxidant. ROS: Reactive Oxygen Species; TNF-α: Tumor Necrosis Factor-alpha; NF-κB: transcription factor nuclear kappa b; IL-1β: Interleukin 1 beta; COX-2: Cyclooxygenase 2; MDA: Malondialdehyde; MPO: Myeloperoxidase; GSH: Reduced glutathione. Arrows green (stimulate / increase), red arrows (inhibit).

4. Materials and Methods

4.1. Animals

The animals were obtained from the Department of Surgery of the Federal University of Ceara (UFC) were used. The male Swiss mice (25–30 g) were housed in polypropylene cages, lined with wood, in a controlled environment with a temperature of 23 ± 2 °C, in a cycle of 12 h light/12 h dark, with free access to water and standard feed. The procedures and experimental protocols were approved by the Ethics Committee on Animal Use (n° 208/16) from the Federal University of Piaui (CEUA/UFPI).

4.2. Drugs and Plant Materials

Two drug drugs were used for mucositis induction and treatment, respectively: 5-FU (FauldFluor®, Libbs, Sao Paulo, Brazil) celecoxib (CLX- Celebra®, Pfizer, Sao Paulo, Brazil). Raw samples of CG were collected in 2013 by the Biotechnology and Biodiversity Center Research–BIOTEC, Parnaíba, Brazil, from the trunk of native cashew trees (*A. occidentale* L.) in Ilha Grande de Santa Isabel, Piauí, Brazil (Latitude, decimal degrees S-2.8242; Longitude, decimal degrees W-41.7331). The tree was identified and a voucher specimen, voucher number 52, was deposited at the HDELTA herbarium (Federal University of Piauí, Parnaíba, Piauí, Brazil).

4.3. Extraction and Purification of Cashew Gum

The CG was purified with sodium salt, as previously described [60]. Bark free nodules were selected and dissolved at a final concentration of 5% (*w*/*v*) in distilled water. The pH of the solution was adjusted to approximately 7.0. The clear solution was successively filtered through sintered glass and the heteropolysaccharide was precipitated with ethanol [61,62].

4.4. Induction of Experimental Intestinal Mucositis

The experimental intestinal mucositis model in Swiss Mice was induced as described by Soares et al. [39]. The 5-FU (450 mg/kg) was given intraperitoneally (i.p) in a single dose on the first day of the experimental protocol. Three days of treatment with CG were performed. The mice were pretreated daily with oral CG (30, 60, 90 mg/kg), 1h before the injection of 5- FU, after then the same oral doses were performed once a day. After four days of treatment, the animals were euthanized by ketamine (270 mg/kg) and xylazine (15 mg/kg) and the intestinal samples were collected. The body weight of mice was measured daily before the treatment administered to confirm the experimental model of intestinal mucositis induced by 5-FU. In this study, the mice was randomly allocated in seven groups (n = 6): Saline (NaCl 0.9%), 5-FU (5-FU + NaCl 0.9%), CG 30 (5-FU + CG 30 mg/kg), CG 60 (5-FU + CG 60 mg/kg), CG 90 (5-FU + CG 90 mg/kg), CLX (5-FU + celecoxib 7.5 mg/kg, i.p), CLX + CG 90 (5-FU + celecoxib 7.5 mg/kg, i.p + CG 90 mg/kg). To investigate the participation of COX-2 on the effects of treatment with CG during intestinal mucositis induced by 5-FU, COX-2 was blocked by celecoxib in an independent experiment. The mice were treated with celecoxib and CG 90 in combination or alone for three days.

4.5. Histopathological and Morphometric Analysis

After euthanasia, duodenum samples were obtained and fixed in 10% formaldehyde for performing the histopathological and morphometric analysis [63,64]. These samples were embedded in paraffin, sectioned at 4 μm and stained with hematoxylin and eosin (H&E). A blinded and randomized histopathological analysis was performed by an experienced histopathologist to assess the severity of mucositis using a scores system [65], the tissues were ranging from 0 (absence of lesion/normal histological findings) to 3 (maximum lesion degree), indicating shortened villi with vacuolized cells, necrosis of crypts, intense infiltration of inflammatory cells, vacuolization and edema in the mucosal layer and muscular layer with edema, vacuolization and neutrophil infiltrate. The effective concentration of CG in the treatment of mucositis was determined following the histological analysis.

4.6. Leukocyte Count

Mice were anesthetized with a combination of anesthetics (xylazine 10m/kg and ketamine 80 mg/kg) and, a peripheral blood sample was collected from the ocular artery, and was diluted in the liquid of Turk at a ratio of 20 μL of blood to 380 μL of solution. The total leukocytes were counted using a Neubauer chamber [66], and the results were expressed as a total number of leukocytes per mm3 of blood.

4.7. Dosage of Malondialdehyde (MDA)

The MDA is a product of lipid peroxidation frequently used as a marker of oxidative stress. Briefly, the intestinal samples were homogenized (10%) with potassium phosphate buffer (1.15%). Then, were added phosphoric acid (1%) and thiobarbituric acid (0.6%) to the homogenates and incubated at (100 °C, for 45 min) followed by the addition of 1.5 mL n-butanol. The supernatant was obtained and measured after centrifugation (5000 rpm, for 10 min). The results were expressed as nMol of MDA/mg of tissue by 535 nm absorbance measure [67,68].

4.8. Concentration of Glutathione (GSH)

The concentration of GSH in the duodenal samples was performed according to the method described by Sedlak and Lindsay [69]. The levels of nonprotein sulfhydryl groups (NPSH) were determined from 50 to 100 mg of the intestinal mucosa of each animal. The tissues were homogenized in 1 mL of 0.02M EDTA for each sample. Aliquots of 100 μL of the homogenate were mixed with 80 μL of distilled water and 20 μL of 50% trichloroacetic acid (TCA) for precipitation of proteins. The tubes were centrifuged for 15 min at 3000 rpm at 4 °C. A total of 100 μL of the supernatant was added to 200 μL of 0.4 M Tris buffer (pH 8.9) and 5 μL of 0.01 M 5,5-dithiobis-(2-nitrobenzoic acid) (DTNB, Sigma Aldrich, St. Louis, Missouri, USA). The mixture was then homogenate for 3 min and the absorbance was read at 412 nm. Results were expressed as micrograms of NPSH groups per milliliter of homogenate (μg/mL).

4.9. *Myeloperoxidase Assay (MPO)*

MPO activity was determined by the technique described by Bradley et al [70]. Briefly, the duodenum segments (50–100 mg) were homogenized in 1 mL of potassium buffer containing 0.5% hexadecyltrimethylammonium bromide (HTAB), then centrifuged (4000 rpm, 7 min, 4 °C). The MPO activity was analyzed by measuring the absorbance at 450 nm using diisocyanate dihydrochloride and 1% hydrogen peroxide in the resuspended pellet. The results were recorded as MPO units per mg tissue.

4.10. *Mast Cell Analysis*

The paraffin blocks with duodenum samples were processed for toluidine blue staining to identified mast cells, according to Michalany [71]. The slides were deparaffinized with xylene, incubated for 3 min with toluidine blue solution (1 g of toluidine blue dissolved in 70% ethanol), washed three times in distilled water, dehydrated, and mounted. The total number of mast cells were counted manually, considering four specimens per group and ten fields per slide. The results were expressed as the mean of 10 fields in each group.

4.11. *Immunohistochemistry for the Detection of COX-2 and IL-1β*

Duodenal sections were deparaffinized with oven insertion (60 °C) and three cycles of xylol immersion for 5 min each. Then, the sections were rehydrated in decreasing alcohol concentrations (100, 90, 80 and 70%). The histological sections were then washed with distilled water for 10 min and the antigenic recovery in citrate buffer (pH 7.0, DAKO®, Sao Paulo, Brazil) was carried out for 20 min in the water bath (95 °C). The slides were then washed with phosphate-buffered saline solution (PBS) for 5 min at room temperature. Following, endogenous peroxidase blockade with 3% hydrogen peroxide solution (H_2O_2) was performed for 30 min. The sections were then incubated overnight with goat anti-COX-2 primary antibody (SantaCruz®, Dallas, TX, USA), and rabbit anti-IL-1β (SantaCruz®, Dallas, TX, USA) diluted in antibody diluent (1:100) for 60 min, respectively. After the slides were washed with PBS and incubated with rabbit IgG (GBI Labs®, Bothell, WA, USA) secondary antibody diluted (1:400) for 30 min. For revelation, the sections were incubated with the streptavidin conjugated peroxidase complex (ABC complex) for 30 min and chromogen 3,3′diaminobenzidine peroxide, DAB (DAKO®, Sao Paulo, Brazil), followed by counterstaining with hematoxylin (DAKO®, Sao Paulo, Brazil), for 10 min. Negative controls were processed simultaneously as described above, with the primary antibody being replaced for antibody diluent. The procedures were performed in an automated manner using Autostainer Plus (DAKO®, Sao Paulo, Brazil). To assess COX-2 immunostaining, quantification was performed by immunolabelled cells with the aid of Image J software. For IL-1β immunostaining images, quantification was performed by measuring the % immunolabelled area with the aid of Adobe Photoshop 10. All images were captured with the aid of an optical microscope to the image acquisition system (LEICA, Wetzlar, HE, Germany).

4.12. *Statistical Analysis*

Quantitative results were expressed as mean ± standard error of the mean (SEM) and the qualitative data (histological scores) were pointed scores and expressed by the median ± minimum and maximum. The results with a parametric distribution were analyzed by Analysis of Variance (ANOVA) followed by post hoc test Tuckey through the program GraphPad Prism version 6.0 (GraphPad Software Inc., La Jolla, CA, USA). The data obtained from non-parametric distribution were analyzed using Kruskal-Wallis test followed by Dunn's (multiple comparisons). Values of p-value < 0.05 were considered statistically significant.

5. Conclusions

In summary, CG decreased inflammation, oxidative stress, and intestinal injury induced by 5-FU in the duodenum. The effects of CG were found to be related to COX-2 pathway. The concomitant administration of CG and CLX completely reverted COX-2 and IL-1β immunostaining markers and intestinal injury induced by 5-FU. Thus, we suggest that CG has potential application in the development of novel drugs against intestinal mucositis due to antineoplastic agents. Additionally, we recommend further studies to elucidate the molecular mechanisms related to the effects of GC under pro-inflammatory cytokines expression as well as other possible mechanisms of action involved in the protective effect of CG on chemotherapy-induced intestinal mucositis.

Author Contributions: J.A.L.M., L.K.M.S., J.A.R., A.P.F.F., and G.S.C. conceived and designed the experiments; J.A.L.M., J.E.F.B., D.S.M., P.V.S.P., D.V.S.C., R.R.S., C.N.C.L., A.G.S., R.F.C.L., and D.A.S. performed the experiments; J.A.L.M., D.S.M., D.V.S.C., G.A.C.B., J.V.R.M. and G.S.C. analyzed the data; J.A.L.M., R.R.S., D.V.S.C. and G.S.C. wrote the paper.

Acknowledgments: This research was supported by Conselho Nacional de Desenvolvimento Científico e Tecnológico–CNPq, Coordenação de Aperfeiçoamento de Pessoal de Nıvel Superior–CAPES, Fundação Cearense de Apoio ao Desenvolvimento Científico e Tecnológico–FUNCAP. We thank Microscopy and Image Processing Core (NEMPI) at Federal University of Ceará.

References

1. Kumar, V.; Abbas, A.K.; Aster, J.C. *Robbins Basic Pathology E-Book*, 9th ed.; Elsevier Health Sciences: Rio de Janeiro, Brazil, 2013.
2. Ferreira, J.E.V.; de Figueiredo, A.F.; Barbosa, J.P.; Pinheiro, J.C. Chemometric study on molecules with anticancer properties. In *Chemometrics in Practical Applications*; IntechOpen: London, UK, 2012; pp. 185–186.
3. Organization, W.H. Cancer. Available online: http://www.who.int/cancer/en/ (accessed on 17 August 2018).
4. Chang, C.-T.; Ho, T.-Y.; Lin, H.; Liang, J.-A.; Huang, H.-C.; Li, C.-C.; Lo, H.-Y.; Wu, S.-L.; Huang, Y.-F.; Hsiang, C.-Y. 5-Fluorouracil induced intestinal mucositis via nuclear factor-κB activation by transcriptomic analysis and in vivo bioluminescence imaging. *PLoS ONE* **2012**, *7*, e31808. [CrossRef]
5. Udofot, O.; Affram, K.; Bridg'ette Israel, E.A. Cytotoxicity of 5-fluorouracil-loaded pH-sensitive liposomal nanoparticles in colorectal cancer cell lines. *Integr. Cancer Sci. Ther.* **2015**, *2*, 245–252. [CrossRef] [PubMed]
6. Wilhelm, M.; Mueller, L.; Miller, M.C.; Link, K.; Holdenrieder, S.; Bertsch, T.; Kunzmann, V.; Stoetzer, O.J.; Suttmann, I.; Braess, J. Prospective, multicenter study of 5-fluorouracil therapeutic drug monitoring in metastatic colorectal cancer treated in routine clinical practice. *Clin. Colorectal Cancer* **2016**, *15*, 381–388. [CrossRef] [PubMed]
7. Kawashima, R.; Fujimaki, M.; Ikenoue, Y.; Danjo, K.; Koizumi, W.; Ichikawa, T. Influence of an elemental diet on 5-fluorouracil-induced morphological changes in the mouse salivary gland and colon. *Support. Care Cancer* **2016**, *24*, 1609–1616. [CrossRef] [PubMed]
8. Kawashima, R.; Kawakami, F.; Maekawa, T.; Yamamoto, H.; Koizumi, W.; Ichikawa, T. Elemental diet moderates 5-fluorouracil-induced gastrointestinal mucositis through mucus barrier alteration. *Cancer Chemother. Pharmacol.* **2015**, *76*, 269–277. [CrossRef]
9. Kobuchi, S.; Ito, Y.; Sakaeda, T. Population Pharmacokinetic–Pharmacodynamic Modeling of 5-Fluorouracil for Toxicities in Rats. *Eur. J. Drug Metab. Pharmacokinet.* **2017**, *42*, 707–718. [CrossRef]
10. Peterson, D.; Bensadoun, R.-J.; Roila, F.; Group, E.G.W. Management of oral and gastrointestinal mucositis: ESMO Clinical Practice Guidelines. *Ann. Oncol.* **2011**, *22*, 78–84. [CrossRef]
11. Kim, H.J.; Kim, J.H.; Moon, W.; Park, J.; Park, S.J.; Am Song, G.; Han, S.H.; Lee, J.H. Rebamipide attenuates 5-fluorouracil-induced small intestinal mucositis in a mouse model. *Biol. Pharm. Bull.* **2015**, *38*, 179–183. [CrossRef]
12. Ofori-Kwakye, K.; Amekyeh, H.; El-Duah, M.; Kipo, S.L. Mechanical and tablet coating properties of cashew tree (Anacardium occidentale l) gum-based films. *Asian J. Pharm. Clin. Res.* **2012**, *5*, 62–68.
13. Olusola, A.; Toluwalope, G.; Olutayo, O. Carboxymethylation of Anacardium occidentale L. exudate gum: Synthesis and characterization. *Sch. Acad. J. Pharm.* **2014**, *3*, 213–216.

14. Schirato, G.V.; Monteiro, F.M.F.; Silva, F.d.O.; Luís, d.L.F.J.; Leão, A.M.d.A.C.; Porto, A.L.F. O polissacarídeo do Anacardium occidentale L. na fase inflamatória do processo cicatricial de lesões cutâneas. *Ciência Rural* **2006**, *36*, 149–154. [CrossRef]
15. Kumar, A.; Moin, A.; Ahmed, A.; Shivakumar, H.G. Cashew gum a versatile hydrophyllic polymer: A review. *Curr. Drug Ther.* **2012**, *7*, 2–12. [CrossRef]
16. Quelemes, P.V.; Araruna, F.B.; de Faria, B.E.; Kuckelhaus, S.A.; da Silva, D.A.; Mendonça, R.Z.; Eiras, C.; dos S Soares, M.J.; Leite, J.R.S. Development and antibacterial activity of cashew gum-based silver nanoparticles. *Int. J. Mol. Sci.* **2013**, *14*, 4969–4981. [CrossRef]
17. Araújo, T.S.; Costa, D.S.; Sousa, N.A.; Souza, L.K.; de Araújo, S.; Oliveira, A.P.; Sousa, F.B.M.; Silva, D.A.; Barbosa, A.L.; Leite, J.R.S. Antidiarrheal activity of cashew GUM, a complex heteropolysaccharide extracted from exudate of Anacardium occidentale L. in rodents. *J. Ethnopharmacol.* **2015**, *174*, 299–307. [CrossRef] [PubMed]
18. AlRashdi, A.S.; Salama, S.M.; Alkiyumi, S.S.; Abdulla, M.A.; Hadi, A.H.A.; Abdelwahab, S.I.; Taha, M.M.; Hussiani, J.; Asykin, N. Mechanisms of gastroprotective effects of ethanolic leaf extract of Jasminum sambac against HCl/ethanol-induced gastric mucosal injury in rats. *Evid.Based Complement. Altern. Med.* **2012**, *2012*, 786426. [CrossRef]
19. Bonacorsi, C.; Da Fonseca, L.M.; Raddi, M.S.G.; Kitagawa, R.R.; Vilegas, W. Comparison of Brazilian plants used to treat gastritis on the oxidative burst of Helicobacter pylori-stimulated neutrophil. *Evid. Based Complement. Altern. Med.* **2013**, *2013*, 851621. [CrossRef] [PubMed]
20. Reddy, S.C.; Shetty, B.V.; Rao, G.M. Oral Ingestion of Spondias pinnata Bark Extract Trim Down Severity of Small Intestinal Mucositis in Etoposide Treated Rats. *Cancer Sci. Ther.* **2015**, *7*, 030–033. [CrossRef]
21. Chikezie, P.C. Sodium metabisulfite–induced polymerization of sickle cell hemoglobin incubated in the extracts of three medicinal plants (Anacardium occidentale, Psidium guajava, and Terminalia catappa). *Pharmacogn. Mag.* **2011**, *7*, 126–132. [CrossRef]
22. Okpashi, V.E.; Bayim, B.P.-R.; Obi-Abang, M. Comparative effects of some medicinal plants: Anacardium occidentale, Eucalyptus globulus, Psidium guajava, and Xylopia aethiopica extracts in alloxan-induced diabetic male Wistar albino rats. *Biochem. Res. Int.* **2014**, *2014*. [CrossRef]
23. Jaiswal, Y.; Tatke, P.; Gabhe, S.; Vaidya, A. Antidiabetic activity of extracts of Anacardium occidentale Linn. leaves on n-streptozotocin diabetic rats. *J. Tradit. Complement. Med.* **2017**, *7*, 421–427. [CrossRef]
24. Souza, N.C.; de Oliveira, J.M.; Morrone, M.d.S.; Albanus, R.D.O.; Amarante, M.d.S.M.; Camillo, C.d.S.; Langassner, S.M.Z.; Gelain, D.P.; Moreira, J.C.F.; Dalmolin, R.J.S. Antioxidant and anti-inflammatory properties of Anacardium occidentale leaf extract. *Evid. Based Complement. Altern. Med.* **2017**, *2017*, 2787308. [CrossRef] [PubMed]
25. Silva, J.G.d.; Souza, I.A.; Higino, J.S.; Siqueira-Junior, J.P.; Pereira, J.V.; Pereira, M.d.S.V. Atividade antimicrobiana do extrato de Anacardium occidentale Linn. em amostras multiresistentes de Staphylococcus aureus. *Rev. Bras. Farmacogn.* **2007**, *17*, 572–577. [CrossRef]
26. Tchikaya, F.O.; Bantsielé, G.B.; Kouakou-Siransy, G.; Datté, J.Y.; Datté, P.; Zirihi, N.G.; Offoumou, M.A. Anacardium occidentale Linn.(Anacardiaceae) stem bark extract induces hypotensive and cardio-inhibitory effects in experimental animal models. *Afr. J. Tradit. Complement. Altern. Med.* **2011**, *8*, 452–461. [CrossRef]
27. Cardoso Palheta, I.; Caldeira Tavares-Martins, A.C.; Araujo Lucas, F.C.; Goncalves Jardim, M.A. Ethnobotanical study of medicinal plants in urban home gardens in the city of Abaetetuba, Pará state, Brazil. *Boletín Latinoamericano y del Caribe de Plantas Medicinales y Aromáticas* **2017**, *16*, 206–262.
28. Vasconcelos, M.d.S.; Rochette, N.F.G.; de Oliveira, M.L.M.; Nunes-Pinheiro, D.C.S.; Tomé, A.R.; Maia de Sousa, F.Y.; Pinheiro, F.G.M.; Moura, C.F.H.; Miranda, M.R.A.; Mota, E.F. Anti-inflammatory and wound healing potential of cashew apple juice (Anacardium occidentale L.) in mice. *Exp. Biol. Med.* **2015**, *240*, 1648–1655. [CrossRef]
29. Yeung, C.-Y.; Chan, W.-T.; Jiang, C.-B.; Cheng, M.-L.; Liu, C.-Y.; Chang, S.-W.; Chiau, J.-S.C.; Lee, H.-C. Amelioration of chemotherapy-induced intestinal mucositis by orally administered probiotics in a mouse model. *PLoS ONE* **2015**, *10*, e0138746. [CrossRef]
30. Carvalho, R.D.; Breyner, N.; Menezes-Garcia, Z.; Rodrigues, N.M.; Lemos, L.; Maioli, T.U.; Souza, D.G.; Carmona, D.; Faria, A.M.; Langella, P. Secretion of biologically active pancreatitis-associated protein I (PAP) by genetically modified dairy Lactococcus lactis NZ9000 in the prevention of intestinal mucositis. *Microb. Cell Factories* **2017**, *16*, 27. [CrossRef]

31. Li, Y.; Liu, M.; Zuo, Z.; Liu, J.; Yu, X.; Guan, Y.; Zhan, R.; Han, Q.; Zhang, J.; Zhou, R. TLR9 Regulates the NF-κB–NLRP3–IL-1β Pathway Negatively in Salmonella-Induced NKG2D-Mediated Intestinal Inflammation. *J. Immunol.* **2017**, *199*, 761–773. [CrossRef]
32. Gerhard, D.; Sousa, F.J.D.S.S.; Andraus, R.A.C.; Pardo, P.E.; Nai, G.A.; Neto, H.B.; Messora, M.R.; Maia, L.P. Probiotic therapy reduces inflammation and improves intestinal morphology in rats with induced oral mucositis. *Braz. Oral Res.* **2017**, *31*, 1–11. [CrossRef]
33. De Araújo, A.A.; Borba, P.B.; de Souza, F.H.D.; Nogueira, A.C.; Saldanha, T.S.; Araújo, T.E.F.; Silva, A.I.; de Araújo Júnior, R.F. In a methotrexate-induced model of intestinal mucositis, olmesartan reduced inflammation and induced enteropathy characterized by severe diarrhea, weight loss, and reduced sucrose activity. *Biol. Pharm. Bull.* **2015**, *38*, 746–752. [CrossRef]
34. De Barros, P.A.V.; Andrade, M.E.R.; de Vasconcelos Generoso, S.; Miranda, S.E.M.; dos Reis, D.C.; Leocádio, P.C.L.; e Souza, É.L.d.S.; dos Santos Martins, F.; da Gama, M.A.S.; Cassali, G.D. Conjugated linoleic acid prevents damage caused by intestinal mucositis induced by 5-fluorouracil in an experimental model. *Biomed. Pharmacother.* **2018**, *103*, 1567–1576. [CrossRef] [PubMed]
35. Al-Asmari, A.K.; Khan, A.Q.; Al-Asmari, S.A.; Al-Rawi, A.; Al-Omani, S. Alleviation of 5-fluorouracil-induced intestinal mucositis in rats by vitamin E via targeting oxidative stress and inflammatory markers. *J. Complement. Integr. Med.* **2016**, *13*, 377–385. [CrossRef] [PubMed]
36. Han, X.; Wu, Z.; Di, J.; Pan, Y.; Zhang, H.; Du, Y.; Cheng, Z.; Jin, Z.; Wang, Z.; Zheng, Q. CXCL9 attenuated chemotherapy-induced intestinal mucositis by inhibiting proliferation and reducing apoptosis. *Biomed. Pharmacother.* **2011**, *65*, 547–554. [CrossRef]
37. Zhang, S.; Liu, Y.; Xiang, D.; Yang, J.; Liu, D.; Ren, X.; Zhang, C. Assessment of dose-response relationship of 5-fluorouracil to murine intestinal injury. *Biomed. Pharmacother.* **2018**, *106*, 910–916. [CrossRef] [PubMed]
38. Kumar, S.; Aninat, C.; Michaux, G.; Morel, F. Anticancer drug 5-fluorouracil induces reproductive and developmental defects in Caenorhabditis elegans. *Reprod. Toxicol.* **2010**, *29*, 415–420. [CrossRef] [PubMed]
39. Soares, P.M.; Mota, J.M.S.; Gomes, A.S.; Oliveira, R.B.; Assreuy, A.M.S.; Brito, G.A.C.; Santos, A.A.; Ribeiro, R.A.; Souza, M.H. Gastrointestinal dysmotility in 5-fluorouracil-induced intestinal mucositis outlasts inflammatory process resolution. *Cancer Chemother. Pharmacol.* **2008**, *63*, 91–98. [CrossRef]
40. Quaresma, M.P. *Lactobacillus spp. e Bifidobacterium sp. Attenuate Experimental Intestinal Mucositis Induced by 5-Fluorouracil in Mice*; Federal University of Ceará: Fortaleza, Brazil, 2016.
41. Sonis, S.T. A biological approach to mucositis. *J. Support. Oncol.* **2004**, *2*, 21–32.
42. Guabiraba, R.; Besnard, A.; Menezes, G.; Secher, T.; Jabir, M.; Amaral, S.; Braun, H.; Lima-Junior, R.C.; Ribeiro, R.; Cunha, F. IL-33 targeting attenuates intestinal mucositis and enhances effective tumor chemotherapy in mice. *Mucosal Immunol.* **2014**, *7*, 1079–1093. [CrossRef]
43. Bastos, C.C.C.; de Ávila, P.H.M.; dos Santos Filho, E.X.; de Ávila, R.I.; Batista, A.C.; Fonseca, S.G.; Lima, E.M.; Marreto, R.N.; de Mendonca, E.F.; Valadares, M.C. Use of Bidens pilosa L.(Asteraceae) and Curcuma longa L.(Zingiberaceae) to treat intestinal mucositis in mice: Toxico-pharmacological evaluations. *Toxicol. Rep.* **2016**, *3*, 279–287. [CrossRef] [PubMed]
44. Justino, P.F.; Melo, L.F.; Nogueira, A.F.; Costa, J.V.; Silva, L.M.; Santos, C.M.; Mendes, W.O.; Costa, M.R.; Franco, A.X.; Lima, A.A.; et al. Treatment with Saccharomyces boulardii reduces the inflammation and dysfunction of the gastrointestinal tract in 5-fluorouracil-induced intestinal mucositis in mice. *Br. J. Nutr.* **2014**, *111*, 1611–1621. [CrossRef] [PubMed]
45. De Ávila, P.H.M.; de Ávila, R.I.; dos Santos Filho, E.X.; Bastos, C.C.C.; Batista, A.C.; Mendonca, E.F.; Serpa, R.C.; Marreto, R.N.; da Cruz, A.F.; Lima, E.M. Mucoadhesive formulation of Bidens pilosa L.(Asteraceae) reduces intestinal injury from 5-fluorouracil-induced mucositis in mice. *Toxicol. Rep.* **2015**, *2*, 563–573. [CrossRef]
46. Al-Asmari, A.; Al-Zahrani, A.; Khan, A.; Al-Shahrani, H.; Ali Al Amri, M. Taurine ameliorates 5-flourouracil-induced intestinal mucositis, hepatorenal and reproductive organ damage in Wistar rats: A biochemical and histological study. *Hum. Exp. Toxicol.* **2016**, *35*, 10–20. [CrossRef] [PubMed]
47. Heber, D. Oxidative Stress Markers and Inflammation: The Role of Spices and Herbs. *Nutr. Today* **2014**, *49*, S4–S5. [CrossRef]
48. Nogueira, L.T.; Costa, D.V.; Gomes, A.S.; Martins, C.S.; Silva, A.M.; Coelho-Aguiar, J.M.; Castelucci, P.; Lima-Júnior, R.C.; Leitão, R.F.; Moura-Neto, V.; et al. The involvement of mast cells in the irinotecan-induced enteric neurons loss and reactive gliosis. *J. Neuroinflamm.* **2017**, *14*, 79. [CrossRef]

49. Hamilton, M.J.; Frei, S.M.; Stevens, R.L. The multifaceted mast cell in inflammatory bowel disease. *Inflamm. Bowel Dis.* **2014**, *20*, 2364–2378. [CrossRef] [PubMed]
50. De Winter, B.Y.; van den Wijngaard, R.M.; de Jonge, W.J. Intestinal mast cells in gut inflammation and motility disturbances. *Biochim. Biophys. Acta Mol. Basis Dis.* **2012**, *1822*, 66–73. [CrossRef]
51. Theoharides, T.C.; Alysandratos, K.-D.; Angelidou, A.; Delivanis, D.-A.; Sismanopoulos, N.; Zhang, B.; Asadi, S.; Vasiadi, M.; Weng, Z.; Miniati, A.; et al. Mast cells and inflammation. *Biochim. Biophys. Acta Mol. Basis Dis.* **2012**, *1822*, 21–33. [CrossRef]
52. Ramsay, D.B.; Stephen, S.; Borum, M.; Voltaggio, L.; Doman, D.B. Mast cells in gastrointestinal disease. *Gastroenterol. Hepatol.* **2010**, *6*, 772–777.
53. Bischoff, S.C. Mast cells in gastrointestinal disorders. *Eur. J. Pharmacol.* **2016**, *778*, 139–145. [CrossRef]
54. Short, S.S.; Wang, J.; Castle, S.L.; Fernandez, G.E.; Smiley, N.; Zobel, M.; Pontarelli, E.M.; Papillon, S.C.; Grishin, A.V.; Ford, H.R. Low doses of celecoxib attenuate gut barrier failure during experimental peritonitis. *Lab. Investig.* **2013**, *93*, 1265–1275. [CrossRef] [PubMed]
55. Javle, M.M.; Cao, S.; Durrani, F.A.; Pendyala, L.; Lawrence, D.D.; Smith, P.F.; Creaven, P.J.; Noel, D.C.; Iyer, R.V.; Rustum, Y.M. Celecoxib and mucosal protection: Translation from an animal model to a phase I clinical trial of celecoxib, irinotecan, and 5-fluorouracil. *Clin. Cancer Res.* **2007**, *13*, 965–971. [CrossRef] [PubMed]
56. Verri Jr, W.A.; Cunha, T.M.; Parada, C.A.; Poole, S.; Cunha, F.Q.; Ferreira, S.H. Hypernociceptive role of cytokines and chemokines: Targets for analgesic drug development? *Pharmacol. Ther.* **2006**, *112*, 116–138. [CrossRef] [PubMed]
57. Al-Azri, A.R.; Gibson, R.J.; Bowen, J.M.; Stringer, A.M.; Keefe, D.M.; Logan, R.M. Involvement of matrix metalloproteinases (MMP-3 and MMP-9) in the pathogenesis of irinotecan-induced oral mucositis. *J. Oral Pathol. Med.* **2015**, *44*, 459–467. [CrossRef]
58. Ribeiro, R.A.; Wanderley, C.W.; Wong, D.V.; Mota, J.M.S.; Leite, C.A.; Souza, M.H.; Cunha, F.Q.; Lima-Junior, R.C. Irinotecan-and 5-fluorouracil-induced intestinal mucositis: Insights into pathogenesis and therapeutic perspectives. *Cancer Chemother. Pharmacol.* **2016**, *78*, 881–893. [CrossRef]
59. Al-Dasooqi, N.; Sonis, S.T.; Bowen, J.M.; Bateman, E.; Blijlevens, N.; Gibson, R.J.; Logan, R.M.; Nair, R.G.; Stringer, A.M.; Yazbeck, R.; et al. Emerging evidence on the pathobiology of mucositis. *Support. Care Cancer* **2013**, *21*, 2075–2083. [CrossRef]
60. De Paula, R.; Santana, S.; Rodrigues, J. Composition and rheological properties of Albizia lebbeck gum exudate. *Carbohydr. Polym.* **2001**, *44*, 133–139. [CrossRef]
61. Silva, D.A.; Feitosa, J.P.; Maciel, J.S.; Paula, H.C.; de Paula, R.C. Characterization of crosslinked cashew gum derivatives. *Carbohydr. Polym.* **2006**, *66*, 16–26. [CrossRef]
62. Da Silva, D.A.; Feitosa, J.P.; Paula, H.C.; de Paula, R.C. Synthesis and characterization of cashew gum/acrylic acid nanoparticles. *Mater. Sci. Eng. C* **2009**, *29*, 437–441. [CrossRef]
63. Soares, P.M.; Mota, J.M.S.; Souza, E.P.; Justino, P.F.; Franco, A.X.; Cunha, F.Q.; Ribeiro, R.A.; Souza, M.H. Inflammatory intestinal damage induced by 5-fluorouracil requires IL-4. *Cytokine* **2013**, *61*, 46–49. [CrossRef]
64. Dos Santos Filho, E.X.; Ávila, P.H.M.; Bastos, C.C.C.; Batista, A.C.; Naves, L.N.; Marreto, R.N.; Lima, E.M.; Mendonca, E.F.; Valadares, M.C. Curcuminoids from Curcuma longaL. reduced intestinal mucositis induced by 5-fluorouracil in mice: Bioadhesive, proliferative, anti-inflammatory and antioxidant effects. *Toxicol. Rep.* **2016**, *3*, 55–62. [CrossRef]
65. MacPherson, B.; Pfeiffer, C. Experimental production of diffuse colitis in rats. *Digestion* **1978**, *17*, 135–150. [CrossRef] [PubMed]
66. Moura, R.; Wada, C.; Purchio, A.; Almeida, T. *Studies of the Figurative Elements of Blood*, 3rd ed.; Atheneu: São Paulo, Brazil, 1998.
67. Bradford, M.M. A rapid and sensitive method for the quantitation of microgram quantities of protein utilizing the principle of protein-dye binding. *Anal. Biochem.* **1976**, *72*, 248–254. [CrossRef]
68. Ohkawa, H.; Ohishi, N.; Yagi, K. Assay for lipid peroxides in animal tissues by thiobarbituric acid reaction. *Anal. Biochem.* **1979**, *95*, 351–358. [CrossRef]

69. Sedlak, J.; Lindsay, R.H. Estimation of total, protein-bound, and nonprotein sulfhydryl groups in tissue with Ellman's reagent. *Anal. Biochem.* **1968**, *25*, 192–205. [CrossRef]

70. Bradley, P.P.; Priebat, D.A.; Christensen, R.D.; Rothstein, G. Measurement of cutaneous inflammation: Estimation of neutrophil content with an enzyme marker. *J. Investig. Dermatol.* **1982**, *78*, 206–209. [CrossRef] [PubMed]

71. Michalany, J. *Histological Technique Pathological Anatomy: With Instructions for the Surgeon, Nurse, Cytotechnician*, 3rd ed.; Michalany: São Paulo, Brazil, 2008.

10

Cyclooxygenase-1 (COX-1) and COX-1 Inhibitors in Cancer

Alessandra Pannunzio and Mauro Coluccia *

Department of Pharmacy-Drug Sciences, University of Bari "Aldo Moro", Via E. Orabona 4, I-70125 Bari, Italy; alessandra.pannunzio@uniba.it

* Correspondence: mauro.coluccia@uniba.it;

Abstract: Prostaglandins and thromboxane are lipid signaling molecules deriving from arachidonic acid by the action of the cyclooxygenase isoenzymes COX-1 and COX-2. The role of cyclooxygenases (particularly COX-2) and prostaglandins (particularly PGE_2) in cancer-related inflammation has been extensively investigated. In contrast, COX-1 has received less attention, although its expression increases in several human cancers and a pathogenetic role emerges from experimental models. COX-1 and COX-2 isoforms seem to operate in a coordinate manner in cancer pathophysiology, especially in the tumorigenesis process. However, in some cases, exemplified by the serous ovarian carcinoma, COX-1 plays a pivotal role, suggesting that other histopathological and molecular subtypes of cancer disease could share this feature. Importantly, the analysis of functional implications of COX-1-signaling, as well as of pharmacological action of COX-1-selective inhibitors, should not be restricted to the COX pathway and to the effects of prostaglandins already known for their ability of affecting the tumor phenotype. A knowledge-based choice of the most appropriate tumor cell models, and a major effort in investigating the COX-1 issue in the more general context of arachidonic acid metabolic network by using the systems biology approaches, should be strongly encouraged.

Keywords: cyclooxygenase-1; cyclooxygenase-2; cancer; inflammation; tumorigenesis; COX-1 inhibitor

---

1. Introduction

Already in 1863, the German pathologist Rudolf C. Virchow had observed that some cancers were inherently associated with white blood cell infiltration [1]. However, it was only at the end of 20th century that an increasing body of research led to propose chronic inflammation as one of the enabling characteristics of cancer development [2,3], and the complex inflammatory network in premalignant and frankly malignant disease is now actively explored with the aim of translating epidemiological and experimental evidence into clinical practice [4].

Cancer may originate in the chronic inflammation setting associated with persistent infections, immune-mediated damage, or prolonged exposure to irritants. On the other hand, the genetic and epigenetic alterations underlying the cancerogenesis process inevitably modify the tissue homeostasis and may induce a chronic inflammatory response. Irrespective of the presumed primary or secondary nature of the process, inflammatory cells and mediators can be detected in most tumor tissues, where they act on both tumor and stromal cells and contribute to determine a tumor-promoting microenvironment [5].

In the general complexity of the inflammatory response (hundreds of chemical mediators have been identified, but how they function in a coordinated manner is still not fully understood), the arachidonic acid (AA) metabolites play a relevant role which appears intertwined with their functions in cell and tissue homeostasis [6]. Prostaglandins (PGs), including PGD_2, PGE_2, PGF_{2a},

PGI_2 and thromboxane (TX)A_2 (collectively known also as prostanoids) are produced from arachidonic acid by sequential actions of cyclooxygenases (COX-1 or COX-2) and specific synthases, and they exert their effects in autocrine and/or paracrine manner mainly through G protein-coupled receptors (GPCRs) at the cell surface [7].

The involvement of prostaglandins in cancer was first evidenced in human esophageal carcinoma cells, when their invasive and metastatic potential in nude mice was found to be related to PGE_2 and PGF_{2a} production [8]. Elevated levels of PGE_2 have been found in numerous cancers, and its effects on multiple cell signaling pathways involved in tumor malignant phenotype induction and maintenance have been thereafter demonstrated [9–13]. However, PGE_2 is not the only PG involved in carcinogenesis. PGD_2 potentially contributes to the colon cancer risk in ulcerative colitis [14]; more recently, (TX)A_2 was found to be involved in colorectal cancer pathophysiology [15,16], as well as in multiple myeloma [17] and lung [18] cancer cell proliferation.

The committed step of PG biosynthesis is catalyzed by COX-1 and COX-2 isoforms. These enzymes display many similarities in structure and catalytic properties and yield the same product, PGH_2. However, COX-1 and COX-2 are different in their regulation of expression, tissue distribution, and associated synthases, thus subserving distinct biological tasks. COX-1 is constitutively expressed in most tissues (e.g., platelets, lung, prostate, brain, gastrointestinal tract, kidney, liver and spleen), where the COX-1-derived prostanoids are involved in homeostatic functions. It is generally accepted that COX-1 activity maintains the prostanoid production at a basal rate, and allows a rapid increase when cell membrane remodeling produces a rise of free AA. In contrast, COX-2 is generally considered as the inducible isoform, responsible for enhanced prostanoid production in response to inflammatory stimuli and growth factors during inflammation and various pathological conditions, including cancer [19,20]. It should be noted, however, that the concept of "constitutive" and "inducible" isoforms has been challenged by growing evidence indicating that both isoforms are present in normal tissues and can be up-regulated in various pathological conditions [21]. Both the expression and regulation of COX isoforms have been intensively investigated, and reviews about transcriptional regulatory mechanisms [22], and the regulation of gene expression at the co- or post-transcriptional level [23] have been recently published.

The role of cyclooxygenases (in particular COX-2) and prostaglandin products (in particular PGE_2) in cancer-related inflammation has been extensively investigated in many neoplastic diseases, including esophageal [24], gastrointestinal [25,26] and pancreatic [27] cancers, breast [28] and cervical [29] cancers, renal [30], prostate [31], and bladder [32] cancers, skin [33,34] and head and neck [35] cancers, hematological tumors [36], and mesothelioma [37]. Tumor cells are often characterized by COX-2 aberrant expression [38,39], resulting from transcriptional and/or post-transcriptional alterations and contributing to tumor diseases, such as in colorectal cancer [40]. Importantly, the tumor-associated aberrant expression of COX-2 is often related to epigenetic alterations affecting COX-2 gene (PTGS2) as well as other genes involved into biosynthesis and signaling of its main prostaglandin products [41].

Epidemiological data are convincingly supported by various in vivo experimental systems, including chemically induced or transgenic models of colorectal, breast, and other types of cancer [42]. Finally, the therapeutic potential of aspirin, traditional nonsteroidal anti-inflammatory drugs (NSAIDs) and COX-2-selective inhibitors (coxibs) in human cancer has also been widely explored. A very large body of research, including about 2000 relevant publications only for aspirin, proposes that the anticancer activity of these drugs depends upon their ability to interfere with multiple pro-tumorigenic signaling pathways, some of them COX-dependent [38] and others COX-independent [43].

Unlike COX-2, the role of COX-1 in cancer has generally received less attention. Being usually considered as the constitutively expressed isoform that is involved in homeostatic cell and tissue functions, COX-1 was thought not be involved in carcinogenesis. However, increased levels of COX-1 expression have been occasionally reported in several cancers [44], and it has been shown that the genetic disruption of COX-1 is as effective as COX-2 disruption in reducing intestinal [45] and skin tumorigenesis [46] in mouse models, thus suggesting that both COX isoforms could cooperate in the cancerogenesis process. In the following, an overview of the available evidence about COX-1 expression and involvement in different neoplastic diseases will be presented. The objective of this review is to go through the COX-1-relevant literature in oncology and medicinal chemistry, thus attempting to fill the existing gap and highlighting the potential future studies.

2. COX-1 Involvement in Neoplastic Diseases

Renal cell carcinoma. The pathophysiological relevance of COX-2 in renal cell carcinoma (RCC) is generally acknowledged, and recently, it has been shown that COX-2 inhibition enhances the efficacy of immunotherapy and tyrosine kinase inhibitor-based treatment [30]. COX-1 expression, however, has been practically unexplored, except for a report on COX-1 mRNA overexpression in an RCC rat model [47]. Interestingly, two recent immunohistochemical investigations have shown a correlation between COX-1 overexpression and poor prognosis in RCC [48], and the validity of the combined use of COX-1 and VEGF in RCC histopathologic prognosis [49].

Skin cancer. The role of cyclooxygenase-dependent signaling in skin pathophysiology and non-melanoma carcinogenesis has been recently reviewed [33]. There is accumulating evidence that cyclooxygenase-2 may be involved in the pathogenesis of non-melanoma skin cancer, whereas COX-1 expression appears unaltered with respect to healthy tissue. At preclinical level, however, genetic studies show that the activity of both COX isoforms is mechanistically involved in the basal cell carcinoma pathogenesis [50,51].

Head and neck cancer. There are few data regarding COX-1 in head and neck cancer. A comparison of cyclooxygenase-1 expression levels between cancerous tissue from head and neck cancer patients and normal mucosa was performed by immunohistochemistry, Western blotting, and real-time RT-PCR (reverse transcription polymerase chain reaction), showing COX-1 overexpression in cancer cells and no expression in normal mucosa [52]. A progression-associated up-regulation of COX-1 expression was detected by immunohistochemistry in patients with hyperplasia, dysplasia, and carcinoma of oral mucosa [53] and a major expression of either COX-1 or COX-2 was reported in patients with oral squamous cell carcinoma with respect to normal mucosa [54]. More recently, tumor samples from patients with sebaceous gland carcinoma, an aggressive tumor commonly localized at Meibomian or Zeis glands, were examined by high-throughput tissue microarray for the expression of proteins involved in angiogenesis, inflammation, apoptosis, cell proliferation, cell-to-cell contact, and carcinogenesis. High expression of COX-1 and COX-2 was reported in 97% and 82% of patients, respectively [55]. Interesting implications on the COX-1 role derive also from in vitro investigations in head and neck squamous cell carcinoma (HNSCC) cell lines, in which the effects of pharmacologic inhibitors of cyclooxygenases were compared to those of small-interfering RNA as far as cell-growth, vascular endothelial growth factor (VEGF) production, and intracellular signaling are concerned [56,57]. The results showed that COX-2 inhibition blocked VEGF productions in some HNSCC cells; in contrast, other COX-2 (and PGE_2) expressing HNSCC cells showed little response to COX-2 inhibition, this effect depending upon a differential expression of COX-1.

Esophageal cancer. Barrett's esophagus, a complication of the chronic gastro-esophageal reflux disease, represents the best-known risk factor for esophageal adenocarcinoma development. Esophageal cancer prevention strategies [58], the role of inflammatory mediators in the disease pathophysiology [24], as well as encouraging experimental and epidemiological data on chemoprophylaxis with NSAIDs in patients with Barrett's esophagus have been recently reviewed [59], along with a body of evidence supporting a role for COX-2 in the pathogenetic sequence leading to esophageal adenocarcinoma [60,61]. Interestingly, a possible involvement of COX-1 in the disease pathophysiology had already been suggested by the co-expression of both COX isoforms and angiogenic (VEGF-A) and lymphangiogenic (VEGF-C) growth factors in primary human tumor samples [62]. More recently, a possible cooperation of COX-1 and COX-2 isoforms has been suggested in an investigation of the PGE_2 pathway in a rat model of esophageal adenocarcinoma induced by gastroduodenal reflux resulting from esophagojejunostomy [63], as well as by the finding that in the same experimental model indomethacin (a dual COX-1/COX-2 inhibitor) reduced the inflammatory lesions and tumor development, whereas a selective COX-2 inhibitor (MF-tricyclic) was ineffective [64]. Interestingly, a recent meta-analysis of nine observational studies has shown that both low-dose aspirin and non-aspirin COX inhibitor use is associated with a reduced risk of developing esophageal adenocarcinoma in patients with Barrett's esophagus [65].

Colorectal cancer. In the colorectal carcinogenesis, the long-term transition process from normal mucosa to benign adenoma and final carcinoma provides the possibility to adopt preventive measures. Many evidences exist underlying the pathophysiological link between chronic inflammation and colorectal cancer [66], and the role of COX-2 in the carcinogenesis process has been extensively investigated [67,68]. COX-1 and COX-2 mRNA expression profiles were examined in tumor tissue in comparison to normal mucosa in stage III (Dukes' C) colorectal cancer patients by Church et al. [69]. In contrast to the general opinion that constitutive COX-1 was not subject to variable expression, an altered regulation of COX-1 expression between normal and malignant tissues was reported, consistent with a COX-1 role in tumorigenesis. A significant correlation between levels of mRNA for COX-1, COX-2, TGF-beta1 and PGES, and those for proangiogenic factors VEGF-A and VEGF-C were also found in primary adenocarcinomas of the small intestine, thus suggesting a role for these factors in the propagation this rare neoplasia [70]. Interestingly, experimental mouse studies using genetic disruption of COX-1 or COX-2 plus *Apc* genes already 15 years ago suggested that both isoforms were involved in intestinal polyp formation [45]. Moreover, up-regulation of COX-1 protects intestinal stem cells from the DNA-damaging effect of azoxymethane and may play a key role in the early phase of intestinal tumorigenesis [71]. Furthermore, analysis of the expression levels of COX-1, COX-2, and mPGES (the downstream prostaglandin E synthase) in COX-$1^{-/-}$ and COX-$2^{-/-}$ ApcΔ716 double-knockout mice revealed that COX-1 was required from the early stage of intestinal polyp development, and that additional expression of COX-2 together with mPGES was necessary for subsequent accelerated growth of polyps [72]. On this basis, a mechanistic cooperation between COX-1 in the early stage of tumorigenesis and COX-2 in the subsequent polyp growth was proposed. In early stage of intestinal carcinogenesis, COX-1-PGE_2 signaling associated with a suppression of the PG-catabolizing enzyme, 15-prostaglandin-dehydrogenase (15-PGDH), has been proposed to occur before COX-2 induction [73]. Recent studies have also shown that COX-1 is required for the maintenance of anchorage-independent growth ability of colon cancer cells (a key feature of malignant phenotype), as well as for tumor promoter-induced transformation of preneoplastic cells [74]. Interestingly, Li et al. in the same work identified a novel selective COX-1 inhibitor, 6-C-(E-phenylethenyl)-naringenin, a derivative of the flavonoid naringenin, also showing its chemopreventive efficacy in a colon cancer xenograft model.

Breast cancer. In the breast cancer microenvironment, there is a complex interplay between tumor and stromal cells, and a relevant contribute of COX-2-derived prostanoids is generally acknowledged [24,75,76]. However, both isoforms are expressed in breast cancer clinical samples, COX-1 being primarily localized in stromal cells [77,78]. Up-regulation of COX-1 gene expression in tumor tissues compared to normal tissue has been demonstrated also by whole genome expression analysis of breast carcinomas [79]. Moreover, induction of cell growth arrest and apoptosis are induced in MCF-7 human breast cell line in vitro by the COX-1 inhibitor FR122047 [80], and additive effects on tumor cell growth by COX-1 and COX-2 inhibitors are induced in vitro [81] and in vivo [82].

Cervical cancer. Human papilloma virus (HPV) infection of the cervical epithelium is well regarded as the main cause of cervical cancer [83], and a link between HPV E6 and E7 oncoproteins and COX-2 transcription has been established [84,85]. However, current data supporting a benefit for NSAIDs in the treatment of cervical intraepithelial neoplasia—the premalignant cervical lesion—are uncertain [86]. COX-1 up-regulation in cervical carcinoma was reported more than 10 years ago, and COX-1-dependent autocrine/paracrine regulation of COX-2, PGE_2 receptors, and angiogenic factors was demonstrated in vitro [87]. Interestingly, it has been recently demonstrated that seminal plasma can promote cervical tumor cell growth in vitro and in vivo through the activation of inflammatory pathways involving both COX isoforms [88] and the expression of angiogenic chemokines [89]. Moreover, in an in vitro investigation of the co-regulation of COX-1 and downstream prostaglandin E synthases (mPGES-1, mPGES-2 and cPGES) in several tumor cell lines including cervical cancer, it was found that COX-1 and mPGES-1 messenger RNA (mRNA) are co-regulated and functionally coupled in basal PGE_2 synthesis [90]. Although few clinical investigations of COX isoforms expression in cervical cancer are available [91,92], these experimental results, along with previous findings on the relationships between COX isoforms expression and radiosensitivity of cervical cancer cell lines [93] suggest that also the COX-1 role in cervical cancer prevention and treatment could be reevaluated [94].

Endometrial cancer. It is generally accepted that production of prostaglandins by endometrial epithelial cells under resting conditions is regulated through the constitutive expression of COX-1, whereas under stimulated conditions prostaglandin production is a result of the up-regulation of COX-2. A critical role for COX-2 isoform in the maintenance of endometrial tissue during the menstrual cycle as well as in the progression of endometrial cancer has been already observed [95,96], along with the potential clinical benefit of a selective COX-2 inhibitor in COX-2 positive endometrial cancers [97]. However, a possible involvement of COX-1 in the early stage of endometrial cancer development has been suggested, based on a higher COX-1 mRNA expression in patients with WHO (World Health Organization)-grade G1 and G2 endometrial cancer [98]. Moreover, a possible role for COX-1 in endometrial cancerogenesis has been suggested [99]. In a mechanistic investigation of the oxytocin ability of modulating the invasive properties of human endometrial carcinoma cells, the results showed that the hormone increased the invasive properties of tumor cells through the activation of PIK3/AKT pathway; this in turn led to up-regulation of both COX isoforms and subsequent PGE_2 production. Interestingly, both COX isoforms were necessary and acted cooperatively for the oxytocin-induced invasion, COX-1 triggering the pro-invasive matrix metalloproteinase (MMP)-14 (a major MMP-2 activator), and COX-2 up-regulating MMP-2 expression. Importantly, an over-expression of oxytocin receptor was detected in endometrial cancer patients, thus indicating the clinical relevance of the oxytocin pathway in endometrial cancer progression.

Ovarian cancer. Epithelial ovarian cancer (EOC), the most lethal gynecological malignancy mainly occurring in older (postmenopausal) woman, is a highly heterogeneous disease [100], and includes distinct histological subtypes. A number of inflammatory cells and mediators are involved in EOC development and progression, and accumulating clinical and experimental evidence strongly suggests that inflammation might represent a unifying pathophysiological mechanism of ovarian carcinogenesis [101,102]. Interestingly, COX-1 was first identified as ovarian cancer marker two decades ago [103]. Since then, COX-1 over-expression has been reported by several groups in multiple human, mouse, as well as hen models of ovarian cancer [104–109]. COX-1 has been suggested as the major enzyme regulating PGE_2 production in ovarian cancer cells [110], and along with COX-2 it plays an essential role in gonadotropin-induced tumor cell migration and invasion [111]. Thus, it is not surprising that both COX-1 and COX-2 have been included in a panel of inflammatory markers that characterize the rapidly growing and highly aggressive (type II) ovarian carcinomas [112]. Accordingly, the expression of COX-1 is higher in ovarian cancer patients with low CD8+ (cytotoxic T cells) and high CD1a+ (dendritic cells) cell density than in those with high CD8+ cell density [113], and COX-1 overexpression is the characterizing element in a cluster of ovarian cancer patients in which the poor prognosis is associated with an immunosuppressive status [114]. However, a role for COX-2 isoform in ovarian cancer has been also reported in clinical [115], as well as experimental investigations [116,117]. A major contribution for clarifying this apparent controversy comes from a very recent large-scale quantitative analysis of the expression of COX isoforms through The Cancer Genome Atlas (TCGA) dataset [118]. This study revealed markedly higher COX-1 expression than COX-2 in high-grade serous ovarian cancer (HGSOC)—the most aggressive EOC histotype—along with higher COX-1 expression in HGSOC tumors than 10 other tumor types in TCGA. Interestingly, a similar or higher expression of COX-2 isoform was instead observed for endometrioid, mucinous and clear cell tumors in an independent tissue microarray, thus suggesting a more relevant role for COX-2 in other EOC histotypes. Importantly, genetic knockdown of COX-1 in ovarian cancer cell lines resulted in down-regulation of both PG signaling and multiple pro-tumorigenic pathways, thus strongly encouraging further development of methods to selectively target COX-1 in the management of HGSOC tumors. The COX-1 relevance in ovarian cancer is also indirectly witnessed by the major efficacy of aspirin, a stronger COX-1 than COX-2 inhibitor, in COX-1-overexpressing in vitro and in vivo models of ovarian cancer [119–122].

Hematological tumors. COX-2 expression in hematological malignancies, including chronic lymphocytic leukemia, chronic myeloid leukemia, lymphoma, and multiple myeloma, favors tumor cell growth and survival, and represents a poor prognostic indicator [36]. As for myeloid and lymphoid acute leukemia, the transcription of both COX-1 and COX-2 isoforms in human leukemic blast cells from acute myeloid (AML) and acute lymphoid (ALL) patients has been well documented, but only COX-1 protein is expressed and active. COX-1-derived PGE_2 stimulates the spontaneous growth of AML leukemic blasts in vitro [123]. Among the various COX-derived metabolites, only PGE_2 appears to be endowed with a stimulating effect on the growth of leukemic blast cells in vitro [124], this suggesting a potential benefit stemming from COX-1 selective inhibition. COX-1, but not COX-2, is expressed and enzymatically active also in primary blasts from patients affected by acute promyelocytic leukemia (APL), a distinct AML subtype characterized by the t(15;17) translocation involving the PML gene on chromosome 15 and the retinoic acid receptor-alpha (RAR-alpha) gene on chromosome 17. A major component of APL therapy is all-*trans* retinoic acid (ATRA), based on its ability of activating gene transcription and tumor cell differentiation [125]. The ATRA-induced cell differentiation program is very complex, as shown by systems analysis of transcriptome and proteome [126], and includes also COX-1, but not COX-2, upregulation [127]. In this respect, it should be noted that the COX-1 selective inhibitor SC-560, as well as the non-selective indomethacin, impair both PGE_2 production and ATRA-dependent differentiation of NB4 leukemic cells, a model of acute promyelocytic leukemia, thus suggesting that COX-1-inhibiting NSAIDs should be avoided in APL patients under ATRA treatment [128].

COX-1 and cancer stem cells. According to the cancer stem cell (CSC) model, tumor tissues are hierarchically organized as normal tissues, the cancer stem cells being able to fuel or reinitiate tumor growth, giving rise to the progeny which constitutes the bulk of tumor mass. The CSC niche homeostasis is regulated by a complex system of molecular signals, which include also the COX-derived AA metabolites [129,130]. In more detail, COX-2 is up-regulated in CSCs isolated from distinct tumor histotypes (e.g., in breast, colon and bone tumors), is co-expressed with stemness molecular markers, and promotes CSC growth in vitro systems, as recently reviewed by Pang L.Y. et al. [131]. This is not surprising, considering the relevance of COX-2-PGE_2 system in stem cell biology of normal tissues [132], as well as the well-known relevance of COX-2 in cancer. However, some experimental evidence of COX-1 involvement in CSC biology also exists. In the azoxymethane (AOM) murine colon cancer model, the early molecular response of intestinal stem cells to genotoxic insult is driven by COX-1-PGE_2 signaling, and results in increased stem cell survival [71]. In breast CSCs, isolated from primary cultures of spontaneous tumors from HER2/Neu transgenic mice, and characterized by proteomic analysis, both COX-1 and COX-2 genes are overexpressed with respect to non-CSCs. Moreover, both COX isoforms belong to an eight-gene signature that correlates with breast cancer patient survival, thus suggesting a role of both isoforms in breast cancers with HER2 overexpression [133]. More recently, the development of anticancer drug resistance has been demonstrated to depend also upon the activation of mesenchymal stem cells (MSCs), which are able of modulating in many ways the response to chemotherapy [134]. A peculiar occurrence after cisplatin treatment is the secretion of specific polyunsaturated fatty acids (12-oxo-5,8,10-heptadecatrienoic acid and hexadeca-4,7,10,13-tetraenoic acid) that are able to confer resistance to various anticancer drugs. Interestingly, the central enzymes involved in the synthesis of MSC-derived chemoprotective factors are COX-1 and thromboxane synthase [135], thus suggesting that enzyme inhibition could restore cancer cell sensitivity.

To summarize, there is a rich body of evidence suggesting that also COX-1 is involved in multiple aspects of cancer pathophysiology. In most cases, it seems that COX-1 and COX-2 isoforms operate in a coordinated manner, while in specific conditions a prominent role for COX-1 has been demonstrated. Functional consequences of COX-1 activation have been poorly investigated as compared to COX-2 activation, even though the effects of COX-1-PGE_2 signaling on tumor cell phenotype have been described. However, a proper consideration should be given to the distinct functional modifications associated to COX-1 (or COX-2) expression [136], as shown also by a very recent genomic, lipidomic and metabolomic analysis of cyclooxygenase-null murine fibroblasts [137]. This study, which describes the common and dissimilar functional interactions of the COX isoforms at the cellular level by using a systems biology approach, demonstrates that COX-1 up-regulation results in a distinct "eicosanoid storm" along with an "anti-inflammatory, proinflammatory, and redox-activated" signatures. Even though fibroblasts are not cancer cells, these results suggest that COX-1 activity, when placed in pivotal position, can affect cell behavior even beyond eicosanoid metabolism.

3. Antitumor Activity of COX-1 Selective Inhibitors

Specific inhibition of COX-2 has been extensively investigated, and many highly selective COX-2 inhibitors are available [138]. In contrast, relatively few COX-1-selective inhibitors have been described [139], and only some of them have been investigated for anticancer activity (Figure 1).

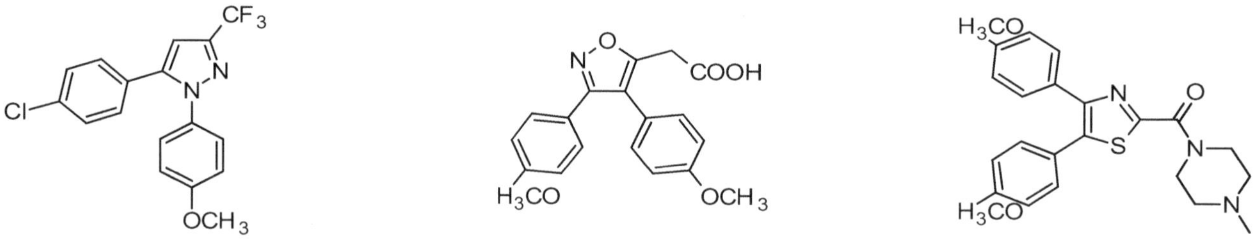

SC-560 mofezolac FR122047

Figure 1. COX-1-selective inhibitors investigated for anticancer properties. SC-560,5-(4-chlorophenyl)-1-(4-methoxyphenyl)-3-(trifluoromethyl)pyrazole; mofezolac, (3,4-bis(4-methoxyphenyl)-5-isoxazolyl)acetic acid; FR122047, 1-((4,5-bis(4-methoxyphenyl)-2-thiazoyl)carbonyl)-4-methylpiperazine.

SC-560. SC-560 is a member of diaryl heterocycle class of COX inhibitors, discovered during the COX-2 inhibitor programs, and originally used as a pharmacologic tool to analyze the role of COX-1-derived prostaglandins in inflammation and pain [140]. The pharmacological action of SC-560 has been explored in various pathological conditions, and its antitumor activity has been investigated in multiple in vitro and in vivo experimental models of ovarian cancer and colorectal cancer, as well as other tumor histotypes, as described in the following.

Based upon a peculiar histopathological pattern showing elevated levels of COX-1 (not COX-2) in the epithelial compartment of ovarian tumor tissue undergoing extensive angiogenesis, the pharmacological action of SC-560 in ovarian cancer models was first investigated by Gupta R.A. et al. [104]. On ovarian cancer cell lines characterized for COX isoforms expression and activity, SC-560 showed in vitro antiproliferative effects similar to those of indomethacin and celecoxib (non-COX isoform selective and COX-2-selective, respectively), and only at doses 50–100 times greater than those achieved in in vivo systems [140]. In contrast, only SC-560 was found to inhibit arachidonic acid-induced VEGF secretion at low doses, an effect that was dose-dependently reverted by PGE_2. The in vivo tumor growth inhibitory efficacy of SC-560 was then demonstrated by Daikoku T. et al. in genetically engineered ovarian cancer murine models, in which COX-1 overexpression was common to various disease-associated genetic alterations [105,106]. As far as COX-1 downstream targets are concerned, experimental evidence for PPARδ–ERK signaling involvement was provided in murine, as well as in human ovarian cancer [119]. The in vivo activity of SC-560 alone or in various combination protocols has been extensively investigated by Li W. et al. in the SKOV-3 xenograft model [141–147]. In this model, SKOV-3 cells predominantly express the COX-1 isoform, as determined by immunohistochemical analysis of tumor samples [142], and SC-560 treatment at COX-1-specific inhibitory dosages produced a slight to moderate reduction of tumor growth. Interestingly, combination treatment of SC-560 with cisplatin [147] or taxol [144–147] generally provided greater efficacy than individual agents on various pharmacological end-points, including angiogenesis, proliferation and apoptosis. Not surprisingly, a combination of SC-560 with the non-selective inhibitor ibuprofen [141] or the COX-2-selective celecoxib [143] also showed major efficacy in the SKOV-3 system, suggesting that the inhibition of both COX-1 and COX-2 could overcome a potential compensation between the two isoforms in the SKOV-3 xenograft biology. From a mechanistic point of view, the in vivo effects of SC-560 in the SKOV-3 system may be related to the treatment-dependent reduction of PGE_2 production and to the associated inhibition of angiogenesis. However, a clear evidence for an exclusive or prevailing COX-1 dependence of prostaglandin production in SKOV-3 cells is lacking. Moreover, it cannot be excluded that in in vivo systems SC-560 could inhibit also COX-2 [148], and that COX-independent effects could contribute to antitumor activity. Some concern is partly due to the SKOV-3 cell line itself, which in some cases is reported as negative for COX-1 expression [104]. This is not actually unusual in the cyclooxygenase literature; the contrasting results variably depend upon a different source of the cell line, antibody cross-reactivity or other technical issues [149], and distinct experimental conditions (i.e., in vitro versus in vivo). Interestingly, SC-560 increases also paclitaxel sensitivity of taxane-resistant ovarian cancer cell lines characterized by MDR1/P-glycoprotein upregulation. A similar effect was produced by the COX-2 selective inhibitor NS398, not modified by PGE_2 addition, thus suggesting a prostaglandin- and COX-independent mechanism [150]. The concrete possibility that SC-560 could represent a promising lead for ovarian cancer treatment is also suggested by the SC-560 belonging to a group of small molecule compounds that are potentially able to target ovarian cancer stem cell (OVCSC)-specific genes [151]. This interesting feature has been recently discovered through the characterization of OVCSC-specific gene expression profiling and a co-expression extrapolation with CMAP, a massive repository of gene expression data that provides information on gene expression modification of several cell lines treated with >1000 bioactive compounds [152].

In vitro and in vivo activity of SC-560 in comparison to celecoxib against colorectal cancer cells was investigated by Grosch S. et al. [153], by evaluating their effects on survival, cell cycle progression, and apoptosis of colon cancer cell characterized for COX-1 and COX-2 expression. Independently from COX status, both SC-560 and celecoxib affected in vitro cell survival and induced a G0/G1 block, whereas only celecoxib induced apoptosis. In vivo, both compounds were active towards a HCT-15 (COX-2 deficient) xenograft, but devoid of significant effect on HT-29 (COX-2 expressing) tumors, overall indicating a COX-independent mechanism of action. The effects of SC-560 on HT-29 colon cancer cells have been investigated also by Wu W. K. et al. [154], showing that the growth inhibitory effect was accompanied by G1-S transition arrest and phosphoinositide 3-kinase (PI3K)-induced autophagy. Proliferation inhibition and cell-cycle progression arrest induced in vitro by SC-560 has been investigated also on HCT-116 colon cancer cells, which had been previously characterized by a total absence of COX expression and activity [155]. Lee et al. showed that the growth inhibitory effect towards HCT-116 cells was affected by the cell cycle regulator protein p21CIP1 [156]. Moreover, Sakoguchi-Okada N. et al. showed that the growth inhibitory and apoptotic effect of SC-560 (and other non-selective and COX-2-selective inhibitors) on HCT-116 cells was associated with inhibition of survivin expression and Wnt/beta-catenin signaling pathway [157]. With the aim of identifying possible COX-independent mechanisms of action of NSAIDs, treatment-induced gene expression modifications of HCT-116 cells were investigated by using suppression subtractive hybridization [158]. Interestingly, two cancer-related genes, NAG-1 (officially known as GDF15), and thymosin β-4 (TMSB4X), were induced by SC-560, thus suggesting potentially contrasting effects on its antitumor activity. NAG-1 codes indeed for a pleiotropic cytokine of the TGF-β superfamily expressed in a broad range of cell types and involved in the cellular stress response program. NAG-1 induction effect may either be tumor-growth suppressive or enhancing, depending upon its induction pattern (acute or sustained) and pathophysiological context [159]. The induction of thymosin β-4 too could potentially compromise the anticancer activity of SC-560, being thymosin β-4 mechanistically involved in the metastatic process [160,161] and associated with poor prognosis in CRC [162]. Cyclooxygenase- and prostaglandin-independent growth inhibitory effects of SC-560 have been reported in vitro in cells representing various other tumor histotypes. The growth and cell-cycle progression of human A549, H460, and H358 lung cancer cells is affected by SC-560 at doses that are definitely higher than those required for COX-inhibiting activity. Interestingly, the growth suppression induced by SC-560, but not celecoxib treatment, was associated with reactive oxygen species production [163]. Multiple myeloma cell proliferation is also inhibited by SC-560 at doses that are 10 times higher than those necessary for enzymatic inhibition [164]. SC-560 treatment of HuH-6 and HA22T/VGH human hepatocellular carcinoma cell lines, expressing both COX isoforms at mRNA and protein level, led to growth inhibition and apoptosis, and inhibited anchorage-independent growth of HuH-6 cells in soft agar, an in vitro marker for malignancy of cancer cells [165]. From a mechanistic point of view, treatment of tumor cells with SC-560, as well as with the coxib CAY10404, was associated with activation of ERK1/2 signaling pathway.

Mofezolac. Among the few selective COX-1 inhibitors investigated as potential analgesics and anti-platelet agents, mofezolac has been developed and marketed in Japan as a powerful pain killer [166], and its anticancer activity has been investigated almost exclusively in colorectal cancer experimental models. In vitro treatment of a COX-1-expressing RGMI cell line (non-transformed cells derived from rat gastric mucosa) by mofezolac induces a weak apoptotic effect, substantially prostaglandin-synthesis independent, with respect to indomethacin or sodium diclofenac [167], and a similar behavior was also observed in AGS gastric adenocarcinoma cells, treated at concentrations that were similar to those found at gastric mucosa after oral administration [168]. With regard to in vivo models of colorectal cancer, mofezolac treatment suppresses the development of aberrant crypt foci (putative preneoplastic lesions) induced by azoxymethane (AOM) and reduces the number of intestinal polyps in Apc knockout mice. In both murine models, the efficacy of mofezolac was similar to that of nimesulide, this indicating a tumorigenic role for both cyclooxygenase isoforms in this experimental model [169]. Accordingly, a combination treatment with COX-1- and COX-2-selective inhibitors more effectively suppressed polyp growth than either of the single treatments alone in Apc knockout mice [170]. Besides inhibiting preneoplastic lesions, mofezolac significantly reduces the incidence, multiplicity and volume of azoxymethane-induced rat colon carcinomas [171], thus confirming the COX-1 pathophysiological role in the AOM-induced intestinal carcinogenesis. Interestingly, Mofezolac is also effective in suppressing beef tallow-promoted colon carcinogenesis in rats, thus suggesting a potential benefit for populations with high fat intake [172].

FR122047. The COX-1-selective inhibitor, 4,5-bis(4-methoxyphenyl)-2-[(1-methylpiperazin-4-yl) carbonyl]thiazole (FR122047) was originally developed as antiplatelet agent devoid of ulcerogenic effects [173], and investigated as analgesic agent [174], or used as tool for studying the involvement of COX-1 as well as the role of prostanoids generated along the COX-1 and COX-2 pathways in various models of inflammation [175,176]. The antitumor activity of FR122047 has been investigated in vitro on MCF-7 breast cancer cells [80]. FR122047 treatment inhibits in vitro cell growth of MCF-7 cells, and induces apoptotic cell death that is mechanistically independent from treatment-associated ROS production, as well as from PGE_2 production inhibition. Mechanisms of MCF-7 cell death induced by FR12207 were further investigated by the same group [177], showing that FR122047 treatment induces caspase-mediated apoptosis and at the same time stimulates a defensive autophagic response of MCF-7 cells. Interestingly, the inhibition of caspase-9 blocks the cytoprotective autophagic process, thus increasing the susceptibility of MCF-7 cells to FR-122047-induced cell death.

In general, in vitro and in vivo antitumor properties of COX-1-selective inhibitors resemble those of other NSAIDs and coxibs; in some cases, COX-dependent, and in others, COX-independent mechanisms having been reported. Preliminary screening of the anticancer properties of COX inhibitors is usually performed by investigating the in vitro effect upon cell proliferation and cell cycle progression of tumor cells characterized for COX expression and activity. COX-1-selective inhibitors, not different from other NSAIDs or coxibs, impair cell growth and proliferation, this biological end-point being most often associated with cell cycle G1-phase arrest and cell death. These effects are usually observed at compound concentrations that are much higher than those of common cytotoxic drugs [178], and very often higher than clinically relevant COX-inhibitor concentrations. The true effective concentration of COX inhibitors in in vitro systems could actually be lower than that indicated, owing to a subtractive interaction with the serum proteins of culture medium [179]. However, whilst considering the protein interaction caveat, it is not surprising that COX-1 inhibitors (as well as traditional NSAIDs and coxibs) have weak antiproliferative effects related to enzymatic inhibition. This probably reflects the weak impact of COX-derived PGs in the maintenance of in vitro growth and proliferation condition. In the various inflammatory pathological conditions in which the PG activity has been investigated, these molecules do not operate as primary signals of homeostasis modification, but rather as amplification signals at the tissue level [19]. There is no reason to believe that in vitro tumor cell proliferation could be a different situation, as shown also by the lack of efficacy of COX inhibitors against resting tumor cells [180]. Therefore, to obtain more useful information from a basic antitumor assay such as cell growth and proliferation inhibition, it would be preferable to use tumor cells that increase their proliferation rate as a result of PG addition, and to demonstrate that this effect is impaired by the COX inhibitor under investigation. In this context, it would be preferable to integrate the COX expression and activity data into a more general knowledge of genes and gene products that are associated with AA metabolism in the tumor cells under investigation. This information is available to the scientific community in public databases, e.g., the Cancer Cell Line Encyclopedia [181], and it is essential for a reasoned choice of tumor cells to be used, also in relation to their suitability as models of human clinical disease [182]. The elegant paper of Wilson A.J. et al. [118] on the relevance of COX-1 in HGSOC witnesses the effectiveness of this strategy. Moreover, treatment effects upon cell cycle progression and the cell survival–death homeostasis could be more conveniently investigated in the same experimental setting by using modern multiparametric imaging technologies [183], thereby obtaining a comprehensive picture of treatment-associated phenotypic modifications. In in vitro systems again, specific investigations could be planned by using 3D tumor cell models enriched with stromal cells, to more closely mimic the tissue-like condition in which PGs usually operate. As far as other tumor phenotype hallmarks potentially affected by COX-derived PGs, such as angiogenesis, invasion and metastasis, and immune effects, they all would only be observed in in vivo systems, although some useful indication can be provided by in vitro assays measuring cell adhesion properties, migration, invasion, and colony formation [178]. As far as the COX-independent mechanism, which are often described for COX-1-selective inhibitors, they could also be of interest. Unlike what occurred with the COX-independent pharmacological actions of coxibs [184], which gave rise to substantial research and development activity [43], the results so far reported for COX-1-selective inhibitors have not triggered systematic research on this topic. This is not surprising, considering the small number COX-1-selective compounds available. On the other hand, a COX-independent mechanism occurs in an unpredictable manner, and sometimes in a different context, as in the case of the ability of mofezolac to interact with c-myc oncoprotein [185].

4. Conclusions

The involvement of COX-1 activity in cancer seems to have, in most cases, a pathophysiological role that is consistent and coordinated with COX-2, as in other inflammation-associated pathological conditions. However, in some cases, as exemplified by serous ovarian carcinoma, COX-1 overexpression plays a pivotal role, stimulating more in-depth studies on its function in this specific condition, and suggesting that other histopathological and molecular subtypes of cancer disease could share this feature. However, it seems clear that the analysis of functional implications of COX-1-signaling, as well as of the pharmacological action of COX-1-selective inhibitors, should not be restricted to the COX pathway, and to the effects of prostaglandins that are already known for their ability to affect the tumor phenotype. A knowledge-based choice of the most appropriate tumor cell models, and a major effort in investigating the COX-1 issue in the more general context of the arachidonic acid metabolic network by using systems biology approaches, should be strongly encouraged.

Author Contributions: Conceptualization, M.C.; Writing–Original draft, M.C. and A.P.; Writing–Review and Editing, M.C. and A.P.; Funding Acquisition, M.C.

Acknowledgments: The authors thank Federica Campanella for her help in the literature research.

References

1. Balkwill, F.; Mantovani, A. Inflammation and cancer: Back to Virchow? *Lancet* **2001**, *357*, 539–545. [CrossRef]
2. Hanahan, D.; Weinberg, R.A. Hallmarks of cancer: The next generation. *Cell* **2011**, *144*, 646–674. [CrossRef] [PubMed]
3. Ben-Neriah, Y.; Karin, M. Inflammation meets cancer, with NF-κB as the matchmaker. *Nat. Immunol.* **2011**, *12*, 715–723. [CrossRef] [PubMed]
4. Crusz, S.M.; Balkwill, F.R. Inflammation and cancer: Advances and new agents. *Nat. Rev. Clin. Oncol.* **2015**, *12*, 584–596. [CrossRef] [PubMed]
5. Coussens, L.M.; Zitvogel, L.; Palucka, A.K. Neutralizing tumor-promoting chronic inflammation: A magic bullet? *Science* **2013**, *339*, 286–291. [CrossRef] [PubMed]
6. Dennis, E.A.; Norris, P.C. Eicosanoid storm in infection and inflammation. *Nat. Rev. Immunol.* **2015**, *15*, 511–523. [CrossRef] [PubMed]
7. Hirata, T.; Narumiya, S. Prostanoid receptors. *Chem. Rev.* **2011**, *111*, 6209–6230. [CrossRef] [PubMed]
8. Botha, J.H.; Bobinson, K.M.; Ramchurren, N.; Reddi, K.; Norman, R.J. Human esophageal carcinoma cell lines: Prostaglandin production, biological properties, and behavior in nude mice. *J. Natl. Cancer Inst.* **1986**, *76*, 1053–1056. [PubMed]
9. Wang, D.; Dubois, R.N. Eicosanoids and cancer. *Nat. Rev. Cancer* **2010**, *10*, 181–193. [CrossRef] [PubMed]
10. Nakanishi, M.; Rosenberg, D.W. Multifaceted roles of PGE2 in inflammation and cancer. *Semin. Immunopathol.* **2013**, *35*, 123–137. [CrossRef] [PubMed]
11. Sha, W.; Brüne, B.; Weigert, A. The multi-faceted roles of prostaglandin E2 in cancer-infiltrating mononuclear phagocyte biology. *Immunobiology* **2012**, *217*, 1225–1232. [CrossRef] [PubMed]
12. Oshima, H.; Oshima, M. The inflammatory network in the gastrointestinal tumor microenvironment: Lessons from mouse models. *J. Gastroenterol.* **2012**, *47*, 97–106. [CrossRef] [PubMed]
13. Kalinski, P. Regulation of immune responses by prostaglandin E2. *J. Immunol.* **2012**, *188*, 21–28. [CrossRef] [PubMed]
14. Vong, L.; Ferraz, J.G.; Panaccione, R.; Beck, P.L.; Wallace, J.L. A pro-resolution mediator, prostaglandin D(2), is specifically up-regulated in individuals in long-term remission from ulcerative colitis. *Proc. Natl. Acad. Sci. USA* **2010**, *107*, 12023–12027. [CrossRef] [PubMed]
15. Li, H.; Liu, K.; Boardman, L.A.; Zhao, Y.; Wang, L.; Sheng, Y.; Oi, N.; Limburg, P.J.; Bode, A.M.; Dong, Z. Circulating prostaglandin biosynthesis in colorectal cancer and potential clinical significance. *EBioMedicine* **2015**, *2*, 165–171. [CrossRef] [PubMed]
16. Dovizio, M.; Tacconelli, S.; Ricciotti, E.; Bruno, A.; Maier, T.J.; Anzellotti, P.; Di Francesco, L.; Sala, P.; Signoroni, S.; Bertario, L.; et al. Effects of celecoxib on prostanoid biosyntesis and circulating angiogenesis proteins in familial adenomatous polyposis. *J. Pharmacol. Exp. Ther.* **2012**, *341*, 242–250. [CrossRef] [PubMed]

17. Liu, Q.; Tao, B.; Liu, G.; Chen, G.; Zhu, Q.; Yu, Y.; Yu, Y.; Xiong, H. Thromboxane A2 receptor inhibition suppresses multiple myeloma cell proliferation by inducing p38/c-Jun N-terminal Kinase (JNK) Mitogen-activated Protein Kinase (MAPK)-mediated G2/M progression delay and cell apoptosis. *J. Biol. Chem.* **2016**, *291*, 4779–4792. [CrossRef] [PubMed]
18. Li, X.; Tai, H.H. Activation of thromboxane A(2) receptors induces orphan nuclear receptor Nurr1 expression and stimulates cell proliferation in human lung cancer cells. *Carcinogenesis* **2009**, *30*, 1606–1613. [CrossRef] [PubMed]
19. Ricciotti, E.; FitzGerald, G.A. Prostaglandins and inflammation. *Arterioscler. Thromb. Vasc. Biol.* **2011**, *31*, 986–1000. [CrossRef] [PubMed]
20. Smith, W.L.; DeWitt, D.L.; Garavito, R.M. Cyclooxygenases: Structural, cellular, and molecular biology. *Annu. Rev. Biochem.* **2000**, *69*, 145–182. [CrossRef] [PubMed]
21. Zidar, N.; Odar, K.; Glavac, D.; Jerse, M.; Zupanc, T.; Stajer, D. Cyclooxygenase in normal human tissues—Is COX-1 really a constitutive isoform, and COX-2 an inducible isoform? *J. Cell. Mol. Med.* **2009**, *13*, 3753–3763. [CrossRef] [PubMed]
22. Kang, Y.J.; Mbonye, U.R.; DeLong, C.J.; Wada, M.; Smith, W.L. Regulation of intracellular cyclooxygenase levels by gene transcription and protein degradation. *Prog. Lipid Res.* **2007**, *46*, 108–125. [CrossRef] [PubMed]
23. Lutz, C.S.; Cornett, A.L. Regulation of genes in the arachidonic acid metabolic pathway by RNA processing and RNA-mediated mechanisms. *Wiley Interdiscip. Rev. RNA* **2013**, *4*, 593–605. [CrossRef] [PubMed]
24. Zhang, M.; Zhou, S.; Zhang, L.; Ye, W.; Wen, Q.; Wang, J. Role of cancer-related inflammation in esophageal cancer. *Crit. Rev. Eukaryot. Gene Expr.* **2013**, *23*, 27–35. [CrossRef] [PubMed]
25. Cheng, J.; Fan, X.M. Role of cyclooxygenase-2 in gastric cancer development and progression. *World J. Gastroenterol.* **2013**, *19*, 7361–7368. [CrossRef] [PubMed]
26. Cathcart, M.C.; O'Byrne, K.J.; Reynolds, J.V.; O'Sullivan, J.; Pidgeon, G.P. COX-derived prostanoid pathways in gastrointestinal cancer development and progression: Novel targets for prevention and intervention. *Biochim. Biophys. Acta* **2012**, *1825*, 49–63. [CrossRef] [PubMed]
27. Knab, L.M.; Grippo, P.J.; Bentrem, D.J. Involvement of eicosanoids in the pathogenesis of pancreatic cancer: The roles of cyclooxygenase-2 and 5-lipoxygenase. *World J. Gastroenterol.* **2014**, *20*, 10729–10739. [CrossRef] [PubMed]
28. Glover, J.A.; Hughes, C.M.; Cantwell, M.M.; Murray, L.J. A systematic review to establish the frequency of cyclooxygenase-2 expression in normal breast epithelium, ductal carcinoma in situ, microinvasive carcinoma of the breast and invasive breast cancer. *Br. J. Cancer* **2011**, *105*, 13–17. [CrossRef] [PubMed]
29. Parida, S.; Mandal, M. Inflammation induced by human papillomavirus in cervical cancer and its implication in prevention. *Eur. J. Cancer Prev.* **2014**, *23*, 432–448. [CrossRef] [PubMed]
30. Kaminska, K.; Szczylik, C.; Lian, F.; Czarnecka, A.M. The role of prostaglandin E2 in renal cell cancer development: Future implications for prognosis and therapy. *Future Oncol.* **2014**, *10*, 2177–2187. [CrossRef] [PubMed]
31. Shao, N.; Feng, N.; Wang, Y.; Mi, Y.; Li, T.; Hua, L. Systematic review and meta-analysis of COX-2 expression and polymorphisms in prostate cancer. *Mol. Biol. Rep.* **2012**, *39*, 10997–11004. [CrossRef] [PubMed]
32. Gakis, G. The role of inflammation in bladder cancer. *Adv. Exp. Med. Biol.* **2014**, *816*, 183–196. [CrossRef] [PubMed]
33. Elmets, C.A.; Ledet, J.J.; Athar, M. Cyclooxygenases: Mediators of UV-induced skin cancer and potential targets for prevention. *J. Investig. Dermatol.* **2014**, *134*, 2497–2502. [CrossRef] [PubMed]
34. Rundhaug, J.E.; Simper, M.S.; Surh, I.; Fischer, S.M. The role of the EP receptors for prostaglandin E2 in skin and skin cancer. *Cancer Metastasis Rev.* **2011**, *30*, 465–480. [CrossRef] [PubMed]
35. Mendes, R.A.; Carvalho, J.F.; van der Waal, I. An overview on the expression of cyclooxygenase-2 in tumors of the head and neck. *Oral Oncol.* **2009**, *45*, e124–e128. [CrossRef] [PubMed]
36. Ramon, S.; Woeller, C.F.; Phipps, R.P. The influence of Cox-2 and bioactive lipids on hematological cancers. *Curr. Angiogenes.* **2013**, *2*, 135–142. [CrossRef] [PubMed]
37. Nuvoli, B.; Galati, R. Cyclooxygenase-2, epidermal growth factor receptor, and aromatase signaling in inflammation and mesothelioma. *Mol. Cancer Ther.* **2013**, *12*, 844–852. [CrossRef] [PubMed]
38. Greenhough, A.; Smartt, H.J.; Moore, A.E.; Roberts, H.R.; Williams, A.C.; Paraskeva, C.; Kaidi, A. The COX-2/PGE2 pathway: Key roles in the hallmarks of cancer and adaptation to the tumour microenvironment. *Carcinogenesis* **2009**, *30*, 377–386. [CrossRef] [PubMed]

39. Harris, R.E. Cyclooxygenase-2 (cox-2) and the inflammogenesis of cancer. *Subcell. Biochem.* **2007**, *42*, 93–126. [CrossRef] [PubMed]
40. Dixon, D.A.; Blanco, F.F.; Bruno, A.; Patrignani, P. Mechanistic aspects of COX-2 expression in colorectal neoplasia. *Recent Results Cancer Res.* **2013**, *191*, 7–37. [CrossRef] [PubMed]
41. Cebola, I.; Peinado, M.A. Epigenetic deregulation of the COX pathway in cancer. *Prog. Lipid Res.* **2012**, *51*, 301–313. [CrossRef] [PubMed]
42. Fischer, S.M.; Hawk, E.T.; Lubet, R.A. Coxibs and other nonsteroidal anti-inflammatory drugs in animal models of cancer chemoprevention. *Cancer Prev. Res.* **2011**, *4*, 1728–1735. [CrossRef] [PubMed]
43. Gurpinar, E.; Grizzle, W.E.; Piazza, G.A. NSAIDs inhibit tumorigenesis, but how? *Clin. Cancer Res.* **2014**, *20*, 1104–1113. [CrossRef] [PubMed]
44. Rouzer, C.A.; Marnett, L.J. Cyclooxygenases: Structural and functional insights. *J. Lipid Res.* **2009**, *50*, S29–S34. [CrossRef] [PubMed]
45. Chulada, P.C.; Thompson, M.B.; Mahler, J.F.; Doyle, C.M.; Gaul, B.W.; Lee, C.; Tiano, H.F.; Morham, S.G.; Smithies, O.; Langenbach, R. Genetic disruption of Ptgs-1, as well as Ptgs-2, reduces intestinal tumorigenesis in Min mice. *Cancer Res.* **2000**, *60*, 4705–4708. [PubMed]
46. Tiano, H.F.; Loftin, C.D.; Akunda, J.; Lee, C.A.; Spalding, J.; Sessoms, A.; Dunson, D.B.; Rogan, E.G.; Morham, S.G.; Smart, R.C.; et al. Deficiency of either cyclooxygenase (COX)-1 or COX-2 alters epidermal differentiation and reduces mouse skin tumorigenesis. *Cancer Res.* **2002**, *62*, 3395–3401. [PubMed]
47. Okamoto, T.; Hara, A.; Hino, O. Down-regulation of cyclooxygenase-2 expression but up-regulation of cyclooxygenase-1 in renal carcinomas of the Eker (TSC2 gene mutant) rat model. *Cancer Sci.* **2003**, *94*, 22–25. [CrossRef] [PubMed]
48. Yu, Z.H.; Zhang, Q.; Wang, Y.D.; Chen, J.; Jiang, Z.M.; Shi, M.; Guo, X.; Qin, J.; Cui, G.H.; Cai, Z.M.; et al. Overexpression of cyclooxygenase-1 correlates with poor prognosis in renal cell carcinoma. *Asian Pac. J. Cancer Prev.* **2013**, *14*, 3729–3734. [CrossRef] [PubMed]
49. Osman, W.M.; Youssef, N.S. Combined use of COX-1 and VEGF immunohistochemistry refines the histopathologic prognosis of renal cell carcinoma. *Int. J. Clin. Exp. Pathol.* **2015**, *8*, 8165–8177. [PubMed]
50. Tang, J.Y.; Aszterbaum, M.; Athar, M.; Barsanti, F.; Cappola, C.; Estevez, N.; Hebert, J.; Hwang, J.; Khaimskiy, Y.; Kim, A.; et al. Basal cell carcinoma chemoprevention with nonsteroidal anti-inflammatory drugs in genetically predisposed PTCH1+/− humans and mice. *Cancer Prev. Res.* **2010**, *3*, 25–34. [CrossRef] [PubMed]
51. Müller-Decker, K. Cyclooxygenase-dependent signaling is causally linked to non-melanoma skin carcinogenesis: Pharmacological, genetic, and clinical evidence. *Cancer Metastasis Rev.* **2011**, *30*, 343–361. [CrossRef] [PubMed]
52. Erovic, B.M.; Woegerbauer, M.; Pammer, J.; Selzer, E.; Grasl, M.C.; Thurnher, D. Strong evidence for up-regulation of cyclooxygenase-1 in head and neck cancer. *Eur. J. Clin. Investig.* **2008**, *38*, 61–66. [CrossRef] [PubMed]
53. Mauro, A.; Lipari, L.; Leone, A.; Tortorici, S.; Burruano, F.; Provenzano, S.; Gerbino, A.; Buscemi, M. Expression of cyclooxygenase-1 and cyclooxygenase-2 in normal and pathological human oral mucosa. *Folia Histochem. Cytobiol.* **2010**, *48*, 555–563. [CrossRef] [PubMed]
54. Pannone, G.; Sanguedolce, F.; De Maria, S.; Farina, E.; Lo Muzio, L.; Serpico, R.; Emanuelli, M.; Rubini, C.; De Rosa, G.; Staibano, S.; et al. Cyclooxygenase isozymes in oral squamous cell carcinoma: A real-time RT-PCR study with clinic pathological correlations. *Int. J. Immunopathol. Pharmacol.* **2007**, *20*, 317–324. [CrossRef] [PubMed]
55. Erovic, B.M.; Al Habeeb, A.; Harris, L.; Goldstein, D.P.; Kim, D.; Ghazarian, D.; Irish, J.C. Identification of novel target proteins in sebaceous gland carcinoma. *Head Neck* **2013**, *35*, 642–648. [CrossRef] [PubMed]
56. Park, S.W.; Kim, H.S.; Hah, J.H.; Kim, K.H.; Heo, D.S.; Sung, M.W. Differential effects between cyclooxygenase-2 inhibitors and siRNA on vascular endothelial growth factor production in head and neck squamous cell carcinoma cell lines. *Head Neck* **2010**, *32*, 1534–1543. [CrossRef] [PubMed]
57. Park, S.W.; Kim, H.S.; Choi, M.S.; Kim, J.E.; Jeong, W.J.; Heo, D.S.; Sung, M.W. The influence of cyclooxygenase-1 expression on the efficacy of cyclooxygenase-2 inhibition in head and neck squamous cell carcinoma cell lines. *Anticancer Drugs* **2011**, *22*, 416–423. [CrossRef] [PubMed]

58. Akiyama, J.; Alexandre, L.; Baruah, A.; Buttar, N.; Chandra, R.; Clark, A.B.; Hart, A.R.; Hawk, E.; Kandioler, D.; Kappel, S.; et al. Strategy for prevention of cancers of the esophagus. *Ann. N. Y. Acad. Sci.* **2014**, *1325*, 108–126. [CrossRef] [PubMed]
59. Tsibouris, P.; Vlachou, E.; Isaacs, P.E. Role of chemoprophylaxis with either NSAIDs or statins in patients with Barrett's esophagus. *World J. Gastrointest. Pharmacol. Ther.* **2014**, *5*, 27–39. [CrossRef] [PubMed]
60. Morris, C.D.; Armstrong, G.R.; Bigley, G.; Green, H.; Attwood, S.E. Cyclooxygenase-2 expression in the Barrett's metaplasia–dysplasia–adenocarcinoma sequence. *Am. J. Gastroenterol.* **2001**, *96*, 990–996. [CrossRef] [PubMed]
61. Taddei, A.; Fabbroni, V.; Pini, A.; Lucarini, L.; Ringressi, M.N.; Fantappiè, O.; Bani, D.; Messerini, L.; Masini, E.; Bechi, P. Cyclooxygenase-2 and inflammation mediators have a crucial role in reflux-related esophageal histological changes and Barrett's esophagus. *Dig. Dis. Sci.* **2014**, *59*, 949–957. [CrossRef] [PubMed]
62. Von Rahden, B.H.; Stein, H.J.; Pühringer, F.; Koch, I.; Langer, R.; Piontek, G.; Siewert, J.R.; Höfler, H.; Sarbia, M. Coexpression of cyclooxygenases (COX-1, COX-2) and vascular endothelial growth factors (VEGF-A, VEGF-C) in esophageal adenocarcinoma. *Cancer Res.* **2005**, *65*, 5038–5044. [CrossRef] [PubMed]
63. Piazuelo, E.; Santander, S.; Cebrián, C.; Jiménez, P.; Pastor, C.; García-González, M.A.; Esteva, F.; Esquivias, P.; Ortego, J.; Lanas, A. Characterization of the prostaglandin E2 pathway in a rat model of esophageal adenocarcinoma. *Curr. Cancer Drug Targets* **2012**, *12*, 132–143. [CrossRef] [PubMed]
64. Esquivias, P.; Morandeira, A.; Escartín, A.; Cebrián, C.; Santander, S.; Esteva, F.; García-González, M.A.; Ortego, J.; Lanas, A.; Piazuelo, E. Indomethacin but not a selective cyclooxygenase-2 inhibitor inhibits esophageal adenocarcinogenesis in rats. *World J. Gastroenterol.* **2012**, *18*, 4866–4874. [CrossRef] [PubMed]
65. Zhang, S.; Zhang, X.Q.; Ding, X.W.; Yang, R.K.; Huang, S.L.; Kastelein, F.; Bruno, M.; Yu, X.J.; Zhou, D.; Zou, X.P. Cyclooxygenase inhibitors use is associated with reduced risk of esophageal adenocarcinoma in patients with Barrett's esophagus: A meta-analysis. *Br. J. Cancer* **2014**, *110*, 2378–2388. [CrossRef] [PubMed]
66. Janakiram, N.B.; Rao, C.V. The role of inflammation in colon cancer. *Adv. Exp. Med. Biol.* **2014**, *816*, 25–52. [CrossRef] [PubMed]
67. Arber, N.; Eagle, C.J.; Spicak, J.; Rácz, I.; Dite, P.; Hajer, J.; Zavoral, M.; Lechuga, M.J.; Gerletti, P.; Tang, J.; et al. PreSAP Trial Investigators. Celecoxib for the prevention of colorectal adenomatous polyps. *N. Engl. J. Med.* **2006**, *355*, 885–895. [CrossRef] [PubMed]
68. Kraus, S.; Naumov, I.; Arber, N. COX-2 active agents in the chemoprevention of colorectal cancer. *Recent Results Cancer Res.* **2013**, *191*, 95–103. [CrossRef] [PubMed]
69. Church, R.D.; Yu, J.; Fleshman, J.W.; Shannon, W.D.; Govindan, R.; McLeod, H.L. RNA profiling of cyclooxygenases 1 and 2 in colorectal cancer. *Br. J. Cancer* **2004**, *91*, 1015–1018. [CrossRef] [PubMed]
70. Von Rahden, B.H.; Brücher, B.L.; Langner, C.; Siewert, J.R.; Stein, H.J.; Sarbia, M. Expression of cyclo-oxygenase 1 and 2, prostaglandin E synthase and transforming growth factor beta1, and their relationship with vascular endothelial growth factors A and C, in primary adenocarcinoma of the small intestine. *Br. J. Surg.* **2006**, *93*, 1424–1432. [CrossRef] [PubMed]
71. Riehl, T.E.; George, R.J.; Sturmoski, M.A.; May, R.; Dieckgraefe, B.; Anant, S.; Houchen, C.W. Azoxymethane protects intestinal stem cells and reduces crypt epithelial mitosis through a COX-1 dependent mechanism. *Am. J. Physiol. Gastrointest. Liver Physiol.* **2006**, *291*, G1062–G1070. [CrossRef] [PubMed]
72. Takeda, H.; Sonoshita, M.; Oshima, H.; Sugihara, K.; Chulada, P.C.; Langenbach, R.; Oshima, M.; Taketo, M.M. Cooperation of cyclooxygenase 1 and cyclooxygenase 2 in intestinal polyposis. *Cancer Res.* **2003**, *63*, 4872–4877. [PubMed]
73. Smartt, H.J.; Greenhough, A.; Ordóñez-Morán, P.; Talero, E.; Cherry, C.A.; Wallam, C.A.; Parry, L.; Al Kharusi, M.; Roberts, H.R.; Mariadason, J.M.; et al. β-catenin represses expression of the tumour suppressor 15-prostaglandin dehydrogenase in the normal intestinal epithelium and colorectal tumour cells. *Gut* **2012**, *61*, 1306–13014. [CrossRef] [PubMed]
74. Li, H.; Zhu, F.; Chen, H.; Cheng, K.W.; Zykova, T.; Oi, N.; Lubet, R.A.; Bode, A.M.; Wang, M.; Dong, Z. 6-C-(E-phenylethenyl)-naringenin suppresses colorectal cancer growth by inhibiting cyclooxygenase-1. *Cancer Res.* **2014**, *74*, 243–252. [CrossRef] [PubMed]
75. Vona-Davis, L.; Rose, D.P. The obesity-inflammation-eicosanoid axis in breast cancer. *J. Mammary Gland Biol. Neoplasia* **2013**, *18*, 291–307. [CrossRef] [PubMed]

76. Hoellen, F.; Kelling, K.; Dittmer, C.; Diedrich, K.; Friedrich, M.; Thill, M. Impact of cyclooxygenase-2 in breast cancer. *Anticancer Res.* **2011**, *31*, 4359–4367. [PubMed]
77. Hwang, D.; Scollard, D.; Byrne, J.; Levine, E. Expression of cyclooxygenase-1 and cyclooxygenase-2 in human breast cancer. *J. Natl. Cancer Inst.* **1998**, *90*, 455–460. [CrossRef] [PubMed]
78. Fahlén, M.; Zhang, H.; Löfgren, L.; Masironi, B.; von Schoultz, E.; von Schoultz, B.; Sahlin, L. Expression of cyclooxygenase-1 and cyclooxygenase-2, syndecan-1 and connective tissue growth factor in benign and malignant breast tissue from premenopausal women. *Gynecol. Endocrinol.* **2017**, *33*, 353–358. [CrossRef] [PubMed]
79. Haakensen, V.D.; Bjøro, T.; Lüders, T.; Riis, M.; Bukholm, I.K.; Kristensen, V.N.; Troester, M.A.; Homen, M.M.; Ursin, G.; Børresen-Dale, A.L.; et al. Serum estradiol levels associated with specific gene expression patterns in normal breast tissue and in breast carcinomas. *BMC Cancer* **2011**, *11*, 332. [CrossRef] [PubMed]
80. Jeong, H.S.; Kim, J.H.; Choi, H.Y.; Lee, E.R.; Cho, S.G. Induction of cell growth arrest and apoptotic cell death in human breast cancer MCF-7 cells by the COX-1 inhibitor FR122047. *Oncol. Rep.* **2010**, *24*, 351–356. [CrossRef] [PubMed]
81. McFadden, D.W.; Riggs, D.R.; Jackson, B.J.; Cunningham, C. Additive effects of Cox-1 and Cox-2 inhibition on breast cancer in vitro. *Int. J. Oncol.* **2006**, *29*, 1019–1023. [CrossRef] [PubMed]
82. Kundu, N.; Fulton, A.M. Selective cyclooxygenase (COX)-1 or COX-2 inhibitors control metastatic disease in a murine model of breast cancer. *Cancer Res.* **2002**, *62*, 2343–2346. [PubMed]
83. Boccardo, E.; Lepique, A.P.; Villa, L.L. The role of inflammation in HPV carcinogenesis. *Carcinogenesis* **2010**, *31*, 1905–1912. [CrossRef] [PubMed]
84. Subbaramaiah, K.; Dannenberg, A.J. Cyclooxygenase-2 transcription is regulated by human papillomavirus 16 E6 and E7 oncoproteins: Evidence of a corepressor/coactivator exchange. *Cancer Res.* **2007**, *67*, 3976–3985. [CrossRef] [PubMed]
85. Young, J.L.; Jazaeri, A.A.; Darus, C.J.; Modesitt, S.C. Cyclooxygenase-2 in cervical neoplasia: A review. *Gynecol. Oncol.* **2008**, *109*, 140–145. [CrossRef] [PubMed]
86. Grabosch, S.M.; Shariff, O.M.; Wulff, J.L.; Helm, C.W. Non-steroidal anti-inflammatory agents to induce regression and prevent the progression of cervical intraepithelial neoplasia. *Cochrane Database Syst. Rev.* **2014**, CD004121. [CrossRef] [PubMed]
87. Sales, K.J.; Katz, A.A.; Howard, B.; Soeters, R.P.; Millar, R.P.; Jabbour, H.N. Cyclooxygenase 1 is up-regulated in cervical carcinomas: Autocrine/paracrine regulation of cyclooxygenase-2, prostaglandin E receptors and angiogenic factors by Cyclooxygenase-1. *Cancer Res.* **2002**, *62*, 424–432. [PubMed]
88. Sutherland, J.R.; Sales, K.J.; Jabbour, H.N.; Katz, A.A. Seminal plasma enhances cervical adenocarcinoma cell proliferation and tumour growth in vivo. *PLoS ONE* **2012**, *7*, e33848. [CrossRef] [PubMed]
89. Sales, K.J.; Sutherland, J.R.; Jabbour, H.N.; Katz, A.A. Seminal plasma induces angiogenic chemokine expression in cervical cancer cells and regulates vascular function. *Biochim. Biophys. Acta* **2012**, *1823*, 1789–1795. [CrossRef] [PubMed]
90. Radilova, H.; Libra, A.; Holasova, S.; Safarova, M.; Viskova, A.; Kunc, F.; Buncek, M. COX-1 is coupled with mPGES-1 and ABCC4 in human cervix cancer cells. *Mol. Cell. Biochem.* **2009**, *330*, 131–140. [CrossRef] [PubMed]
91. Jung, Y.W.; Kim, S.W.; Kim, S.; Kim, J.H.; Cho, N.H.; Kim, J.W.; Kim, Y.T. Prevalence and clinical relevance of cyclooxygenase-1 and -2 expression in stage IIB cervical adenocarcinoma. *Eur. J. Obstet. Gynecol. Reprod. Biol.* **2010**, *148*, 62–66. [CrossRef] [PubMed]
92. Athavale, R.; Clooney, K.; O'Hagan, J.; Shawki, H.; Clark, A.H.; Green, J.A. COX-1 and COX-2 expression in stage I and II invasive cervical carcinoma: Relationship to disease relapse and long-term survival. *Int. J. Gynecol. Cancer* **2006**, *16*, 1303–1308. [CrossRef] [PubMed]
93. Jeon, Y.T.; Song, Y.C.; Kim, S.H.; Wu, H.G.; Kim, I.H.; Park, I.A.; Kim, J.W.; Park, N.H.; Kang, S.B.; Lee, H.P.; et al. Influences of cyclooxygenase-1 and -2 expression on the radiosensitivities of human cervical cancer cell lines. *Cancer Lett.* **2007**, *256*, 33–38. [CrossRef] [PubMed]
94. Kim, H.S.; Kim, T.; Kim, M.K.; Suh, D.H.; Chung, H.H.; Song, YS. Cyclooxygenase-1 and -2: Molecular targets for cervical neoplasia. *J. Cancer Prev.* **2013**, *18*, 123–134. [CrossRef] [PubMed]
95. Ohno, S.; Ohno, Y.; Suzuki, N.; Inagawa, H.; Kohchi, C.; Soma, G.; Inoue, M. Multiple roles of cyclooxygenase-2 in endometrial cancer. *Anticancer Res.* **2005**, *25*, 3679–3687. [PubMed]

96. Nasir, A.; Boulware, D.; Kaiser, H.E.; Lancaster, J.M.; Coppola, D.; Smith, P.V.; Hakam, A.; Siegel, S.E.; Bodey, B. Cyclooxygenase-2 (COX-2) expression in human endometrial carcinoma and precursor lesions and its possible use in cancer chemoprevention and therapy. *In Vivo* **2007**, *21*, 35–43. [PubMed]
97. Hasegawa, K.; Torii, Y.; Ishii, R.; Oe, S.; Kato, R.; Udagawa, Y. Effects of a selective COX-2 inhibitor in patients with uterine endometrial cancers. *Arch. Gynecol. Obstet.* **2011**, *284*, 1515–1521. [CrossRef] [PubMed]
98. Sugimoto, T.; Koizumi, T.; Sudo, T.; Yamaguchi, S.; Kojima, A.; Kumagai, S.; Nishimura, R. Correlative expression of cyclooxygenase-1 (Cox-1) and human epidermal growth factor receptor type-2 (Her-2) in endometrial cancer. *Kobe J. Med. Sci.* **2007**, *53*, 177–187. [PubMed]
99. Déry, M.C.; Chaudhry, P.; Leblanc, V.; Parent, S.; Fortier, A.M.; Asselin, E. Oxytocin increases invasive properties of endometrial cancer cells through phosphatidylinositol 3-kinase/AKT-dependent up-regulation of cyclooxygenase-1, -2, and X-linked inhibitor of apoptosis protein. *Biol. Reprod.* **2011**, *85*, 1133–1142. [CrossRef] [PubMed]
100. Vaughan, S.; Coward, J.I.; Bast, R.C., Jr.; Berchuck, A.; Berek, J.S.; Brenton, J.D.; Coukos, G.; Crum, C.C.; Drapkin, R.; Etemadmoghadam, D.; et al. Rethinking ovarian cancer: Recommendations for improving outcomes. *Nat. Rev. Cancer* **2011**, *11*, 719–725. [CrossRef] [PubMed]
101. Shan, W.; Liu, J. Inflammation, a hidden path to breaking the spell of ovarian cancer. *Cell Cycle* **2009**, *8*, 3107–3111. [CrossRef] [PubMed]
102. Macciò, A.; Madeddu, C. Inflammation and ovarian cancer. *Cytokine* **2012**, *58*, 133–147. [CrossRef] [PubMed]
103. Lee, G.; Ng, H.T. Clinical evaluations of a new ovarian cancer marker, COX-1. *Int. J. Gynaecol. Obstet.* **1995**, *49*, S27–S32. [CrossRef]
104. Gupta, R.A.; Tejada, L.V.; Tong, B.J.; Das, S.K.; Morrow, J.D.; Dey, S.K.; DuBois, R.N. Cyclooxygenase-1 is overexpressed and promotes angiogenic growth factor production in ovarian cancer. *Cancer Res.* **2003**, *63*, 906–911. [PubMed]
105. Daikoku, T.; Wang, D.; Tranguch, S.; Morrow, J.D.; Orsulic, S.; DuBois, R.N.; Dey, S.K. Cyclooxygenase-1 is a potential target for prevention and treatment of ovarian epithelial cancer. *Cancer Res.* **2005**, *65*, 3735–3744. [CrossRef] [PubMed]
106. Daikoku, T.; Tranguch, S.; Trofimova, I.N.; Dinulescu, D.M.; Jacks, T.; Nikitin, A.Y.; Connolly, D.C.; Dey, S.K. Cyclooxygenase-1 is overexpressed in multiple genetically engineered mouse models of epithelial ovarian cancer. *Cancer Res.* **2006**, *66*, 2527–2531. [CrossRef] [PubMed]
107. Hales, D.B.; Zhuge, Y.; Lagman, J.A.; Ansenberger, K.; Mahon, C.; Barua, A.; Luborsky, J.L.; Bahr, J.M. Cyclooxygenases expression and distribution in the normal ovary and their role in ovarian cancer in the domestic hen (*Gallus domesticus*). *Endocrine* **2008**, *33*, 235–244. [CrossRef] [PubMed]
108. Urick, M.E.; Johnson, P.A. Cyclooxygenase 1 and 2 mRNA and protein expression in the *Gallus domesticus* model of ovarian cancer. *Gynecol. Oncol.* **2006**, *103*, 673–678. [CrossRef] [PubMed]
109. Eilati, E.; Pan, L.; Bahr, J.M.; Hales, D.B. Age dependent increase in prostaglandin pathway coincides with onset of ovarian cancer in laying hens. *Prostaglandins Leukot. Essent. Fat. Acids* **2012**, *87*, 177–184. [CrossRef] [PubMed]
110. Kino, Y.; Kojima, F.; Kiguchi, K.; Igarashi, R.; Ishizuka, B.; Kawai, S. Prostaglandin E2 production in ovarian cancer cell lines is regulated by cyclooxygenase-1, not cyclooxygenase-2. *Prostaglandins Leukot. Essent. Fat. Acids* **2005**, *73*, 103–111. [CrossRef] [PubMed]
111. Lau, M.T.; Wong, A.S.; Leung, P.C. Gonadotropins induce tumor cell migration and invasion by increasing cyclooxygenases expression and prostaglandin E(2) production in human ovarian cancer cells. *Endocrinology* **2010**, *151*, 2985–2993. [CrossRef] [PubMed]
112. Ali-Fehmi, R.; Semaan, A.; Sethi, S.; Arabi, H.; Bandyopadhyay, S.; Hussein, Y.R.; Diamond, M.P.; Saed, G.; Morris, R.T.; Munkarah, A.R. Molecular typing of epithelial ovarian carcinomas using inflammatory markers. *Cancer* **2011**, *117*, 301–309. [CrossRef] [PubMed]
113. Liu, M.; Matsumura, N.; Mandai, M.; Li, K.; Yagi, H.; Baba, T.; Suzuki, A.; Hamanishi, J.; Fukuhara, K.; Konishi, I. Classification using hierarchical clustering of tumor-infiltrating immune cells identifies poor prognostic ovarian cancers with high levels of COX expression. *Mod. Pathol.* **2009**, *22*, 373–384. [CrossRef] [PubMed]
114. Hamanishi, J.; Mandai, M.; Abiko, K.; Matsumura, N.; Baba, T.; Yoshioka, Y.; Kosaka, K.; Konishi, I. The comprehensive assessment of local immune status of ovarian cancer by the clustering of multiple immune factors. *Clin. Immunol.* **2011**, *141*, 338–347. [CrossRef] [PubMed]

115. Lee, J.Y.; Myung, S.K.; Song, Y.S. Prognostic role of cyclooxygenase-2 in epithelial ovarian cancer: A meta-analysis of observational studies. *Gynecol. Oncol.* **2013**, *129*, 613–619. [CrossRef] [PubMed]
116. Kim, H.J.; Yim, G.W.; Nam, E.J.; Kim, Y.T. Synergistic effect of COX-2 inhibitor on paclitaxel-induced apoptosis in the human ovarian cancer cell line OVCAR-3. *Cancer Res. Treat.* **2014**, *46*, 81–92. [CrossRef] [PubMed]
117. Guo, F.J.; Tian, J.Y.; Jin, Y.M.; Wang, L.; Yang, R.Q.; Cui, M.H. Effects of cyclooxygenase-2 gene silencing on the biological behavior of SKOV3 ovarian cancer cells. *Mol. Med. Rep.* **2015**, *11*, 59–66. [CrossRef] [PubMed]
118. Wilson, A.J.; Fadare, O.; Beeghly-Fadiel, A.; Son, D.S.; Liu, Q.; Zhao, S.; Saskowski, J.; Uddin, M.J.; Daniel, C.; Crews, B.; et al. Aberrant over-expression of COX-1 intersects multiple pro-tumorigenic pathways in high-grade serous ovarian cancer. *Oncotarget* **2015**, *6*, 21353–21368. [CrossRef] [PubMed]
119. Daikoku, T.; Tranguch, S.; Chakrabarty, A.; Wang, D.; Khabele, D.; Orsulic, S.; Morrow, J.D.; Dubois, R.N.; Dey, S.K. Extracellular signal-regulated kinase is a target of cyclooxygenase-1-peroxisome proliferator-activated receptor-delta signaling in epithelial ovarian cancer. *Cancer Res.* **2007**, *67*, 5285–5292. [CrossRef] [PubMed]
120. Sonnemann, J.; Hüls, I.; Sigler, M.; Palani, C.D.; Hong, L.T.T.; Völker, U.; Kroemer, H.K.; Beck, J.F. Histone deacetylase inhibitors and aspirin interact synergistically to induce cell death in ovarian cancer cells. *Oncol. Rep.* **2008**, *20*, 219–224. [CrossRef] [PubMed]
121. Cho, M.; Kabir, S.M.; Dong, Y.; Lee, E.; Rice, V.M.; Khabele, D.; Son, D.S. Aspirin blocks EGF-stimulated cell viability in a COX-1 dependent manner in ovarian cancer cells. *J. Cancer* **2013**, *4*, 671–678. [CrossRef] [PubMed]
122. Son, D.S.; Wilson, A.J.; Parl, A.K.; Khabele, D. The effects of the histone deacetylase inhibitor romidepsin (FK228) are enhanced by aspirin (ASA) in COX-1 positive ovarian cancer cells through augmentation of p21. *Cancer Biol. Ther.* **2010**, *9*, 928–935. [CrossRef] [PubMed]
123. Truffinet, V.; Donnard, M.; Vincent, C.; Faucher, J.L.; Bordessoule, D.; Turlure, P.; Trimoreau, F.; Denizot, Y. Cyclooxygenase-1, but not -2, in blast cells of patients with acute leukemia. *Int. J. Cancer* **2007**, *121*, 924–927. [CrossRef] [PubMed]
124. Fiancette, R.; Vincent-Fabert, C.; Guerin, E.; Trimoreau, F.; Denizot, Y. Lipid mediators and human leukemic blasts. *J. Oncol.* **2011**, *2011*, 389021. [CrossRef] [PubMed]
125. McCulloch, D.; Brown, C.; Iland, H. Retinoic acid and arsenic trioxide in the treatment of acute promyelocytic leukemia: Current perspectives. *Onco Targets Ther.* **2017**, *10*, 1585–1601. [CrossRef] [PubMed]
126. Zhou, G.B.; Li, G.; Chen, S.J.; Chen, Z. From dissection of disease pathogenesis to elucidation of mechanisms of targeted therapies: Leukemia research in the genomic era. *Acta Pharmacol. Sin.* **2007**, *28*, 1434–1449. [CrossRef] [PubMed]
127. Rocca, B.; Morosetti, R.; Habib, A.; Maggiano, N.; Zassadowski, F.; Ciabattoni, G.; Chomienne, C.; Papp, B.; Ranelletti, F.O. Cyclooxygenase-1, but not -2, is upregulated in NB4 leukemic cells and human primary promyelocytic blasts during differentiation. *Leukemia* **2004**, *18*, 1373–1379. [CrossRef] [PubMed]
128. Habib, A.; Hamade, E.; Mahfouz, R.; Nasrallah, M.S.; de Thé, H.; Bazarbachi, A. Arsenic trioxide inhibits ATRA-induced prostaglandin E2 and cyclooxygenase-1 in NB4 cells, a model of acute promyelocytic leukemia. *Leukemia* **2008**, *22*, 1125–1130. [CrossRef] [PubMed]
129. Lau, E.Y.; Ho, N.P.; Lee, T.K. Cancer stem cells and their microenvironment: Biology and therapeutic implications. *Stem Cells Int.* **2017**, *2017*, 3714190. [CrossRef] [PubMed]
130. Peitzsch, C.; Tyutyunnykova, A.; Pantel, K.; Dubrovska, A. Cancer stem cells: The root of tumor recurrence and metastases. *Semin. Cancer Biol.* **2017**, *44*, 10–24. [CrossRef] [PubMed]
131. Pang, L.Y.; Hurst, E.A.; Argyle, D.J. Cyclooxygenase-2: A role in cancer stem cell survival and repopulation of cancer cells during therapy. *Stem Cells Int.* **2016**, *2016*, 2048731. [CrossRef] [PubMed]
132. Goessling, W.; North, T.E.; Loewer, S.; Lord, A.M.; Lee, S.; Stoick-Cooper, C.L.; Weidinger, G.; Puder, M.; Daley, G.Q.; Moon, R.T.; et al. Genetic interaction of PGE2 and Wnt signaling regulates developmental specification of stem cells and regeneration. *Cell* **2009**, *136*, 1136–1147. [CrossRef] [PubMed]
133. Kanojia, D.; Zhou, W.; Zhang, J.; Jie, C.; Lo, P.K.; Wang, Q.; Chen, H. Proteomic profiling of cancer stem cells derived from primary tumors of HER2/Neu transgenic mice. *Proteomics* **2012**, *12*, 3407–3415. [CrossRef] [PubMed]
134. Lazennec, G.; Lam, P.Y. Recent discoveries concerning the tumor—Mesenchymal stem cell interactions. *Biochim. Biophys. Acta* **2016**, *1866*, 290–299. [CrossRef] [PubMed]

135. Roodhart, J.M.; Daenen, L.G.; Stigter, E.C.; Prins, H.J.; Gerrits, J.; Houthuijzen, J.M.; Gerritsen, M.G.; Schipper, H.S.; Backer, M.J.; van Amersfoort, M.; et al. Mesenchymal stem cells induce resistance to chemotherapy through the release of platinum-induced fatty acids. *Cancer Cell* **2011**, *20*, 370–383. [CrossRef] [PubMed]
136. Loftin, C.D.; Tiano, H.F.; Langenbanch, R. Phenotypes of the COX-deficient mice indicate physiological and pathophysiological roles for COX-1 and COX-2. *Prostaglandins Other Lipid Mediat.* **2002**, *68–69*, 177–185. [CrossRef]
137. Islam, A.B.; Dave, M.; Amin, S.; Jensen, R.V.; Amin, A.R. Genomic, lipidomic and metabolomic analysis of cyclooxygenase-null cells: Eicosanoid storm, cross talk, and compensation by COX-1. *Genom. Proteom. Bioinform.* **2016**, *14*, 81–93. [CrossRef] [PubMed]
138. Tortorella, M.D.; Zhang, Y.; Talley, J. Desirable Properties for 3rd Generation Cyclooxygenase-2 Inhibitors. *Mini Rev. Med. Chem.* **2016**, *16*, 1284–1289. [CrossRef] [PubMed]
139. Vitale, P.; Panella, A.; Scilimati, A.; Perrone, M.G. COX-1 inhibitors: Beyond structure toward therapy. *Med. Res. Rev.* **2016**, *36*, 641–671. [CrossRef] [PubMed]
140. Smith, C.J.; Zhang, Y.; Koboldt, C.M.; Muhammad, J.; Zweifel, B.S.; Shaffer, A.; Talley, J.J.; Masferrer, J.L.; Seibert, K.; Isakson, P.C. Pharmacological analysis of cyclooxygenase-1 in inflammation. *Proc. Natl. Acad. Sci. USA* **1998**, *95*, 13313–13318. [CrossRef] [PubMed]
141. Li, W.; Xu, R.J.; Lin, Z.Y.; Zhuo, G.C.; Zhang, H.H. Effects of a cyclooxygenase-1-selective inhibitor in a mouse model of ovarian cancer, administered alone or in combination with ibuprofen, a nonselective cyclooxygenase inhibitor. *Med. Oncol.* **2009**, *26*, 170–177. [CrossRef] [PubMed]
142. Li, W.; Ji, Z.L.; Zhuo, G.C.; Xu, R.J.; Wang, J.; Jiang, H.R. Effects of a selective cyclooxygenase-1 inhibitor in SKOV-3 ovarian carcinoma xenograft-bearing mice. *Med. Oncol.* **2010**, *27*, 98–104. [CrossRef] [PubMed]
143. Li, W.; Wang, J.; Jiang, H.R.; Xu, X.L.; Zhang, J.; Liu, M.L.; Zhai, L.Y. Combined effects of cyclooxygenase-1 and cyclooxygenase-2 selective inhibitors on ovarian carcinoma in vivo. *Int. J. Mol. Sci.* **2011**, *12*, 668–681. [CrossRef] [PubMed]
144. Li, W.; Liu, M.L.; Cai, J.H.; Tang, Y.X.; Zhai, L.Y.; Zhang, J. Effect of the combination of a cyclooxygenase-1 selective inhibitor and taxol on proliferation, apoptosis and angiogenesis of ovarian cancer in vivo. *Oncol. Lett.* **2012**, *4*, 168–174. [CrossRef] [PubMed]
145. Li, W.; Cai, J.H.; Zhang, J.; Tang, Y.X.; Wan, L. Effects of cyclooxygenase inhibitors in combination with taxol on expression of cyclin D1 and Ki-67 in a xenograft model of ovarian carcinoma. *Int. J. Mol. Sci.* **2012**, *13*, 9741–9753. [CrossRef] [PubMed]
146. Li, W.; Tang, Y.X.; Wan, L.; Cai, J.H.; Zhang, J. Effects of combining Taxol and cyclooxygenase inhibitors on the angiogenesis and apoptosis in human ovarian cancer xenografts. *Oncol. Lett.* **2013**, *5*, 923–928. [CrossRef] [PubMed]
147. Li, W.; Wan, L.; Zhai, L.Y.; Wang, J. Effects of SC-560 in combination with cisplatin or taxol on angiogenesis in human ovarian cancer xenografts. *Int. J. Mol. Sci.* **2014**, *5*, 19265–19280. [CrossRef] [PubMed]
148. Brenneis, C.; Maier, T.J.; Schmidt, R.; Hofacker, A.; Zulauf, L.; Jakobsson, P.J.; Scholich, K.; Geisslinger, G. Inhibition of prostaglandin E2 synthesis by SC-560 is independent of cyclooxygenase 1 inhibition. *FASEB J.* **2006**, *20*, 1352–1360. [CrossRef] [PubMed]
149. Saed, G.M. Immunohistochemical staining of cyclooxygenases with monoclonal antibodies. *Methods Mol. Biol.* **2008**, *477*, 219–228. [CrossRef] [PubMed]
150. Lee, J.P.; Hahn, H.S.; Hwang, S.J.; Choi, J.Y.; Park, J.S.; Lee, I.H.; Kim, T.J. Selective cyclooxygenase inhibitors increase paclitaxel sensitivity in taxane-resistant ovarian cancer by suppressing P-glycoprotein expression. *J. Gynecol. Oncol.* **2013**, *24*, 273–279. [CrossRef] [PubMed]
151. Huang, Y.; Ju, B.; Tian, J.; Liu, F.; Yu, H.; Xiao, H.; Liu, X.; Liu, W.; Yao, Z.; Hao, Q. Ovarian cancer stem cell-specific gene expression profiling and targeted drug prescreening. *Oncol. Rep.* **2014**, *31*, 1235–1248. [CrossRef] [PubMed]
152. Lee, J.K.; Havaleshko, D.M.; Cho, H.; Weinstein, J.N.; Kaldjian, E.P.; Karpovich, J.; Grimshaw, A.; Theodorescu, D. A strategy for predicting the chemosensitivity of human cancer and its application to drug discovery. *Proc. Natl. Acad. Sci. USA* **2007**, *104*, 13086–13091. [CrossRef] [PubMed]
153. Grösch, S.; Tegeder, I.; Niederberger, E.; Bräutigam, L.; Geisslinger, G. COX-2 independent induction of cell cycle arrest and apoptosis in colon cancer cells by the selective COX-2 inhibitor celecoxib. *FASEB J.* **2001**, *15*, 2742–2744. [CrossRef] [PubMed]

154. Wu, W.K.; Sung, J.J.; Wu, Y.C.; Li, H.T.; Yu, L.; Li, Z.J.; Cho, C.H. Inhibition of cyclooxygenase-1 lowers proliferation and induces macroautophagy in colon cancer cells. *Biochem. Biophys. Res. Commun.* **2009**, *382*, 79–84. [CrossRef] [PubMed]
155. Sheng, H.; Shao, J.; Kirkland, S.C.; Isakson, P.; Coffey, R.J.; Morrow, J.; Beauchamp, R.D.; DuBois, R.N. Inhibition of human colon cancer cell growth by selective inhibition of cyclooxygenase-2. *J. Clin. Investig.* **1997**, *99*, 2254–2259. [CrossRef] [PubMed]
156. Lee, E.; Choi, M.K.; Han, I.O.; Lim, S.J. Role of p21CIP1 as a determinant of SC560 response in human HCT116 colon carcinoma cells. *Exp. Mol. Med.* **2006**, *38*, 325–331. [CrossRef] [PubMed]
157. Sakoguchi-Okada, N.; Takahashi-Yanaga, F.; Fukada, K.; Shiraishi, F.; Taba, Y.; Miwa, Y.; Morimoto, S.; Iida, M.; Sasaguri, T. Celecoxib inhibits the expression of survivin via the suppression of promoter activity in human colon cancer cells. *Biochem. Pharmacol.* **2007**, *73*, 1318–1329. [CrossRef] [PubMed]
158. Jain, A.K.; Moore, S.M.; Yamaguchi, K.; Eling, T.E.; Baek, S.J. Selective nonsteroidal anti-inflammatory drugs induce thymosin beta-4 and alter actin cytoskeletal organization in human colorectal cancer cells. *J. Pharmacol. Exp. Ther.* **2004**, *311*, 885–891. [CrossRef] [PubMed]
159. Moon, Y. NSAID-activated gene 1 and its implications for mucosal integrity and intervention beyond NSAIDs. *Pharmacol. Res.* **2017**, *121*, 122–128. [CrossRef] [PubMed]
160. Wang, W.S.; Chen, P.M.; Hsiao, H.L.; Wang, H.S.; Liang, W.Y.; Su, Y. Overexpression of the thymosin beta-4 gene is associated with increased invasion of SW480 colon carcinoma cells and the distant metastasis of human colorectal carcinoma. *Oncogene* **2004**, *23*, 6666–6671. [CrossRef] [PubMed]
161. Piao, Z.; Hong, C.S.; Jung, M.R.; Choi, C.; Park, Y.K. Thymosin β4 induces invasion and migration of human colorectal cancer cells through the ILK/AKT/β-catenin signaling pathway. *Biochem. Biophys. Res. Commun.* **2014**, *452*, 858–864. [CrossRef] [PubMed]
162. Gemoll, T.; Strohkamp, S.; Schillo, K.; Thorns, C.; Habermann, J.K. MALDI-imaging reveals thymosin beta-4 as an independent prognostic marker for colorectal cancer. *Oncotarget* **2015**, *6*, 43869–43880. [CrossRef] [PubMed]
163. Lee, E.; Choi, M.K.; Youk, H.J.; Kim, C.H.; Han, I.O.; Yoo, B.C.; Lee, M.K.; Lim, S.J. 5-(4-chlorophenyl)-1-(4-methoxyphenyl)-3-trifluoromethylpyrazole acts in a reactive oxygen species-dependent manner to suppress human lung cancer growth. *J. Cancer Res. Clin. Oncol.* **2006**, *132*, 223–233. [CrossRef] [PubMed]
164. Ding, J.; Tsuboi, K.; Hoshikawa, H.; Goto, R.; Mori, N.; Katsukawa, M.; Hiraki, E.; Yamamoto, S.; Abe, M.; Ueda, N. Cyclooxygenase isozymes are expressed in human myeloma cells but not involved in anti-proliferative effect of cyclooxygenase inhibitors. *Mol. Carcinog.* **2006**, *45*, 250–259. [CrossRef] [PubMed]
165. Lampiasi, N.; Foderà, D.; D'Alessandro, N.; Cusimano, A.; Azzolina, A.; Tripodo, C.; Florena, A.M.; Minervini, M.I.; Notarbartolo, M.; Montalto, G.; et al. The selective cyclooxygenase-1 inhibitor SC-560 suppresses cell proliferation and induces apoptosis in human hepatocellular carcinoma cells. *Int. J. Mol. Med.* **2006**, *17*, 245–252. [CrossRef] [PubMed]
166. Goto, K.; Ochi, H.; Yasunaga, Y.; Matsuyuki, H.; Imayoshi, T.; Kusuhara, H.; Okumoto, T. Analgesic effect of mofezolac, a non-steroidal anti-inflammatory drug, against phenylquinone-induced acute pain in mice. *Prostaglandins Other Lipid Mediat.* **1998**, *56*, 245–254. [CrossRef]
167. Kusuhara, H.; Matsuyuki, H.; Matsuura, M.; Imayoshi, T.; Okumoto, T.; Matsui, H. Induction of apoptotic DNA fragmentation by nonsteroidal anti-inflammatory drugs in cultured rat gastric mucosal cells. *Eur. J. Pharmacol.* **1998**, *360*, 273–280. [CrossRef]
168. Kusuhara, H.; Komatsu, H.; Sumichika, H.; Sugahara, K. Reactive oxygen species are involved in the apoptosis induced by nonsteroidal anti-inflammatory drugs in cultured gastric cells. *Eur. J. Pharmacol.* **1999**, *383*, 331–337. [CrossRef]
169. Kitamura, T.; Kawamori, T.; Uchiya, N.; Itoh, M.; Noda, T.; Matsuura, M.; Sugimura, T.; Wakabayashi, K. Inhibitory effects of mofezolac, a cyclooxygenase-1 selective inhibitor, on intestinal carcinogenesis. *Carcinogenesis* **2002**, *23*, 1463–1466. [CrossRef] [PubMed]
170. Kitamura, T.; Itoh, M.; Noda, T.; Matsuura, M.; Wakabayashi, K. Combined effects of cyclooxygenase-1 and cyclooxygenase-2 selective inhibitors on intestinal tumorigenesis in adenomatous polyposis coli gene knockout mice. *Int. J. Cancer* **2004**, *109*, 576–580. [CrossRef] [PubMed]

171. Niho, N.; Kitamura, T.; Takahashi, M.; Mutoh, M.; Sato, H.; Matsuura, M.; Sugimura, T.; Wakabayashi, K. Suppression of azoxymethane-induced colon cancer development in rats by a cyclooxygenase-1 selective inhibitor, mofezolac. *Cancer Sci.* **2006**, *97*, 1011–1014. [CrossRef] [PubMed]
172. Miao, L.; Shiraishi, R.; Fujise, T.; Kuroki, T.; Kakimoto, T.; Sakata, Y.; Takashima, T.; Iwakiri, R.; Fujimoto, K.; Shi, R.; et al. Chemopreventive effect of mofezolac on beef tallow diet/azoxymethane-induced colon carcinogenesis in rats. *Hepatogastroenterology* **2011**, *58*, 81–88. [PubMed]
173. Tanaka, A.; Sakai, H.; Motoyama, Y.; Ishikawa, T.; Takasugi, H. Antiplatelet agents based on cyclooxygenase inhibition without ulcerogenesis. Evaluation and synthesis of 4,5-bis(4-methoxyphenyl)-2-substituted-thiazoles. *J. Med. Chem.* **1994**, *37*, 1189–1199. [CrossRef] [PubMed]
174. Ochi, T.; Motoyama, Y.; Goto, T. The analgesic effect profile of FR122047, a selective cyclooxygenase-1 inhibitor, in chemical nociceptive models. *Eur. J. Pharmacol.* **2000**, *391*, 49–54. [CrossRef]
175. Ochi, T.; Goto, T. Differential effect of FR122047, a selective cyclo-oxygenase-1 inhibitor, in rat chronic models of arthritis. *Br. J. Pharmacol.* **2002**, *135*, 782–788. [CrossRef] [PubMed]
176. Ochi, T.; Ohkubo, Y.; Mutoh, S. Role of cyclooxygenase-2, but not cyclooxygenase-1, on type II collagen-induced arthritis in DBA/1J mice. *Biochem. Pharmacol.* **2003**, *66*, 1055–1060. [CrossRef]
177. Jeong, H.S.; Choi, H.Y.; Lee, E.R.; Kim, J.H.; Jeon, K.; Lee, H.J.; Cho, S.G. Involvement of caspase-9 in autophagy-mediated cell survival pathway. *Biochim. Biophys. Acta* **2011**, *1813*, 80–90. [CrossRef] [PubMed]
178. Boccarelli, A.; Pannunzio, A.; Coluccia, M. The Challenge of Establishing Reliable Screening Tests for Selecting Anticancer Metal Compounds. In *Bioinorganic Medicinal Chemistry*; Alessio, E., Ed.; Wiley-VCH Verlag GmbH & Co., KGaA: Weinheim, Germany, 2011; pp. 175–196. ISBN 978-3-527-32631-0.
179. Lin, J.H.; Cocchetto, D.M.; Duggan, D.E. Protein binding as a primary determinant of the clinical pharmacokinetic properties of non-steroidal anti-inflammatory drugs. *Clin. Pharmacokinet.* **1987**, *12*, 402–432. [CrossRef] [PubMed]
180. Duan, W.; Zhang, L. Cyclooxygenase inhibitors not inhibit resting lung cancer A549 cell proliferation. *Prostaglandins Leukot. Essent. Fat. Acids.* **2006**, *74*, 317–321. [CrossRef] [PubMed]
181. Cancer Cell Line Encyclopedia (CCLE). Available online: http://www.broadinstitute.org/ccle (accessed on 4 September 2018).
182. Domcke, S.; Sinha, R.; Levine, D.A.; Sander, C.; Schultz, N. Evaluating cell lines as tumour models by comparison of genomic profiles. *Nat. Commun.* **2013**, *4*, 2126. [CrossRef] [PubMed]
183. Bray, M.A.; Singh, S.; Han, H.; Davis, C.T.; Borgeson, B.; Hartland, C.; Kost-Alimova, M.; Gustafsdottir, S.M.; Gibson, C.C.; Carpenter, A.E. Cell Painting a high-content image-based assay for morphological profiling using multiplexed fluorescent dyes. *Nat. Protoc.* **2016**, *11*, 1757–1774. [CrossRef] [PubMed]
184. Grösch, S.; Maier, T.J.; Schiffmann, S.; Geisslinger, G. Cyclooxygenase-2 (COX-2)-independent anticarcinogenic effects of selective COX-2 inhibitors. *J. Natl. Cancer Inst.* **2006**, *98*, 736–747. [CrossRef] [PubMed]
185. National Center for Biotechnology Information. PubChem BioAssay Database, AID=624141. Available online: https://pubchem.ncbi.nlm.nih.gov/bioassay/624141 (accessed on 4 September 2018).

11

Design, Synthesis and Biological Evaluation of Pyridineamide Derivatives Containing a 1,2,3-Triazole Fragment as Type II c-Met Inhibitors

Hehua Xiong †, Jianxin Cheng †, Jianqing Zhang, Qian Zhang, Zhen Xiao, Han Zhang, Qidong Tang * and Pengwu Zheng *

School of Pharmacy, Jiangxi Science & Technology Normal University, Nanchang 330013, China; 18296154955@163.com (H.X.); cjx3159@163.com (J.C.); zhang1405474771@163.com (J.Z.); 15797966937@163.com (Q.Z.); xz950420@163.com (Z.X.); zbl1045762244@163.com (H.Z.)

* Correspondence: tangqidongcn@126.com (Q.T.); zhengpw@jxstnu.edu.cn (P.Z.);

† These authors contribute equally to this work.

Academic Editor: Qiao-Hong Chen

Abstract: A series of 4-(pyridin-4-yloxy)benzamide derivatives containing a 1,2,3-triazole fragment were designed, synthesized, and their inhibitory activity against A549, HeLa, and MCF-7 cancer cell lines was evaluated. Most compounds exhibited moderate to potent antitumor activity against the three cell lines. Among them, the promising compound **B26** showed stronger inhibitory activity than Golvatinib, with IC_{50} values of 3.22, 4.33, and 5.82 μM against A549, HeLa, and MCF-7 cell lines, respectively. The structure–activity relationships (SARs) demonstrated that the modification of the terminal benzene ring with a single electron-withdrawing substituent (fluorine atom) and the introduction of a pyridine amide chain with a strong hydrophilic group (morpholine) to the hinge region greatly improved the antitumor activity. Meanwhile, the optimal compound **B26** showed potent biological activity in some pharmacological experiments in vitro, such as cell morphology study, dose-dependent test, kinase activity assay, and cell cycle experiment. Finally, the molecular docking simulation was performed to further explore the binding mode of compound **B26** with c-Met.

Keywords: 4-(pyridin-4-yloxy)benzamide; 1,2,3-triazole; c-Met; inhibitor

1. Introduction

Cancer has become a serious threat to human life and health [1,2]. c-Met tyrosine kinase is a kind of type III tyrosine kinase, which is closely related to cellular activities [3] such as growth, reproduction, metastasis, etc. However, abnormal expression of c-Met kinases in cells usually triggers the occurrence, invasion, and metastasis of various cancer diseases [4]. c-Met kinase has been found overexpressed in various cancer cells and has become an attractive target for cancer treatment [5,6]. Nowadays, developing small molecule c-Met kinase inhibitors has become a hotspot in the treatment of human cancer [7].

c-Met inhibitors are classified as type I and type II inhibitors according to the binding mode of inhibitors with c-Met. Usually, c-Met inhibitors of type I are single-target inhibitors that bind to the hinge region of the ATP pocket, and c-Met inhibitors of type II are multitarget inhibitors that bind to the hinge region and an extra hydrophobic pocket [8,9]. With the development of biology and pharmacology, the intracellular mechanisms have been elucidated, and research in small molecule inhibitors has made significant progress. Type II c-Met inhibitors possess more potent inhibitory activity and better tolerance to drug resistance through binding to kinases of multiple types. Cabozantinib, a c-Met inhibitor of type II, was approved by the FDA for treatment of prostate cancer in 2012. Some representative c-Met inhibitors (type II) in the clinical trial phase are listed in Figure 1, including

Golvatinib, BMS-777607, Altriatinib, and TAS-115 [10–12]. Furthermore, according to the structure characteristics of inhibitors, the skeleton of c-Met inhibitor (type II) was summarized into blocks A, B, C, and D by our research group, as shown in Figure 1 [13].

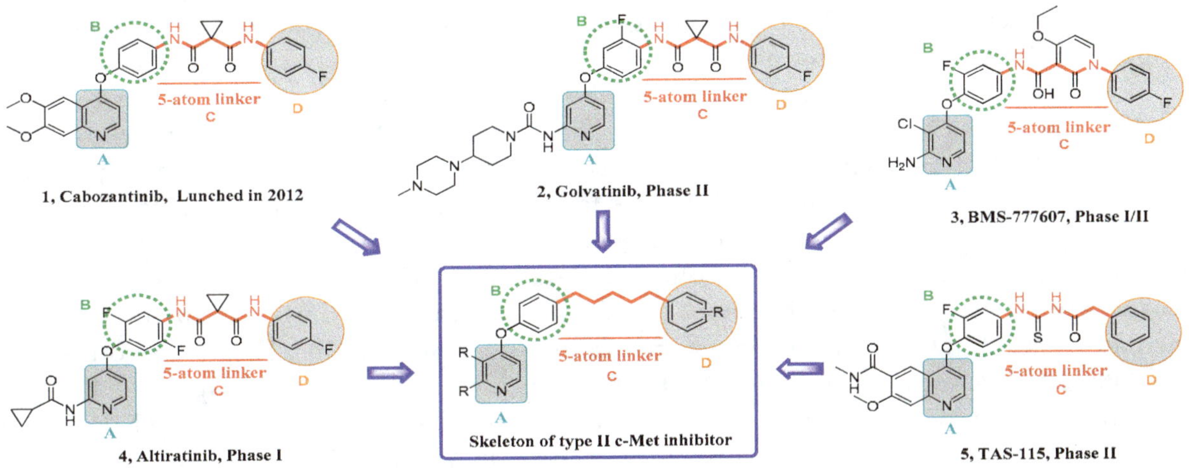

Figure 1. Some representative c-Met inhibitors of type II and the summarized skeleton.

We explored the SARs of c-Met inhibitors (type II) bearing pyridinamide structure using Golvatinib as a lead compound in this study. In order to guide our modification of the lead compound, a molecular docking simulation of Golvatinib and c-Met protein was performed, as shown in Figure 2. The docking results indicated that blocks A and C, which possessed hydrogen bonding interactions with residues Met1160, Asp1222, and Lys1110, played a key role in maintaining the inhibitory activity against c-Met. Therefore, the modification was mainly concentrated on blocks A and C. Firstly, a pyridylamide structure in block A, including hydrogen bond donor and hydrogen bond acceptor atoms, was introduced into the meta position of pyridine in order to enhance the interaction with the hinge region residues, and then some alkyl chains bearing morpholine or thiophene groups were connected to the terminal of the pyridine amide structure for better water solubility of compounds. Then, a 1,2,3-triazole fragment with good biological activity and two hydrogen bond acceptor atoms was introduced to block C for more tight combination between the compounds and c-Met. In addition, considering the steric hindrance problem [14], H/F atoms and different substituents were introduced in blocks B and D, respectively, to explore their effects on biological activity of target compounds. Finally, a series of small molecule inhibitors containing the 1,2,3-triazole fragment were designed, synthesized, and biologically evaluated.

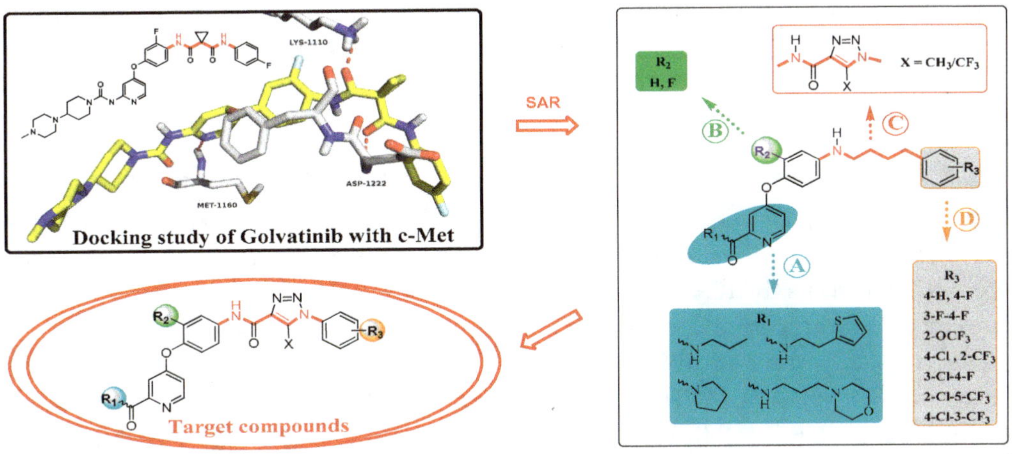

Figure 2. Design strategy of target compounds based on the molecular simulation and structure–activity relationships (SARs).

2. Results and Discussion

2.1. Chemistry

The synthesis route of target compounds **B1–B27** is shown in Scheme 1. Firstly, the commercially available pyridinecarboxylic acid **6** was reacted with $SOCl_2$ using NaBr as catalyst to yield 4-chloropicolinoyl chloride **7**, which was then converted into ethyl 4-chloropicolinate **8** with ethanol. Next, 4-chloropicolinate **8** was subjected to nucleophilic substitute with *p*-nitrophenol or 2-fluoro-4-nitrophenol using chlorobenzene as solvent to give picolinate analogues **9a–9b**, which were then dissolved in 1,4-dioxane and hydrolyzed with NaOH aqueous solution to obtain picolinic acid analogues **10a–10b**. Intermediates **10a–10b** were reacted with $SOCl_2$ to get the corresponding acyl chlorides and then connected with amines (including propan-1-amine, 2-(thiophen-2-yl)ethan-1-amine, pyrrolidine and 3-morpholinopropan-1-amine) to obtain picolinamide analogues **11a–11e**. Finally, the key intermediates **12a–12e** were produced by the reduction of **11a–11e** with hydrazine hydrate as reducing agent. Other intermediates **13a–13i**, which have been reported in our previous research [15], were combined with intermediates **12a–12e** by a nucleophilic substitute reaction to get the target compounds **B1–B27**.

The structural information of the target compounds was confirmed by ^{1}H-NMR, ^{13}C-NMR, and TOF MS (ES+), which were consistent with the structures depicted.

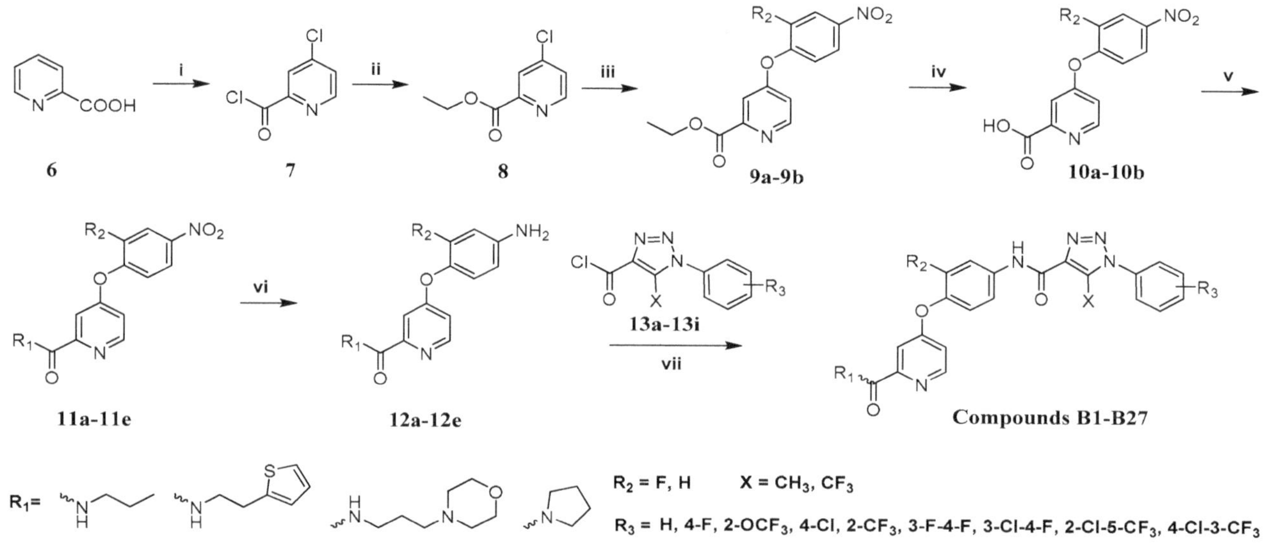

Scheme 1. The synthetic route for target compounds **B1–B27**. Reagents and conditions: (i) NaBr, $SOCl_2$, 85 °C, 18 h; (ii) triethylamine, dichloromethane (DCM), EtOH, 0 °C, 1 h; (iii) *p*-nitrophenol or 2-fluoro-4-nitrophenol, chlorobenzene, 135 °C, 4 h; (iv) 1,4-dioxane, sodium hydroxide (10%), r.t., 0.5 h; (v) $SOCl_2$, amines, Et_3N, DCM, 0–85 °C, 1 h; (vi) EtOH, activated carbon, $FeCl_3{\cdot}6H_2O$, hydrazine hydrate (80%), 90 °C, 4 h. (vii) EtOH, activated carbon, $FeCl_3{\cdot}6H_2O$, hydrazine hydrate (80%), 90 °C, 4 h; (vii) DCM, $NaHCO_3$, 0 °C, 1 h.

2.2. Antitumor Activity of Compounds **B1–B27** Against A549, HeLa, and MCF-7 Cell Lines and SAR Analysis

The antitumor activity of target compounds against A549, HeLa, and MCF-7 cell lines was evaluated to investigate their inhibitory activity against cancer cells [16]. The antitumor activities of compounds were displayed as the IC_{50} (half-inhibitory concentration) values, as shown in Tables 1 and 2. Most compounds exhibited moderate to potent antitumor activity against three cell lines. Compounds **B25–B27** possessed more potent inhibitory activity than Golvatinib, as shown in Table 2, with IC_{50} values in the range of 3.22–13.60 μM. The optimal compound **B26** showed excellent inhibitory activity against A549, HeLa, and MCF-7 cell lines with IC_{50} values of 3.22 ± 0.12, 4.33 ± 0.09, and 5.82 ± 0.09 μM, respectively, which were more efficient than Golvatinib (8.14 ± 0.45, 15.17 ± 0.17, and 16.91 ± 0.29 μM).

Table 1. Antitumor activities of the target compounds **B1–B18** against A549, HeLa, and MCF-7 cell lines.

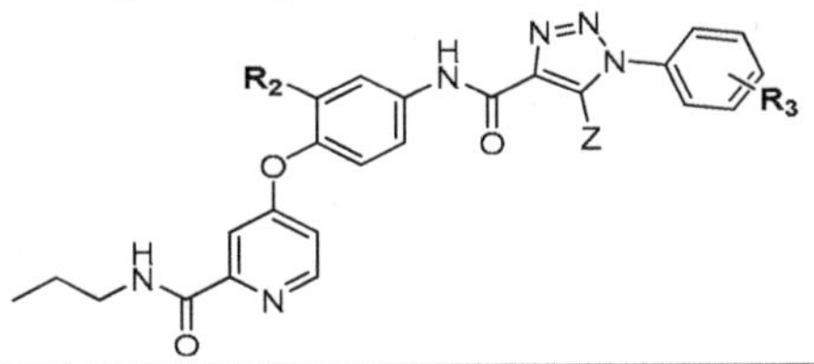

Compd.	R_2	R_3	Z	IC_{50} (μM) ± SD		
				A549	HeLa	MCF-7
B1		4-H	CH_3	46.55 ± 1.90	52.31 ± 5.42	63.05 ± 2.44
B2		4-F	CH_3	21.30 ± 0.66	42.06 ± 6.03	32.13 ± 0.86
B3		2-OCF_3	CH_3	32.67 ± 1.16	53.94 ± 4.23	48.71 ± 3.26
B4		4-Cl	CF_3	56.26 ± 2.26	48.23 ± 1.59	120.76 ± 1.25
B5	H	2-CF_3	CF_3	35.57 ± 1.03	59.55 ± 2.94	270.40 ± 12.35
B6		3-F-4-F	CF_3	256.30 ± 10.37	170.38 ± 13.69	NA [a]
B7		3-Cl-4-F	CF_3	221.98 ± 21.46	295.65 ± 15.37	NA
B8		2-Cl-5-CF_3	CF_3	238.07 ± 17.84	NA	NA
B9		4-Cl-3-CF_3	CF_3	357.24 ± 14.50	NA	NA
B10		4-H	CH_3	33.31 ± 1.25	41.55 ± 2.26	60.50 ± 3.99
B11		4-F	CH_3	19.70 ± 0.89	46.57 ± 1.59	29.11 ± 1.30
B12		2-OCF_3	CH_3	24.24 ± 0.71	53.04 ± 1.11	42.26 ± 1.09
B13		4-Cl	CF_3	46.13 ± 3.59	55.43 ± 2.30	82.48 ± 2.34
B14	F	2-CF_3	CF_3	32.94 ± 2.33	40.68 ± 1.09	84.45 ± 12.34
B15		3-F-4-F	CF_3	123.07 ± 10.23	240.60 ± 22.49	332.01 ± 20.08
B16		3-Cl-4-F	CF_3	150.58 ± 12.21	270.24 ± 13.56	NA
B17		2-Cl-5-CF_3	CF_3	223.34 ± 10.89	NA	NA
B18		4-Cl-3-CF_3	CF_3	246.70 ± 21.23	NA	NA
Golvatinib [b]				8.14 ± 0.45	15.17 ± 0.17	16.91 ± 0.29

[a] NA: Low inhibitory activity, [b] Used as the positive control.

Table 2. Antitumor activities of the target compounds **B10–B12** and **B19–B27** against A549, HeLa, and MCF-7 cell lines.

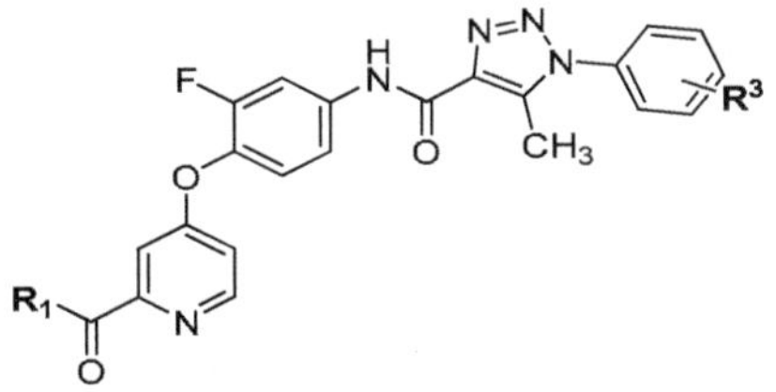

Compd.	R_1	R_3	IC_{50} (μM) ± SD		
			A549	HeLa	MCF-7
B10		4-H	33.31 ± 1.25	41.55 ± 2.26	60.50 ± 3.99
B11	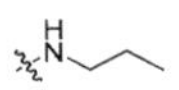	4-F	19.70 ± 0.89	46.57 ± 1.59	29.11 ± 1.30
B12		2-OCF_3	24.24 ± 0.71	53.04 ± 1.11	42.26 ± 1.09
B19		4-H	27.25 ± 0.79	32.31 ± 2.11	39.08 ± 0.97
B20	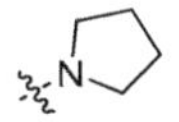	4-F	12.10 ± 0.31	21.84 ± 1.93	19.12 ± 0.21
B21		2-OCF_3	17.72 ± 0.42	29.55 ± 2.04	41.10 ± 1.21
B22		4-H	19.88 ± 0.75	45.18 ± 3.89	33.80 ± 1.11
B23	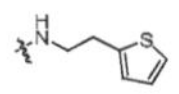	4-F	12.52 ± 0.37	15.19 ± 0.96 [a]	35.11 ± 3.05
B24		2-OCF_3	13.34 ± 0.58	19.73 ± 0.83	44.82 ± 2.96
B25		4-H	6.43 ± 0.21	10.51 ± 0.68	13.60 ± 0.86
B26	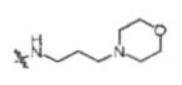	4-F	3.22 ± 0.12	4.33 ± 0.09	5.82 ± 0.09
B27		2-OCF_3	4.91 ± 0.09	5.72 ± 0.17	9.34 ± 0.52
Golvatoinib [b]			8.14 ± 0.45	15.17 ± 0.17	16.91 ± 0.29

[a] Bold values show the IC_{50} values of the target compounds lower than the values of the positive control; [b] Used as the positive control.

According to the antitumor activity of compounds **B1–B27** listed in Tables 1 and 2, the SARs were summarized as follows. Overall, the F atom on the meta-central benzene ring provided stronger inhibitory activity against cancer cells than H atom, for example, compounds **B1–B8** displayed less inhibitory activity than compounds **B9–B18**. A single substitution (such as H/F/OCF_3/Cl/CF_3) linked to the terminal benzene ring was favorable for maintaining the biological activity, such as compounds **B1–B5** and **B10–B15** that possessed moderate antitumor activity with IC_{50} values less than 60 μM against A549 and HeLa cell lines. However, the double substituents connected to the terminal benzene ring obviously impaired the inhibitory activity of compounds **B6–B9** and **B15–B18,** whose IC_{50} values were more than 120 μM against three cell lines. A possible explanation would be that the introduction of two substituents to the terminal benzene ring may create steric hindrance, which made it difficult for compounds to extend into the hydrophobic pocket and to bind tightly to c-Met kinase.

Inspired by the inhibitory activity of compounds **B1–B3** and **B10–B12**, as shown in Table 1, the F atom of the central benzene ring and the single group (H, F, or OCF_3) of the terminal benzene ring were reserved to perform a SAR study of the pyridine amide moiety. Hydrophilic groups, including morpholine or thiophene groups attached to the terminal of pyridine amide, have a great contribution to inhibitory activity of the compounds **B22–B27** (with IC_{50} values in the range of 3.22–45.18 μM).

In summary, introducing morpholino groups and F atoms to the pyridylpropyl amide and the terminal benzene ring, respectively, made significant advances in the inhibitory activity.

2.3. *Dose-Dependent Test of Compound* ***B26*** *Against A549 Cells*

To explore the relationship between concentrations and antitumor activity of compound **B26**, we carried out a dose-dependent test based on the MTT method [16], in which A549 cells were treated with seven different concentrations of compound **B26** (0.137, 0.411, 1.234, 3.704, 11.11, 33.33, and 100 μM), using Golvatinib as a positive control, as seen in Figure 3. The results revealed that compound **B26** could effectively inhibit cancer cells in a dose-dependent manner. Notably, compound **B26** inhibited A549 cells more than 50% at the concentration of 3.704 μM, while the inhibitory rate of Golvatinib was less than 40% at the same concentration.

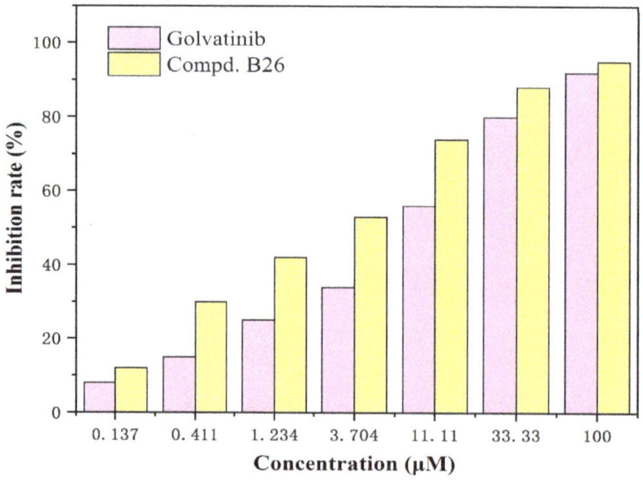

Figure 3. Relationship between concentration and inhibition rate of compound **B26** against A549 cells.

2.4. *Cell Cycle Study of A549 Cells Treated with Compound* ***B26***

To further investigate the inhibitory pattern of compound **B26** on the growth of cancer cells, cell cycle distribution analysis [17] was carried out on A549 cells, as shown in Figure 4. Compound **B26** at concentrations of 5, 10, and 15 μM and Golvatinib at a concentration of 5 μM were delivered to A549 cells for 24 h, as shown in Figure 4. With the increased concentration of compound **B26**, the percentage of cells blocked in G_0/G_1 phase was increased from 65.44% to 79.18%, while the percentage in the S phase decreased from 21.91% to 16.56%. There was no significant change in G_2/M phase. The result showed that compound **B26** (74.41%) and Golvatinib (74.77%) had the same inhibitory effect on A549 cells at the concentration of 5 μM, both of which could block cells in the G_0/G_1 phase.

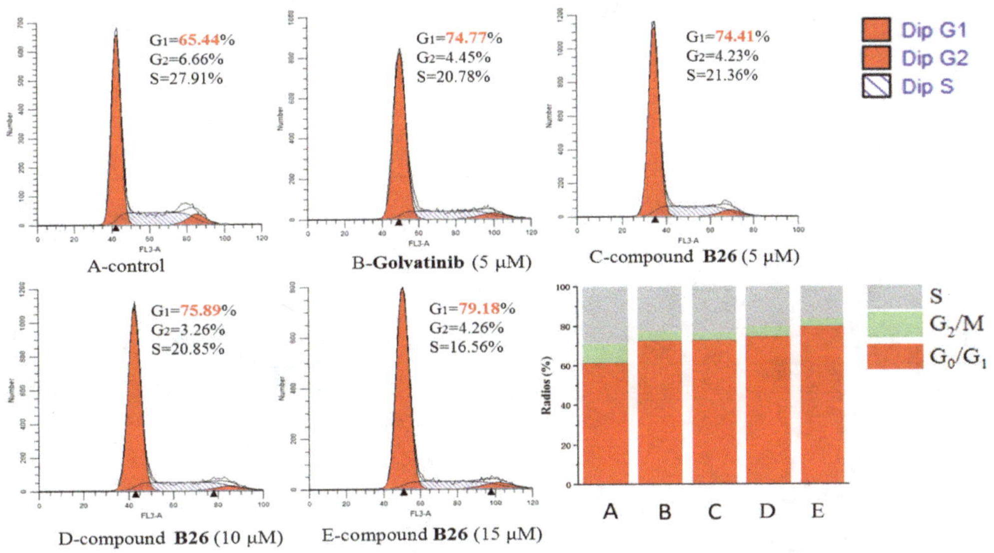

Figure 4. Cell cycle study of A549 cells treated with compound **B26** and Golvatinib.

2.5. c-Met Enzyme Assay of Compounds B25–B27 and Staurosporine

Compounds **B25**, **B26**, and **B27**, possessing potent antitumor activity against A549, HeLa, and MCF-7 cell lines, were selected to investigate their c-Met kinase assay by mobility shift assay method [18] with staurosporine as a positive control, which was used to insure the reliability of the experimental data. Compound **B26** exhibited potent inhibitory activity against c-Met with an inhibition rate of 36% at the concentration of 0.625 μM, as shown in Table 3.

Table 3. c-Met kinase activity of selected compounds **B25**, **B26**, **B27**, and staurosporine.

Compound (0.625 μM)	Rates (%)
B25	4.3
B26	36.0
B27	23.8
Staurosporine	87.3

2.6. Molecular Docking Simulation of Compounds (B26 and Golvatinib) and c-Met

Next, we further explored the binding mode of compound **B26** and Golvatinib with c-Met kinase (PDB: 3LQ8, extracted from the PDB database) through molecule docking simulation using AutoDock 4.2 software [19], as shown in Figure 5. The docking results indicated that compound **B26** and Golvatinib in an extended conformation formed strong hydrogen bonding interactions with residues Met1160, Asp1222, and Lys1110, as shown in Figure 5a–d. Interestingly, the pyridylamide structure of compound **B26** formed a bidentate hydrogen bond with residue Met1160, as shown in Figure 5a,b, which may offer a stronger ability of compound **B26** to bind with c-Met. Compound **B26** formed more hydrogen bonding interactions with Met1160 than Golvatinib, which may explain the better antitumor activity of compound **B26**.

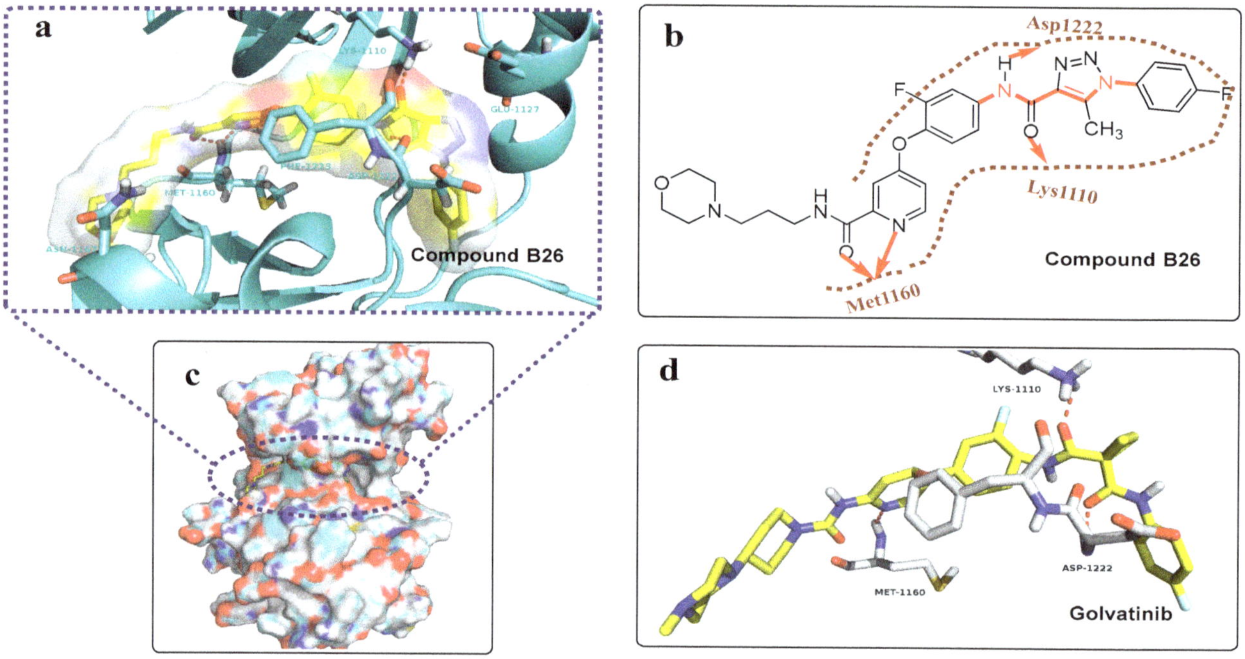

Figure 5. Figure 5a, 5b, and 5c are partial views, two-dimensional partial views, and integral cavity views of the docking results of c-Met (PDB code: 3LQ8) and compound **B26**, respectively. Figure 5d shows partial views of c-Met and Golvatinib. The c-Met protein and compounds are displayed by cartoons and sticks, respectively. Hydrogen bonding interactions between compounds and c-Met are indicated with dashed lines or arrows in red.

3. Experimental Section

3.1. Chemistry

Unless specifically required, all reagents used in the experiments were purchased as commercial analytical grade and used without further purification. Frequently used solvents (dichloromethane, ethyl acetate, tetrahydrofuran, 1,4-dioxane, methanol, ethanol, etc.) were absolutely anhydrous. Flash column chromatography was performed on silica gel (300 mesh) using a mixture of petroleum ether (PE) and ethyl acetate (EA). The reaction process was monitored by thin-layer chromatography (TLC, SH-GH254) and spots were visualized with ultraviolet analyzer (light in 254 or 365 nm). ^{1}H-NMR and ^{13}C-NMR spectra analysis of compounds was implemented in Bruker 400 MHz spectrometer (Bruker Bioscience, Billerica, MA, USA) using tetramethylsilane (TMS) as an internal standard at room temperature. Mass spectrometry (MS) of target compounds was carried out Waters High Resolution Quadrupole Time of Flight Tandem Mass Spectrometry (Waters, Xevo G2-XS Tof). The melting point of the compounds was measured by SGW X-4 micro melting point instrument. The purity of compounds was determined by an Agilent 1260 liquid chromatograph equipped with an Inertex-C18 column, and all were more than 95%.

3.1.1. Preparation of 4-Chloropicolinoyl Chloride (7)

Pyridinecarboxylic acid **6** (10.00 g, 0.081 mol), NaBr (0.10 g, 0.001 mol), and a drop of *N,N*-dimethylformamide (DMF) were added in thionyl chloride ($SOCl_2$, 50 mL) and stirred at 85 °C for 18 h. The reaction was monitored by TLC. After completion of the reaction, the solvent was removed under vacuum to obtain a yellow liquid, which was dissolved in DCM for further use.

3.1.2. Preparation of Ethyl 4-Chloropicolinate (8)

Dichloromethane (30 mL), ethanol (16.43 g, 0.170 mol), and triethylamine (17.17 g, 0.170 mol) were successively added to a beaker and stirred at 0 °C for 0.5 h. Subsequently, a mixture of

4-chloropicolinoyl chloride **7** (16.43 g, 0.110 mol) and DCM (5 mL) was added dropwise, stirred at 0 °C for 0.5 h, and monitored by TLC. After completion of the reaction, NaOH solution was added to the mixture to adjust the pH value 9–10. Ultimately, the organic layers were combined and dried to obtain a brown liquid.

3.1.3. Preparation of Ethyl 4-(4-Nitrophenoxy)picolinate (**9a**) and Ethyl4-(2-Fluoro-4-Nitrophenoxy) picolinate (**9b**)

Intermediate **8** (13.22 g, 0.071 mol) and *p*-nitrophenol or 2-fluoro-4-nitrophenol (0.026 mol) were dissolved in chlorobenzene (40 mL) and then stirred at 130 °C for 4 h. The completion of the reaction was monitored by TLC. After completion of the reaction, the cold petroleum ether (100 mL) was poured into the reaction solvent and stirred at room temperature for 0.5 h. Next, petroleum ether (100 mL) was poured off to give a viscous liquid, which was then dissolved in DCM (300 mL) and extracted with aqueous solution of NaOH. The organic layer was combined, dried, and concentrated under vacuum to get a pale yellow solid.

3.1.4. Preparation of 4-(4-Nitrophenoxy)picolinic Acid (**10a**) and 4-(2-Fluoro-4-Nitrophenoxy)picolinic Acid (**10b**)

Intermediates **9a–9b** (0.035 mol) were dissolved in 1,4-dioxane (50 mL) and stirred at room temperature for 0.5 h. A solution of 10% NaOH (2.28 mL, 0.057 mol) was then added dropwise to the above mixture, stirred at room temperature for 0.5 h, and monitored by TLC. After completion of the reaction, the solvent was evaporated under vacuum to give a white solid. The white solid was then dissolved in saturated NaCl solution (500 mL) and stirred at room temperature for 10 h. Subsequently, after the pH of the solution was adjusted to 2–3 by 75% hydrochloric acid (HCl), a yellow solid was precipitated, filtered, and dried.

3.1.5. Preparation of 4-(4-Nitrophenoxy)picolinamide or 4-(2-Fluoro-4-Nitrophenoxy)picolinamide Analogues (**11a–11e**)

Intermediates **10a–10b** (0.020 mol) and one drop of DMF were successively dissolved in $SOCl_2$ (50 mL) and stirred at 85 °C for 0.5 h. Then reaction solvent was concentrated in vacuum, dissolved in DCM (8 mL), and added dropwise to a mixture of DCM (50 mL), ammonia analogs (0.020 mol), and triethylamine (0.020 mol). The reaction solution was stirred at 0 °C for 0.5 h, and monitored by TLC. Finally, a gray slid was obtained by the same post-treatment method as that used for preparation of ethyl 4-chloropicolinate **8**.

3.1.6. Preparation of 4-(4-Aminophenoxy)picolinamide or 4-(2-Fluoro-4-aminophenoxy)picolinamide Analogues (**12a–12e**)

Intermediates **11a–11e** (0.016 mol), activated carbon (1.92 g, 0.160 mol), and $FeCl_3{\cdot}6H_2O$ (0.43 g, 0.016 mol) were dissolved in ethanol (30 mL) and stirred at 90 °C for 0.5 h. Then, 80% hydrazine hydrate (8.00 g, 0.128 mol) was added dropwise and stirred for 3.5 h. The reaction was monitored by TLC. After completion of the reaction, the solution was filtered, concentrated, and recrystallized to give a green solid.

3.1.7. Preparation of 5-Methyl-1-Phenyl-1H-1,2,3-Triazole-4-Carbonyl Chloride or 1-Phenyl-5-(trifluoromethyl)-1H-1,2,3-Triazole-4-Carbonyl Chloride Analogues (**13i–13e**)

The preparation of intermediates **13a–13i** was carried out according to our previous research [15].

3.1.8. Preparation of Target Compounds **B1–B27**

Intermediates **12a–12e** (0.002 mol) and sodium bicarbonate (4.20 g, 0.005 mol) were dissolved in DCM and stirred at 0 °C for 0.5 h. The solution of intermediates **13a–13i** (0.002 mol) and DCM were added dropwise to the above mixture, and stirred at 0 °C for 0.5 h. The reaction was monitored by TLC. After completion of the reaction, the solution was extracted with a mixture of DCM/NaOH (500 mL) three times and then the organic layers were combined, dried over sodium sulfate, evaporated, and purified by chromatographic column to possess a light yellow or white solid.

4-(4-(5-methyl-1-phenyl-1H-1,2,3-triazole-4-carboxamido)phenoxy)-N-propylpicolinamide (**B1**) Light yellow solid; Yield: 78.5%; m.p.: 116.8–117.1 °C; ^{1}H-NMR (400 MHz, DMSO-d_6, ppm) δ 10.75 (s, 1H), 8.82 (s, 1H), 8.52 (d, J = 5.5 Hz, 1H), 8.03 (s, 1H), 8.01 (s, 1H), 7.67 (s, 2H), 7.64 (d, J = 6.4 Hz, 2H), 7.43 (s, 1H), 7.23 (d, J = 8.4 Hz, 2H), 7.18 (d, J = 4.5 Hz, 1H), 3.22 (dd, J = 12.8, 6.3 Hz, 2H), 2.59 (s, 3H), 1.50 (dt, J = 14.1, 7.0 Hz, 2H), 0.84 (t, J = 7.2 Hz, 3H). TOF MS ES+ (m/z): $[M + H]^+$, calcd for $C_{25}H_{24}N_6O_3$: 457.1988, found, 457.1986.

4-(4-(1-(4-fluorophenyl)-5-methyl-1H-1,2,3-triazole-4-carboxamido)phenoxy)-N-propylpicolinamide (**B2**) Light yellow solid; Yield: 59.3%; m.p.: 110.4–110.8 °C; ^{1}H-NMR (400 MHz, DMSO-d_6, ppm) δ 10.64 (s, 1H), 8.71 (s, 1H), 8.40 (d, J = 5.6 Hz, 1H), 7.91 (s, 1H), 7.89 (s, 1H), 7.65 (d, J = 4.8 Hz, 1H), 7.63 (d, J = 4.6 Hz, 1H), 7.39 (t, J = 8.7 Hz, 2H), 7.31 (d, J = 2.1 Hz, 1H), 7.11 (d, J = 8.8 Hz, 2H), 7.06 (d, J = 3.1 Hz, 1H), 3.10 (dd, J = 13.3, 6.6 Hz, 2H), 2.46 (s, 3H), 1.38 (dt, J = 14.2, 7.1 Hz, 2H), 0.72 (t, J = 7.3 Hz, 3H). TOF MS ES+ (m/z): $[M + H]^+$, calcd for $C_{25}H_{23}FN_6O_3$: 475.1894, found, 475.1896.

4-(4-(5-methyl-1-(2-(trifluoromethoxy)phenyl)-1H-1,2,3-triazole-4-carboxamido)phenoxy)-N-propylpicolinamide (**B3**) White solid; Yield: 78.2%; m.p.: 97.7–98.0 °C; ^{1}H-NMR (400 MHz, DMSO-d_6, ppm) δ 10.81 (s, 1H), 8.81 (s, 1H), 8.52 (d, J = 5.3 Hz, 1H), 8.03 (s, 1H), 8.01 (s, 1H), 7.88 (d, J = 7.7 Hz, 1H), 7.84 (d, J = 7.6 Hz, 1H), 7.78 (d, J = 7.7 Hz, 1H), 7.72 (t, J = 7.2 Hz, 1H), 7.42 (s, 1H), 7.23 (d, J = 8.6 Hz, 2H), 7.18 (d, J = 0.8 Hz, 1H), 3.22 (d, J = 6.2 Hz, 2H), 2.46 (s, 3H), 1.51 (dd, J = 14.0, 7.0 Hz, 2H), 0.84 (t, J = 7.2 Hz, 3H). TOF MS ES+ (m/z): $[M + H]^+$, calcd for $C_{26}H_{23}F_3N_6O_4$: 541.1811, found, 541.1813.

4-(4-(1-(4-chlorophenyl)-5-(trifluoromethyl)-1H-1,2,3-triazole-4-carboxamido)phenoxy)-N-propylpicolinamide (**B4**) White solid; Yield: 66.4%; m.p.: 159.0–159.2 °C; ^{1}H-NMR (400 MHz, DMSO-d_6, ppm) δ 11.19 (s, 1H), 8.80 (s, 1H), 8.52 (d, J = 5.5 Hz, 1H), 7.99 (s, 1H), 7.97 (d, J = 1.2 Hz, 1H), 7.79 (d, J = 4.4 Hz, 3H), 7.75 (d, J = 8.7 Hz, 1H), 7.42 (s, 1H), 7.27 (d, J = 8.7 Hz, 2H), 7.19 (d, J = 5.5 Hz, 1H), 3.23 (dd, J = 13.2, 6.7 Hz, 2H), 1.57–1.47 (m, 2H), 0.84 (t, J = 7.4 Hz, 3H). ^{13}C-NMR (100 MHz, DMSO-d_6, ppm) δ 165.73, 163.13, 156.58, 152.54, 150.36(2,C), 149.46, 142.31, 136.19, 135.84, 134.09, 129.70(2,C), 128.22(2,C), 122.40(2,C), 121.33(2,C), 114.18(2,C), 108.95, 40.58, 22.34, 11.27. TOF MS ES+ (m/z): $[M + H]^+$, calcd for $C_{25}H_{20}ClF_3N_6O_3$: 545.1316, found, 545.1317.

N-propyl-4-(4-(5-(trifluoromethyl)-1-(2-(trifluoromethyl)phenyl)-1H-1,2,3-triazole-4-carboxamido)phenoxy) picolinamide (**B5**) White yellow solid; Yield: 69.4%; m.p.: 163.4–163.7 °C; ^{1}H-NMR (400 MHz, DMSO-d_6, ppm) δ 11.26 (s, 1H), 8.80 (s, 1H), 8.53 (d, J = 5.2 Hz, 1H), 8.15–8.09 (m, 2H), 8.05 (d, J = 7.2 Hz, 1H), 8.00 (d, J = 7.7 Hz, 3H), 7.43 (s, 1H), 7.27 (d, J = 8.5 Hz, 2H), 7.18 (d, J = 2.7 Hz, 1H), 3.23 (dd, J = 12.4, 6.0 Hz, 2H), 1.57–1.47 (m, 2H), 0.84 (t, J = 7.3 Hz, 3H). ^{13}C-NMR (100 MHz, DMSO-d_6, ppm) δ 165.72, 163.14, 156.20, 152.53, 150.36(2,C), 149.53, 141.89, 135.72, 134.28(2,C), 132.86, 132.02, 130.02(2,C), 127.71, 122.60(2,C), 121.29(2,C), 114.17(2,C), 108.96, 40.57, 22.33, 11.24. TOF MS ES+ (m/z): $[M + H]^+$, calcd for $C_{26}H_{20}F_6N_6O_3$: 579.1580, found, 579.1573.

4-(4-(1-(3,4-difluorophenyl)-5-(trifluoromethyl)-1H-1,2,3-triazole-4-carboxamido)phenoxy)-N-propylpicolinamide (**B6**) Light yellow solid; Yield: 85.0%; m.p.: 97.6–97.8 °C; ^{1}H-NMR (400 MHz, DMSO-d_6, ppm) δ 11.21 (s, 1H), 8.80 (s, 1H), 8.52 (d, J = 4.9 Hz, 1H), 8.12 (s, 1H), 7.98 (d, J = 6.9 Hz, 2H), 7.81 (d, J = 8.9 Hz, 1H), 7.74 (s, 1H), 7.41 (s, 1H), 7.27 (d, J = 6.9 Hz, 2H), 7.20 (d, J = 2.3 Hz, 1H), 3.26–3.19 (m, 2H), 1.52 (dd, J = 13.7, 6.8 Hz, 2H), 0.84 (t, J = 7.1 Hz, 3H). ^{13}C-NMR (100 MHz, DMSO-d_6, ppm) δ 165.73, 163.13, 156.48, 152.54, 150.36(2,C), 149.48, 142.09, 135.81, 131.59, 124.44, 122.46(2,C), 121.32(2,C), 118.63, 118.44, 117.06, 116.86, 114.19(2,C), 108.93, 40.58, 22.34, 11.26. TOF MS ES+ (m/z): $[M + H]^+$, calcd for $C_{25}H_{19}F_5N_6O_3$: 547.1517, found, 547.1517.

4-(4-(1-(3-chloro-4-fluorophenyl)-5-(trifluoromethyl)-1H-1,2,3-triazole-4-carboxamido)phenoxy)-N-propylpicolinamide (**B7**) White solid; Yield: 81.6%; m.p.: 153.6–153.9 °C; ^{1}H-NMR (400 MHz, DMSO-d_6, ppm) δ 11.23 (s,

1H), 8.80 (t, J = 5.9 Hz, 1H), 8.52 (d, J = 5.6 Hz, 1H), 7.99 (s, 1H), 7.97 (s, 1H), 7.79 (d, J = 4.0 Hz, 3H), 7.42 (s, 1H), 7.27 (d, J = 8.6 Hz, 2H), 7.18 (d, J = 3.8 Hz, 1H), 3.23 (dd, J = 13.3, 6.5 Hz, 2H), 1.57–1.47 (m, 2H), 0.84 (t, J = 7.3 Hz, 3H). ^{13}C-NMR (100 MHz, DMSO-d_6, ppm) δ 165.73, 163.15, 156.61, 152.52, 150.33(2,C), 149.45, 142.38, 136.20, 135.87, 134.06, 129.69(2,C), 128.18(2,C), 122.39(2,C), 121.29(2,C), 114.13(2,C), 108.99, 40.58, 22.34, 11.25. TOF MS ES+ (*m/z*): $[M + H]^+$, calcd for $C_{25}H_{19}ClF_4N_6O_3$: 563.1222, found, 563.1216.

4-(4-(1-(2-chloro-5-(trifluoromethyl)phenyl)-5-(trifluoromethyl)-1H-1,2,3-triazole-4-carboxamido)phenoxy)-N-propylpicolinamide (**B8**) White solid; Yield: 56.7%; m.p.: 143.3–143.7 °C; ^{1}H-NMR (400 MHz, DMSO-d_6, ppm) δ 11.30 (s, 1H), 8.81 (s, 1H), 8.65 (s, 1H), 8.53 (d, J = 4.9 Hz, 1H), 8.21 (d, J = 8.0 Hz, 1H), 8.15 (d, J = 7.9 Hz, 1H), 8.00 (d, J = 8.4 Hz, 2H), 7.42 (s, 1H), 7.27 (d, J = 8.5 Hz, 2H), 7.19 (d, J = 2.1 Hz, 1H), 3.22 (dd, J = 12.2, 6.0 Hz, 2H), 1.52 (dq, J = 13.9, 7.1 Hz, 2H), 0.84 (t, J = 7.1 Hz, 3H). ^{13}C-NMR (100 MHz, DMSO-d_6, ppm) δ 165.72, 163.14, 156.13, 152.54, 150.37(2,C), 149.56, 141.97, 135.71, 135.05, 133.58, 131.78(2,C), 131.49, 130.44, 127.03, 122.63(2,C), 121.28(2,C), 114.18(2,C), 108.96, 40.58, 22.33, 11.25. TOF MS ES+ (*m/z*): $[M + H]^+$, calcd for $C_{26}H_{19}ClF_6N_6O_3$: 613.1190, found, 613.1189.

4-(4-(1-(4-chloro-3-(trifluoromethyl)phenyl)-5-(trifluoromethyl)-1H-1,2,3-triazole-4-carboxamido)phenoxy)-N-propylpicolinamide (**B9**) Light yellow solid; Yield: 66.3%; m.p.: 155.5–155.8 °C; ^{1}H-NMR (400 MHz, DMSO-d_6, ppm) δ 11.21 (s, 1H), 8.81 (s, 1H), 8.53 (d, J = 5.3 Hz, 1H), 8.44 (s, 1H), 8.17 (d, J = 8.1 Hz, 1H), 8.10 (d, J = 8.4 Hz, 1H), 7.99 (d, J = 8.7 Hz, 2H), 7.41 (s, 1H), 7.27 (d, J = 8.6 Hz, 2H), 7.19 (d, J = 2.9 Hz, 1H), 3.22 (dd, J = 12.8, 6.2 Hz, 2H), 1.52 (dq, J = 14.8, 7.4 Hz, 2H), 0.84 (t, J = 7.3 Hz, 3H). TOF MS ES+ (*m/z*): $[M + H]^+$, calcd for $C_{26}H_{19}ClF_6N_6O_3$: 613.1190, found, 613.1188.

4-(2-fluoro-4-(5-methyl-1-phenyl-1H-1,2,3-triazole-4-carboxamido)phenoxy)-N-propylpicolinamide (**B10**) White solid; Yield: 76.8%; m.p.: 143.3–143.7 °C; ^{1}H-NMR (400 MHz, DMSO-d_6, ppm) δ 10.96 (s, 1H), 8.83 (s, 1H), 8.54 (d, J = 5.4 Hz, 1H), 8.11 (d, J = 13.2 Hz, 1H), 7.86 (d, J = 8.7 Hz, 1H), 7.67 (d, J = 2.6 Hz, 5H), 7.48–7.39 (m, 2H), 7.23 (d, J = 4.7 Hz, 1H), 3.23 (dd, J = 12.9, 6.3 Hz, 2H), 2.59 (s, 3H), 1.57–1.47 (m, 2H), 0.84 (t, J = 7.3 Hz, 3H). ^{13}C-NMR (100 MHz, DMSO-d_6, ppm) δ 165.66, 163.43, 160.15, 153.09, 150.87(2,C), 138.46, 138.29, 135.61, 130.48, 130.09(3,C), 125.84(3,C), 124.07, 117.64, 113.82, 109.37, 108.46, 41.02, 22.73, 11.67, 9.86. TOF MS ES+ (*m/z*): $[M + H]^+$, calcd for $C_{25}H_{23}FN_6O_3$: 475.1894, found, 475.1894.

4-(2-fluoro-4-(1-(4-fluorophenyl)-5-methyl-1H-1,2,3-triazole-4-carboxamido)phenoxy)-N-propylpicolinamide (**B11**) White solid; Yield: 65.1%; m.p.: 143.5–143.8 °C; ^{1}H-NMR (400 MHz, DMSO-d_6, ppm) δ 10.95 (s, 1H), 8.82 (s, 1H), 8.54 (d, J = 5.1 Hz, 1H), 8.10 (d, J = 12.7 Hz, 1H), 7.86 (d, J = 8.6 Hz, 1H), 7.76 (s, 2H), 7.51 (t, J = 8.4 Hz, 2H), 7.44 (d, J = 12.9 Hz, 2H), 7.22 (d, J = 2.5 Hz, 1H), 3.22 (d, J = 6.0 Hz, 2H), 2.58 (s, 3H), 1.51 (dd, J = 13.9, 6.9 Hz, 2H), 0.84 (t, J = 7.2 Hz, 3H). ^{13}C-NMR (100 MHz, DMSO-d_6, ppm) δ 165.65, 164.20, 163.42, 161.74, 160.11, 153.08, 150.88, 138.75, 138.22, 131.99, 128.44, 128.35, 124.08, 117.65, 117.18(2,C), 116.95, 113.83, 109.60, 109.38, 108.44, 41.01, 22.73, 11.67, 9.78. TOF MS ES+ (*m/z*): $[M + H]^+$, calcd for $C_{25}H_{22}F_2N_6O_3$: 493.1800, found, 493.1797.

4-(2-fluoro-4-(5-methyl-1-(2-(trifluoromethoxy)phenyl)-1H-1,2,3-triazole-4-carboxamido)phenoxy)-N-propylpicolinamide (**B12**) Light yellow solid; Yield: 63.2%; m.p.: 132.6–132.9 °C; ^{1}H-NMR (400 MHz, DMSO-d_6, ppm) δ 10.99 (s, 1H), 8.82 (s, 1H), 8.55 (d, J = 5.6 Hz, 1H), 8.10 (d, J = 13.2 Hz, 1H), 7.88 (d, J = 7.5 Hz, 1H), 7.85 (d, J = 8.0 Hz, 2H), 7.79 (d, J = 8.4 Hz, 1H), 7.73 (t, J = 7.5 Hz, 1H), 7.46 (d, J = 9.0 Hz, 1H), 7.41 (d, J = 2.5 Hz, 1H), 7.23 (dd, J = 5.5, 2.6 Hz, 1H), 3.26–3.20 (m, 2H), 2.46 (s, 3H), 1.58–1.47 (m, 2H), 0.85 (t, J = 7.4 Hz, 3H). TOF MS ES+ (*m/z*): $[M + H]^+$, calcd for $C_{26}H_{22}F_4N_6O_4$: 559.1717, found, 559.1717.

4-(4-(1-(4-chlorophenyl)-5-(trifluoromethyl)-1H-1,2,3-triazole-4-carboxamido)-2-fluorophenoxy)-N-propylpicolinamide (**B13**) Light yellow solid; Yield: 76.3%; m.p.: 176.5–176.8 °C; ^{1}H-NMR (400 MHz, DMSO-d_6, ppm) δ 11.37 (s, 1H), 8.81 (s, 1H), 8.55 (d, J = 5.3 Hz, 1H), 8.06 (d, J = 12.8 Hz, 1H), 7.79 (d, J = 7.4 Hz, 5H), 7.48 (d, J = 8.9 Hz, 1H), 7.44 (s, 1H), 7.27–7.20 (m, 1H), 3.23 (d, J = 6.1 Hz, 2H), 1.52 (dd, J = 14.1, 7.1 Hz, 2H), 0.84 (t, J = 7.3 Hz, 3H). TOF MS ES+ (*m/z*): $[M + H]^+$, calcd for $C_{25}H_{19}ClF_4N_6O_3$: 563.1222, found, 563.1216.

4-(2-fluoro-4-(5-(trifluoromethyl)-1-(2-(trifluoromethyl)phenyl)-1H-1,2,3-triazole-4-carboxamido)phenoxy)-N-propylpicolinamide (**B14**) Light yellow solid; Yield: 79.6%; m.p.: 172.8–173.1 °C; ^{1}H-NMR (400 MHz, DMSO-d_6, ppm) δ 11.43 (s, 1H), 8.82 (s, 1H), 8.55 (d, *J* = 5.3 Hz, 1H), 8.12 (s, 1H), 8.09 (d, *J* = 4.7 Hz, 1H), 8.05 (s, 1H), 8.00 (d, *J* = 9.1 Hz, 2H), 7.84 (d, *J* = 8.3 Hz, 1H), 7.49 (d, *J* = 8.9 Hz, 1H), 7.44 (s, 1H), 7.24 (d, *J* = 2.5 Hz, 1H), 3.23 (d, *J* = 5.6 Hz, 2H), 1.55–1.49 (m, 2H), 0.84 (t, *J* = 7.2 Hz, 3H). ^{13}C-NMR (100 MHz, DMSO-d_6, ppm) δ 165.15, 163.01, 156.39, 152.70, 150.48(2,C), 141.52, 134.25(2,C), 134.18, 132.86, 132.00, 129.99(2,C), 127.65, 123.86(2,C), 117.59, 113.43(2,C), 109.61, 109.39, 108.12, 40.60, 22.31, 11.21. TOF MS ES+ (*m/z*): $[M + H]^+$, calcd for $C_{26}H_{22}F_4N_6O_3$: 543.1614, found, 543.1616.

4-(4-(1-(3,4-difluorophenyl)-5-(trifluoromethyl)-1H-1,2,3-triazole-4-carboxamido)-2-fluorophenoxy)-N-propylpicolinamide (**B15**) White solid; Yield: 55.4%; m.p.: 134.4–134.8 °C; ^{1}H-NMR (400 MHz, DMSO-d_6, ppm) δ 11.40 (s, 1H), 8.83 (s, 1H), 8.55 (d, *J* = 5.4 Hz, 1H), 8.13 (d, *J* = 9.0 Hz, 1H), 8.06 (d, *J* = 13.0 Hz, 1H), 7.82 (d, *J* = 7.0 Hz, 2H), 7.74 (s, 1H), 7.48 (t, *J* = 8.8 Hz, 1H), 7.42 (s, 1H), 7.25 (d, *J* = 2.0 Hz, 1H), 3.22 (d, *J* = 6.2 Hz, 2H), 1.52 (d, *J* = 7.1 Hz, 2H), 0.84 (t, *J* = 7.1 Hz, 3H). TOF MS ES+ (*m/z*): $[M + H]^+$, calcd for $C_{26}H_{19}F_7N_6O_3$: 597.1485, found, 597.1486.

4-(4-(1-(3-chloro-4-fluorophenyl)-5-(trifluoromethyl)-1H-1,2,3-triazole-4-carboxamido)-2-fluorophenoxy)-N-propylpicolinamide (**B16**) White solid; Yield: 59.7%; m.p.: 163.3–163.5 °C; ^{1}H-NMR (400 MHz, DMSO-d_6, ppm) δ 11.39 (s, 1H), 8.82 (t, *J* = 5.8 Hz, 1H), 8.56 (d, *J* = 5.6 Hz, 1H), 8.23 (d, *J* = 4.8 Hz, 1H), 8.06 (d, *J* = 12.9 Hz, 1H), 7.88 (d, *J* = 8.5 Hz, 1H), 7.83 (d, *J* = 8.8 Hz, 1H), 7.77 (t, *J* = 8.9 Hz, 1H), 7.48 (t, *J* = 9.0 Hz, 1H), 7.42 (s, 1H), 7.25 (d, *J* = 5.4 Hz, 1H), 3.23 (dd, *J* = 13.3, 6.5 Hz, 2H), 1.53 (dt, *J* = 14.5, 7.4 Hz, 2H), 0.85 (t, *J* = 7.4 Hz, 3H). TOF MS ES+ (*m/z*): $[M + H]^+$, calcd for $C_{25}H_{18}ClF_5N_6O_3$: 581.1127, found, 581.1128.

4-(4-(1-(2-chloro-5-(trifluoromethyl)phenyl)-5-(trifluoromethyl)-1H-1,2,3-triazole-4-carboxamido)-2-fluorophenoxy)-N-propylpicolinamide (**B17**) White solid; Yield: 64.5%; m.p.: 154.1–154.4 °C; ^{1}H-NMR (400 MHz, DMSO-d_6, ppm) δ 11.48 (s, 1H), 8.83 (s, 1H), 8.65 (s, 1H), 8.55 (d, *J* = 5.0 Hz, 1H), 8.21 (d, *J* = 7.8 Hz, 1H), 8.15 (d, *J* = 8.2 Hz, 1H), 8.07 (d, *J* = 12.9 Hz, 1H), 7.84 (d, *J* = 8.6 Hz, 1H), 7.49 (t, *J* = 8.8 Hz, 1H), 7.43 (s, 1H), 7.25 (d, *J* = 1.4 Hz, 1H), 3.23 (d, *J* = 6.0 Hz, 2H), 1.52 (dd, *J* = 13.9, 6.9 Hz, 2H), 0.84 (t, *J* = 7.3 Hz, 3H). TOF MS ES+ (m/z): $[M + H]^+$, calcd for $C_{26}H_{18}ClF_7N_6O_3$: 631.1089, found, 631.1089.

4-(4-(1-(4-chloro-3-(trifluoromethyl)phenyl)-5-(trifluoromethyl)-1H-1,2,3-triazole-4-carboxamido)-2-fluorophenoxy)-N-propylpicolinamide (**B18**) White solid; Yield: 55.9%; m.p.: 153.4–153.7 °C; ^{1}H-NMR (400 MHz, DMSO-d_6, ppm) δ 11.41 (s, 1H), 8.83 (s, 1H), 8.56 (d, *J* = 5.3 Hz, 1H), 8.45 (s, 1H), 8.18 (d, *J* = 8.4 Hz, 1H), 8.12–8.01 (m, 2H), 7.84 (d, *J* = 8.4 Hz, 1H), 7.48 (t, *J* = 8.9 Hz, 1H), 7.42 (s, 1H), 7.25 (s, 1H), 3.26–3.19 (m, 2H), 1.52 (dq, *J* = 14.4, 7.0 Hz, 2H), 0.84 (t, *J* = 7.2 Hz, 3H). TOF MS ES+ (m/z): $[M + H]^+$, calcd for $C_{26}H_{18}ClF_7N_6O_3$: 631.1089, found, 631.1096.

N-(3-fluoro-4-((2-(pyrrolidine-1-carbonyl)pyridin-4-yl)oxy)phenyl)-5-methyl-1-phenyl-1H-1,2,3-triazole-4-carboxamide (**B19**) Light yellow solid; Yield: 63.2%; m.p.: 169.7–170.0 °C; ^{1}H-NMR (400 MHz, DMSO-d_6, ppm) δ 10.94 (s, 1H), 8.50 (d, *J* = 4.4 Hz, 1H), 8.09 (d, *J* = 12.9 Hz, 1H), 7.84 (d, *J* = 8.4 Hz, 1H), 7.65 (d, *J* = 14.4 Hz, 5H), 7.42 (t, *J* = 8.6 Hz, 1H), 7.13 (d, *J* = 14.2 Hz, 2H), 3.59 (s, 2H), 3.45 (s, 2H), 2.59 (s, 3H), 1.82 (s, 4H). TOF MS ES+ (*m/z*): $[M + H]^+$, calcd for $C_{26}H_{23}FN_6O_3$: 487.1897, found, 487.1902.

N-(3-fluoro-4-((2-(pyrrolidine-1-carbonyl)pyridin-4-yl)oxy)phenyl)-1-(4-fluorophenyl)-5-methyl-1H-1,2,3-triazole-4-carboxamide (**B20**) Light yellow solid; Yield: 66.4%; m.p.: 164.3–164.7 °C; ^{1}H-NMR (400 MHz, DMSO-d_6, ppm) δ 10.94 (s, 1H), 8.51 (d, *J* = 5.3 Hz, 1H), 8.09 (d, *J* = 13.2 Hz, 1H), 7.84 (d, *J* = 8.4 Hz, 1H), 7.75 (d, *J* = 3.2 Hz, 2H), 7.51 (t, *J* = 8.4 Hz, 2H), 7.42 (t, *J* = 8.9 Hz, 1H), 7.18 (s, 1H), 7.12 (d, *J* = 4.6 Hz, 1H), 3.59 (s, 2H), 3.45 (s, 2H), 2.57 (s, 3H), 1.81 (s, 4H). TOF MS ES+ (*m/z*): $[M + H]^+$, calcd for $C_{26}H_{22}F_2N_6O_3$: 505.1800, found, 505.1807.

N-(3-fluoro-4-((2-(pyrrolidine-1-carbonyl)pyridin-4-yl)oxy) phenyl)-5-methyl-1-(2-(trifluoromethoxy)phenyl)-1H-1,2,3-triazole-4-carboxamide (**B21**) White solid; Yield: 66.5%; m.p.: 176.3–176.6 °C; ^{1}H-NMR (400 MHz,

DMSO-d$_6$, ppm) δ 11.00 (s, 1H), 8.51 (d, *J* = 4.9 Hz, 1H), 8.09 (d, *J* = 12.8 Hz, 1H), 7.89 (d, *J* = 7.3 Hz, 1H), 7.85 (d, *J* = 8.0 Hz, 2H), 7.79 (d, *J* = 8.2 Hz, 1H), 7.75–7.70 (m, 1H), 7.43 (t, *J* = 8.6 Hz, 1H), 7.16 (s, 1H), 7.11 (d, *J* = 1.9 Hz, 1H), 3.60 (s, 2H), 3.46 (s, 2H), 2.46 (s, 3H), 1.82 (s, 4H). TOF MS ES+ (m/z): $[M + H]^+$, calcd for $C_{27}H_{22}F_4N_6O_4$: 571.1717, found, 571.1722.

4-(2-fluoro-4-(5-methyl-1-phenyl-1H-1,2,3-triazole-4-carboxamido)phenoxy)-N-(2-(thiophen-2-yl)ethyl)picolinamide (**B22**) Light yellow solid; Yield: 61.9%; m.p.: 124.6–125.0 °C; ^{1}H NMR (400 MHz, DMSO-*d*$_6$, ppm) δ 10.97 (s, 1H), 8.98 (t, *J* = 5.9 Hz, 1H), 8.55 (d, *J* = 5.6 Hz, 1H), 8.11 (d, *J* = 13.2 Hz, 1H), 7.86 (d, *J* = 8.8 Hz, 1H), 7.67 (d, *J* = 2.3 Hz, 5H), 7.48–7.41 (m, 2H), 7.32 (d, *J* = 4.9 Hz, 1H), 7.24 (d, *J* = 3.0 Hz, 1H), 6.96-6.91 (m, 1H), 6.89 (d, *J* = 2.6 Hz, 1H), 3.54 (dd, *J* = 13.4, 6.8 Hz, 2H), 3.06 (t, *J* = 7.1 Hz, 2H), 2.59 (s, 3H). TOF MS ES+ (*m/z*): $[M + H]^+$, calcd for $C_{28}H_{23}FN_6O_3S$: 543.1614, found, 543.1616.

4-(2-fluoro-4-(1-(4-fluorophenyl)-5-methyl-1H-1,2,3-triazole-4-carboxamido)phenoxy)-N-(2-(thiophen-2-yl)ethyl)picolinamide (**B23**) White solid; Yield: 51.7%; m.p.: 110.4–110.8 °C; ^{1}H-NMR (400 MHz, DMSO-*d*$_6$, ppm) δ 10.99 (s, 1H), 9.00 (t, *J* = 5.7 Hz, 1H), 8.57 (d, *J* = 5.6 Hz, 1H), 8.13 (d, *J* = 13.2 Hz, 1H), 7.88 (d, *J* = 8.8 Hz, 1H), 7.79 (d, *J* = 4.8 Hz, 1H), 7.77 (d, *J* = 4.8 Hz, 1H), 7.54 (t, *J* = 8.7 Hz, 2H), 7.47 (d, *J* = 9.1 Hz, 1H), 7.43 (d, *J* = 2.1 Hz, 1H), 7.34 (d, *J* = 4.6 Hz, 1H), 7.26 (d, *J* = 2.4 Hz, 1H), 6.98–6.94 (m, 1H), 6.91 (s, 1H), 3.55 (dd, *J* = 13.3, 6.8 Hz, 2H), 3.08 (t, *J* = 7.1 Hz, 2H), 2.60 (s, 3H). TOF MS ES+ (*m/z*): $[M + H]^+$, calcd for $C_{28}H_{22}F_2N_6O_3S$: 561.1520, found, 561.1529.

4-(2-fluoro-4-(5-methyl-1-(2-(trifluoromethoxy)phenyl)-1H-1,2,3-triazole-4-carboxamido)phenoxy)-N-(2-(thiophen-2-yl)ethyl)picolinamide (**B24**) White solid; Yield: 56.6%; m.p.: 103.4–103.7 °C; ^{1}H-NMR (400 MHz, DMSO-d$_6$, ppm) δ 10.98 (s, 1H), 8.94 (s, 1H), 8.55 (d, *J* = 5.3 Hz, 1H), 8.10 (d, *J* = 13.2 Hz, 1H), 7.88 (d, *J* = 6.4 Hz, 2H), 7.84 (d, *J* = 7.0 Hz, 1H), 7.78 (d, *J* = 8.1 Hz, 1H), 7.72 (t, *J* = 7.4 Hz, 1H), 7.44 (t, *J* = 8.8 Hz, 2H), 7.31 (d, *J* = 4.1 Hz, 1H), 7.23 (d, *J* = 2.3 Hz, 1H), 6.96–6.92 (m, 1H), 6.90 (s, 1H), 3.55 (d, *J* = 6.2 Hz, 2H), 3.07 (t, *J* = 6.9 Hz, 2H), 2.47 (s, 3H). TOF MS ES+ (m/z): $[M + H]^+$, calcd for $C_{29}H_{22}F_4N_6O_4S$: 627.1437, found, 627.1439.

4-(2-fluoro-4-(5-methyl-1-phenyl-1H-1,2,3-triazole-4-carboxamido)phenoxy)-N-(3-morpholinopropyl)picolinamide (**B25**) White solid; Yield: 42.6%; m.p.: 108.3–108.6 °C; ^{1}H-NMR (400 MHz, DMSO-*d*$_6$, ppm) δ 10.67 (s, 1H), 9.05 (s, 1H), 8.53 (s, 1H), 8.03 (d, *J* = 7.5 Hz, 2H), 7.67 (s, 5H), 7.45 (s, 1H), 7.23 (d, *J* = 7.6 Hz, 1H), 7.17 (s, 1H), 3.64 (s, 4H), 3.36 (s, 2H), 2.60 (s, 3H), 2.44 (s, 6H), 1.72 (s, 2H). ^{13}C-NMR (100 MHz, DMSO-*d*$_6$, ppm) δ 166.25, 163.53, 159.92, 152.85, 150.72, 149.29, 138.56, 138.11, 136.82, 135.67, 130.44, 130.10(2,C), 125.83(2,C), 122.70(2,C), 121.51(2,C), 114.53, 109.30, 66.25(2,C), 56.81, 53.53(2,C), 38.36, 25.59, 9.85. TOF MS ES+ (*m/z*): $[M + H]^+$, calcd for $C_{29}H_{30}FN_7O_4$: 560.2421, found, 560.2416.

4-(2-fluoro-4-(1-(4-fluorophenyl)-5-methyl-1H-1,2,3-triazole-4-carboxamido)phenoxy)-N-(3-morpholinopropyl)picolinamide (**B26**) White solid; Yield: 39.3%; m.p.: 108.5–108.9 °C; ^{1}H-NMR (400 MHz, DMSO-*d*$_6$, ppm) δ 10.73 (s, 1H), 9.10 (s, 1H), 8.52 (d, *J* = 3.7 Hz, 1H), 8.03 (d, *J* = 7.9 Hz, 2H), 7.76 (s, 2H), 7.52 (d, *J* = 6.9 Hz, 2H), 7.43 (s, 1H), 7.23 (d, *J* = 7.9 Hz, 2H), 3.61 (s, 4H), 3.35 (s, 2H), 2.59 (s, 3H), 2.34 (s, 6H), 1.68 (s, 2H). ^{13}C-NMR (100 MHz, DMSO-*d*$_6$, ppm) δ 166.25, 163.48, 159.87, 152.90, 150.69, 149.33, 138.38, 136.78, 132.06, 128.39, 128.30, 122.71(2,C), 121.46(2,C), 117.16(2,C), 116.93(2,C), 114.50, 109.32, 66.54(2,C), 57.08, 53.77(2,C), 38.55, 25.80, 9.74. TOF MS ES+ (*m/z*): $[M + H]^+$, calcd for $C_{29}H_{29}F_2N_7O_4$: 578.2327, found, 578.2347.

4-(2-fluoro-4-(5-methyl-1-(2-(trifluoromethoxy)phenyl)-1H-1,2,3-triazole-4-carboxamido)phenoxy)-N-(3-morpholinopropyl)picolinamide (**B27**) White solid; Yield: 41.0%; m.p.: 97.6–97.9 °C; ^{1}H-NMR (400 MHz, DMSO-d$_6$, ppm) δ 10.78 (s, 1H), 9.05 (s, 1H), 8.54 (s, 1H), 7.99 (d, *J* = 5.2 Hz, 2H), 7.86 (d, *J* = 3.8 Hz, 2H), 7.79 (s, 1H), 7.73 (s, 1H), 7.41 (s, 1H), 7.23 (d, *J* = 6.1 Hz, 2H), 3.91 (d, *J* = 8.3 Hz, 2H), 3.85 (d, *J* = 11.1 Hz, 2H), 3.36 (d, *J* = 5.0 Hz, 2H), 3.06 (s, 4H), 2.45 (s, 2H), 1.98 (s, 2H). TOF MS ES+ (m/z): $[M + H]^+$, calcd for $C_{30}H_{29}F_4N_7O_5$: 643.1059, found, 643.1094.

^{1}H-NMR spectra of representative target compounds (**B1**, **B6**, **B12**, **B13**, **B20**, **B25**, and **B26**), ^{13}C-NMR spectra of representative target compounds (**B6**, **B7**, **B10**, **B11**, **B14**, **B25**, and **B26**), and TOF-MS spectra of representative target compounds (**B13**, **B17**, **B19**, **B21**, **B22**, **B25**, and **B26**) can be seen in the Supplementary Materials.

3.2. Antitumority Assay

The antitumor activities of target compounds were determined by the MTT method using Golvatinib as a positive control. All cancer cell lines (A549, HeLa, and MCF-7) were cultured with Dulbecco Modified Eagle Medium (DMEM) or Roswell Park Memorial Institute (1640) containing 10% fetal bovine serum and 0.1% penicillin–streptomycin, under ambient conditions of 5% CO_2 and 37 °C. Cells were digested with an appropriate amount of Trypsin–EDTA solution to obtain the cell suspension, which was diluted with medium and inoculated into 96-well plates at $5*10^4$ cells per well. After cells were incubated for 24 h, the target compounds diluted by medium to suitable concentrations were added into 96-well plates, and the cells were cultured continue for 72 h. Next, the medium was removed, and then thiazolyl blue tetrazolium bromide (MTT) was added to each well to treat cells for 3.5 h. Ultimately, dimethyl sulfoxide (DMSO) was added to each well after removal of MTT and the absorbance values were measured with the ELISA (enzyme-linked immunosorbent assay) reader. All antitumor activities were tested for three times. The IC_{50} values were the average of three measurements and were calculated using the Bacus Laboratories Incorporated Slide Scanner (Bliss) software.

3.3. Dose-Dependent Test

The dose-dependent effect of compound **B26** on A549 cells was tested by the MTT method using Golvatinib as a positive control. The experimental procedure was identical to that of the cytotoxic activity, wherein the concentration of the test compound was configured to be seven and the cytotoxic activity was five. Seven different concentrations of compound **B26** treated on A549 cells to obtain the corresponding inhibition rates. Experimental data was obtained by Orange (2018 64 bit) software based on the inhibition rate.

3.4. Cell Morphology Studies

Cell morphology studies aimed to explore the morphological changes of A549 cells with and without treatment with compound **B26**, and the cell morphology was visualized by acridine orange (AO) staining. The culture environment of A549 cells was consistent with that in the antitumor activity experiments. Cells were digested with Trypsin–EDTA solution to get the cell suspension, which was diluted with 1640 medium and inoculated into a 24-well plate at $2*10^4$ cells per well. After incubating for 12 h, compound **B26** diluted to suitable concentrations by 1640 medium was added into a 24-well plate, and cell culture was continued for 12 h. Then, the 1640 medium in the well plate was removed and every well were washed three times with phosphate buffer saline (PBS). After washing with PBS three times, A549 cells were treated with AO for 15 min. A549 cells were washed three times with PBS again, and the cell morphology distribution was observed directly by a fluorescence microscope. Ultimately, the picture is exported via computer.

3.5. Cell Cycle Study

A549 cells were seeded into six-well plates at $1*10^5$ cells per well and incubated for 24 h. Then, the medium containing DMEM (control, without compound) or compound **B26** with different concentrations was added to the culture plate, and A549 cells were further cultured for 24 h. Then, A549 cells were collected into a centrifuge tube and fixed with a small amount of ice-cold 70% ethanol at 4 °C for 6–12 h. Cells washed three times with PBS were incubated with Rnase (1 mg/mL, diluted with PBS) for 30 min at room temperature. Finally, propidium iodide (PI) was added to staining without light for 30 min at room temperature, and the DNA content was measured by flow cytometry within 1 h. Experimental data was obtained by Modify software.

3.6. c-Met Kinase Assay

The kinase assay was implemented through Mobility shift assay. The Mixture the configured available Brij-35 (0.0015%) and 50 mM HEPES (pH = 7.5) to get a kinase buffer base. Then, compounds **B25**, **B26**, and **B27** were configured to five concentrations using dimethyl sulfoxide. The kinase buffer containing the compounds or dimethyl sulfoxide was added to 96-well plates and mixed on the shaker for fifteen minutes. Next, the solution was transferred in duplicate from a 96-well plate to a 384-well plate, and then an enzyme solution (c-Met kinase mixed with kinase buffer) was added to each well. After incubation of the 384-well plate for 10 min at room temperature, a 2.5*peptide solution (formed by the addition of FAM-labeled peptide and ATP to the kinase base buffer) was added to each well. After incubation at 28 °C for a certain period of time, a stop buffer was added to each well for stop the reaction. The inhibition value is obtained by converting the conversion data on the caliper. The formula is that percent inhibition = (max − conversion) / (max − min) * 100. Among them, "max" stands for DMSO control, "min" stands for low control. Finally, the IC_{50} values were obtained by fitting the inhibition rate data using the XLFit excel add-in version software.

3.7. Molecular Docking Study

All the molecular docking simulations were performed by the AutoDock 4.2 software. The crystal structure of c-Met (PDB code: 3LQ8) used in the docking was downloaded from http://www.rcsb.org/. The preparation process of the protein for docking mainly involves the addition of hydrogen atoms and charges, elimination of unrelated water molecules, immobilization of exact residues, and removal of endogenous ligands (Foretinib), etc. The preparation process of the molecules for docking mainly includes the addition of hydrogen atoms and charges. Then the prepared molecules (target compounds) were docked to the certified binding site of c-Met protein. Subsequently, the genetic algorithm was used for energy optimization. All the docking results were modified and processed by PyMOL 1.8.x software (https://pymol.org).

4. Conclusions

In conclusion, a series of 4-(pyridin-4-yloxy)benzamide derivatives bearing a triazole fragment were designed and synthesized. In addition, we evaluated them for antitumor activity against three cancer cell lines and c-Met kinase activity (only for compounds **B25–B27**) in vitro. The pharmacological results indicated that most compounds showed moderate antitumor activity against the three cancer cell lines. In particular, compound **B26** showed excellent inhibitory activity with IC_{50} values of 3.22, 4.33, and 5.82 μM against A549, HeLa, and MCF-7 cell lines, which were more potent than Golvatinib, respectively. The SARs study indicated that the introduction of a morpholino group in the hydrophilic region was more favorable than an alkane chain in terms of antitumor activity, and a single electron-withdrawing substituent (such as a fluorine atom) on the terminal phenyl ring improved the inhibitory activity of the target compounds. Further studies will be carried out in the near future.

Author Contributions: P.Z., Q.T. and J.C. conceived and designed the experiments; H.X., J.Z., Q.Z., Z.X. and H.Z. performed the experiments and statistics analysis; J.C. and H.X. completed the molecular docking simulation and H.X. started the project and wrote the paper. All authors have read and agreed to the published version of the manuscript.

References

1. Miller, K.D.; Nogueira, L.; Mariotto, B.; Rowland, J.H.; Yabroff, K.R.; Alfano, C.M.; DVM, J.A.; Kramer, J.L.; Siegel, R.L. Cancer Treatment and Survivorship Statistics. *CA Cancer J. Clin.* **2016**, *66*, 271–289. [CrossRef] [PubMed]

2. Luo, T.; Zhang, S.G.; Zhu, L.F.; Zhang, F.X.; Li, W.; Zhao, K.; Wen, X.X.; Yu, M.; Zhan, Y.Q.; Chen, H.; et al. A Selective c-Met and Trks Inhibitor Indo5 Suppresses Hepatocellular Carcinoma Growth. *J. Exp. Clin. Canc. Res.* **2019**, *38*, 130–143. [CrossRef] [PubMed]
3. Moslehi, J.J.; Michael, D. Tyrosine Kinase Inhibitor–Associated Cardiovascular Toxicity in Chronic Myeloid Leukemia. *J. Clin. Oncol.* **2015**, *33*, 4210–4222. [CrossRef] [PubMed]
4. Bouattour, M.; Raymond, E.; Qin, S.; Cheng, A.L.; Stammberger, U.; Locatelli, G.; Faivre, S. Recent Developments of c-Met as a Therapeutic Target in Hepatocellular Carcinoma. *Hepatology* **2018**, *67*, 1132–1149. [CrossRef] [PubMed]
5. Kim, H.J.; Kang, S.K.; Kwon, W.S.; Kim, S.T.; Jeong, I.; Jeung, H.C.; Kragh, M.; Horak, I.D.; Chung, H.C.; Rha, S.Y. Forty-Nine Gastric Cancer Cell Lines with Integrative Genomic Profiling for Development of c-Met Inhibitor. *Nt. J. Cancer* **2018**, *143*, 151–159. [CrossRef] [PubMed]
6. Hong, D.S.; LoRusso, P.; Hamid, O.; Janku, F.; Kittaneh, M.; Catenacci, D.V.T.; Chan, E.; Bekaii-Saab, T.; Gadgeel, S.M.; Loberg, R.T.; et al. Phase I Study of AMG 337, a Highly Selective Small-Molecule Met Inhibitor, in Patients with Advanced Solid Tumors. *Clin. Cancer Res.* **2019**, *25*, 2403–2413. [CrossRef] [PubMed]
7. Liu, Y.; Jin, S.Y.; Peng, X.; Lu, D.; Zeng, L.M.; Sun, Y.M.; Ai, J.; Geng, M.Y.; Hu, Y.H. Pyridazinone Derivatives Displaying Highly Potent and Selective Inhibitory Activities Against c-Met Tyrosine Kinase. *Eur. J. Med. Chem.* **2016**, *108*, 322–333. [CrossRef] [PubMed]
8. Li, M.J.; Wu, G.Z.; Kaas, Q.; Jiang, T.; Yu, R.L. Development of Efficient Docking Strategies and Structure–Activity Relationship Study of the c-Met Type II Inhibitors. *J. Mol. Graph Model* **2017**, *75*, 241–249. [CrossRef] [PubMed]
9. Zhao, Y.M.; Zhang, J.K.; Zhuang, R.X.; He, R.Y.; Xi, J.J.; Pan, X.W.; Shao, Y.D.; Pan, Y.M.; Sun, J.J.; Cai, Z.B.; et al. Synthesis and Evaluation of a Series of Pyridine and Pyrimidine Derivatives as Type II c-Met Inhibitors. *Bioorgan. Med. Chem.* **2017**, *25*, 3195–3205. [CrossRef] [PubMed]
10. Nakazawa, Y.; Kawano, S.; Matsui, J.; Funahashi, Y.; Tohyama, Q.; Muto, H.; Nakagawa, T.; Matsushima, T. Multitargeting Strategy Using Lenvatinib and Golvatinib: Maximizing Anti-Angiogenesis Activity in a Preclinical Cancer Model. *Cancer Sci.* **2015**, *106*, 201–207. [CrossRef] [PubMed]
11. Parikh, P.K.; Ghate, M.D. Recent Advances in the Discovery of Small Molecule c-Met Kinase Inhibitors. *Eur. J. Med. Chem.* **2018**, *143*, 1103–1138. [CrossRef] [PubMed]
12. Darwish, H.W.; Abdelhameed, A.S.; Bakheit, A.H.; Alanazi, A.M. A New Method to Determine the New C-Met Inhibitor "Cabozantinib" in Dosage Form and Human Plasma via Micelle-Enhanced Spectrofluorimetry. *RSC Adv.* **2015**, *5*, 40484–40490. [CrossRef]
13. Tang, Q.D.; Duan, Y.L.; Wang, L.X.; O'Yang, Y.Q.; Wang, C.L.; Mei, H.; Tang, S.; Xiong, Y.H.; Zheng, P.W.; Gong, P.; et al. Synthesis and Antiproliferative Activity of Pyrrolo[2, 3-b]pyridine Derivatives Bearing the 1, 8-Naphthyridin-2-One Moiety. *Eur. J. Med. Chem.* **2018**, *143*, 266–275. [CrossRef] [PubMed]
14. Zhang, L.; Zhao, J.Y.; Zhang, B.C.; Lu, T.; Chen, Y.D. Discovery of [1, 2, 4] triazolo [3, 4-b][1, 3, 4] thiadiazole Derivatives as Novel, Potent and Selective c-Met Kinase Inhibitors: Synthesis, SAR Study, and Biological Activity. *Eur. J. Med. Chem.* **2018**, *150*, 809–816. [CrossRef] [PubMed]
15. Wang, L.X.; Xu, S.; Liu, X.B.; Chen, X.Y.; Xiong, H.H.; Hou, S.S.; Zou, W.S.; Tang, Q.D.; Zheng, P.W.; Zhu, W.F. Discovery of Thinopyrimidine-Triazole Conjugates as c-Met Targeting and Apoptosis Inducing Agents. *Bioorg. Chem.* **2018**, *77*, 370–380. [CrossRef] [PubMed]
16. Dadashpour, S.; Küçükkılınç, T.T.; Ayazgök, B.; Hosseinimehr, S.J.; Chippindale, A.M.; Foroumadi, A.; Irannejad, H. Discovery of Novel 1, 2, 4-Triazolo-1, 2, 4-Triazines with Thiomethylpyridine Hinge Binders as Potent c-Met Kinase Inhibitors. *Future Med. Chem.* **2019**, *11*, 1119–1136. [CrossRef] [PubMed]
17. Olmez, I.; Zhang, Y.; Manigat, L.; Benamar, M.; Brenneman, B.; Nakano, I.; Godlewski, J.; Bronisz, A.; Lee, J.; Abbas, T.; et al. Combined c-Met/Trk Inhibition Overcomes Resistance to CDK4/6 Inhibitors in Glioblastoma. *Cancer Res.* **2018**, *78*, 4360–4369. [CrossRef] [PubMed]
18. Liu, X.B.; Kou, J.L.; Xiao, Z.; Tian, F.J.; Hu, J.Y.; Zheng, P.W.; Zhu, W.F. Design, Synthesis and Biological Evaluation of 6, 7-Disubstituted-4-Phenoxyquinoline Derivatives Bearing Pyridazinone Moiety as c-Met Inhibitors. *Molecules* **2018**, *23*, 1543. [CrossRef] [PubMed]
19. Ahmed, E.M.; Khalil, N.A.; Taher, A.T.; Refaey, R.H.; Nissan, Y.M. Triazolopyridazine Derivatives: Synthesis, Cytotoxic Evaluation, c-Met Kinase Activity and Molecular Docking. *Bioorg. Chem.* **2019**, *92*, 103272–103281. [CrossRef] [PubMed]

12

Design, Synthesis and Mechanism of Dihydroartemisinin–Coumarin Hybrids as Potential Anti-Neuroinflammatory Agents

Haonan Yu [1,†], Zhuang Hou [1,†], Xiaoguang Yang [1], Yanhua Mou [2,*] and Chun Guo [1,*]

1 School of Pharmaceutical Engineering, Shenyang Pharmaceutical University, Shenyang 110016, China; yhna380@hotmail.com (H.Y.); houzhuang8@sina.com (Z.H.); Xiaog_yang@163.com (X.Y.)

2 School of Life Sciences and Biological Pharmacy, Shenyang Pharmaceutical University, Shenyang 110016, China

* Correspondence: mu_hua_jj@sina.com (Y.M.); chunguo@syphu.edu.cn (C.G.);

† These authors contributed equally to this work.

Abstract: Cancer patients frequently suffer from cancer-related fatigue (CRF), which is a complex syndrome associated with weakness and depressed mood. Neuroinflammation is one of the major inducers of CRF. The aim of this study is to find a potential agent not only on the treatment of cancer, but also for reducing CRF level of cancer patients. In this study, total-thirty new Dihydroartemisinin–Coumarin hybrids (DCH) were designed and synthesized. The *in vitro* cytotoxicity against cancer cell lines (HT-29, MDA-MB-231, HCT-116, and A549) was evaluated. Simultaneously, we also tested the anti-neuroinflammatory activity of DCH. DCH could inhibit the activated microglia N9 release of NO, TNF-α, and IL-6. The docking analysis was shown that MD-2, the coreceptor of TLR4, might be one of the targets of DCH.

Keywords: anticancer; anti-neuroinflammation; coumarin; dihydroartemisinin

1. Introduction

Chemotherapy is an important method in the therapy of cancer, but the adverse side effects of anticancer agents should also be focused on. Gastrointestinal injury induced by chemotherapeutic agents could result in bacterial/endotoxin translocation from the gut to the systemic blood circulation [1,2]. The released endotoxin would cause a systemic inflammatory response including neuroinflammation [3]. Cancer patients frequently suffer from cancer-related fatigue (CRF), which is a complex syndrome associated with weakness and depressed mood. Diana M., Norden et al. demonstrated that the neuroinflammation is one of the major reasons which induce CRF [4]. Currently, there were no effective method to reduce CRF [5]. The aim of this study is to find a potential anti-neuroinflammatory agents which might reduce CRF of cancer patients.

Central nervous system (CNS) consists of two major types of cells, nerve cells and glial cells. Microglia is a major glial cell and plays an important role as the resident macrophage population in the CNS [6,7]. There has been wide recognition that the fully activated microglial cells are neurotoxic. They release reactive oxygen species, nitric oxide (NO), tumor necrosis factor-alpha (TNF-α), and other potentially cytotoxic molecules [8,9]. It means that activation of microglia could induce neuroinflammation.

Lipopolysaccharide (LPS), also known as endotoxin, is a natural Toll-like receptor 4 (TLR4) ligand and it is also a potent microglial activator that can trigger the production of inflammatory mediators. TLR-4, a transmembrane receptor, plays a vital role in the initiation and acceleration of the inflammatory response induced by LPS [10,11]. TLR4 alone does not directly bind LPS and needs the coreceptor MD-2 [12]. MD-2 is linked with the extracellular domain of TLR4 and is indispensable for LPS recognition [13]. MD-2 is a member of the MD-2-related lipid-recognition protein family [14]. MD-2 directly binds to LPS in its hydrophobic cavity with high affinity [15].

Artemisinin and its derivatives have been the first-line antimalarial drug since the late 1990s. Dihydroartemisinin (DHA) is the primary bioactive metabolite of artemisinin and its derivatives, but not artemisinin per se [16]. Additionally, DHA has higher bioavailability and less side effects than artemisinin [17]. Recent research showed that besides antimalarial activity, DHA also exhibits anticancer and anti-inflammatory activity [18–21]. As the anti-inflammatory agent, DHA could decrease LPS-induced protein expression of TLR4 [22].

Coumarins are widely distributed in different parts of plants. There are various pharmacological activities of coumarins, which includes anti-inflammatory [23,24] and anticancer activity [25,26]. As the anticancer agents, coumarins were reported to exhibit negligible or mild side effects [27,28]. Substitution at the C-3 or C-4 position of coumarins exhibit good cytotoxic activity in various cancer cell lines [26,29–31]. Additionally, as anti-inflammatory agents, some kinds of coumarins could also target TLR4/MD-2 complex [32,33].

In our previous study, Dihydroartemisinin–Coumarin hybrids (DCH) were designed and synthesized referring to the principle of hybridization [34,35]. Each of them contains coumarin moiety, DHA moiety and a linker. DCH could inhibit HT-29 cells proliferation and arrest the G_0/G_1 phase of HT-29 cells [35]. They could also suppress cancer cell migration, and induce apoptosis and ferroptosis of HT-29 cancer cells [35]. It also has been confirmed that the DCH having 1,2,3-triazole linker generally exhibit better cytotoxicity exhibition than the others [35].

With this background, total-thirty new DCH were designed and synthesized, and the synthetic approaches were shown in Figure 1. All of them contained 1,2,3-triazole linker. We focused on the modifications of positions 3 and 4 of the coumarin moiety. Due to the new synthesized DCH were for the cancer patients, we evaluated the in vitro cytotoxicity against cancer cell lines (HT-29, MDA-MB-231, HCT-116, and A549). In addition, DCH could inhibit the activated N9 cell release of NO, TNF-α and IL-6. Furthermore, to investigate the mechanism of the anti-neuroinflammatory activity, docking analysis was applied. The results might support that the anti-neuroinflammatory activity was related to inhibiting TLR4/MD-2 complex.

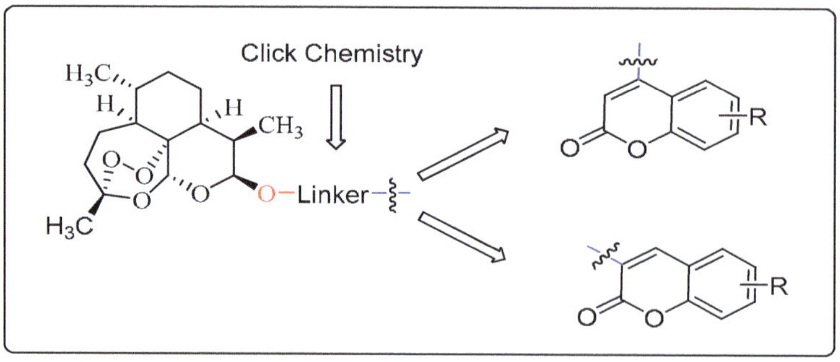

Figure 1. Structures of new designed Dihydroartemisinin–Coumarin hybrids.

2. Results and Discussion

2.1. Chemistry

The synthesis of the intermediates **a–p** and **I–IV** is presented in Scheme 1. The intermediates **I** and **II** were obtained by 2-bromoethanol or 3-bromo-1-propanol, with dihydroartemisinin (DHA), respectively, followed by treating the product with sodium azide. The intermediates **III** and **IV** were synthesized by propargyl alcohol or 3-butyn-1-ol with DHA, respectively. The required 3-methylcoumarin derivatives were obtained by substitution of salicylaldehyde with propionic anhydride in the presence of sodium propionate and triethylamine. The substituted-3-bromomethylcoumarins were prepared by the radical bromination of 3-methylcoumarin derivatives through the reaction with

N-Bromosuccinimide (NBS) in the presence of dibenzoylperoxide [36]. The intermediates **a–e** were synthesized by substituted-3-bromomethylcoumarins via azidation reaction. The required substituted-4-chloromethylcoumarins were prepared by the Pechmann cyclisation [37] of substituted phenols with 4-chloroethylacetoacetate using sulfuric acid as the condensing agent. The intermediates **f–i** were synthesized by substituted-4-chloromethylcoumarin via azidation reaction. To synthesize the intermediates **j–p**, several substituted-4-hydroxycoumarin were prepared by condensing the substituted phenol with malonic acid [38]. Then the products were treated with 3-bromo-1-propyne in the presence of potassium carbonate.

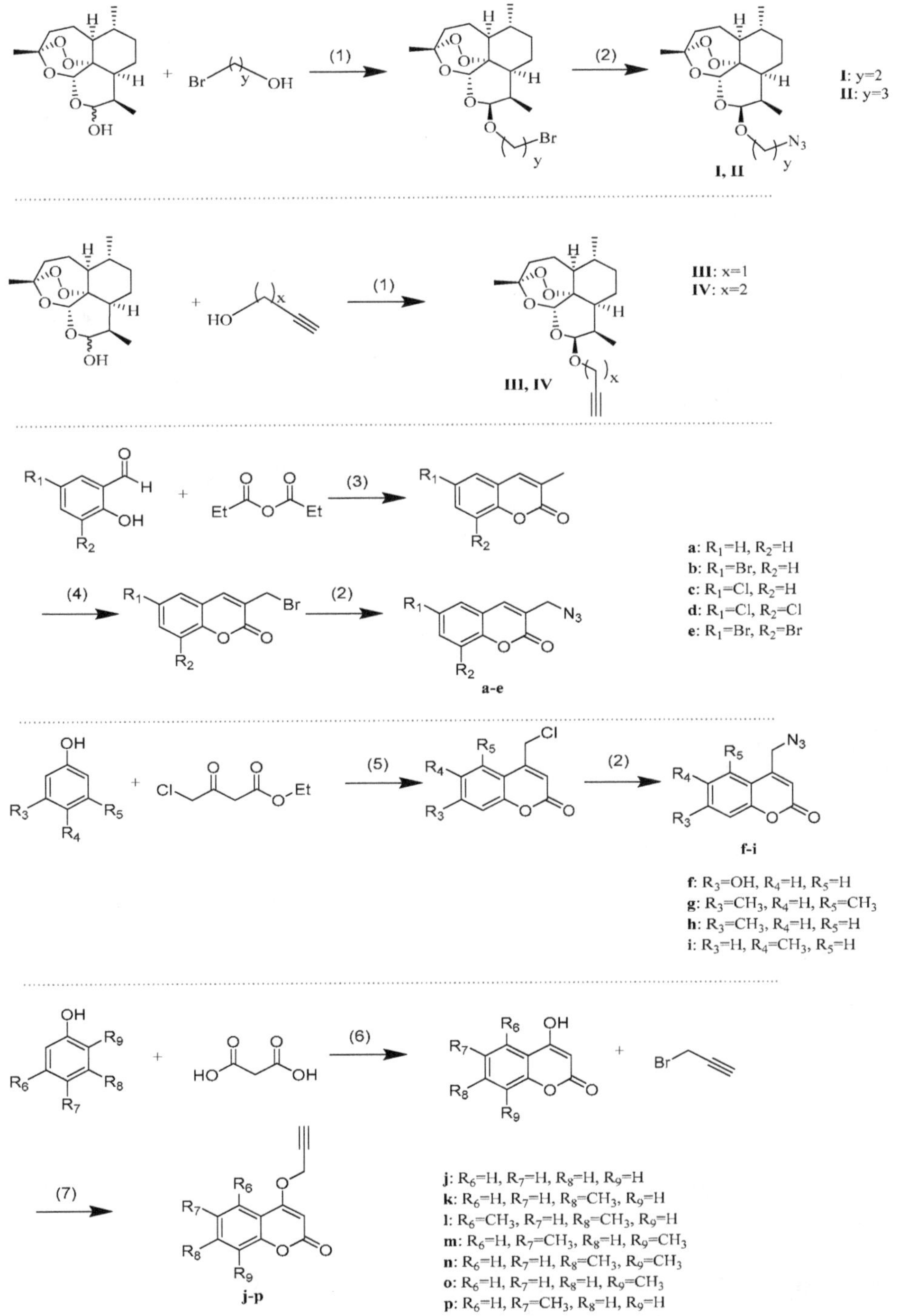

Scheme 1. Synthetic routes of intermediates. Reagents and conditions: (1) $BF_3{\cdot}Et_2O$, CH_2Cl_2, 0 °C; (2) NaN_3, DMF, 60 °C; (3) CH_3CH_2COONa, Et_3N, reflux; (4) NBS, BPO, CCl_4, reflux; (5) 70% H_2SO_4, r.t.; (6) $ZnCl_2$, $POCl_3$, 65 °C; and (7) K_2CO_3, DMF, 60 °C.

The synthesis of the desired new compounds was presented in Scheme 2. The target compounds **1a–1e** and **2a–2e** were obtained by the reaction of the intermediates **III** or **IV** with **a–e** via click chemistry, respectively. The target compounds **3f–3i** and **4f–4i** were synthesized by intermediates **III** or **IV** with **f–i** via click chemistry, respectively. The target compounds **5j**, **5l–5o**, and **6j–6p** were prepared by the reaction of the intermediates **I** or **II** with **j–p** via click chemistry, respectively.

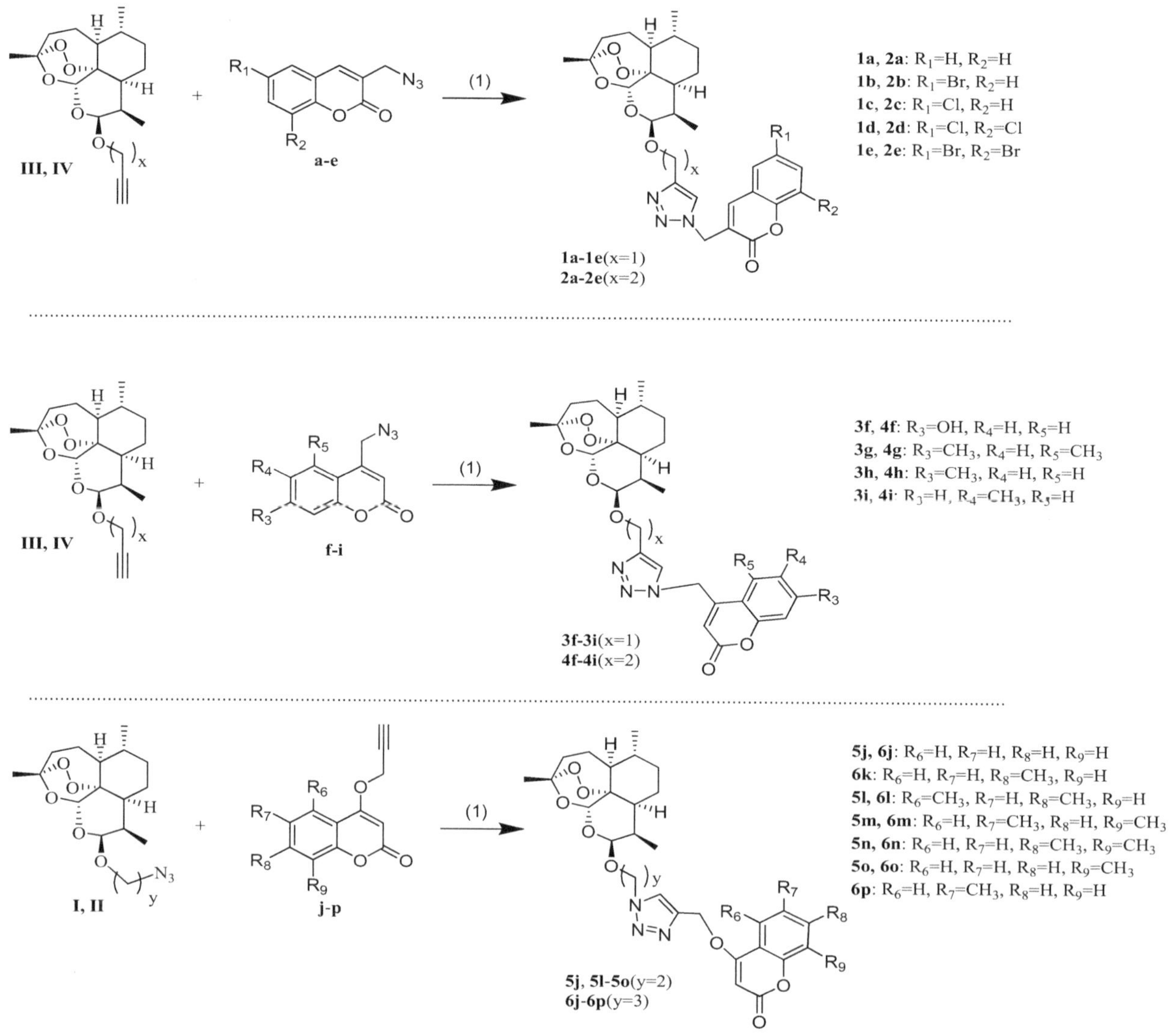

Scheme 2. Synthetic routes of target compounds. Reagents and conditions: (1) CuI, triethylamine, dichloromethane, r.t.

2.2. *Biological Assay*

2.2.1. In Vitro Cytotoxic Activity of the Compounds

As the anti-neuroinflammatory agents for cancer patients, all newly synthesized compounds were evaluated in vitro for antitumor activity against human breast cancer cell line MDA-MB-231, colorectal cancer cells HT-29 and HCT-116, and lung cancer cell line A549 by using the standard MTT method, respectively. Doxorubicin (DOX) and DHA were used as the reference standard. Additionally, owing to the rapid proliferation, the tumor cells actually was always in hypoxia condition. Therefore, the in vitro cytotoxicity was evaluated in two different conditions (hypoxia and normoxia). All data are summarized in Table 1. Most of the target compounds exhibited moderate activities against the tested cell lines and they showed a general promotion under hypoxia conditions.

The structure–activity relationship was evaluated: (i) the series of compounds **5** and **6** generally exhibited better cytotoxicity activity than that of the series of compounds **3** and **4**, which indicated that the 4-oxygen group in the coumarin moiety as a part of linker could improve the antitumor activity; (ii) although compounds **3** and **4** did not exhibit good activity against three cell lines (MDA-MB-231, HCT-116, and A549), they showed good activity against HT-29 like the other derivatives. Therefore, 4-methyl group in the coumarin moiety could improve the selectivity of DCH against HT-29.

In addition, almost all of the target compounds exhibited good cytotoxicity activity against HT-29. Therefore, HT-29 was selected for the next explorations.

Table 1. IC_{50} (μM) of tested samples in MDA-MB-231, HT-29, HCT-116, and A549 cell lines.

	HT-29		**MDA-MB-231**		**HCT-116**		**A549**	
	Hypoxia	**Normoxia**	**Hypoxia**	**Normoxia**	**Hypoxia**	**Normoxia**	**Hypoxia**	**Normoxia**
DOX	<0.1	0.11	0.69	1.37	>2	1.29	>2	>2
DHA	11.74	51.10	45.93	>100	25.89	10.33	>100	>100
1a	14.29	18.40	30.47	64.97	49.79	48.90	53.87	83.48
1b	13.14	21.35	>100	>100	>100	>100	>100	>100
1c	26.37	35.41	32.26	>100	40.38	60.30	48.70	73.49
1d	13.34	14.94	33.93	68.85	48.61	60.01	45.42	53.34
1e	26.95	15.32	45.46	77.89	>100	54.45	59.75	>100
2a	19.42	>100	>100	>100	>100	>100	>100	>100
2b	12.09	9.75	36.86	37.74	>100	55.99	60.16	>100
2c	19.61	17.46	32.47	43.98	64.37	49.48	66.87	87.15
2d	30.81	19.54	47.92	88.46	46.51	53.19	69.67	96.48
2e	13.92	38.52	44.14	>100	86.49	94.16	79.37	>100
3f	15.46	37.83	63.07	>100	67.74	>100	98.00	>100
3g	15.86	23.89	>100	>100	>100	>100	>100	>100
3h	32.04	>100	>100	>100	>100	>100	>100	>100
3i	8.57	16.36	22.81	>100	>100	64.99	62.27	>100
4f	11.30	32.30	78.79	>100	>100	>100	>100	>100
4g	9.33	13.85	22.71	>100	25.65	34.50	>100	>100
4h	56.35	>100	>100	>100	>100	>100	>100	>100
4i	39.02	>100	>100	>100	>100	>100	>100	>100
5j	12.25	30.03	69.41	100.00	>100	77.20	>100	>100
5l	3.76	2.78	>100	>100	>100	>100	>100	>100
5m	5.89	12.88	13.04	14.17	44.81	62.82	1.282	2.670
5n	8.90	10.19	11.68	11.04	32.92	25.64	2.443	2.107
5o	21.25	16.09	16.54	37.41	38.49	29.69	45.06	50.37
6j	7.42	10.49	33.40	67.42	32.84	25.90	49.03	53.37
6k	5.32	6.85	14.46	38.56	33.70	28.13	9.49	14.92
6l	3.40	8.41	6.85	1.17	27.92	26.90	9.78	6.88
6m	5.90	22.43	18.74	24.64	93.53	42.05	20.14	27.87
6n	4.19	9.16	10.84	13.35	33.74	22.51	0.039	30.40
6o	29.02	81.57	18.57	47.65	42.35	12.09	39.92	78.07
6p	12.48	7.49	10.33	22.08	38.05	35.33	18.82	18.85

2.2.2. Morphological Changes and Effect of Compound 5n on Cell Viability

As shown in A–F of Figure 2, there showed a concentration-dependent cell death after treatment with compound **5n** for 48 h. As the concentration up to 100 μM, the compound **5n** could obviously inhibit the proliferation of HT-29. As shown in the (G) of Figure 2, after HT-29 cells were treated with different concentrations of **5n** for 48 h, the cell viability decreased in a dose-dependent manner.

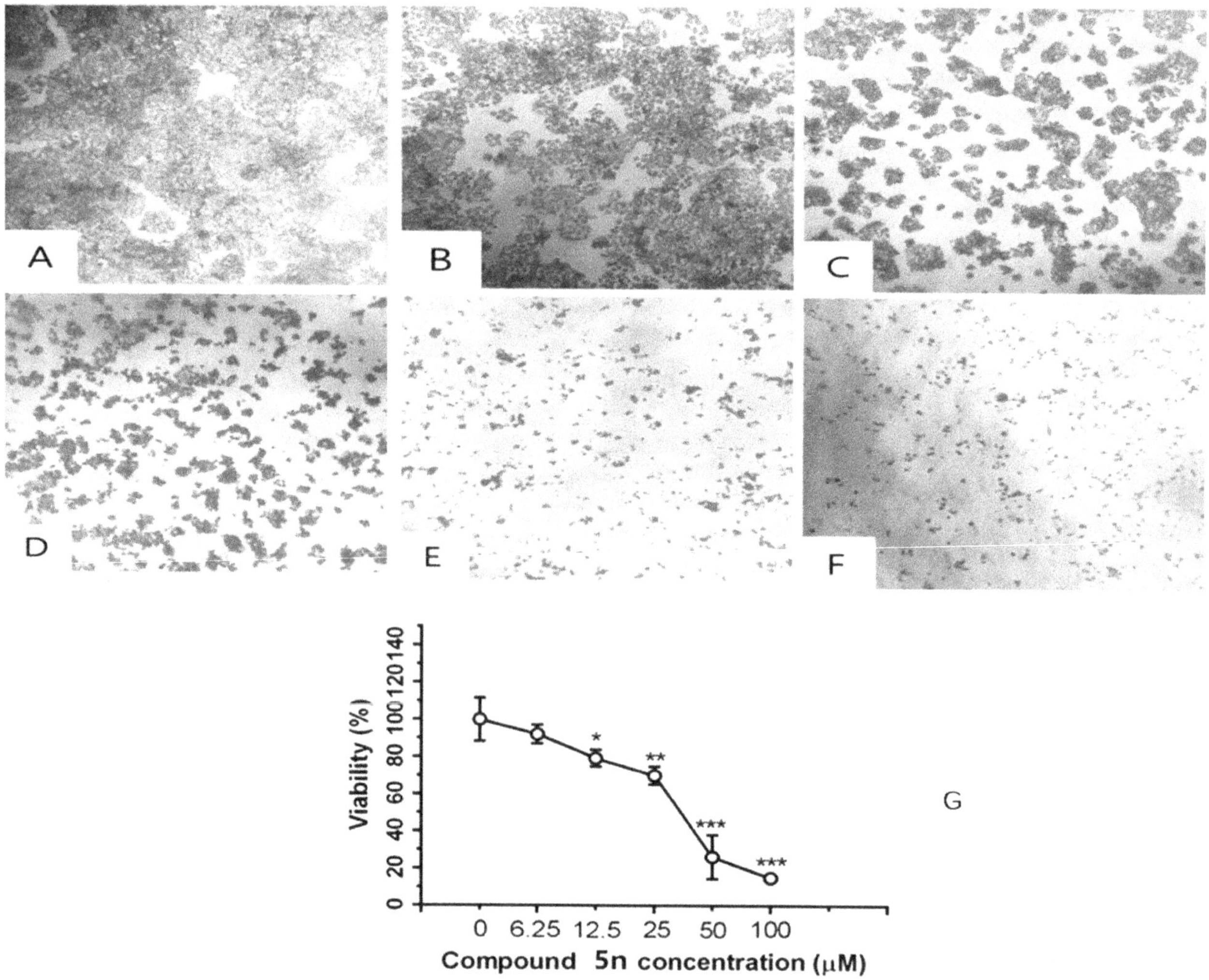

Figure 2. Inhibition of compound **5n** on cell viability in HT-29 cells by MTT staining. Cells were treated with (**A**) 0 μM, (**B**) 6.25 μM, (**C**) 12.5 μM, (**D**) 25.0 μM, (**E**) 50.0 μM, and (**F**) 100.0 μM compound **5n** for 48 h. Representative images were shown; 200×. (**G**) Cells were treated with 6.25, 12.5, 25, 50, and 100 μM compound **5n** for 48 h. Data were shown as mean ± SD. * $p < 0.05$, ** $p < 0.01$ and *** $p < 0.001$ compared with group 0 μM.

2.2.3. Anti-Neuroinflammatory Activity

The anti-neuroinflammatory activity of DCH was evaluated and then the representative compounds were selected for the further study. As shown in Table 2, murine microglial N9 cells were treated with 1 μg/mL LPS for 48 h and the NO level in the medium was measured as the preliminary screening. Most of the tested compounds exhibited good anti-inflammatory activity, and especially the IC_{50} of some compounds were even less than 1 μM. Among them, compound **5n** had the best activity and the IC_{50} reached 0.22 μM. In addition, in order to exclude the death influence, MTT-IC20 of all the compounds were measured. The results showed that DCH did not exhibit cytotoxic activity in N9 cells. The exact reason was still unclear, but we supposed that it might be related to the homeostasis of cells. The tumor cells actually were always in hypoxia condition, in which DCH could promote the cytotoxic activity against tumor cells. In brief, DCH could reduce the release of NO caused by LPS-induced microglial cells.

Table 2. IC_{50} of tested samples in LPS-induced N9 cells for the inhibition of NO; IC_{20} of tested samples in N9 cells for cytotoxic activity.

Compound.	NO-IC_{50} (μM)	MTT-IC_{20} (μM)
1a	1.46	>10
1b	>10	>10
1c	5.33	>10
1d	1.60	>10
1e	0.48	>10
2a	0.97	>10
2b	0.64	>10
2c	2.66	>10
2d	1.35	>10
2e	0.94	>10
3f	0.37	>10
3g	>10	>10
3h	>10	>10
3i	0.72	>10
4f	2.03	>10
4g	1.36	>10
4h	5.69	>10
4i	>10	>10
5j	1.59	>10
5l	3.36	7.13
5m	1.08	1.04
5n	0.22	2.44
5o	0.57	>10
6j	0.29	>10
6k	1.91	>10
6l	0.52	>10
6m	5.80	>10
6n	1.13	6.53
6o	1.43	>10
6p	1.42	>10
DHA	1.58	>10
Minocycline	>10	>10

NO Capture Capability

Sodium nitroprusside (SNP) is a NO donor. In this experiment, the reason of the DCH reducing NO level was preliminary explored. As shown in Figure 3, the results showed that the compounds only partially reduced NO levels by direct NO capture. That means the main reason of the NO level reduction is due to species-specific effect.

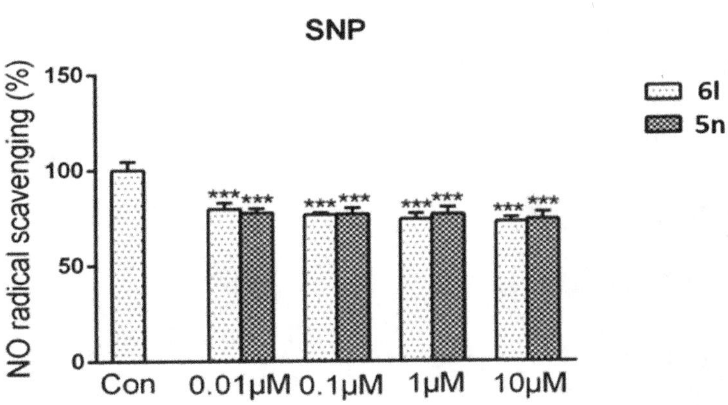

Figure 3. Compound 6l and 5n had NO radical scavenging activity. 6l (0.01 μM, 0.1 μM, 1 μM, and 10 μM) or **5n** (0.01 μM, 0.1 μM, 1 μM, and 10 μM) was added to a concentration of 0.5 mM SNP solution. After reacted for 1 h under normal sun light at room temperature, Griess reagent was added and the optical density was observed at 540 nm. Data were shown as mean ± SD. *** $p < 0.001$ compared with control group.

Effect of Representative Compounds on TNF-α and IL-6 Release

As shown in Table 3, four kinds of DCH were involved to measure the effect on the release of TNF-α and IL-6 from the microglia cells which induced by LPS for 48 h. The results showed that compounds **2b**, **2c**, **5n**, and **6p** could inhibit the release of TNF-α with the inhibition rate of 22% to 32% and the release of IL-6 with the inhibition rate of 26% to 43%. The results indicated that the inhibition effect of DCH on NO release was not only by nonspecific effects, but also by slightly influencing the synthesis and release of upstream inflammatory pathway.

Table 3. The inhibition of compounds (1 μM) on cytokines release (48 h) of the murine microglial cell line N9 induced by lipopolysaccharide (LPS) (1 μg/mL).

Group	TNF-α (pg/mL)	Inhibition (%)	IL-6 (pg/mL)	Inhibition (%)
Con	155.54 ± 79.61	–	0	–
LPS	4455.87 ± 518.24 #	–	1154.44 ± 148.48 #	–
2b	3285.99 ± 1062.40	27.20	797.52 ± 140.74 *	30.92
2c	3077.03 ± 375.48	32.06	850.24 ± 112.47	26.35
5n	3508.08 ± 368.72	22.04	656.75 ± 79.49 **	43.11
6p	3451.29 ± 646.50	23.36	747.80 ± 125.56 *	35.22

# $p < 0.001$ compared with control group, * $p < 0.05$ ** $p < 0.01$ compared with LPS group.

Docking Analysis

Toll-like receptor 4 (TLR4) and its coreceptor—MD-2—are the target of LPS, which could influence innate immune response to release potentially cytotoxic molecules. MD-2 is linked with the extracellular domain of TLR4 and is indispensable for LPS recognition [13]. Therefore, this docking analysis was applied to explore whether or not the target compounds inhibit MD-2 to reduce the release of inflammatory mediators. Umeharu Ohto et al. [39] had revealed the crystal structure of mouse TLR4/MD-2/LPS complex, which was shown in Figure 4. In their study, MD-2 directly bound to LPS in its hydrophobic cavity with high affinity. With this background, compound **5n** was used as the ligand to explore the relationship between DCH and TLR4/MD-2/LPS complex. As shown in Figure 5, compound **5n** could integrate closely with the hydrophobic cavity of MD-2, which is the important TLR4/MD-2/LPS binding position. That means the DCH might disturb the interactions between LPS and TLR4/MD-2 complex. The minimum binding energy of (ΔG) is −10.08 kcal/mol. Given to this result, we supposed TLR4/MD-2 complex is likely to be one of the drug targets of DCH.

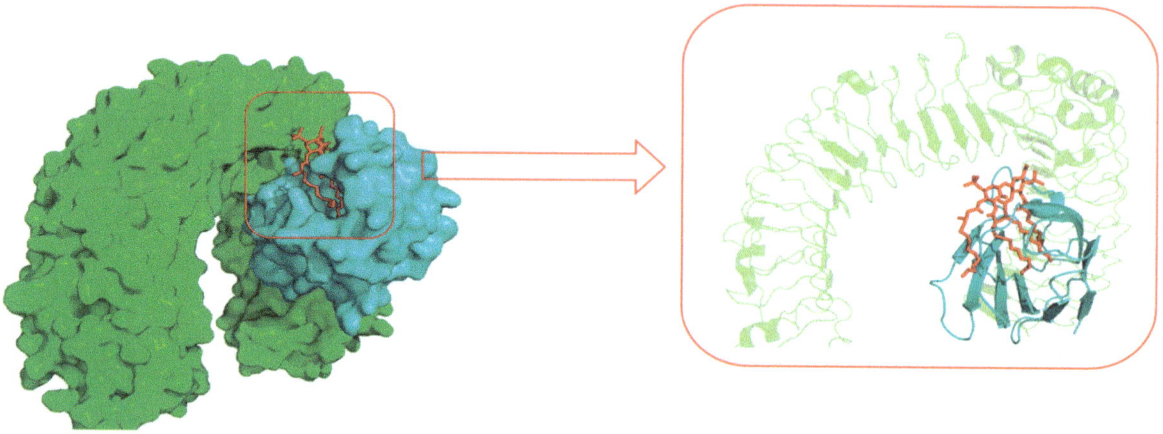

Figure 4. The surface representation of LPS (red) and Toll-like receptor 4 (TLR4) (green)/MD-2 (cyan) binding pocket (PDB: 3VQ2).

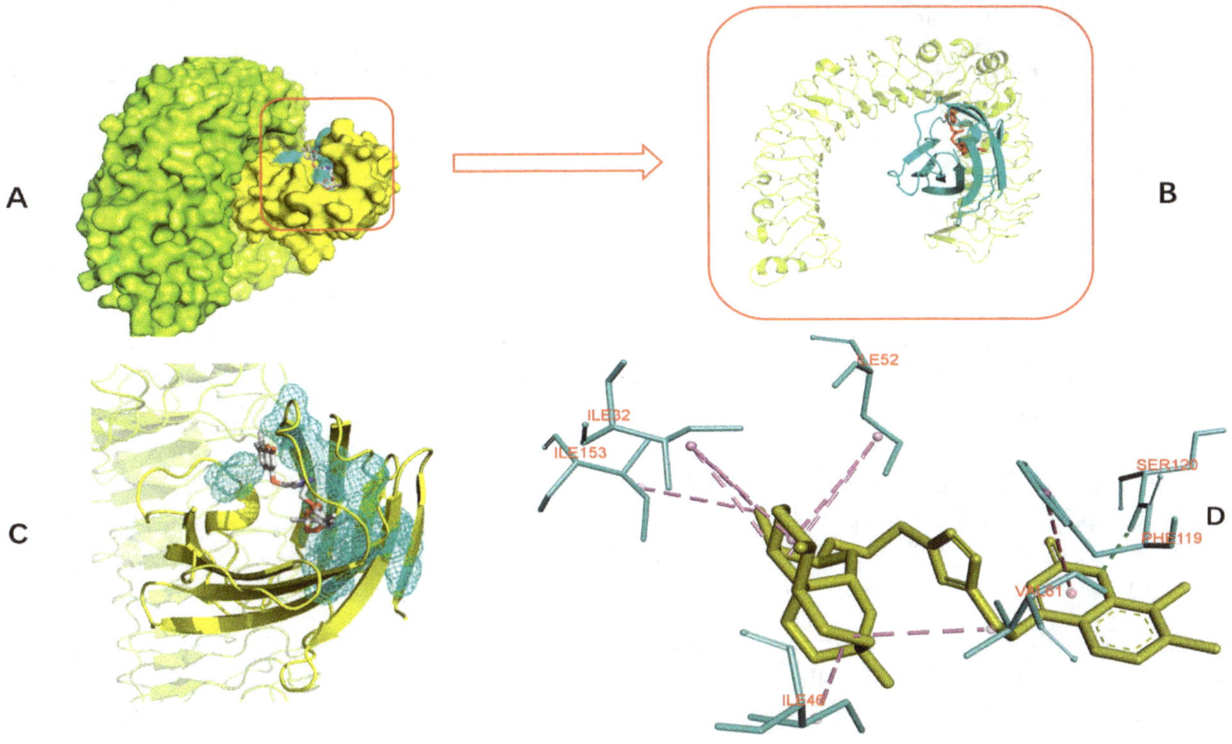

Figure 5. Interaction diagrams of the selected docked conformations of compound 5n to TLR4/MD-2 complex. (**A**) The surface representation of compound **5n** and TLR4 (limon)/MD-2 (yellow) binding pocket. (**B**) The magnified representation of compound **5n** (red) and TLR4 (limon)/MD-2 (cyan) binding pocket. (**C**) The interface of compound **5n** and TLR4/MD-2 complex; (**D**) 3D ligand interactions diagram. Dotted line; pink: alkyl hydrophobic; blue: pi hydrophobic; green: hydrogen bond.

3. Conclusions

Total-thirty new DCH were designed and synthesized. Most of the target compounds exhibited moderate activities against the tested cell lines and they showed a general promotion under hypoxia conditions. Meanwhile, the new potential activity of DCH was found that DCH could exhibit anti-neuroinflammatory activity. DCH could inhibit the release of NO, TNF-α, and IL-6, which were induced by LPS. The docking analysis was shown that MD-2, the coreceptor of TLR4, might be one of the targets of DCH. Additionally, DCH could also reduce NO levels by direct NO capture. In brief, DCH were the potential anti-neuroinflammatory agents which might reduce CRF of cancer patients.

4. Experimental Section

4.1. Chemistry

Unless otherwise specified, all solvents and reagents were commercially available and used without further purification. Analytical TLC was performed using silica gel precoated GF254 plates. The ^{1}H-NMR and ^{13}C-NMR spectra were recorded at 600 MHz and 150 MHZ on a Bruker AV-400 spectrometer (Bruker Bioscience, Billerica, MA, USA), using $CDCl_3$ as solvent with tetramethylsilane as the internal standard. NMR spectra were analyzed using MestReNova. High-resolution mass spectra (HRMS) were measured using an Agilent Accurate-Mass Q-TOF 6530 (Agilent, Santa Clara, CA, USA) instrument in ESI mode. The ^{1}H-NMR and ^{13}C-NMR spectra of synthesized compounds, please see the supplementary materials.

4.1.1. General Procedure for the Synthesis of Compounds **1a–1e** and **2a–2e**

Substituted coumarin (**a–e**) (10 mmol), substituted DHA (**III** or **IV**) (10 mmol), and triethylamine (10 mmol) were dissolved in 20 mL CH_2Cl_2. In addition, CuI (100 mg) was added and the reaction mixture was stirred at room temperature for 8 h under the protection of nitrogen. The mixture was filtered, washed with water, dried over Na_2SO_4 and evaporated to dryness. The crude product was purified through column chromatography.

3-((4-((10S)-dihydroartemisininoxy)methyl-1H-1,2,3-triazol-1-yl)-methyl)-2H-1-chromen-2-one (**1a**) White solid; m.p. 73–75 °C; yield 52%; ^{1}H NMR (600 MHz, $CDCl_3$) δ (ppm): 7.77 (s, 1H), 7.68 (s, 1H), 7.56 (t, *J* = 7.9 Hz, 1H), 7.47 (d, *J* = 7.7 Hz, 1H), 7.34 (d, *J* = 8.4 Hz, 1H), 7.30 (t, *J* = 7.6 Hz, 1H), 5.47 (s, 2H), 5.39 (s, 1H), 4.94 (d, *J* = 12.6 Hz, 1H), 4.92 (d, *J* = 3.5 Hz, 1H), 4.68 (d, *J* = 12.6 Hz, 1H), 2.67–2.60 (m, 1H), 2.38–2.31 (m, 1H), 2.01–1.97 (m, 1H), 1.85–1.81 (m, 1H), 1.77–1.68 (m, 3H), 1.59 (dd, *J* = 13.2, 3.4 Hz, 1H), 1.46–1.43 (m, 1H), 1.41 (s, 3H), 1.31–1.18 (m, 1H), 1.26–1.16 (m, 2H), 0.91 (d, *J* = 6.3 Hz, 3H), 0.88 (d, *J* = 7.3 Hz, 3H); ^{13}C NMR (150 MHz, $CDCl_3$) δ (ppm): 159.64, 152.65, 144.62, 141.31, 131.46, 127.30, 123.92, 122.67, 121.84, 117.53, 115.71, 103.10, 100.77, 86.93, 80.06, 76.22, 76.01, 75.80, 60.70, 51.47, 47.97, 43.33, 36.33, 35.36, 33.52, 29.78, 25.09, 23.59, 23.41, 19.30, 11.99; ESI-HRMS $[M + Na]^+$: (*m/z*) Calcd. for $C_{28}H_{33}N_3O_7Na$: 546.2216. Found: 546.2181.

6-bromo-3-((4-((10S)-dihydroartemisininoxy)methyl-1H-1,2,3-triazol-1-yl)-methyl)-2H-1-chromen-2-one (**1b**) White solid; m.p. 78–80 °C; yield 48%; ^{1}H NMR (600 MHz, $CDCl_3$) δ (ppm): 7.75 (s, 1H), 7.64 (dd, *J* = 8.8, 2.3 Hz, 1H), 7.61 (d, *J* = 2.3 Hz, 1H), 7.55 (s, 1H), 7.24 (d, *J* = 8.8 Hz, 1H), 5.47 (s, 2H), 5.39 (s, 1H), 4.94 (d, *J* = 12.7 Hz, 1H), 4.93 (d, *J* = 3.5 Hz, 1H), 4.69 (d, *J* = 12.8 Hz, 1H), 2.67–2.63 (m, 1H), 2.38–2.33 (m, 1H), 2.03–1.99 (m, 1H), 1.86–1.82 (m, 1H), 1.75–1.70 (m, 2H), 1.62–1.58 (m, 2H), 1.42 (s, 3H), 1.31–1.19 (m, 4H), 0.92 (d, *J* = 6.3 Hz, 3H), 0.89 (d, *J* = 7.4 Hz, 3H); ^{13}C NMR (150 MHz, $CDCl_3$) δ (ppm): 158.90, 151.42, 144.74, 139.67, 134.18, 129.51, 123.17, 122.67, 119.00, 117.43, 116.53, 103.12, 100.87, 86.95, 80.06, 76.20, 75.99, 75.78, 60.76, 51.46, 47.82, 43.32, 36.36, 35.36, 33.52, 29.79, 25.10, 23.62, 23.42, 19.30, 12.00; ESI-HRMS $[M + Na]^+$: (*m/z*) Calcd. for $C_{28}H_{32}BrN_3O_7Na$: 624.1321. Found: 624.1264.

6-chloro-3-((4-((10S)-dihydroartemisininoxy)methyl-1H-1,2,3-triazol-1-yl)-methyl)-2H-1-chromen-2-one (**1c**) White solid; m.p. 93–95 °C; yield 41%; ^{1}H NMR (600 MHz, $CDCl_3$) δ (ppm): 7.75 (s, 1H), 7.56 (s, 1H), 7.51 (dd, *J* = 8.8, 2.5 Hz, 1H), 7.45 (d, *J* = 2.4 Hz, 1H), 7.30 (d, *J* = 8.9 Hz, 1H), 5.47 (s, 2H), 5.39 (s, 1H), 4.95 (d, *J* = 12.7 Hz, 1H), 4.93 (d, *J* = 3.6 Hz, 1H), 4.69 (d, *J* = 12.6 Hz, 1H), 2.68–2.62 (m, 1H), 2.35 (td, *J* = 14.0, 4.0 Hz, 1H), 2.03–1.99 (m, 1H), 1.87–1.82 (m, 1H), 1.75–1.71 (m, 2H), 1.62–1.59 (m, 1H), 1.48–1.43 (m, 2H), 1.42 (s, 3H), 1.31–1.19 (m, 3H), 0.92 (d, *J* = 6.3 Hz, 3H), 0.89 (d, *J* = 7.4 Hz, 3H); ^{13}C NMR (150 MHz, $CDCl_3$) δ (ppm): 158.96, 150.95, 144.73, 139.79, 131.37, 129.27, 126.46, 123.19, 122.67, 118.51, 117.16, 103.12, 100.86, 86.95, 80.06, 76.21, 75.99, 75.78, 60.75, 51.47, 47.84, 43.33, 36.36, 35.36, 33.52, 29.79, 25.10, 23.62, 23.42, 19.30, 12.00; ESI-HRMS $[M + Na]^+$: (*m/z*) Calcd. for $C_{28}H_{32}ClN_3O_7Na$: 580.1826. Found: 580.1788.

6,8-dichloro-3-((4-((10S)-dihydroartemisininoxy)methyl-1H-1,2,3-triazol-1-yl)-methyl)-2H-1-chromen-2-one (**1d**) White solid; m.p. 113–115 °C; yield 60%; ^{1}H NMR (600 MHz, $CDCl_3$) δ (ppm): 7.75 (s, 1H), 7.61 (d, *J* = 2.3 Hz, 1H), 7.55 (s, 1H), 7.37 (d, *J* = 2.4 Hz, 1H), 5.48 (s, 2H), 5.37 (s, 1H), 4.96–4.92 (m, 2H), 4.70 (d, *J* = 12.7 Hz, 1H), 2.69–2.62 (m, 1H), 2.38–2.33 (m, 1H), 2.04–1.99 (m, 1H), 1.87–1.82 (m, 1H), 1.76–1.72 (m, 3H), 1.62–1.59 (m, 1H), 1.42 (s, 3H), 1.32–1.18 (m, 4H), 0.92 (d, *J* = 6.3 Hz, 3H), 0.89 (d, *J* = 7.3 Hz, 3H); ^{13}C NMR (150 MHz, $CDCl_3$) δ (ppm): 157.92, 146.92, 144.86, 139.45, 131.36, 129.12, 125.03, 124.04, 122.68, 121.71, 119.30, 103.13, 100.95, 86.94, 80.04, 76.20, 75.99, 75.78, 60.80, 51.44, 47.63, 43.31, 36.37, 35.35, 33.51, 29.79, 25.09, 23.61, 23.42, 19.28, 12.00; ESI-HRMS $[M + Na]^+$: (*m/z*) Calcd. for $C_{28}H_{31}Cl_2N_3O_7Na$: 614.1437. Found: 614.1428.

6,8-dibromo-3-((4-((10S)-dihydroartemisininoxy)methyl-1H-1,2,3-triazol-1-yl)-methyl)-2H-1-chromen-2-one (**1e**) White solid; m.p. 103–105 °C; yield 61%; ^{1}H NMR (600 MHz, $CDCl_3$) δ (ppm): 7.90 (d, *J* = 2.2 Hz, 1H), 7.75 (s, 1H), 7.56 (d, *J* = 2.2 Hz, 1H), 7.52 (s, 1H), 5.48 (s, 2H), 5.37 (s, 1H), 4.96–4.92 (m, 2H), 4.70 (d, *J* = 12.7 Hz, 1H), 2.67–2.63 (m, 1H), 2.38–2.33 (m, 1H), 2.03–1.99 (m, 1H), 1.87–1.82 (m, 1H),

1.76–1.72 (m, 2H), 1.62–1.58 (m, 4H), 1.42 (s, 3H), 1.25–1.19 (m, 2H), 0.92 (d, J = 6.3 Hz, 3H), 0.90 (d, J = 7.4 Hz, 3H); ^{13}C NMR (150 MHz, $CDCl_3$) δ (ppm): 158.01, 148.45, 144.87, 139.36, 136.89, 128.75, 123.97, 122.67, 119.74, 116.48, 110.29, 103.13, 100.97, 86.95, 80.04, 76.20, 75.99, 75.78, 60.82, 51.45, 47.56, 43.31, 36.37, 35.35, 33.51, 29.79, 25.09, 23.62, 23.42, 19.30, 12.00; ESI-HRMS $[M + Na]^+$: (m/z) Calcd. for $C_{28}H_{31}Br_2N_3O_7Na$: 702.0426. Found: 702.0421.

3-((4-(2-((10S)-dihydroartemisininoxy)ethyl)-1H-1,2,3-triazol-1-yl)-methyl)-2H-1-chromen-2-one (**2a**) White solid; m.p. 143–145 °C; yield 66%; ^{1}H NMR (600 MHz, $CDCl_3$) δ (ppm): 7.65 (s, 1H), 7.63 (s, 1H), 7.56 (ddd, J = 8.7, 7.3, 1.6 Hz, 1H), 7.47 (dd, J = 7.8, 1.6 Hz, 1H), 7.35 (d, J = 8.4 Hz, 1H), 7.30 (td, J = 7.5, 1.1 Hz, 1H), 5.44 (s, 2H), 5.29 (d, J = 9.7 Hz, 1H), 4.78 (d, J = 3.6 Hz, 1H), 4.13–4.09 (m, 1H), 3.69–3.65 (m, 1H), 3.07–2.97 (m, 2H), 2.61–2.55 (m, 1H), 2.33 (td, J = 14.0, 4.0 Hz, 1H), 2.01–1.97 (m, 1H), 1.85–1.81 (m, 1H), 1.71–1.67 (m, 2H), 1.59–1.56 (m, 1H), 1.41 (s, 3H), 1.40–1.38 (m, 1H), 1.28–1.16 (m, 3H), 0.91 (d, J = 6.3 Hz, 3H), 0.89–0.83 (m, 1H), 0.80 (d, J = 7.3 Hz, 3H); ^{13}C NMR (150 MHz, $CDCl_3$) δ (ppm): 159.65, 152.64, 144.77, 141.15, 131.43, 127.30, 123.90, 121.98, 121.78, 117.52, 115.70, 103.03, 100.92, 86.84, 80.02, 76.21, 76.00, 75.78, 66.18, 51.47, 47.86, 43.28, 36.34, 35.36, 33.55, 29.79, 25.57, 25.14, 23.62, 23.34, 19.33, 11.93; ESI-HRMS $[M + Na]^+$: (m/z) Calcd. for $C_{29}H_{35}N_3O_7Na$: 560.2373. Found: 560.2417.

6-bromo-3-((4-(2-((10S)-dihydroartemisininoxy)ethyl)-1H-1,2,3-triazol-1-yl)-methyl)-2H-1-chromen-2-one (**2b**) White solid; m.p. 138–140 °C; yield 52%; ^{1}H NMR (600 MHz, $CDCl_3$) δ (ppm): 7.64 (dd, J = 8.8, 2.3 Hz, 1H), 7.61 (d, J = 2.3 Hz, 1H), 7.60 (s, 1H), 7.52 (s, 1H), 7.23 (d, J = 8.8 Hz, 1H), 5.43 (s, 2H), 5.28 (s, 1H), 4.79 (d, J = 3.5 Hz, 1H), 4.13–4.09 (m, 1H), 3.70–3.66 (m, 1H), 3.07–2.98 (m, 2H), 2.62–2.57 (m, 1H), 2.34 (td, J = 14.0, 4.0 Hz, 1H), 2.01–1.98 (m, 1H), 1.86–1.81 (m, 1H), 1.71–1.67 (m, 2H), 1.60–1.56 (m, 1H), 1.42 (s, 3H), 1.40–1.37 (m, 1H), 1.27–1.17 (m, 3H), 0.92 (d, J = 6.2 Hz, 3H), 0.89–0.85 (m, 1H), 0.82 (d, J = 7.3 Hz, 3H); ^{13}C NMR (150 MHz, $CDCl_3$) δ (ppm): 158.90, 151.40, 144.86, 139.50, 134.15, 129.51, 123.31, 121.76, 118.99, 117.41, 116.51, 103.06, 100.92, 86.85, 80.00, 76.20, 75.99, 75.78, 66.18, 51.45, 47.72, 43.26, 36.37, 35.35, 33.55, 29.78, 25.56, 25.14, 23.63, 23.35, 19.32, 11.95; ESI-HRMS $[M + Na]^+$: (m/z) Calcd. for $C_{29}H_{34}BrN_3O_7Na$: 638.1478. Found: 638.1508.

6-chloro-3-((4-(2-((10S)-dihydroartemisininoxy)ethyl)-1H-1,2,3-triazol-1-yl)-methyl)-2H-1-chromen-2-one (**2c**) White solid; m.p. 138–140 °C; yield 52%; ^{1}H NMR (600 MHz, $CDCl_3$) δ (ppm): 7.60 (s, 1H), 7.53 (s, 1H), 7.50 (dd, J = 8.8, 2.5 Hz, 1H), 7.45 (d, J = 2.4 Hz, 1H), 7.29 (d, J = 8.8 Hz, 1H), 5.43 (d, J = 1.1 Hz, 2H), 5.28 (s, 1H), 4.79 (d, J = 3.6 Hz, 1H), 4.13–4.09 (m, 1H), 3.70–3.66 (m, 1H), 3.05–2.99 (m, 2H), 2.61–2.58 (m, 1H), 2.37–2.31 (m, 1H), 2.01–1.98 (m, 1H), 1.86–1.81 (m, 1H), 1.70–1.68 (m, 2H), 1.60–1.56 (m, 1H), 1.42 (s, 3H), 1.41–1.36 (m, 1H), 1.26–1.17 (m, 3H), 0.92 (d, J = 6.2 Hz, 3H), 0.89–0.85 (m, 1H), 0.82 (d, J = 7.3 Hz, 3H); ^{13}C NMR (150 MHz, $CDCl_3$) δ (ppm): 158.97, 150.93, 144.87, 139.62, 131.34, 129.25, 126.47, 123.35, 121.76, 118.51, 117.14, 103.06, 100.93, 86.85, 80.00, 76.20, 75.99, 75.78, 66.19, 51.45, 47.72, 43.27, 36.37, 35.35, 33.56, 29.79, 25.57, 25.14, 23.63, 23.35, 19.32, 11.95; ESI-HRMS $[M + Na]^+$: (m/z) Calcd. for $C_{29}H_{34}ClN_3O_7Na$: 594.1983. Found: 594.2002.

6,8-dichloro-3-((4-(2-((10S)-dihydroartemisininoxy)ethyl)-1H-1,2,3-triazol-1-yl)-methyl)-2H-1-chromen-2-one (**2d**) White solid; m.p. 101–103 °C; yield 50%; ^{1}H NMR (600 MHz, $CDCl_3$) δ (ppm): 7.60 (d, J = 2.2 Hz, 2H), 7.52 (s, 1H), 7.37 (d, J = 2.3 Hz, 1H), 5.45 (s, 2H), 5.27 (s, 1H), 4.79 (d, J = 3.5 Hz, 1H), 4.13–4.08 (m, 1H), 3.71–3.67 (m, 1H), 3.04–3.01 (m, 2H), 2.61–2.59 (m, 1H), 2.34 (td, J = 14.0, 4.0 Hz, 1H), 2.02–1.98 (m, 1H), 1.85–1.82 (m, 1H), 1.71–1.68 (m, 2H), 1.60–1.58 (m, 1H), 1.42 (s, 3H), 1.41–1.36 (m, 1H), 1.26–1.17 (m, 3H), 0.92 (d, J = 6.1 Hz, 3H), 0.90–0.85 (m, 1H), 0.82 (d, J = 7.3 Hz, 3H); ^{13}C NMR (150 MHz, $CDCl_3$) δ (ppm): 157.93, 146.90, 144.92, 139.29, 131.34, 129.12, 125.04, 124.16, 121.82, 121.70, 119.30, 103.07, 100.94, 86.86, 79.99, 76.20, 75.99, 75.78, 66.17, 51.44, 47.57, 43.26, 36.39, 35.35, 33.55, 29.78, 25.53, 25.13, 23.63, 23.35, 19.32, 11.95; ESI-HRMS $[M + Na]^+$: (m/z) Calcd. for $C_{29}H_{33}Cl_2N_3O_7Na$: 628.1593. Found: 628.1360.

6,8-dibromo-3-((4-(2-((10S)-dihydroartemisininoxy)ethyl)-1H-1,2,3-triazol-1-yl)-methyl)-2H-1-chromen-2-one (**2e**) White solid; m.p. 93–95 °C; yield 44%; ^{1}H NMR (600 MHz, $CDCl_3$) δ (ppm): 7.83 (d, J = 2.1 Hz, 1H), 7.53 (s, 1H), 7.49 (d, J = 2.2 Hz, 1H), 7.42 (s, 1H), 5.38 (s, 2H), 5.21 (s, 1H), 4.73 (d, J = 3.4 Hz, 1H),

4.06–4.02 (m, 1H), 3.64–3.60 (m, 1H), 2.97–2.94 (m, 2H), 2.56–2.51 (m, 1H), 2.30–2.25 (m, 1H), 1.95–1.91 (m, 1H), 1.79–1.75 (m, 1H), 1.64–1.60 (m, 2H), 1.52 (dd, *J* = 13.2, 3.3 Hz, 1H), 1.35 (s, 3H), 1.34–1.29 (m, 1H), 1.19–1.11 (m, 3H), 0.85 (d, *J* = 6.1 Hz, 3H), 0.83–0.78 (m, 1H), 0.75 (d, *J* = 7.4 Hz, 3H); ^{13}C NMR (150 MHz, $CDCl_3$) δ (ppm): 158.01, 148.41, 144.96, 139.16, 136.85, 128.75, 124.12, 121.77, 119.74, 116.47, 110.26, 103.07, 100.93, 86.86, 80.00, 76.21, 76.00, 75.79, 66.19, 51.44, 47.48, 43.26, 36.39, 35.35, 33.55, 29.78, 25.56, 25.13, 23.63, 23.35, 19.33, 11.96; ESI-HRMS [M + Na]$^+$: (*m*/*z*) Calcd. for $C_{29}H_{33}Br_2N_3O_7Na$: 716.0583. Found: 716.0381.

4.1.2. General Procedure for the Synthesis of Compounds **3f–3i** and **4f–4i**

Substituted coumarin (**f–i**) (10 mmol), substituted DHA (**III** or **IV**) (10 mmol) and triethylamine (10 mmol) were dissolved in 20 mL CH_2Cl_2. In addition, CuI (100 mg) was added and the reaction mixture was stirred at room temperature for 8 h under the protection of nitrogen. The mixture was filtered, washed with water, dried over Na_2SO_4 and evaporated to dryness. The crude product was purified through column chromatography.

7-hydroxy-4-((4-((10S)-dihydroartemisininoxy)methyl-1H-1,2,3-triazol-1-yl)-methyl)-2H-1-chromen-2-one (**3f**) White solid; m.p. 165–167 °C; yield 54%; ^{1}H NMR (600 MHz, $CDCl_3$) δ (ppm): 9.61 (s, 1H), 7.68 (d, *J* = 8.8 Hz, 1H), 7.67 (s, 1H), 6.99 (dd, *J* = 8.8, 2.4 Hz, 1H), 6.85 (d, *J* = 2.4 Hz, 1H), 6.15 (s, 1H), 5.76 (d, *J* = 15.4 Hz, 1H), 5.57 (d, *J* = 15.3 Hz, 1H), 5.20 (s, 1H), 4.87 (d, *J* = 1.9 Hz, 1H), 4.86 (d, *J* = 7.4 Hz, 1H), 4.68 (d, *J* = 12.9 Hz, 1H), 2.62–2.60 (m, 1H), 2.34–2.29 (m, 1H), 2.02–1.98 (m, 1H), 1.82–1.78 (m, 1H), 1.66–1.61 (m, 3H), 1.61–1.57 (m, 1H), 1.45–1.42 (m, 1H), 1.40 (s, 3H), 1.20–1.08 (m, 3H), 0.84 (d, *J* = 7.4 Hz, 3H), 0.82 (d, *J* = 6.1 Hz, 3H); ^{13}C NMR (150 MHz, $CDCl_3$) δ (ppm): 160.88, 159.75, 154.96, 146.45, 145.19, 124.19, 122.29, 112.78, 111.57, 108.80, 103.21, 103.04, 101.40, 86.91, 79.92, 76.20, 75.99, 75.78, 60.44, 51.32, 50.16, 43.18, 36.28, 35.26, 33.42, 29.74, 25.00, 23.53, 23.32, 19.26, 11.89; ESI-HRMS [M + Na]$^+$: (*m*/*z*) Calcd. for $C_{28}H_{33}N_3O_8Na$: 562.2165. Found: 562.2172.

5,7-dimethyl-4-((4-((10S)-dihydroartemisininoxy)methyl-1H-1,2,3-triazol-1-yl)-methyl)-2H-1-chromen-2-one (**3g**) White solid; m.p. 133~135 °C; yield 57%; ^{1}H NMR (600 MHz, $CDCl_3$) δ (ppm): 7.56 (s, 1H), 7.07 (s, 1H), 6.95 (s, 1H), 5.90 (d, *J* = 17.0 Hz, 1H), 5.86 (d, *J* = 17.0 Hz, 1H), 5.51 (s, 1H), 5.41 (s, 1H), 4.98 (d, *J* = 12.8 Hz, 1H), 4.93 (d, *J* = 3.5 Hz, 1H), 4.73 (d, *J* = 12.8 Hz, 1H), 2.68 (s, 3H), 2.40 (s, 3H), 2.35 (dd, *J* = 14.0, 4.0 Hz, 1H), 2.05–2.01 (m, 1H), 1.88–1.85 (m, 1H), 1.75–1.70 (m, 2H), 1.60 (dd, *J* = 13.2, 3.4 Hz, 1H), 1.48–1.46 (m, 1H), 1.43 (s, 3H), 1.32–1.20 (m, 5H), 0.93 (d, *J* = 6.3 Hz, 3H), 0.89 (d, *J* = 7.4 Hz, 3H); ^{13}C NMR (150 MHz, $CDCl_3$) δ (ppm): 158.67, 154.26, 149.33, 145.35, 142.10, 133.93, 129.26, 122.10, 115.63, 113.36, 112.80, 103.16, 100.93, 86.98, 80.05, 76.21, 76.00, 75.79, 60.80, 52.05, 51.48, 43.31, 36.34, 35.36, 33.50, 29.78, 25.11, 23.61, 23.44, 23.28, 20.24, 19.31, 12.01; ESI-HRMS [M + Na]$^+$: (*m*/*z*) Calcd. for $C_{30}H_{37}N_3O_7Na$: 574.2539. Found: 574.2553.

7-methyl-4-((4-((10S)-dihydroartemisininoxy)methyl-1H-1,2,3-triazol-1-yl)-methyl)-2H-1-chromen-2-one (**3h**) White solid; m.p. 107–109 °C; yield 50%; ^{1}H NMR (600 MHz, $CDCl_3$) δ (ppm): 7.58 (s, 1H), 7.50 (d, *J* = 8.1 Hz, 1H), 7.19 (s, 1H), 7.11 (d, *J* = 8.1 Hz, 1H), 6.01 (s, 1H), 5.74 (d, *J* = 16.3 Hz, 1H), 5.64 (d, *J* = 16.0 Hz, 1H), 5.30 (s, 1H), 4.92–4.88 (m, 2H), 4.72 (d, *J* = 12.9 Hz, 1H), 2.65–2.61 (m, 1H), 2.45 (s, 3H), 2.34 (td, *J* = 14.0, 4.0 Hz, 1H), 2.04–2.00 (m, 1H), 1.86–1.81 (m, 1H), 1.71–1.66 (m, 2H), 1.58–1.55 (m, 1H), 1.42 (s, 3H), 1.26–1.18 (m, 5H), 0.91 (d, *J* = 5.7 Hz, 3H), 0.86 (d, *J* = 7.3 Hz, 3H); ^{13}C NMR (150 MHz, $CDCl_3$) δ (ppm): 159.01, 152.86, 146.75, 145.42, 143.16, 125.03, 122.23, 121.95, 116.71, 113.56, 113.41, 103.15, 101.10, 86.93, 80.00, 76.21, 75.99, 75.78, 60.90, 51.41, 49.29, 43.27, 36.34, 35.31, 33.47, 29.77, 25.06, 23.58, 23.38, 20.70, 19.30, 11.96; ESI-HRMS [M + Na]$^+$: (*m*/*z*) Calcd. for $C_{29}H_{35}N_3O_7Na$: 560.2373. Found: 560.2375.

6-methyl-4-((4-((10S)-dihydroartemisininoxy)methyl-1H-1,2,3-triazol-1-yl)-methyl)-2H-1-chromen-2-one (**3i**) White solid; m.p. 88–90°C; yield 60%; ^{1}H NMR (600 MHz, $CDCl_3$) δ (ppm): 7.58 (s, 1H), 7.39 (d, *J* = 8.8 Hz, 2H), 7.28 (d, *J* = 8.3 Hz, 1H), 6.01 (s, 1H), 5.75 (d, *J* = 16.3 Hz, 1H), 5.66 (d, *J* = 16.3 Hz, 1H), 5.32 (s, 1H), 4.92 (d, *J* = 12.8 Hz, 1H), 4.90 (d, *J* = 3.5 Hz, 1H), 4.73 (d, *J* = 12.8 Hz, 1H), 2.67–2.60 (m,

1H), 2.41 (s, 3H), 2.34 (td, J = 14.0, 4.0 Hz, 1H), 2.04–1.99 (m, 1H), 1.86–1.81 (m, 1H), 1.72–1.68 (m, 2H), 1.57 (dd, J = 13.2, 3.1 Hz, 1H), 1.42 (s, 3H), 1.26–1.19 (m, 5H), 0.91 (d, J = 5.7 Hz, 3H), 0.86 (d, J = 7.3 Hz, 3H); ^{13}C NMR (150 MHz, $CDCl_3$) δ (ppm): 158.91, 150.87, 146.72, 145.41, 133.69, 132.71, 122.26, 121.95, 116.32, 115.68, 114.29, 103.15, 101.05, 86.94, 80.00, 76.21, 76.00, 75.78, 60.86, 51.42, 49.17, 43.27, 36.34, 35.31, 33.47, 29.76, 25.07, 23.59, 23.39, 20.01, 19.30, 11.96; ESI-HRMS [M + Na]$^+$: (m/z) Calcd. for $C_{29}H_{35}N_3O_7Na$: 560.2373. Found: 560.2403.

7-hydroxy-4-((4-(2-((10S)-dihydroartemisininoxy)ethyl)-1H-1,2,3-triazol-1-yl)-methyl)-2H-1-chromen-2-one (**4f**) White solid; m.p. 121–123 °C; yield 54%; ^{1}H NMR (600 MHz, $CDCl_3$) δ (ppm): 9.98 (s, 1H), 7.68 (d, J = 8.8 Hz, 1H), 7.49 (s, 1H), 7.01 (dd, J = 8.8, 2.4 Hz, 1H), 6.85 (d, J = 2.4 Hz, 1H), 6.16 (s, 1H), 5.68–5.59 (m, 2H), 5.20 (s, 1H), 4.71 (d, J = 3.5 Hz, 1H), 4.08–4.04 (m, 1H), 3.67–3.63 (m, 1H), 3.03–2.94 (m, 2H), 2.56–2.53 (m, 1H), 2.33 (td, J = 14.1, 4.0 Hz, 1H), 2.03–1.99 (m, 1H), 1.86–1.82 (m, 1H), 1.58–1.54 (m, 2H), 1.51–1.48 (m, 1H), 1.40 (s, 3H), 1.40–1.35 (m, 2H), 1.27–1.25 (m, 1H), 1.20–1.16 (m, 2H), 0.88 (d, J = 5.6 Hz, 3H), 0.68 (d, J = 7.3 Hz, 3H); ^{13}C NMR (150 MHz, $CDCl_3$) δ (ppm): 161.02, 159.72, 155.05, 146.56, 145.44, 124.28, 121.23, 112.79, 111.51, 108.74, 103.16, 103.05, 100.88, 86.87, 79.91, 76.20, 75.99, 75.78, 65.75, 51.37, 50.15, 43.11, 36.37, 35.30, 33.45, 29.66, 25.24, 25.09, 23.62, 23.29, 19.29, 11.73; ESI-HRMS [M + Na]$^+$: (m/z) Calcd. for $C_{29}H_{35}N_3O_8Na$: 576.2322. Found: 576.2352.

5,7-dimethyl-4-((4-(2-((10S)-dihydroartemisininoxy)ethyl)-1H-1,2,3-triazol-1-yl)-methyl)-2H-1-chromen-2-one (**4g**) White solid; m.p. 135–137 °C; yield 52%; ^{1}H NMR (600 MHz, $CDCl_3$) δ (ppm): 7.41 (s, 1H), 7.06 (s, 1H), 6.94 (s, 1H), 5.84 (s, 2H), 5.54 (s, 1H), 5.28 (s, 1H), 4.80 (d, J = 3.4 Hz, 1H), 4.15–4.10 (m, 1H), 3.73–3.69 (m, 1H), 3.11–3.00 (m, 2H), 2.66 (s, 3H), 2.61–2.58 (m, 1H), 2.40 (s, 3H), 2.35 (td, J = 14.1, 4.0 Hz, 1H), 2.03–1.99 (m, 1H), 1.89–1.84 (m, 1H), 1.70–1.63 (m, 2H), 1.59–1.55 (m, 1H), 1.49–1.43 (m, 1H), 1.42 (s, 3H), 1.29–1.18 (m, 3H), 0.93 (d, J = 6.3 Hz, 3H), 0.87 (dd, J = 12.4, 4.6 Hz, 1H), 0.80 (d, J = 7.3 Hz, 3H); ^{13}C NMR (150 MHz, $CDCl_3$) δ (ppm): 158.63, 154.30, 149.34, 145.42, 142.09, 133.98, 129.26, 121.15, 115.62, 113.33, 112.98, 103.07, 100.86, 86.87, 80.00, 76.21, 76.00, 75.79, 65.93, 52.03, 51.47, 43.25, 36.36, 35.37, 33.55, 29.76, 25.58, 25.15, 23.66, 23.32, 23.21, 20.24, 19.35, 11.98; ESI-HRMS [M + Na]$^+$: (m/z) Calcd. for $C_{31}H_{39}N_3O_7Na$: 588.2686. Found: 588.2680.

7-methyl-4-((4-(2-((10S)-dihydroartemisininoxy)ethyl)-1H-1,2,3-triazol-1-yl)-methyl)-2H-1-chromen-2-one (**4h**) White solid; m.p. 100–102 °C; yield 53%; ^{1}H NMR (600 MHz, $CDCl_3$) δ (ppm): 7.48 (d, J = 8.1 Hz, 1H), 7.40 (s, 1H), 7.18 (s, 1H), 7.11 (d, J = 8.2 Hz, 1H), 6.00 (s, 1H), 5.68–5.62 (m, 2H), 5.29 (d, J = 12.6 Hz, 1H), 4.76 (d, J = 3.5 Hz, 1H), 4.11–4.08 (m, 1H), 3.69–3.65 (m, 1H), 3.06–2.96 (m, 2H), 2.60–2.54 (m, 1H), 2.45 (s, 3H), 2.34 (td, J = 14.0, 4.0 Hz, 1H), 2.05–1.99 (m, 1H), 1.88–1.83 (m, 1H), 1.66–1.63 (m, 2H), 1.60–1.58 (m, 1H), 1.56–1.53 (m, 1H), 1.41 (s, 3H), 1.27–1.17 (m, 3H), 0.93 (d, J = 6.1 Hz, 3H), 0.89–0.84 (m, 1H), 0.74 (d, J = 7.3 Hz, 3H); ^{13}C NMR (150 MHz, $CDCl_3$) δ (ppm): 158.98, 152.88, 146.91, 145.50, 143.18, 125.06, 122.27, 120.82, 116.69, 113.56, 113.35, 103.08, 100.86, 86.86, 79.97, 76.21, 76.00, 75.78, 65.94, 51.44, 49.21, 43.21, 36.36, 35.35, 33.54, 29.72, 25.55, 25.14, 23.65, 23.31, 20.69, 19.34, 11.86; ESI-HRMS [M + Na]$^+$: (m/z) Calcd. for $C_{30}H_{37}N_3O_7Na$: 574.2529. Found: 574.2567.

6-methyl-4-((4-(2-((10S)-dihydroartemisininoxy)ethyl)-1H-1,2,3-triazol-1-yl)-methyl)-2H-1-chromen-2-one (**4i**) White solid; m.p. 100–102 °C; yield 43%; ^{1}H NMR (600 MHz, $CDCl_3$) δ (ppm): 7.40 (s, 1H), 7.40 (s, 1H), 7.38 (d, J = 1.9 Hz, 1H), 7.28 (d, J = 8.3 Hz, 1H), 6.00 (d, J = 1.2 Hz, 1H), 5.67 (s, 2H), 5.29 (s, 1H), 4.77 (d, J = 3.4 Hz, 1H), 4.13–4.09 (m, 1H), 3.71–3.67 (m, 1H), 3.05–2.99 (m, 2H), 2.61–2.56 (m, 1H), 2.41 (s, 3H), 2.36–2.32 (m, 1H), 2.03–2.00 (m, 1H), 1.88–1.84 (m, 1H), 1.66 (dd, J = 13.7, 3.5 Hz, 1H), 1.61 (d, J = 4.2 Hz, 1H), 1.58–1.53 (m, 2H), 1.42 (s, 3H), 1.24–1.16 (m, 3H), 0.93 (d, J = 6.2 Hz, 3H), 0.88–0.85 (m, 1H), 0.75 (d, J = 7.3 Hz, 3H); ^{13}C NMR (150 MHz, $CDCl_3$) δ (ppm): 158.88, 150.89, 146.89, 145.51, 133.70, 132.73, 122.29, 120.86, 116.31, 115.69, 114.22, 103.09, 100.87, 86.86, 79.98, 76.20, 75.99, 75.78, 65.94, 51.45, 49.06, 43.22, 36.37, 35.35, 33.54, 29.73, 25.57, 25.14, 23.65, 23.31, 20.03, 19.34, 11.86; ESI-HRMS [M + Na]$^+$: (m/z) Calcd. for $C_{30}H_{37}N_3O_7Na$: 574.2529. Found: 574.2558.

4.1.3. General Procedure for the Synthesis of Compounds **5j**,**5l–5o**, and **6j–6p**

Substituted coumarin (**j–p**) (10 mmol), substituted DHA (**I** or **II**) (10 mmol) and triethylamine (10 mmol) were dissolved in 20 mL CH_2Cl_2. In addition, CuI (100 mg) was added and the reaction mixture was stirred at room temperature for 8h under the protection of nitrogen. The mixture was filtered, washed with water, dried over Na_2SO_4 and evaporated to dryness. The crude product was purified through column chromatography.

4-((4-(2-((10S)-dihydroartemisininoxy)ethyl)-1H-1,2,3-triazol-1-yl)-methoxy)-2H-1-chromen-2-one (**5j**) White solid; m.p. 91–93 °C; yield 51%; ^{1}H NMR (600 MHz, $CDCl_3$) δ (ppm): 7.79–7.75 (m, 2H), 7.55 (ddd, *J* = 8.7, 7.3, 1.6 Hz, 1H), 7.33 (d, *J* = 8.3 Hz, 1H), 7.25–7.22 (m, 1H), 5.87 (s, 1H), 5.34 (d, *J* = 2.7 Hz, 2H), 5.16 (s, 1H), 4.77 (d, *J* = 3.6 Hz, 1H), 4.72–4.68 (m, 1H), 4.58–4.54 (m, 1H), 4.32–4.29 (m, 1H), 3.87–3.83 (m, 1H), 2.63–2.60 (m, 1H), 2.33 (td, *J* = 14.0, 4.0 Hz, 1H), 2.01–1.97 (m, 1H), 1.87–1.81 (m, 1H), 1.68–1.64 (m, 1H), 1.58–1.55 (m, 1H), 1.53–1.51 (m, 1H), 1.41 (s, 3H), 1.38 (d, *J* = 11.2 Hz, 1H), 1.26–1.18 (m, 3H), 0.91 (d, *J* = 5.9 Hz, 3H), 0.88–0.83 (m, 1H), 0.78 (d, *J* = 7.4 Hz, 3H); ^{13}C NMR (150 MHz, $CDCl_3$) δ (ppm): 163.90, 161.51, 152.34, 140.45, 131.58, 122.86, 122.85, 122.04, 115.80, 114.40, 103.21, 101.15, 90.15, 86.86, 79.73, 76.20, 75.99, 75.78, 65.36, 61.67, 51.32, 49.57, 42.97, 36.35, 35.25, 33.41, 29.53, 25.06, 23.58, 23.32, 19.29, 11.80; ESI-HRMS [M + Na]$^+$: (*m/z*) Calcd. for $C_{29}H_{35}N_3O_8Na$: 576.2322. Found: 576.2336.

5,7-dimethyl-4-((4-(2-((10S)-dihydroartemisininoxy)ethyl)-1H-1,2,3-triazol-1-yl)-methoxy)-2H-1-chromen-2-one (**5l**) White solid; m.p. 111–113 °C; yield 49%; ^{1}H NMR (600 MHz, $CDCl_3$) δ (ppm): 7.74 (s, 1H), 6.98 (s, 1H), 6.83 (s, 1H), 5.75 (s, 1H), 5.28 (s, 2H), 5.14 (s, 1H), 4.76 (d, J = 3.6 Hz, 1H), 4.70–4.66 (m, 1H), 4.58–4.54 (m, 1H), 4.31–4.27 (m, 1H), 3.87–3.84 (m, 1H), 2.84 (s, 1H), 2.61–2.59 (m, 1H), 2.53 (s, 3H), 2.36 (s, 3H), 2.35–2.30 (m, 1H), 2.04–1.97 (m, 2H), 1.87–1.82 (m, 1H), 1.58–1.54 (m, 1H), 1.52–1.50 (m, 1H), 1.41 (s, 3H), 1.25–1.17 (m, 3H), 0.91 (d, *J* = 5.9 Hz, 3H), 0.88–0.85 (m, 1H), 0.76 (d, *J* = 7.4 Hz, 3H); ^{13}C NMR (150 MHz, $CDCl_3$) δ (ppm): 166.97, 161.69, 153.91, 141.76, 140.42, 135.57, 127.92, 122.68, 114.43, 110.62, 103.21, 101.15, 89.15, 86.85, 79.74, 76.21, 76.00, 75.79, 65.38, 61.48, 51.33, 49.59, 42.97, 36.36, 35.25, 33.42, 29.53, 25.05, 23.58, 23.30, 22.49, 20.35, 19.30, 11.80; ESI-HRMS [M + Na]$^+$: (*m/z*) Calcd. for $C_{31}H_{39}N_3O_8Na$: 604.2635. Found: 604.2645.

6,8-dimethyl-4-((4-(2-((10S)-dihydroartemisininoxy)ethyl)-1H-1,2,3-triazol-1-yl)-methoxy)-2H-1-chromen-2-one (**5m**) White solid; m.p. 111–113 °C; yield 49%; ^{1}H NMR (600 MHz, $CDCl_3$) δ (ppm): 7.77 (s, 1H), 7.39 (s, 1H), 7.22 (s, 1H), 5.83 (s, 1H), 5.32 (d, *J* = 2.5 Hz, 2H), 5.17 (s, 1H), 4.78 (d, *J* = 3.0 Hz, 1H), 4.72–4.68 (m, 1H), 4.59–4.55 (m, 1H), 4.33–4.29 (m, 1H), 3.87–3.83 (m, 1H), 2.64–2.58 (m, 1H), 2.41 (s, 3H), 2.37–2.33 (m, 1H), 2.33 (s, 3H), 2.02–1.98 (m, 1H), 1.88–1.82 (m, 1H), 1.68–1.63 (m, 1H), 1.58–1.53 (m, 1H), 1.53–1.48 (m, 1H), 1.41 (s, 3H), 1.41–1.38 (m, 1H), 1.28–1.16 (m, 3H), 0.91 (d, *J* = 5.9 Hz, 3H), 0.88–0.84 (m, 1H), 0.78 (d, *J* = 7.4 Hz, 3H); ^{13}C NMR (150 MHz, $CDCl_3$) δ (ppm): 165.31, 162.94, 149.91, 141.55, 134.98, 133.03, 125.90, 123.94, 120.25, 114.82, 104.23, 102.18, 90.77, 87.87, 80.76, 77.24, 77.02, 76.81, 66.39, 62.54, 52.35, 50.58, 44.01, 37.37, 36.28, 34.44, 30.57, 26.07, 24.61, 24.35, 20.82, 20.31, 15.65, 12.84; ESI-HRMS [M + Na]$^+$: (*m/z*) Calcd. for $C_{31}H_{39}N_3O_8Na$: 604.2635. Found: 604.2639.

7,8-dimethyl-4-((4-(2-((10S)-dihydroartemisininoxy)ethyl)-1H-1,2,3-triazol-1-yl)-methoxy)-2H-1-chromen-2-one (**5n**) White solid; m.p. 91–93 °C; yield 51%; ^{1}H NMR (600 MHz, $CDCl_3$) δ (ppm): 7.76 (s, 1H), 7.50 (d, *J* = 8.1 Hz, 1H), 7.03 (d, *J* = 8.1 Hz, 1H), 5.79 (s, 1H), 5.32 (d, *J* = 3.0 Hz, 2H), 5.15 (s, 1H), 4.77 (d, *J* = 3.5 Hz, 1H), 4.71–4.67 (m, 1H), 4.58–4.53 (m, 1H), 4.33–4.27 (m, 1H), 3.86–3.82 (m, 1H), 2.63–2.58 (m, 1H), 2.37 (s, 3H), 2.36 (s, 3H), 2.34–2.30 (m, 1H), 2.01–1.97 (m, 1H), 1.86–1.81 (m, 1H), 1.68–1.62 (m, 1H), 1.58–1.53 (m, 1H), 1.51 (dd, *J* = 13.4, 3.5 Hz, 1H), 1.41 (s, 3H), 1.39–1.36 (m, 1H), 1.27–1.15 (m, 3H), 0.91 (d, *J* = 5.8 Hz, 3H), 0.88–0.82 (m, 1H), 0.77 (d, *J* = 7.3 Hz, 3H); ^{13}C NMR (150 MHz, $CDCl_3$) δ (ppm): 165.56, 163.09, 151.58, 142.30, 141.69, 125.34, 124.53, 123.85, 119.71, 113.06, 104.24, 102.18, 89.91, 87.88, 80.78, 77.25, 77.04, 76.82, 66.39, 62.61, 52.37, 50.60, 44.02, 37.37, 36.29, 34.45, 30.58, 26.09, 24.61, 24.35, 20.46, 20.33, 12.85, 11.67; ESI-HRMS [M + Na]$^+$: (*m/z*) Calcd. for $C_{31}H_{39}N_3O_8Na$: 604.2635. Found: 604.2646.

8-methyl-4-((4-(2-((10S)-dihydroartemisininoxy)ethyl)-1H-1,2,3-triazol-1-yl)-methoxy)-2H-1-chromen- 2-one (**5o**) White solid; m.p. 84–86 °C; yield 43%; ^{1}H NMR (600 MHz, $CDCl_3$) δ (ppm): 7.77 (s, 1H), 7.61 (d, J = 7.9 Hz, 1H), 7.39 (d, J = 7.4 Hz, 1H), 7.13 (t, J = 7.7 Hz, 1H), 5.85 (s, 1H), 5.33 (d, J = 2.8 Hz, 2H), 5.15 (s, 1H), 4.77 (d, J = 3.5 Hz, 1H), 4.71–4.67 (m, 1H), 4.58–4.54 (m, 1H), 4.33–4.27 (m, 1H), 3.86–3.82 (m, 1H), 2.62–2.59 (m, 1H), 2.45 (s, 3H), 2.33 (td, J = 14.1, 4.0 Hz, 1H), 2.01–1.97 (m, 1H), 1.86–1.81 (m, 1H), 1.65 (dd, J = 14.0, 3.6 Hz, 1H), 1.58–1.54 (m, 1H), 1.51 (dd, J = 13.4, 3.5 Hz, 1H), 1.41 (s, 3H), 1.40–1.35 (m, 1H), 1.27–1.17 (m, 3H), 0.90 (d, J = 5.8 Hz, 3H), 0.88–0.84 (m, 1H), 0.77 (d, J = 7.3 Hz, 3H); ^{13}C NMR (150 MHz, $CDCl_3$) δ (ppm): 165.30, 162.70, 151.74, 141.60, 133.84, 126.28, 123.84, 123.42, 120.66, 115.15, 104.24, 102.18, 90.88, 87.89, 80.77, 77.25, 77.03, 76.82, 66.39, 62.71, 52.36, 50.60, 44.01, 37.38, 36.28, 34.45, 30.57, 26.09, 24.61, 24.35, 20.33, 15.76, 12.84; ESI-HRMS [M + Na]$^+$: (m/z) Calcd. for $C_{30}H_{37}N_3O_8Na$: 590.2478. Found: 590.2477.

4-((4-(3-((10S)-dihydroartemisininoxy)propyl)-1H-1,2,3-triazol-1-yl)-methoxy)-2H-1-chromen-2-one (**6j**) White solid; m.p. 74–76 °C; yield 47%; ^{1}H NMR (600 MHz, $CDCl_3$) δ (ppm): 7.79 (dd, J = 8.0, 1.6 Hz, 1H), 7.72 (s, 1H), 7.55 (ddd, J = 8.7, 7.4, 1.6 Hz, 1H), 7.32 (dd, J = 8.4, 1.1 Hz, 1H), 7.26–7.23 (m, 1H), 5.86 (s, 1H), 5.41 (s, 1H), 5.34 (s, 2H), 4.79 (d, J = 3.6 Hz, 1H), 4.56–4.46 (m, 2H), 3.93–3.89 (m, 1H), 3.44–3.41 (m, 1H), 2.69–2.63 (m, 1H), 2.39–2.34 (m, 1H), 2.27–2.20 (m, 2H), 2.05–2.01 (m, 1H), 1.91–1.86 (m, 1H), 1.79–1.75 (m, 1H), 1.67–1.64 (m, 1H), 1.51–1.46 (m, 2H), 1.42 (s, 3H), 1.39–1.33 (m, 1H), 1.28–1.22 (m, 2H), 0.96 (d, J = 6.4 Hz, 3H), 0.94 (d, J = 7.4 Hz, 3H); ^{13}C NMR (150 MHz, $CDCl_3$) δ (ppm): 163.96, 161.59, 152.33, 140.41, 131.55, 122.89, 122.40, 122.13, 115.78, 114.42, 103.18, 101.19, 90.16, 86.93, 79.93, 76.21, 76.00, 75.79, 63.62, 61.66, 51.47, 46.73, 43.23, 36.45, 35.33, 33.53, 29.78, 29.43, 25.12, 23.64, 23.54, 19.33, 12.07; ESI-HRMS [M + Na]$^+$: (m/z) Calcd. for $C_{30}H_{37}N_3O_8Na$: 590.2478. Found: 590.2463.

7-methyl-4-((4-(3-((10S)-dihydroartemisininoxy)propyl)-1H-1,2,3-triazol-1-yl)-methoxy)-2H-1-chromen-2-one (**6k**) White solid; m.p. 80–82 °C; yield 51%; ^{1}H NMR (600 MHz, $CDCl_3$) δ (ppm): 7.71 (s, 1H), 7.65 (d, J = 8.1 Hz, 1H), 7.12 (s, 1H), 7.05 (d, J = 8.1 Hz, 1H), 5.80 (s, 1H), 5.41 (s, 1H), 5.32 (s, 2H), 4.79 (d, J = 3.6 Hz, 1H), 4.53–4.46 (m, 2H), 3.93–3.89 (m, 1H), 3.44–3.40 (m, 1H), 2.69–2.64 (m, 1H), 2.44 (s, 3H), 2.37 (td, J = 14.0, 4.0 Hz, 1H), 2.27–2.21 (m, 2H), 2.05–2.01 (m, 1H), 1.91–1.86 (m, 1H), 1.80–1.75 (m, 2H), 1.68–1.64 (m, 1H), 1.51–1.46 (m, 2H), 1.42 (s, 3H), 1.28–1.24 (m, 3H), 0.96 (d, J = 6.4 Hz, 3H), 0.94 (d, J = 7.3 Hz, 3H); ^{13}C NMR (150 MHz, $CDCl_3$) δ (ppm): δ 164.21, 161.95, 152.44, 142.81, 140.51, 124.11, 122.39, 121.82, 115.88, 111.91, 103.19, 101.18, 89.25, 86.93, 79.94, 76.20, 75.99, 75.78, 63.62, 61.55, 51.47, 46.73, 43.24, 36.44, 35.33, 33.53, 29.78, 29.42, 25.12, 23.63, 23.53, 20.72, 19.33, 12.07; ESI-HRMS [M + Na]$^+$: (m/z) Calcd. for $C_{31}H_{39}N_3O_8Na$: 604.2635. Found: 604.2617.

5,7-dimethyl-4-((4-(3-((10S)-dihydroartemisininoxy)propyl)-1H-1,2,3-triazol-1-yl)-methoxy)-2H-1-chromen-2-one (**6l**) White solid; m.p. 86–88 °C; yield 42%; ^{1}H NMR (600 MHz, $CDCl_3$) δ (ppm): 7.68 (s, 1H), 6.98 (s, 1H), 6.83 (s, 1H), 5.74 (s, 1H), 5.40 (s, 1H), 5.28 (s, 2H), 4.78 (d, J = 3.7 Hz, 1H), 4.53–4.48 (m, 2H), 3.91–3.87 (m, 1H), 3.42–3.38 (m, 1H), 2.69–2.64 (m, 1H), 2.53 (s, 3H), 2.40–2.33 (m, 4H), 2.25–2.19 (m, 2H), 2.05–2.01 (m, 1H), 1.91–1.86 (m, 1H), 1.80–1.77 (m, 1H), 1.76–1.73 (m, 1H), 1.67–1.64 (m, 1H), 1.51–1.47 (m, 2H), 1.42 (s, 3H), 1.30–1.21 (m, 3H), 0.96 (d, J = 6.4 Hz, 3H), 0.94 (d, J = 7.4 Hz, 3H); ^{13}C NMR (150 MHz, $CDCl_3$) δ (ppm): 166.99, 161.73, 153.90, 141.72, 140.46, 135.57, 127.92, 122.26, 114.43, 110.63, 103.18, 101.15, 89.14, 86.91, 79.93, 76.21, 76.00, 75.78, 63.49, 61.58, 51.46, 46.66, 43.23, 36.46, 35.33, 33.53, 29.78, 29.42, 25.11, 23.64, 23.54, 22.46, 20.35, 19.33, 12.08; ESI-HRMS [M + Na]$^+$: (m/z) Calcd. for $C_{32}H_{41}N_3O_8Na$: 618.2791. Found: 618.2827.

6,8-dimethyl-4-((4-(3-((10S)-dihydroartemisininoxy)propyl)-1H-1,2,3-triazol-1-yl)-methoxy)-2H-1-chromen-2-one (**6m**) White solid; m.p. 90–92 °C; yield 55%; ^{1}H NMR (600 MHz, $CDCl_3$) δ (ppm): 7.71 (s, 1H), 7.40 (s, 1H), 7.21 (s, 1H), 5.82 (s, 1H), 5.41 (s, 1H), 5.32 (s, 2H), 4.79 (d, J = 3.6 Hz, 1H), 4.55–4.46 (m, 2H), 3.94–3.90 (m, 1H), 3.44–3.40 (m, 1H), 2.69–2.63 (m, 1H), 2.40 (s, 3H), 2.39–2.34 (m, 1H), 2.33 (s, 3H), 2.27–2.21 (m, 2H), 2.06–2.01 (m, 1H), 1.91–1.86 (m, 1H), 1.79–1.77 (m, 1H), 1.76–1.73 (m, 1H), 1.67–1.63 (m, 1H), 1.51–1.45 (m, 2H), 1.42 (s, 3H), 1.37–1.35 (m, 1H), 1.28–1.22 (m, 2H), 0.95 (d, J = 6.4 Hz, 3H), 0.94 (d, J = 7.4 Hz, 3H); ^{13}C NMR (150 MHz, $CDCl_3$) δ (ppm): 165.37, 163.02, 149.90, 141.55,

134.97, 133.07, 125.88, 123.45, 120.35, 114.83, 104.21, 102.21, 90.79, 87.96, 80.97, 77.25, 77.04, 76.83, 64.68, 62.56, 52.51, 47.77, 44.27, 37.47, 36.37, 34.56, 30.82, 30.47, 26.15, 24.67, 24.57, 20.83, 20.36, 15.66, 13.11; ESI-HRMS $[M + Na]^+$: (*m*/*z*) Calcd. for $C_{32}H_{41}N_3O_8Na$: 618.2791. Found: 618.2808.

7,8-dimethyl-4-((4-(3-((10S)-dihydroartemisininoxy)propyl)-1H-1,2,3-triazol-1-yl)-methoxy)-2H-1-chromen-2-one (**6n**) White solid; m.p. 115–117 °C; yield 44%; ^{1}H NMR (600 MHz, $CDCl_3$) δ (ppm): 7.71 (s, 1H), 7.52 (d, *J* = 8.1 Hz, 1H), 7.04 (d, *J* = 8.1 Hz, 1H), 5.80 (s, 1H), 5.40 (s, 1H), 5.32 (s, 2H), 4.79 (d, *J* = 3.5 Hz, 1H), 4.56–4.45 (m, 2H), 3.93–3.89 (m, 1H), 3.44–3.40 (m, 1H), 2.69–2.64 (m, 1H), 2.39–2.34 (m, 7H), 2.27–2.19 (m, 2H), 2.06–2.01 (m, 1H), 1.92–1.86 (m, 1H), 1.81–1.77 (m, 1H), 1.74 (dd, *J* = 13.4, 3.5 Hz, 1H), 1.67–1.63 (m, 1H), 1.52–1.45 (m, 2H), 1.42 (s, 3H), 1.39–1.34 (m, 1H), 1.27–1.24 (m, 2H), 0.96 (d, *J* = 6.4 Hz, 3H), 0.94 (d, *J* = 7.4 Hz, 3H); ^{13}C NMR (150 MHz, $CDCl_3$) δ (ppm): 165.61, 163.15, 151.58, 142.28, 141.66, 125.37, 124.51, 123.38, 119.78, 113.07, 104.21, 102.21, 89.92, 87.96, 80.97, 77.25, 77.04, 76.82, 64.66, 62.60, 52.51, 47.76, 44.27, 37.47, 36.37, 34.56, 30.82, 30.46, 26.15, 24.67, 24.57, 20.46, 20.37, 13.11, 11.67; ESI-HRMS $[M + Na]^+$: (*m*/*z*) Calcd. for $C_{32}H_{41}N_3O_8Na$: 618.2791. Found: 618.2793.

8-methyl-4-((4-(3-((10S)-dihydroartemisininoxy)propyl)-1H-1,2,3-triazol-1-yl)-methoxy)-2H-1-chromen-2-one (**6o**) White solid; m.p. 143–145°C; yield 38%; ^{1}H NMR (600 MHz, $CDCl_3$) δ (ppm): 7.71 (s, 1H), 7.63 (d, *J* = 8.0 Hz, 1H), 7.39 (d, *J* = 7.3 Hz, 1H), 7.14 (t, *J* = 7.7 Hz, 1H), 5.85 (s, 1H), 5.40 (s, 1H), 5.33 (s, 2H), 4.79 (d, *J* = 3.7 Hz, 1H), 4.55–4.46 (m, 2H), 3.93–3.89 (m, 1H), 3.44–3.40 (m, 1H), 2.70–2.63 (m, 1H), 2.45 (s, 3H), 2.37 (td, *J* = 14.0, 3.9 Hz, 1H), 2.28–2.19 (m, 2H), 2.05–2.01 (m, 1H), 1.92–1.86 (m, 1H), 1.81–1.72 (m, 2H), 1.67–1.64 (m, 1H), 1.53–1.46 (m, 2H), 1.42 (s, 3H), 1.39–1.33 (m, 1H), 1.30–1.22 (m, 2H), 0.96 (d, *J* = 6.4 Hz, 3H), 0.94 (d, *J* = 7.4 Hz, 3H); ^{13}C NMR (150 MHz, $CDCl_3$) δ (ppm): 165.35, 162.77, 151.73, 141.56, 133.82, 126.25, 123.45, 123.40, 120.73, 115.17, 104.22, 102.21, 90.89, 87.96, 80.97, 77.24, 77.03, 76.82, 64.65, 62.69, 52.51, 47.76, 44.27, 37.48, 36.37, 34.56, 30.82, 30.46, 26.15, 24.67, 24.57, 20.37, 15.76, 13.11; ESI-HRMS $[M + Na]^+$: (*m*/*z*) Calcd. for $C_{31}H_{39}N_3O_8Na$: 604.2635. Found: 604.2646.

6-methyl-4-((4-(3-((10S)-dihydroartemisininoxy)propyl)-1H-1,2,3-triazol-1-yl)-methoxy)-2H-1-chromen-2-one (**6p**) White solid; m.p. 80–82 °C; yield 45%; ^{1}H NMR (600 MHz, $CDCl_3$) δ (ppm): 7.72 (s, 1H), 7.56 (s, 1H), 7.35 (dd, *J* = 8.5, 2.0 Hz, 1H), 7.21 (d, *J* = 8.4 Hz, 1H), 5.84 (s, 1H), 5.41 (s, 1H), 5.33 (s, 2H), 4.80 (d, *J* = 3.6 Hz, 1H), 4.55–4.47 (m, 2H), 3.94–3.90 (m, 1H), 3.45–3.41 (m, 1H), 2.70–2.64 (m, 1H), 2.40–2.33 (m, 4H), 2.27–2.21 (m, 2H), 2.06–2.01 (m, 1H), 1.91–1.87 (m, 1H), 1.80–1.73 (m, 2H), 1.65 (dd, *J* = 13.3, 3.4 Hz, 1H), 1.53–1.46 (m, 2H), 1.42 (s, 3H), 1.38–1.34 (m, 1H), 1.28–1.22 (m, 2H), 0.96 (d, *J* = 6.4 Hz, 3H), 0.94 (d, *J* = 7.3 Hz, 3H); ^{13}C NMR (150 MHz, $CDCl_3$) δ (ppm): 165.02, 162.88, 151.52, 141.46, 133.69, 133.59, 123.52, 122.80, 116.56, 115.08, 104.22, 102.22, 91.11, 87.97, 80.97, 77.24, 77.03, 76.82, 64.68, 62.60, 52.51, 47.80, 44.27, 37.48, 36.37, 34.57, 30.82, 30.48, 26.15, 24.67, 24.58, 20.90, 20.37, 13.12; ESI-HRMS $[M + Na]^+$: (*m*/*z*) Calcd. for $C_{31}H_{39}N_3O_8Na$: 604.2635. Found: 604.2621.

4.2. Biology

4.2.1. Storage and Preparation of Samples

All the target compounds were dissolved in dimethylsulfoxide and storage under −20 °C. They get to be diluted to different concentration when they will be used.

4.2.2. Cell Culture

After recovery, the cells were cultured in 96-well plates for 24 h at 37 °C in a humidified atmosphere with 95% air and 5% CO_2. After treated with different tested compounds, the hypoxia groups were placed in a sealed hypoxia incubator chamber (Stemcell Technologies, Inc., Vancouver, BC, Canada) filled with 5% CO_2 and 95% N_2 for 24 h, and then transferred to the incubator chamber filled with air for 72 h. On the contrary, the normoxia groups were cultured under air condition for 96h.

Cancer cells HT-29 (Human Colorectal Adenocarcinoma cell line), MDA-MB-231 (Human Breast Cancer cell line), HCT-116 (Human Colorectal Carcinoma cell line), and A549 (Human Lung Adenocarcinomic cell line) were from ATCC.

4.2.3. MTT Assay

When the adherent cells reached 80% confluence, the culture medium was discarded. The cells were digested by trypsin and collected after centrifugation. The fresh culture medium was gently blown into it to form single-cell suspension. Cell suspension will be diluted to 1.5–3 × 10^4 cells/mL. Each hole of 96-well plates was added 100 μL cell suspension and incubated for 24 h (5% CO_2; 37 °C). Then the holes were added different concentrations of tested compounds. The early screening concentration is set to 100 μM, 50 μM, 25 μM, 12.5 μM, and 6.25 μM. Three replicates were made for each concentration of the tested compounds. After the cells were grown for 96h, 20 μL MTT (5 mg/mL) was added to each well and incubated for 4 h. The medium was discarded and each well was added 100 μL DMSO to dissolve the formazan blue. Absorbance was measured at 570 nm with a microplate reader (Synergy-HT, BioTek Instruments, Winooski, VT, USA).

Hypoxia condition: The cells were treated with different concentration of tested compounds, placed in hypoxia chamber (Catalog Number 27310, Stemcell Technologies, Inc., Vancouver, BC, Canada), and incubated for 24 h (5% air; 95% N_2; 37 °C). Then the cells were placed in normoxia condition (5% CO_2; 37 °C) and incubated for 72 h.

4.2.4. Preparation of N9 Cells

The murine microglial cell line N9 was a kind gift from Dr. P. Ricciardi-Castagnoli (Universita Degli Studi di Milano-Bicocca, Milan, Italy).

N9 cells, which were in the logarithmic phase, were incubated for 24 h by adherent culture. Subsequently, the medium was changed to new one without serum. The cells were treated with different concentration of tested compounds. After specific time in the LPS condition, the supernatants were collected and analyzed.

4.2.5. Nitrite Measurement

The nitrite levels in medium were determined by Griess reaction. The absorbance was measured at 540 nm using a microplate reader.

4.2.6. NO Capture Analysis

SNP was dissolved in PBS to prepare the 100 mM stock solution. In this experiment, SNP solution of 25 μL was added to 975 μL PBS solution which included different concentration of tested compounds. After 60 min under r.t. condition, the concentration of NO_2^- was tested using Griess assay.

4.2.7. Evaluation of Inflammatory Mediator

The secreted level of TNF-α and IL-6 was measured using mouse Th1/Th2/Th17 Cytokine Kit, purchased from BD Pharningen. The data was analyzed by FCAP Array v3.0. IL-2, IL-4, IL-10, IL-17A, and IFN-γ were not detected in the experiment.

4.2.8. Molecular Docking Simulations

The crystallographic structure of TLR4/MD-2 complex was retrieved from the Protein DataBank (PDB ID: 3VQ2), which was optimized by removing water molecules, cofactors and heteroatoms. Receptor grid was generally around the MD-2 active site. Docking calculations were accomplished using AutoDock4. The docking results were further analyzed and visually optimized by Discovery Studio 4.0 and PyMOL.

Author Contributions: H.Y. performed experiments, analyzed data, and drafted the manuscript. Z.H. performed experiments, analyzed data, and revised the manuscript. X.Y. performed experiments. Y.M. and C.G. conceived the work, gave critical comments, and revised the manuscript.

Abbreviations

DHA	Dihydroartemisinin
DCH	Dihydroartemisinin–Coumarin hydrids
CRF	Cancer-related fatigue
DOX	Doxorubicin
CNS	Central nervous system
SNP	Sodium nitroprusside
LPS	Lipopolysaccharide
TLR4	Toll-like receptor 4

References

1. Tsuji, E.; Hiki, N.; Nomura, S.; Fukushima, R.; Kojima, J.; Ogawa, T.; Mafune, K.; Mimura, Y.; Kaminishi, M. Simultaneous onset of acute inflammatory response, sepsis-like symptoms and intestinal mucosal injury after cancer chemotherapy. *Int. J. Cancer* **2003**, *107*, 303–308. [CrossRef] [PubMed]
2. Cerci, C.; Ergin, C.; Eroglu, E.; Agalar, C.; Agalar, F.; Cerci, S.; Bulbul, M. Effects of granulocyte-colony stimulating factor on peritoneal defense mechanisms and bacterial translocation after administration of systemic chemotherapy in rats. *World J. Gastroenterol.* **2007**, *13*, 2596–2599. [CrossRef] [PubMed]
3. Rivest, S. Molecular insights on the cerebral innate immune system. *Brain Behav. Immun.* **2003**, *17*, 13–19. [CrossRef]
4. Norden, D.M.; Bicer, S.; Clark, Y.; Jing, R.; Henry, C.J.; Wold, L.E.; Reiser, P.J.; Godbout, J.P.; McCarthy, D.O. Tumor growth increases neuroinflammation, fatigue and depressive-like behavior prior to alterations in muscle function. *Brain Behav. Immun.* **2015**, *43*, 76–85. [CrossRef] [PubMed]
5. Bower, J.E.; Lamkin, D.M. Inflammation and cancer-related fatigue: Mechanisms, contributing factors, and treatment implications. *Brain Behav. Immun.* **2013**, *30*, S48–S57. [CrossRef]
6. Perry, V.H.; Gordon, S. Macrophages and microglia in the nervous system. *Trends Neurosci.* **1988**, *11*, 273–277. [CrossRef]
7. Kreutzberg, G.W. Microglia: A sensor for pathological events in the CNS. *Trends Neurosci.* **1996**, *19*, 312–318. [CrossRef]
8. Colton, C.A.; Gilbert, D.L. Production of superoxide anions by a CNS macrophage, the microglia. *FEBS Lett.* **1987**, *223*, 284–288. [CrossRef]
9. Banati, R.B.; Gehrmann, J.; Schubert, P.; Kreutzberg, G.W. Cytotoxicity of microglia. *Glia* **1993**, *7*, 111–118. [CrossRef]
10. Lissauer, M.E.; Johnson, S.B.; Bochicchio, G.V.; Feild, C.J.; Cross, A.S.; Hasday, J.D.; Whiteford, C.C.; Nussbaumer, W.A.; Towns, M.; Scalea, T.M. Differential expression of toll-like receptor genes: Sepsis compared with sterile inflammation 1 day before sepsis diagnosis. *Shock* **2009**, *31*, 238–244. [CrossRef]
11. Steiner, A.A.; Chakravarty, S.; Rudaya, A.Y.; Herkenham, M.; Romanovsky, A.A. Bacterial lipopolysaccharide fever is initiated via Toll-like receptor 4 on hematopoietic cells. *Blood* **2006**, *107*, 4000–4002. [CrossRef]
12. Shimazu, R.; Akashi, S.; Ogata, H.; Nagai, Y.; Fukudome, K.; Miyake, K.; Kimoto, M. MD-2, a Molecule that Confers Lipopolysaccharide Responsiveness on Toll-like Receptor 4. *J. Exp. Med.* **1999**, *189*, 1777–1782. [CrossRef] [PubMed]
13. Nagai, Y.; Akashi, S.; Nagafuku, M.; Ogata, M.; Iwakura, Y.; Akira, S.; Kitamura, T.; Kosugi, A.; Kimoto, M.; Miyake, K. Essential role of MD-2 in LPS responsiveness and TLR4 distribution. *Nat. Immunol.* **2002**, *3*, 667–672. [CrossRef] [PubMed]
14. Inohara, N.; Nuñez, G. ML—A conserved domain involved in innate immunity and lipid metabolism. *Trends Biochem. Sci.* **2002**, *27*, 219–221. [CrossRef]
15. Viriyakosol, S.; Tobias, P.S.; Kitchens, R.L.; Kirkland, T.N. MD-2 binds to bacterial lipopolysaccharide. *J. Biol. Chem.* **2001**, *276*, 38044–38051. [PubMed]

16. Navaratnam, V.; Mansor, S.M.; Sit, N.W.; Grace, J.; Li, Q.; Olliaro, P. Pharmacokinetics of artemisinin-type compounds. *Clin. Pharmacokinet.* **2000**, *39*, 255–270. [CrossRef] [PubMed]
17. Balint, G.A. Artemisinin and its derivatives: An important new class of antimalarial agents. *Pharmacol. Ther.* **2001**, *90*, 261–265. [CrossRef]
18. Chen, H.; Gu, S.; Dai, H.; Li, X.; Zhang, Z. Dihydroartemisinin Sensitizes Human Lung Adenocarcinoma A549 Cells to Arsenic Trioxide via Apoptosis. *Biol. Trace Elem. Res.* **2017**, *179*, 203–212. [CrossRef]
19. Cao, L.; Duanmu, W.; Yin, Y.; Zhou, Z.; Ge, H.; Chen, T.; Tan, L.; Yu, A.; Hu, R.; Fei, L.; et al. Dihydroartemisinin exhibits anti-glioma stem cell activity through inhibiting p-AKT and activating caspase-3. *Die Pharm.* **2014**, *69*, 752–758.
20. Zhang, Z.; Guo, M.; Zhao, S.; Shao, J.; Zheng, S. ROS-JNK1/2-dependent activation of autophagy is required for the induction of anti-inflammatory effect of dihydroartemisinin in liver fibrosis. *Free Radic. Biol. Med.* **2016**, *101*, 272–283. [CrossRef]
21. Jiang, L.B.; Meng, D.H.; Lee, S.M.; Liu, S.H.; Xu, Q.T.; Wang, Y.; Zhang, J. Dihydroartemisinin inhibits catabolism in rat chondrocytes by activating autophagy via inhibition of the NF-kappaB pathway. *Sci. Rep.* **2016**, *6*, 38979. [CrossRef]
22. Huang, X.; Xie, Z.; Liu, F.; Han, C.; Zhang, D.; Wang, D.; Bao, X.; Sun, J.; Wen, C.; Fan, Y. Dihydroartemisinin inhibits activation of the Toll-like receptor 4 signaling pathway and production of type I interferon in spleen cells from lupus-prone MRL/lpr mice. *Int. Immunopharmacol.* **2014**, *22*, 266–272. [CrossRef]
23. Witaicenis, A.; de Oliveira, E.C.S.; Tanimoto, A.; Zorzella-Pezavento, S.F.G.; de Oliveira, S.L.; Sartori, A.; Di Stasi, L.C. 4-methylesculetin, a coumarin derivative, ameliorates dextran sulfate sodium-induced intestinal inflammation. *Chem. Biol. Interact.* **2018**, *280*, 59–63. [CrossRef] [PubMed]
24. Chougala, B.M.; Samundeeswari, S.; Holiyachi, M.; Naik, N.S.; Shastri, L.A.; Dodamani, S.; Jalalpure, S.; Dixit, S.R.; Joshi, S.D.; Sunagar, V.A. Green, unexpected synthesis of bis-coumarin derivatives as potent anti-bacterial and anti-inflammatory agents. *Eur. J. Med. Chem.* **2018**, *143*, 1744–1756. [CrossRef] [PubMed]
25. Emami, S.; Dadashpour, S. Current developments of coumarin-based anti-cancer agents in medicinal chemistry. *Eur. J. Med. Chem.* **2015**, *102*, 611–630. [CrossRef] [PubMed]
26. Basanagouda, M.; Jambagi, V.B.; Barigidad, N.N.; Laxmeshwar, S.S.; Devaru, V.; Narayanachar. Synthesis, structure-activity relationship of iodinated-4-aryloxymethyl-coumarins as potential anti-cancer and anti-mycobacterial agents. *Eur. J. Med. Chem.* **2014**, *74*, 225–233. [CrossRef]
27. Devji, T.; Reddy, C.; Woo, C.; Awale, S.; Kadota, S.; Carrico-Moniz, D. Pancreatic anticancer activity of a novel geranylgeranylated coumarin derivative. *Bioorg. Med. Chem. Lett.* **2011**, *21*, 5770–5773. [CrossRef] [PubMed]
28. Bronikowska, J.; Szliszka, E.; Jaworska, D.; Czuba, Z.P.; Krol, W. The coumarin psoralidin enhances anticancer effect of tumor necrosis factor-related apoptosis-inducing ligand (TRAIL). *Molecules* **2012**, *17*, 6449–6464. [CrossRef] [PubMed]
29. Reddy, N.S.; Gumireddy, K.; Mallireddigari, M.R.; Cosenza, S.C.; Venkatapuram, P.; Bell, S.C.; Reddy, E.P.; Reddy, M.V. Novel coumarin-3-(N-aryl)carboxamides arrest breast cancer cell growth by inhibiting ErbB-2 and ERK1. *Bioorg. Med. Chem.* **2005**, *13*, 3141–3147. [CrossRef]
30. Harada, K.; Kubo, H.; Tomigahara, Y.; Nishioka, K.; Takahashi, J.; Momose, M.; Inoue, S.; Kojima, A. Coumarins as novel 17beta-hydroxysteroid dehydrogenase type 3 inhibitors for potential treatment of prostate cancer. *Bioorg. Med. Chem. Lett.* **2010**, *20*, 272–275. [CrossRef]
31. Vijay Avin, B.R.; Thirusangu, P.; Lakshmi Ranganatha, V.; Firdouse, A.; Prabhakar, B.T.; Khanum, S.A. Synthesis and tumor inhibitory activity of novel coumarin analogs targeting angiogenesis and apoptosis. *Eur. J. Med. Chem.* **2014**, *75*, 211–221. [CrossRef]
32. Jin, J.; Yu, X.; Hu, Z.; Tang, S.; Zhong, X.; Xu, J.; Shang, P.; Huang, Y.; Liu, H. Isofraxidin targets the TLR4/MD-2 axis to prevent osteoarthritis development. *Food Funct.* **2018**, *9*, 5641–5652. [CrossRef]
33. Liu, J.; Chen, Q.; Jian, Z.; Xiong, X.; Shao, L.; Jin, T.; Zhu, X.; Wang, L. Daphnetin Protects against Cerebral Ischemia/Reperfusion Injury in Mice via Inhibition of TLR4/NF-kappaB Signaling Pathway. *Biomed. Res. Int.* **2016**, *2016*, 2816056. [CrossRef]
34. Tian, Y.; Liang, Z.; Xu, H.; Mou, Y.; Guo, C. Design, Synthesis and Cytotoxicity of Novel Dihydroartemisinin-Coumarin Hybrids via Click Chemistry. *Molecules* **2016**, *21*, 758. [CrossRef]
35. Yu, H.; Hou, Z.; Tian, Y.; Mou, Y.; Guo, C. Design, synthesis, cytotoxicity and mechanism of novel dihydroartemisinin-coumarin hybrids as potential anti-cancer agents. *Eur. J. Med. Chem.* **2018**, *151*, 434–449. [CrossRef]

36. Tan, Y.; Yang, X.-D.; Liu, W.-J.; Sun, X.-W. Novel one-pot asymmetric cascade approach toward densely substituted enantioenriched α-methylene-γ-lactams. *Tetrahedron Lett.* **2014**, *55*, 6105–6108. [CrossRef]
37. Pechmann, H.V. Berichte der deutschen chemischen. *Gesellschaft* **1884**, *17*, 929.
38. Ji, Q.; Ge, Z.; Ge, Z.; Chen, K.; Wu, H.; Liu, X.; Huang, Y.; Yuan, L.; Yang, X.; Liao, F. Synthesis and biological evaluation of novel phosphoramidate derivatives of coumarin as chitin synthase inhibitors and antifungal agents. *Eur. J. Med. Chem.* **2016**, *108*, 166–176. [CrossRef]
39. Ohto, U.; Fukase, K.; Miyake, K.; Shimizu, T. Structural basis of species-specific endotoxin sensing by innate immune receptor TLR4/MD-2. *Proc. Natl. Acad. Sci. USA* **2012**, *109*, 7421–7426. [CrossRef]

Permissions

All chapters in this book were first published by MDPI; hereby published with permission under the Creative Commons Attribution License or equivalent. Every chapter published in this book has been scrutinized by our experts. Their significance has been extensively debated. The topics covered herein carry significant findings which will fuel the growth of the discipline. They may even be implemented as practical applications or may be referred to as a beginning point for another development.

The contributors of this book come from diverse backgrounds, making this book a truly international effort. This book will bring forth new frontiers with its revolutionizing research information and detailed analysis of the nascent developments around the world.

We would like to thank all the contributing authors for lending their expertise to make the book truly unique. They have played a crucial role in the development of this book. Without their invaluable contributions this book wouldn't have been possible. They have made vital efforts to compile up to date information on the varied aspects of this subject to make this book a valuable addition to the collection of many professionals and students.

This book was conceptualized with the vision of imparting up-to-date information and advanced data in this field. To ensure the same, a matchless editorial board was set up. Every individual on the board went through rigorous rounds of assessment to prove their worth. After which they invested a large part of their time researching and compiling the most relevant data for our readers.

The editorial board has been involved in producing this book since its inception. They have spent rigorous hours researching and exploring the diverse topics which have resulted in the successful publishing of this book. They have passed on their knowledge of decades through this book. To expedite this challenging task, the publisher supported the team at every step. A small team of assistant editors was also appointed to further simplify the editing procedure and attain best results for the readers.

Apart from the editorial board, the designing team has also invested a significant amount of their time in understanding the subject and creating the most relevant covers. They scrutinized every image to scout for the most suitable representation of the subject and create an appropriate cover for the book.

The publishing team has been an ardent support to the editorial, designing and production team. Their endless efforts to recruit the best for this project, has resulted in the accomplishment of this book. They are a veteran in the field of academics and their pool of knowledge is as vast as their experience in printing. Their expertise and guidance has proved useful at every step. Their uncompromising quality standards have made this book an exceptional effort. Their encouragement from time to time has been an inspiration for everyone.

The publisher and the editorial board hope that this book will prove to be a valuable piece of knowledge for researchers, students, practitioners and scholars across the globe.

List of Contributors

Charlotte M. Miller, Elaine C. O'Sullivan and Florence O. McCarthy
School of Chemistry, Analytical and Biological Chemistry Research Facility, University College Cork, Western Road, T12 K8AF Cork, Ireland

Hui Wen, Yuke Liu, Shufang Wang, Ting Wang, Gang Zhang, Xiaoguang Chen, Yan Li, Huaqing Cui, Fangfang Lai and Li Sheng
State Key Laboratory of Bioactive Substances and Function of Natural Medicine, Institute of Materia Medica, Peking Union Medical College and Chinese Academy of Medical Sciences, Beijing 100050, China

Mirosława Grymel, Gabriela Pastuch-Gawołek and Monika Krawczyk
Department of Organic Chemistry, Bioorganic Chemistry and Biotechnology, Silesian University of Technology, B. Krzywoustego 4, 44-100 Gliwice, Poland
Biotechnology Center, Silesian University of Technology, B. Krzywoustego 8, 44-100 Gliwice, Poland

Anna Lalik
Biotechnology Center, Silesian University of Technology, B. Krzywoustego 8, 44-100 Gliwice, Poland
Department of Systems Biology and Engineering, Silesian University of Technology, Akademicka 16, 44-100 Gliwice, Poland

Mateusz Zawojak and Seweryn Boczek
Department of Organic Chemistry, Bioorganic Chemistry and Biotechnology, Silesian University of Technology, B. Krzywoustego 4, 44-100 Gliwice, Poland

Karol Erfurt
Department of Chemical Organic Technology and Petrochemistry, Silesian University of Technology, B. Krzywoustego 4, 44-100 Gliwice, Poland

Hana Skoupilova and Roman Hrstka
Research Centre for Applied Molecular Oncology, Masaryk Memorial Cancer Institute, Zluty kopec 7, 656 53 Brno, Czech Republic

Vladimir Rak
Department of Radiation Oncology, Masaryk Memorial Cancer Institute, Zluty kopec 7, 656 53 Brno, Czech Republic

Jiri Pinkas
J. Heyrovský Institute of Physical Chemistry, Academy of Sciences of the Czech Republic, v. v. i., Dolejškova 2155/3, 182 23 Prague 8, Czech Republic

Jindrich Karban
Institute of Chemical Process Fundamentals, Academy of Sciences of the Czech Republic, v. v. i., Rozvojová 135, 165 02 Prague 6, Czech Republic

Bhupender S. Chhikara
Department of Chemistry, Aditi Mahavidyalaya, University of Delhi, Bawana, Delhi 110039, India
Department of Biomedical and Pharmaceutical Sciences, College of Pharmacy, University of Rhode Island, Rhode Island, Kingston, RI 02881, USA

Sajda Ashraf and Zaheer Ul-Haq
Dr. Panjwani Center for Molecular Medicine and Drug Research, ICCBS, University of Karachi, Karachi 75210, Pakistan

Saghar Mozaffari
Center For Targeted Drug Delivery, Department of Biomedical and Pharmaceutical Sciences, Chapman University School of Pharmacy, Harry and Diane Rinker Health Science Campus, California, Irvine, CA 92618, USA

Nicole St. Jeans
Department of Biomedical and Pharmaceutical Sciences, College of Pharmacy, University of Rhode Island, Rhode Island, Kingston, RI 02881, USA

Dindyal Mandal, Rakesh Kumar Tiwari and Keykavous Parang
Department of Biomedical and Pharmaceutical Sciences, College of Pharmacy, University of Rhode Island, Rhode Island, Kingston, RI 02881, USA
Center For Targeted Drug Delivery, Department of Biomedical and Pharmaceutical Sciences, Chapman University School of Pharmacy, Harry and Diane Rinker Health Science Campus, California, Irvine, CA 92618, USA

Mónica Fernández-Cancio and Laura Audí
Growth and Development Research Unit, Vall d'Hebron Research Institute (VHIR), Center for Biomedical Research on Rare Diseases (CIBERER), Instituto de Salud Carlos III, Autonomous University of Barcelona, Barcelona 08035, Spain

Núria Camats
Growth and Development Research Unit, Vall d'Hebron Research Institute (VHIR), Center for Biomedical Research on Rare Diseases (CIBERER), Instituto de Salud Carlos III, Autonomous University of Barcelona, Barcelona 08035, Spain
Pediatric Endocrinology Unit, Department of Paediatrics, University Children's Hospital Bern, Bern 3010, Switzerland
Department of Biomedical Research, University of Bern, Bern 3010, Switzerland

Christa E. Flück, Adam Zalewski and Amit V. Pandey
Pediatric Endocrinology Unit, Department of Paediatrics, University Children's Hospital Bern, Bern 3010, Switzerland
Department of Biomedical Research, University of Bern, Bern 3010, Switzerland

Bernhard Dick and Brigitte M. Frey
Department of Nephrology and Hypertension, University of Bern, Bern 3010, Switzerland

Raquel Monné
Pediatric Service, Hospital Joan XXIII, Tarragona 43005, Spain

Núria Torán
Pathology Department, Hospital Universitari Vall d'Hebron, CIBERER, Barcelona 08035, Spain

Claudia Cava
Institute of Molecular Bioimaging and Physiology, National Research Council (IBFM-CNR), Via F.Cervi 93, 20090 Segrate-Milan, Italy

Isabella Castiglioni
Department of Physics "Giuseppe Occhialini", University of Milan-Bicocca Piazza dell'Ateneo Nuovo, 20126 Milan, Italy

Elisa Roda
Department of Biology and Biotechnology "L. Spallanzani", University of Pavia, 27100 Pavia, Italy
Laboratory of Clinical & Experimental Toxicology, Pavia Poison Centre, National Toxicology Information Centre, Toxicology Unit, Istituti Clinici Scientifici Maugeri IRCCS, 27100 Pavia, Italy

Fabrizio De Luca, Daniela Ratto, Carmine Di Iorio, Maria Grazia Bottone and Paola Rossi
Department of Biology and Biotechnology "L. Spallanzani", University of Pavia, 27100 Pavia, Italy

Carlo Alessandro Locatelli
Laboratory of Clinical & Experimental Toxicology, Pavia Poison Centre, National Toxicology Information Centre, Toxicology Unit, Istituti Clinici Scientifici Maugeri IRCCS, 27100 Pavia, Italy

Elena Savino
Department of Earth and Environmental Science, University of Pavia, 27100 Pavia, Italy

João Antônio Leal de Miranda and Gilberto Santos Cerqueira
Department of Morphology, Faculty of Medicine, Federal University of Ceará, s/n Delmiro de Farias Street, Porangabuçu Campus, Fortaleza 60416-030, Brazil
Biotechnology and Biodiversity Center Research, BIOTEC, Federal University of Piauí, Parnaíba, Piauí 64202-020, Brazil

João Erivan Façanha Barreto, Dainesy Santos Martins, Paulo Vitor de Souza Pimentel, Deiziane Viana da Silva Costa, Ana Paula Fragoso de Freitas, Ariel Gustavo Scafuri, Renata Ferreira de Carvalho Leitão and Gerly Anne de Castro Brito
Department of Morphology, Faculty of Medicine, Federal University of Ceará, s/n Delmiro de Farias Street, Porangabuçu Campus, Fortaleza 60416-030, Brazil

Reyca Rodrigues e Silva, Luan Kelves Miranda de Souza, Durcilene Alves da Silva and Jand Venes Rolim Medeiros
Biotechnology and Biodiversity Center Research, BIOTEC, Federal University of Piauí, Parnaíba, Piauí 64202-020, Brazil

Camila Nayane de Carvalho Lima
Nucleus of Research and Development of Medications (NPDM), Federal University of Ceará, Coronel Nunes de Melo Street, 100, Fortaleza 60430-275, Brazil

Jefferson Almeida Rocha
Research Group in Natural Sciences and Biotechnology, Federal University of Maranhão, s/n Avenue Aurila Maria Santos Barros de Sousa, Frei Alberto Beretta, Grajaú-MA 65940-000, Brazil

Alessandra Pannunzio and Mauro Coluccia
Department of Pharmacy-Drug Sciences, University of Bari "Aldo Moro", Via E. Orabona 4, I-70125 Bari, Italy

Hehua Xiong, Jianxin Cheng, Jianqing Zhang, Qian Zhang, Zhen Xiao, Han Zhang, Qidong Tang and Pengwu Zheng
School of Pharmacy, Jiangxi Science & Technology Normal University, Nanchang 330013, China

Haonan Yu, Zhuang Hou, Xiaoguang Yang and Chun Guo
School of Pharmaceutical Engineering, Shenyang Pharmaceutical University, Shenyang 110016, China

Yanhua Mou
School of Life Sciences and Biological Pharmacy, Shenyang Pharmaceutical University, Shenyang 110016, China

Index